PATHOLOGY OF BONE MARROW

PATHOLOGY OF BONE MARROW

Faramarz Naeim, M.D.
Professor of Pathology and Laboratory Medicine
Head of Hematopathology
UCLA School of Medicine
Los Angeles, California

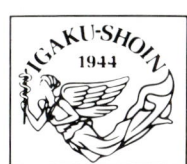

IGAKU-SHOIN New York • Tokyo

Interior design: Lillie McIntyre
Cover design: Wanda Lubelska
Printer/Binder: Arcata Graphics Kingsport
Compositor: Better Graphics
Production Editor: David Lasky

Published and distributed by

IGAKU-SHOIN Medical Publishers, Inc.
One Madison Avenue, New York, N.Y. 10010

IGAKU-SHOIN Ltd.,
5-24-3 Hongo, Bunkyo-ku, Tokyo

Copyright © 1992 by IGAKU-SHOIN Medical Publishers, Inc.
All rights reserved. No part of this book may be translated or reproduced in any
form by print, photo-print, microfilm or any other means without written permission.

Library of Congress Cataloging-in-Publication Data
Pathology of bone marrow / edited by Faramarz Naeim.
    p. cm.
  Includes bibliographical references and index.
  1. Bone marrow—Diseases. 2. Myeloproliferative disorders.
3. Hematopoietic stem cells—Diseases. I. Naeim, Faramarz.
    [DNLM: 1. Bone Marrow—pathology. 2. Bone Marrow Diseases-
-diagnosis. 3. Bone Marrow Diseases—etiology. 4. Bone Marrow
Diseases—pathology. WH 380 P2968]
RC645.7.P38 1991
616.4'1—dc20
  for Library of Congress   91-35311
                                                                                                          CIP

ISBN: 0-89640-209-6 (New York)
ISBN: 4-260-14209-7 (Tokyo)

Printed and bound in the U.S.A.

10 9 8 7 6 5 4 3 2 1

To my parents and to Ester, Arash and Shiva.

PREFACE

The main purpose of this book is to provide physicians in training and those in the practice of pathology or hematology a comprehensive and concise source of information on bone marrow pathology and a means to improve their diagnostic skills. A multidisciplinary approach is applied to the characterization of bone marrow lesions, with the primary emphasis on morphology. Histologic and cytologic findings are correlated with relevant ancillary studies, such as special cytochemical staining, immunophenotyping, biochemistry, DNA hybridization techniques, DNA content analysis, and karyotyping, that often provide essential or additional support in establishing the diagnosis and/or prognosis of bone marrow disorders.

The first three chapters provide basic information covering normal hematopoiesis, the use of special procedures and newly developed techniques, and a general overview of abnormal bone marrow morphology. Chapters four through seven are devoted to the multipotent stem cell disorders and hematopoietic malignancies, covering aplastic anemias, myeloproliferative disorders, myelodysplastic syndromes, leukemias, lymphomas, and plasma cell dyscrasias. Disorders representing monolineage involvement of the three major hematopoietic arms of the bone marrow (white blood cells, red blood cells, and megakaryocytes/platelets) are discussed in chapters eight through ten. Chapter eleven is devoted to bone marrow transplantation. For most disease categories, the general format of discussion includes etiology and pathogenesis, pathologic features and clinical aspects.

Faramarz Naeim, MD

ACKNOWLEDGMENTS

The author is particularly grateful to Dr. Stephen Nimer and Dr. Robert Gale who shared their knowledge and experience and contributed to Chapters one and eleven, respectively. He would like to thank Dr. Wayne Grody and Dr. Richard Gatti for assisting him in preparing Chapter two. He is also indebted to Ms. Janice McDonald for her secretarial assistance and Ms. Carol Appleton for her help in the development and printing of many of the photographs reproduced in this book.

CONTRIBUTORS

Robert Peter Gale, M.D., Ph.D.
Associate Professor of Medicine
UCLA School of Medicine
Los Angeles, California

Stephen Nimer, M.D.
Assistant Professor of Medicine
UCLA School of Medicine
Los Angeles, California

CONTENTS

1. BONE MARROW STRUCTURE AND FUNCTION   1
   Faramarz Naeim and Stephen Nimer

2. BONE MARROW EXAMINATION: SPECIAL PROCEDURES   32

3. ABNORMAL MORPHOLOGY: GENERAL CONSIDERATIONS   72

4. BONE MARROW HYPOPLASIA   102

5. MYELODYSPLASTIC AND MYELOPROLIFERATIVE SYNDROMES   113

6. LEUKEMIAS AND LYMPHOMAS   141

7. PLASMA CELL DYSCRASIA   232

8. WHITE BLOOD CELL DISORDERS   250

9. DISORDERS OF RED BLOOD CELLS: ANEMIAS   287

10. DISORDERS OF MEGAKARYOCYTES AND PLATELETS   325

11. BONE MARROW TRANSPLANTATION   343
    Faramarz Naeim and Robert Peter Gale

    Index   356

1 BONE MARROW STRUCTURE AND FUNCTION

Faramarz Naeim, Stephen Nimer

BONE MARROW STRUCTURE

Bone marrow is a mesenchymal derived tissue which is composed of hematopoietic cells and bone marrow stroma. Bone marrow stroma comprises the skeleton of the bone marrow tissue and the special microenvironment that is necessary for hematopoietic cell growth and differentiation. Stromal cells are composed of several subtypes such as adipocytes, fibroblast-like ("reticulum") cells, endothelial cells, osteoblasts and osteoclasts, each with special functional properties. The fibroblast-like stromal cells and the stromal matrix make up a fine reticulin meshwork which supports hematopoietic cells in the bone marrow space. The extracellular matrix, produced by bone marrow stromal cells, is composed of a variety of substances such as collagen, fibronectin, vitronectin, laminin, thrombospondin, hemonectin and proteoglycans. These substances, in addition to their role in facilitating cell–cell interactions, can bind and present growth factors to the hematopoietic progenitor cells.

The hematopoietic cells are closely associated with the thin-walled venous sinuses.[1-4] The venous sinuses are the most prominent vascular spaces in the bone marrow. They are covered by a layer of endothelial cells on the inside and supported by fibroblast-like stromal cells (parasinal, adventitial) on the outside.[2,4] These sinuses receive blood from two sources.[5,6] One is the nutrient artery, which penetrates the bony shaft, branches into the bone marrow cavity, and forms capillary-venous sinus junctions. The second source of arterial blood is the periosteal capillary network, which connects with the sinuses at the bone-marrow junction through the Haversian canals. The smaller venous sinuses drain into a large, centrally located sinus, which connects with other large sinuses to form the comitant vein. The comitant vein and the nutrient artery course through the bone marrow adjacent to each other in the same vascular canal (Fig 1-1). The nerve fibers of the bone marrow accompany the blood vessels and respond to intermedullary pressure by transmitting signals to the vessel walls for the adjustment of blood flow and

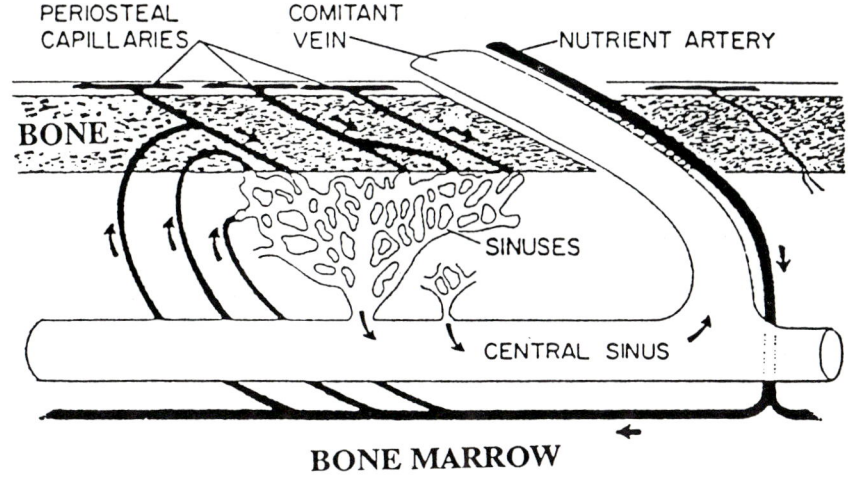

Figure 1-1. Diagram of the microcirculation of bone marrow. From De Bruyn PPH: Structural substrates of bone marrow function. *Semin Hematol* 18:179, 1981, with permission.

release of hematopoietic cells into the circulation. Bone marrow is devoid of lymphatics.[4]

The proportion of hematopoietic cells compared to fatty tissue, in clinicopathological terms, is expressed as bone marrow cellularity. Bone marrow cellularity is defined as the percentage of the bone marrow volume occupied by hematopoietic cells and depends on the age of the individual and the location of the marrow.[7,8] In a middle-aged, healthy person, bone marrow cellularity of the iliac crest is about 50%. Younger individuals show greater than 50% bone marrow cellularity. The proportion of fatty tissue increases with age (Figure 1-2). This increase appears to be the result of an increase in the volume as well as

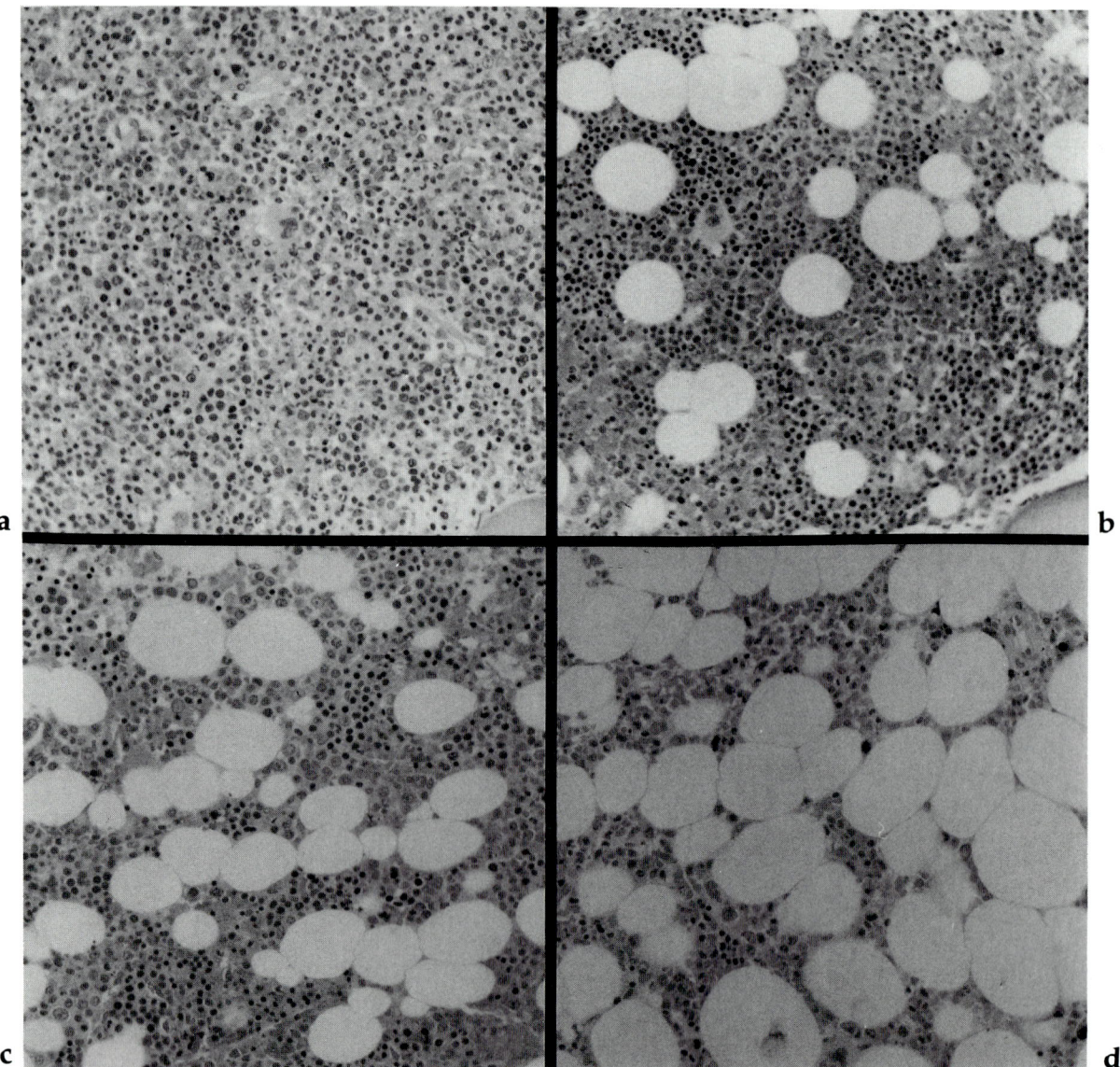

Figure 1-2. Iliac crest bone marrow biopsy sections obtained from a 9-month-old (a), a 25-year-old (b), a 56-year-old (c) and a 78-year-old (d) individual demonstrating bone marrow cellularity at different ages.

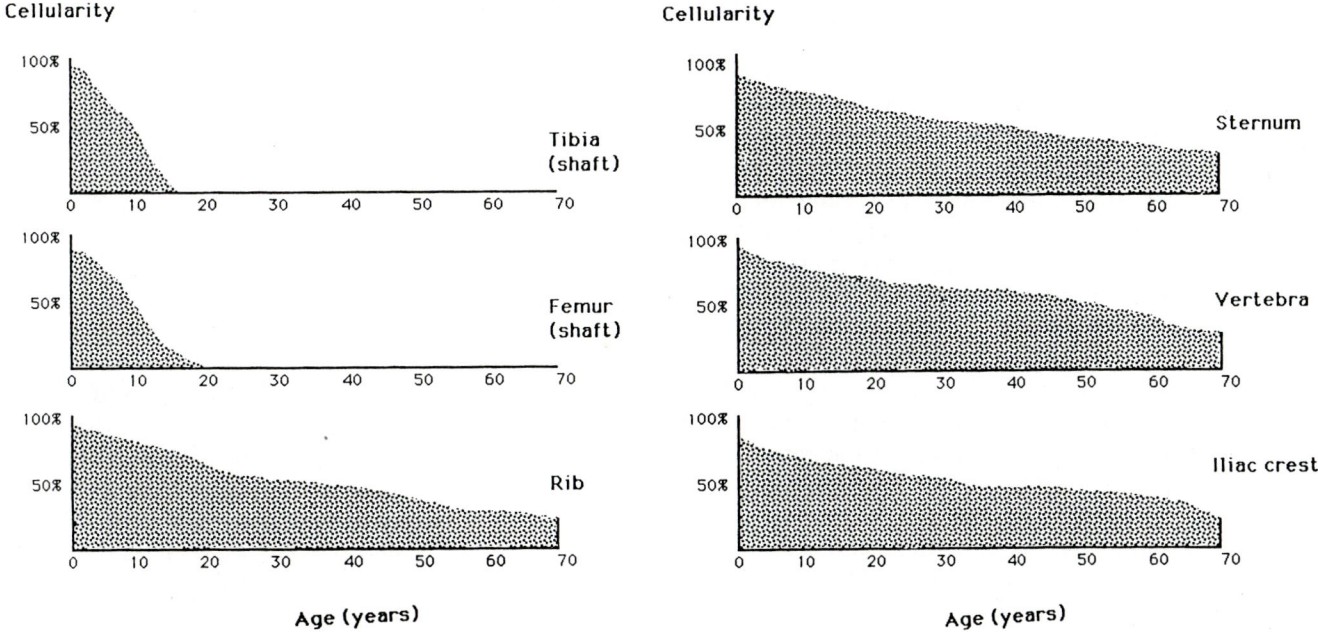

Figure 1-3. Bone marrow cellularity in relation to age and anatomic site. Adapted from Hartsock et al: Normal variations with aging of the amount of hematopoietic tissue in bone marrow from the anterior iliac crest. *Am J Clin Pathol* 43:326, 1965 and Custer RP: *An Atlas of the Blood and Bone Marrow,* ed 2. Philadelphia, WB Saunders, 1974.

the number of adipocytes.[9] Bone marrow cellularity is higher in the vertebrae and lower in the ribs than in the iliac crest and sternum[7,8] (Figure 1-3).

HEMATOPOIESIS AND THE REGULATORY MECHANISMS

Hematopoiesis

Embryonic hematopoiesis begins in the yolk sac when the mesoderm layer is formed at the end of the third week of gestation and declines to an insignificant level by the end of the first trimester.[10-14] At this stage the hematopoietic stem cells derived from yolk sac mesoderm (mesoblasts) differentiate into primitive erythroblasts, which apparently remain in nucleated forms and synthesize embryonic hemoglobins (Hb Portland, Hb Gower I and II). By the end of the first trimester, the liver develops into the most prominent source of hematopoiesis. Hepatic blood cell formation is much more comprehensive than the mesoblastic stage and involves the formation of all hematopoietic elements. Hepatic hematopoietic activity reaches its maximum level around the third month and gradually declines from the seventh month until birth. Hematopoiesis begins to occur in the bone marrow around the fifth month of gestation and continues to increase thereafter. Other sources of blood cell formation during fetal life include the spleen (especially during the second trimester), thymus, and lymph nodes, though the thymus and lymph nodes are primarily involved in lymphocyte production. The bone marrow is the most prominent hematopoietic organ at birth and remains so throughout life. Every day, in normal adult bone marrow, approximately 2.5 billion red cells, 1.0 billion granulocytes and 2.5 billion platelets are produced per kilogram of body weight.[15] The bone marrow's ability to produce blood cells may increase 5- to 10-fold when there is an urgent need for hematopoietic compensation, such as during massive bleeding or infection.

The mechanism(s) of the shift of hematopoiesis from one organ to another during fetal life is not fully understood. It is not clear whether this shift is due to migration of the hematopoietic cells from one organ to another or is the result of activation and differentiation of primitive multipotent mesenchymal cells already present in these organs.[4,14] It is likely that the concentration of growth factors required for the growth of hematopoietic progenitors in the liver or bone marrow changes with time and creates an optimal environment for hematopoiesis first in one organ and then in another. How this is accomplished and where the progenitor cells come from remain unanswered questions.

The bone marrow microenvironment, which consists of stromal cells, extracellular matrix and a variety of growth factors, has an intimate relationship with the hematopoietic cells. Surface membrane adhesion molecules which are expressed on the bone marrow cells facilitate cell–cell and cell–matrix contact and play a role in proliferation, activation, departure and homing of the hematopoietic cells.[16,17] Stromal cells are able to generate certain growth factors, such as granulocyte–macrophage colony–stimulating factor, granulocyte colony–stimulating factor, and macrophage colony–stimulating factor. Proteoglycans such as heparan sulphate, chondroitin sulphate and hyaluronic acid are able to bind a number of growth factors, including granulocyte–macrophage colony–stimulating factor and interleukin-3, and present them in biologically active forms to hematopoietic cells.[18-20] The contact between stromal and hematopoietic cells may initiate the proliferation and differentiation process of stem cells and their progeny by facilitating their exposure to these growth factors[20] or other stromal cell factors.[5,21,22] The different components of the stromal matrix can also contribute to the specificity of cell growth. For example, hemonectin selectively binds cells of granulocytic lineage.[23]

As part of the bone marrow microenvironment, the sinus endothelial cells play a role in selective release of the hematopoietic cells into the circulation. Under normal conditions, only mature cells are able to pass through the walls of the marrow venous sinuses and enter the circulation. During this transmural blood cell passage, mature blood cells penetrate the body of the sinus endothelial cells (by creating a migration pore) to get into the sinus cavity.[2,24-26] This penetration usually occurs close to endothelial cell junctions, where the endothelial cytoplasm is relatively thin. In addition to the transmural migration of mature blood cells into the circulation, the cytoplasm of megakaryocytes penetrates sinus endothelial cells.[26,27] The penetrated portions of the megakaryocytic cytoplasm, which are referred to as "proplatelet processes," are the source of the platelets released into the circulation.

Hematopoietic Stem Cells and Growth Factors

Hematopoietic Stem Cells

All hematopoietic cells, including erythrocytes, granulocytes and macrophages, megakaryocytes and lymphocytes, derive from a multipotent hematopoietic stem cell[10,11,28-31] (Figure 1-4). Stem cells are not morphologically recognizable, but they have the capacity for extensive self-replication, as well as differentiation along all hematopoietic lineages. The earliest stem cells give rise to more restricted stem cells which have less self-renewal capacity and less multipotentiality. With further differentiation, these cells give rise to committed progenitors which can proliferate and mature along only a single pathway. These cells can be grown in vitro to form colonies of cells. A cell capable of giving rise to a hematopoietic cell colony is referred to as a "colony-forming unit (CFU)." The progenitor cell for neutrophilic granulocytes and monocytes (CFU-GM) can give rise to two more restricted stem cells, one which differentiates along the neutrophilic pathway (CFU-G) and another which differentiates only along the monocytic pathway (CFU-M). Progenitors for neutrophilic granulocytes (CFU-G), the monocyte/macrophage system (CFU-M), eosinophils (CFU-Eo), basophils (CFU-Bas), erythrocytes [BFU-E (burst-forming unit–erythroid) and CFU-E] or megakaryocytes (BFU-Meg and CFU-Meg) have been described, and the growth of these committed progenitors in culture has been shown to require the presence of specific colony-stimulating factors (CSF) (see Figure 1-4).

The process by which stem cells choose between self-renewal or terminal differentiation is thought to be stochastic rather than deterministic[32]; that is, the decision occurs randomly rather than being preprogrammed into the cell. Restriction in the differentiation potential of stem cells occurs as the cell becomes committed to a specific lineage, but recent evidence suggests that some committed progenitors may still maintain the ability to form other cell types under different directive influences. The stochastic hypothesis does not preclude directive influences of the microenvironment on the differentiation process. Thus the process of differentiation may involve the

Bone Marrow Structure and Function

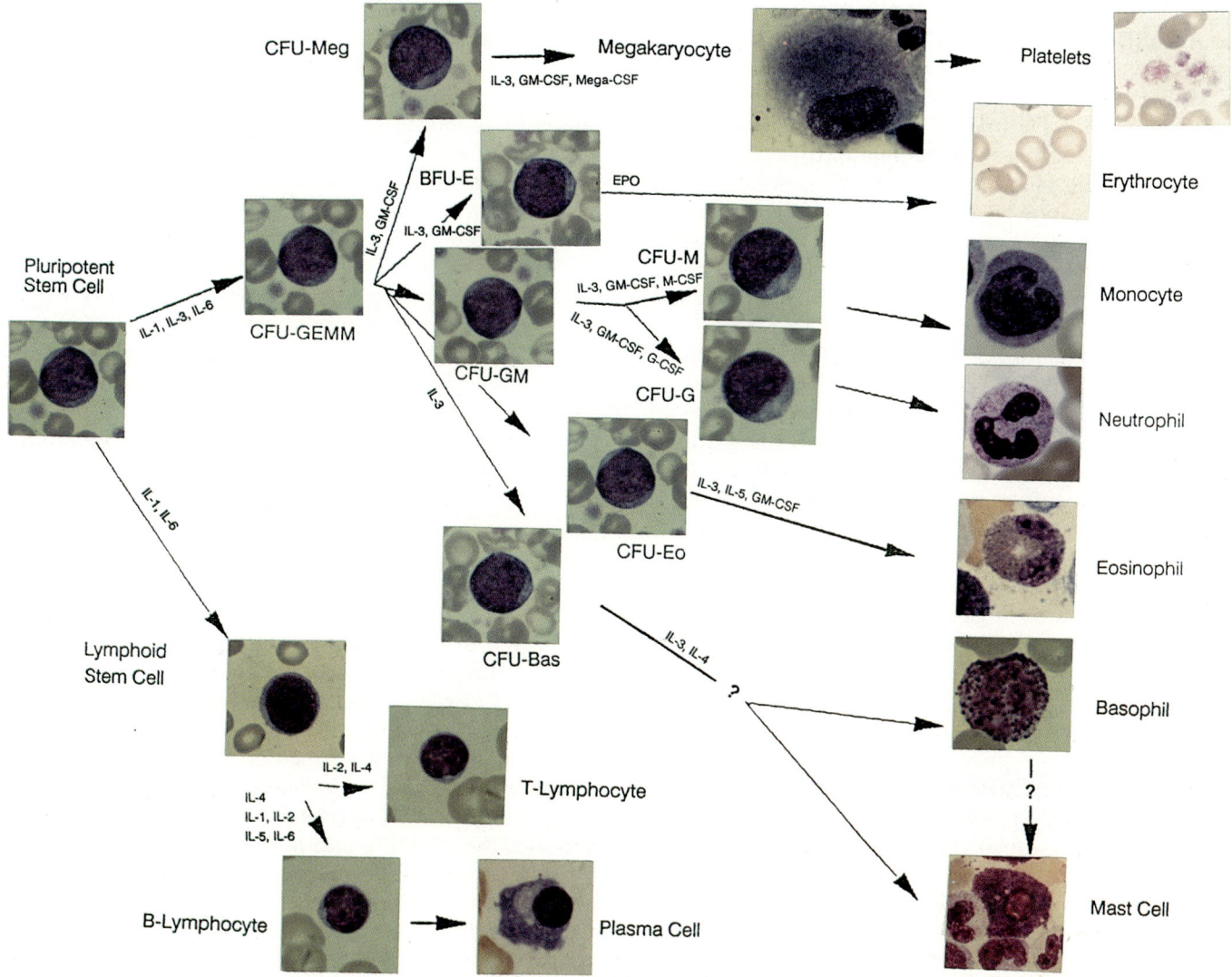

Figure 1-4. Current scheme of hematopoiesis detailing sources of mature blood elements and the stage of development at which various cytokines act.

expression of cellular receptors for specific growth factors which allow the progenitor cells to respond to particular regulatory hormonal signals in the environment. For example, expression of GM-CSF receptors is associated with granulocyte and monuclear phagocyte development, whereas expression of erythropoietin receptors is a characteristic of cells already committed to erythroid differentiation.

Both in vivo and in vitro models have been used to isolate and characterize multipotent stem cells. The first assay used to identify stem cells was based on the ability of these cells to form hematopoietic colonies in the spleens of lethally irradiated mice.[33] This assay, developed by Till and McCulloch, defined the colony-forming unit of the spleen (CFU-S), which is capable of forming erythroid, granulocytic, megakaryocytic and mixed colonies in the spleen. Later studies demonstrated that the discrete splenic nodules formed in these animals arose from single cells, and serial transfer studies proved the capacity of CFU-S to undergo self-renewal.[34]

Since then, a number of investigations have shown that the CFU-S does not have unlimited self-renewal properties and thus does not represent the true multipotent hematopoietic stem cell.[35] Attempts to develop systems capable of identifying stem cells more primitive than CFU-S led to the use of 5-fluorouracil (5-FU) treatment of mice prior to bone marrow harvesting in order to eliminate cycling cells. These studies[36,37] demonstrated that progenitor cells isolated from 5-FU-treated mice have greater proliferative and self-renewal capabilities than CFU-S but are still not the pluripotent stem cell.

The work done in mice provided the basis for human cell culture experiments which demonstrated the presence of hematopoietic stem cells in the bone marrow. The initial development of semisolid culture techniques to grow human bone marrow cells in culture was a major advance that allowed investigators to study the clonal proliferation of hematopoietic progenitors.[38,39] In this system, nonadherent human bone marrow cells are plated on a feeder layer, and colonies of maturing myeloid cells develop from hematopoietic progenitors in response to the presence of CSFs in the feeder layer. Variations of this assay system have been used to identify a primitive myeloid progenitor cell in humans, the CFU-blast, which is characterized by a high in vitro self-renewal capability and complete myeloid potential, yet these cells are also probably not the true pluripotent stem cell.[40]

Recent development of a mouse model to study hematopoiesis has provided a way to isolate what may be the true pluripotent stem cell. Using monoclonal antibodies to isolate specific cell populations, a weakly Thy 1-positive, lineage-negative, Sca 1-positive cell has been shown to repopulate hematopoiesis completely in lethally irradiated mice.[41] This cell constitutes 0.05% of normal bone marrow cells and has unit efficiency in all assays. Injection of 80–100 cells will rescue 100% of lethally irradiated animals, and cells taken from a rescued mouse can rescue a second lethally irradiated mouse. The human equivalent of this murine hematopoietic stem cell has not yet been identified.

Bone marrow transplantation could be a human in vivo assay for the ability of the hematopoietic stem cell to reconstitute the hematopoietic system. A monoclonal antibody that recognizes a cell-surface determinant called CD34 has been used to isolate CD34+ cells from bone marrow.[42,43] The CD34 antigen is present on human stem cells and other hematopoietic precursors, although most CD34+ cells are not pluripotent stem cells. CD34+ bone marrow cells have shown to reconstitute lethally irradiated nonhuman primates, and clinical trials using these cells to reconstitute hematopoiesis are underway. There is considerable controversy about whether the cell capable of rescuing a lethally irradiated individual is the same as the most primitive multipotent stem cells.

Studies in man and mouse demonstrate that the majority of multipotent stem cells are not actively cycling but are resting in the nonproliferating state of the cell cycle (G_0).[36] Various hormonal signals have been identified which can act to stimulate movement of cells from G_0 to G_1; these include interleukin-6 (IL-6),[44] interleukin-1 (IL-1),[45,46] and G-CSF.[47] Two recently described factors, IL-11 and "stem cell factor," have also been shown to stimulate cycling of the pluripotent stem cell. The survival and proliferation of primitive hematopoietic progenitors in culture is growth factor dependent, and interleukin-3 (IL-3) is the CSF most effective in supporting the proliferation of multipotent progenitors, including CFU blasts.[48,49]

Hematopoietic Growth Factors

Advances in molecular biology have led to the identification, purification and molecular cloning of the CSFs, which are glycoproteins that stimulate the formation of specific colonies from bone marrow hematopoietic progenitor cells. Four CSFs were initially identified in the mouse based on the types of colonies that grew in their presence: macrophage CSF (M-CSF), granulocyte-macrophage CSF (GM-CSF), granulocyte CSF (G-CSF), and multi-CSF or IL-3.[50-54] The human equivalents of these molecules have all been cloned and are being used in clinical trials.[55,56] The CSFs share several common features. They have activity on mature effector cells as well as hematopoietic progenitors, are active at picomolar concentrations and bind to low numbers of specific cell surface receptors on target cells. At least one subunit of the receptors for each of these growth factors has now been cloned, allowing the receptor's physiology to be studied more easily. Each CSF will be individually reviewed, but it is important to point out that not only does each CSF have a variety of biological activities, but also that the synergistic effects of the CSFs are quite numerous. In vitro and in vivo synergistic effects have been reported when IL-3 or GM-CSF is combined with IL-1, IL-4, IL-6, G-CSF, erythropoietin or M-CSF.[57-60] Stem cell factor can also synergize with a variety of CSFs. It can also be difficult to identify precisely the activities of a single factor because one factor can induce the release of other growth factors from bone marrow stroma or hematopoietic cells.

In addition to their effects on normal hematopoietic cells, CSFs stimulate the growth of leukemia cells in vitro. Receptors for GM-CSF, G-CSF and IL-3 have been found on fresh myeloid leukemia cells, and myeloid leukemia cell lines have been used extensively for studying the interactions between the CSFs and their receptors.[61,62]

GRANULOCYTE-MACROPHAGE–CSF (GM-CSF): Human GM-CSF is a 22-kD glycoprotein encoded by a gene localized to the long arm of chromosome 5.[63] GM-CSF is produced by activated T lymphocytes, by mesenchymal cells in response to tumor necrosis factor of IL-1 and by activated macrophages.[64-66] Although the natural product is variably glycosylated, bacterially derived recombinant GM-CSF, which lacks carbohydrate, is fully active.

GM-CSF stimulates the formation of neutrophil, macrophage, mixed neutrophil-macrophage and eosinophil colonies in vitro from normal bone marrow. Under certain circumstances, GM-CSF also enhances megakaryocyte and erythroid colony formation in vitro.[53,67-69] GM-CSF can also enhance numerous host defense functions of mature neutrophils, macrophages and eosinophils.

Recombinant human GM-CSF (rhGM-CSF) has been evaluated in several clinical settings, including acquired immunodeficiency syndrome (AIDS), aplastic anemia, myelodysplasia, and following myelotoxic chemotherapy for malignancy.[55,56,70,71] In all these settings, GM-CSF induces a neutrophilic granulocytosis and, variably, monocytosis and eosinophilia. Erythrocyte and platelet numbers are generally unaffected. Bone marrow changes in patients with refractory aplastic anemia treated with rhGM-CSF include increased marrow cellularity with elevated myeloid:erythroid (M:E) ratio and frequent clustering of the myeloid cells close to the bone trabeculae. The paraosteal localization of the myeloid precursors may reflect a high concentration of stem cells and/or stromal cells in the bone marrow adjacent to the bone or a localized higher concentration of GM-CSF[72] (Figure 1-5). Circulating myeloid progenitors are increased following GM-CSF therapy, and combinations of cytotoxic chemotherapy and GM-CSF have been used to isolate large enough numbers of stem cells from peripheral blood for transplantation.

GRANULOCYTE-CSF (G-CSF): G-CSF is a 19.6-kD glycoprotein encoded by a gene located on chromosome 17.[73] G-CSF is produced by monocytes, fibroblasts and endothelial cells and stimulates the in vitro growth of pure neutrophil colonies.[74] Unlike GM-CSF, G-CSF is not species specific and does not directly stimulate progenitors of lineages other than neutrophils. G-CSF can, however, induce pluripotent stem cells to enter the cell cycle and can act synergistically with other growth factors. G-CSF has activities similar to those of GM-CSF on mature neutrophils, but has no effects on macrophages or eosinophils. G-CSF also stimulates differentiation of myeloid progenitors, but this activity is relatively weak.

G-CSF has also been used in many clinical conditions to stimulate white blood cell production. Intravenous or subcutaneous administration of G-CSF stimulates granulocytosis in patients with neutropenia secondary to hairy cell leukemia, idiopathic neutropenia, myelodysplasia and cyclic neutropenia.[75-78] G-CSF can also shorten the period of neutropenia following myelotoxic chemotherapy, which may allow more consistent administration of effective doses of chemotherapy.[79]

MACROPHAGE-CSF (M-CSF): M-CSF is a monocyte/macrophage-specific growth factor originally purified from mouse L cells and human urine.[80] The M-CSF gene has recently been assigned to the long arm of chromosome 1.[81] Unlike GM-CSF, G-CSF and IL-3, which are monomers, M-CSF is a glycosylated homodimer with a molecular weight of 70 to 90 kD. M-CSF is produced by endothelial cells, fibroblasts and monocytes.[82,83] It supports the formation of macrophage colonies and has prominent effects on mature mononuclear phagocytes, stimulating RNA and protein synthesis. M-CSF stimulates production of other monokines (including interferon, IL-1, and tumor necrosis factor), and it enhances macrophage antibody-dependent, cell-mediated cytotoxicity. Human M-CSF is more active on murine bone marrow than on human bone marrow in vitro, suggesting that it may have a lesser role in stimulating hematopoiesis in man than in mice. Clinical trials of M-CSF have been reported in bone marrow transplantation and other myelosuppressive conditions.[84]

INTERLEUKIN-3 (IL-3): IL-3 (also referred to as "multi-CSF") is a 15- to 25-kD glycoprotein produced by activated T lymphocytes which stimulates proliferation of pluripotent myeloid cells.[85] The gene encoding IL-3 is located within 9 kb of the GM-CSF gene, on the long arm of chromosome 5.[86] IL-3 affects earlier progenitors than does GM-CSF, although the activities of these two factors overlap.[87] IL-3 stimulates

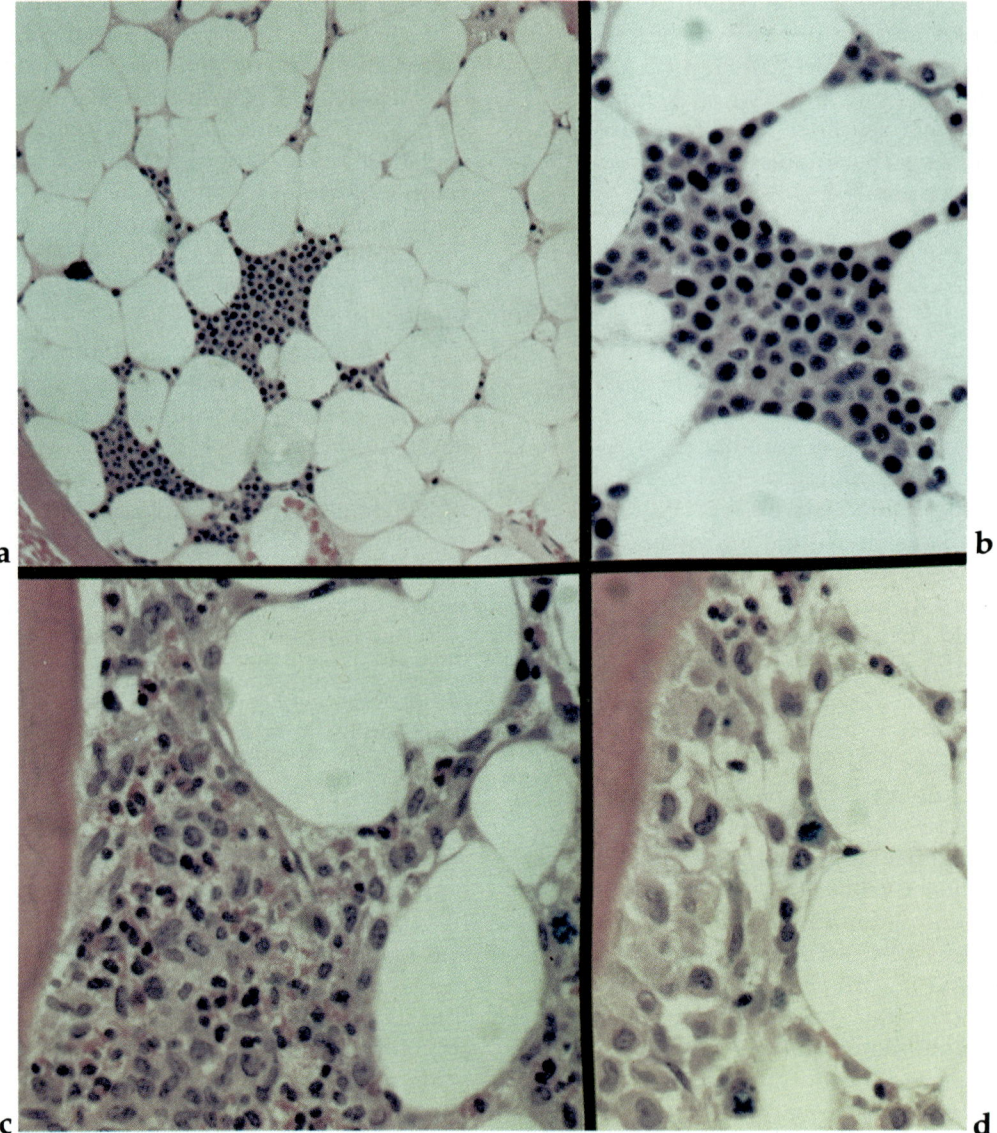

Figure 1-5. The effect of recombinant GM-CSF therapy on patients with severe aplastic anemia. Marked hypocellarity with islands of erythroid cells is demonstrated in a bone marrow biopsy section from a patient with severe aplastic anemia before GM-CSF therapy (a) and (b). After 2–4 weeks of GM-CSF therapy, myelopoiesis is noted, predominantly in the paraosteal areas (c, d).

the formation of neutrophil, macrophage, eosinophil, mast cell, erythroid, and megkaryocytic colonies from human bone marrow. IL-3 can also act synergistically with numerous other growth factors in in vitro assays. IL-3 exerts biological effects on mature monocytes, eosinophils, mast cells and basophils, but it does not bind to mature granulocytes.

Clinical trials with recombinant IL-3 are being initiated in a number of disease settings, including myelodysplasia, bone marrow failure, following cytoxic chemotherapy and after bone marrow transplantation.[88] Preliminary data indicate increases in neutrophils, monocytes, eosinophils, basophils, lymphocytes and, to a much more variable degree, in platelets. The number of circulating red blood cells has occasionally increased.

ERYTHROPOIETIN: Erythropoietin is a 36-kD glycoprotein first purified from the urine of patients with aplastic anemia. It is encoded by a single gene located on chromosome 7, and is produced predominantly in the liver during fetal gestation and in the kidney after birth.[89-91] Erythropoietin stimulates the growth and differentiation of committed erythroid progenitors (CFU-E). It can also stimulate the growth of more primitive erythroid progenitors (burst forming unit-erythroid, BFU-E) in combination with burst-promoting activity (which can be provided by GM-CSF, IL-3 or other molecules).[91,92] In some in vitro systems, erythropoietin, either alone or in combination with other growth factors, can stimulate the proliferation of megakaryocytic progenitors.

Erythropoietin has been given to dialysis patients and patients with end-stage renal disease in an attempt to correct their anemia, which results predominantly from inadequate production of erythropoietin by the kidney.[93] These studies demonstrate a dose-dependent rise in reticulocyte count and hematocrit and a marked decrease in red blood cell transfusion dependency. The efficacy of erythropoietin in this setting has been truly remarkable. Erythropoietin is also being used to treat other types of anemia such as AIDS-associated anemia, anemia of chronic disease (rheumatoid arthritis) and anemia of malignancy.

INTERLEUKIN-1 (IL-1): The IL-1 family of proteins plays an important role in the host defense against infection and in the inflammatory and immunologic processes. IL-1 is produced predominantly by stimulated macrophages and monocytes, but also by fibroblasts, endothelial cells and several other cell types.[94] Two forms of IL-1 have been identified: an acidic form known as IL-1α and a neutral form known as IL-1β.[95] IL-1 has prominent immunologic effects on the differentiation and activation of lymphocytes, which can result in the production of lymphokines. IL-1 also has a variety of nonimmunologic functions, acting as an endogenous pyrogen and as a stimulator of acute phase protein synthesis by the liver.

IL-1, either alone or through the release of IL-6, can potentiate the activity of a variety of growth factors on hematopoietic progenitor cells.[59] In addition, IL-1 can stimulate the production of hematopoietic growth factors (e.g., GM-CSF or G-CSF).

INTERLEUKIN-6 (IL-6): IL-6 is a 26-kD glycoprotein that possesses a broad range of activities. IL-6 was previously known as "B-cell stimulatory factor 2," "beta 2 interferon," "hybridoma growth factor" and "hepatocyte-stimulating factor." IL-6, like IL-1 and G-CSF, promotes the transition of the stem cells from the G_0 to the G_1 phase of their growth cycle and shortens the G_0 phase.[58] Both IL-6 and G-CSF have been referred to as "competence factors"; they promote the transition of stem cells from G_0, but they do not stimulate the proliferation of the cells once they have left G_0. IL-6 therefore acts very early in the differentiation of hematopoietic progenitors. It can also act synergistically with a variety of later acting factors. IL-6 has potent effects on the growth of myeloma cells and may be an important paracrine stimulator of the in vivo growth of these cells.

In vivo administration of IL-6 to mice has been shown to increase platelet numbers, which could be clinically useful. Based upon its in vitro activities, it may be possible to administer IL-6 followed by another CSF in order to stimulate hematopoiesis maximally in humans.[60]

OTHER CYTOKINES: IL-2, -4, -5 and -7 are primarily involved with immunologic functions[54] but have some hematopoietic effects as well. IL-9, IL-11 and stem cell factor (also known as "Steel factor", kit ligand or "mast cell growth factor") are recently identified factors whose activities on hematopoietic progenitor cells are now being characterized.[96-98]

Interleukin-2 (IL-2) was the first fully characterized T-cell growth factor.[54,99] IL-2 is normally produced by activated CD4-positive or CD8-positive T cells and by natural killer (NK) cells. Antigen-stimulated T cells express IL-2 receptors and secrete IL-2. Binding of IL-2 to its receptor is responsible for amplification of the immune response, whereas expression of the IL-2 receptor gives specificity to the response.[99]

Interleukin-4 (Il-4) is another growth factor that has important effects on the immune response, affecting both T and B cells and macrophages.[54,100,101] IL-4, originally designated as "B-cell stimulating factor-1 (BSF-1)," has multiple effects on B-cell functions, including enhancement in production of IgG and IgE, and induction of Class II major histocompatibility complex antigen expression. In addition, IL-4 stimulates the proliferation of thymocytes and T lymphocytes, (an activity previously described as "T-cell growth factor-2" activity). IL-4 can also stimulate the growth of hematopoietic cells such as mast cells, macrophages and megakaryocytes, and can act in concert with erythropoietin to support the growth of erythroid progenitors. IL-4 has also been shown to inhibit the expression of IL-1 and tumor necrosis factor-alpha by peripheral blood monocytes.[102]

Interleukin-5 (IL-5) was originally identified based upon its ability to induce activated B cells to differentiate into immunoglobulin-secreting cells.[54] These activities were originally described as "T-cell replacing factor (TRF)" and "B-cell growth factor-II" activities. Molecular cloning of the TRF cDNA confirmed that a single molecule was responsible for both the TRF and B-cell growth factor-II (BCGF-II) activities, and recent studies have shown that IL-5 is identical to eosinophil differentiation factor (EDF), which stimulates the proliferation, differentiation and function of eosinophils.[103] IL-5 may play a critical role in the eosinophilia that accompanies parasitic infections and the eosinophilia seen after IL-2 therapy. IL-5 may also be responsible for the tissue eosinophilia seen in Hodgkin's disease.

Interleukin-7 (IL-7) is a recently described factor which promotes the proliferation of bone marrow B lymphocytes.[104] IL-7 has some activity on peripheral blood T cells and activated mouse thymocytes, but no activity on prethymic or intrathymic T-cell progenitor clones.[105]

Tumor necrosis factor-alpha and -beta (TNF-α, -β) are produced by monocytes, T cells and NK cells. TNF induces production of several cytokines by bone marrow stromal cells and increases monocyte cytotoxicity and B-cell proliferation.[106] TFN, in concentrations higher than can be achieved in man, can cause tumor necrosis. Much lower concentrations of TNF can cause profound cachexia and weight loss.

MORPHOLOGIC CHARACTERISTICS OF BONE MARROW CELLS

Normal bone marrow consists of a heterogeneous population of cells in various stages of differentiation (Figure 1-6). This characteristic heterogeneity, which is diffusely present throughout the marrow, is altered in many hematologic disorders, particularly hematologic malignancies. In this section, the morphologic features of hematopoietic cells proceeding along their differentiation pathways will be discussed. In addi-

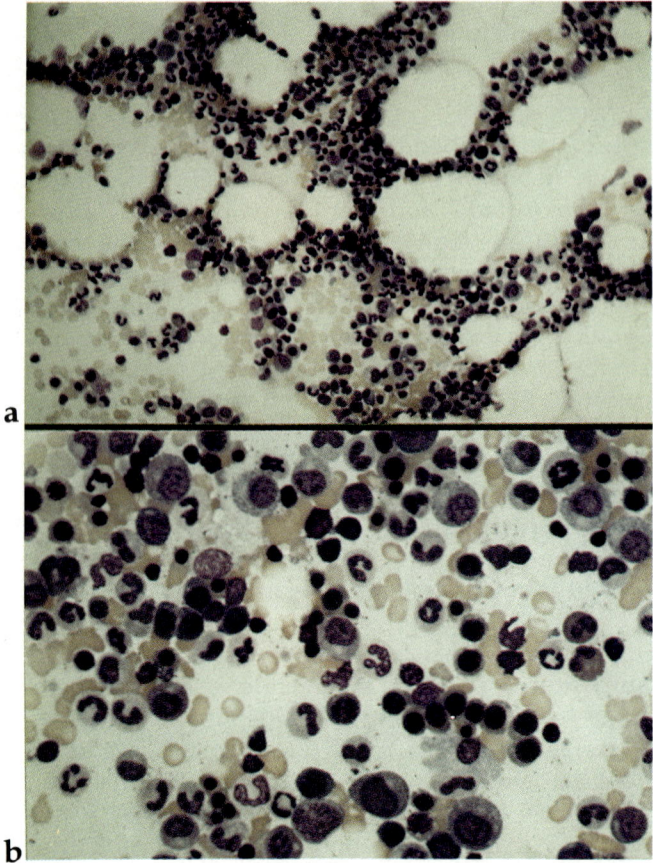

Figure 1-6. A normal bone marrow smear demonstrating various hematopoietic cells in stages of differentiation; low power (a) and high power (b).

tion, bone marrow stromal cells will be morphologically characterized.

Neutrophilic Precursors

Myeloblasts

Myeloblasts are the earliest granulocytic precursors morphologically identified. They range in size from 10 to 20 μm in diameter and have a high nuclear/cytoplasmic ratio, round to oval centrally located nuclei, finely dispersed chromatin and several nucleoli (Figure 1-7). Their cytoplasm has either no granules (Type I myeloblast) or a small number of azurophilic granules (Type II myeloblast). Myeloblasts are strongly positive for HLA-DR, CD13 and CD33 surface antigens.

Bone Marrow Structure and Function

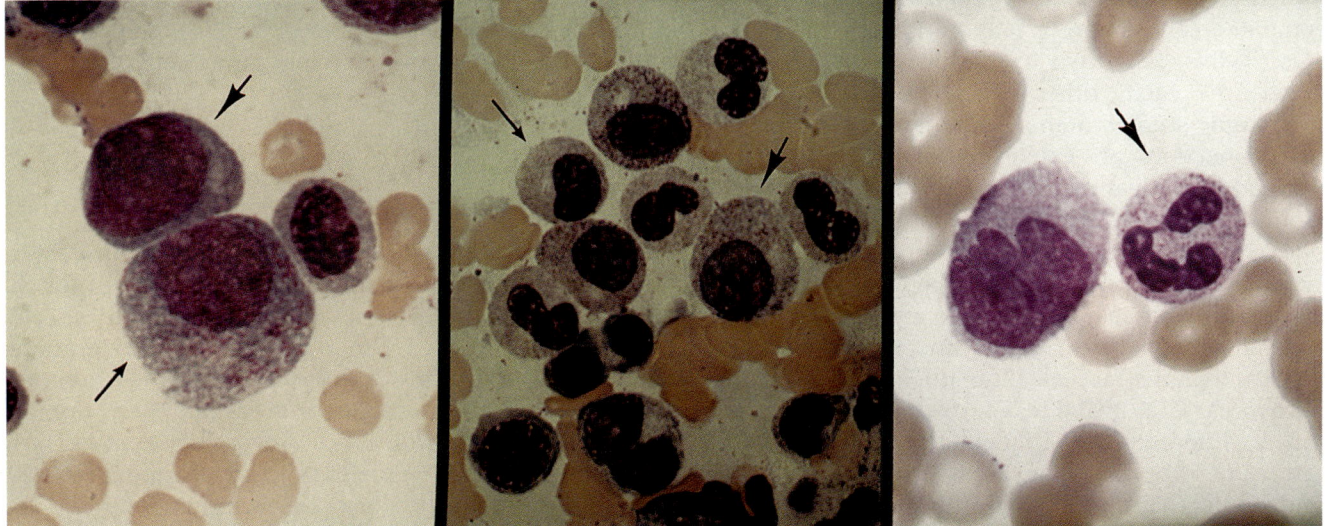

Figure 1-7. Granulocytic lineage: a myeloblast (thick arrow) and a promyelocyte (thin arrow) (a), several neutrophilc myelocytes (thick arrow) and metamyelocytes (thin arrow) (b), and a neutrophilic segmented cell (arrow) adjacent to a monocyte (c).

Promyelocytes

Promyelocytes are usually larger than myeloblasts, ranging from 13 to 25 μm in diameter, with more cytoplasm and more cytoplasmic granules than the myeloblasts (see Figure 1-7). A perinuclear pale area, representing the Golgi system, is usually present. The nuclear/cytoplasmic ratio is high and the nucleus is usually eccentrically located, with a slightly coarser chromatin than that of myeloblasts. Nucleoli are prominent. The cytoplasmic granules are a mixture of primary (azurophilic) and secondary (specific) granules, with a preponderance of the former, especially in younger promyelocytes. The bulk of the primary granules apparently is made during the promyelocytic stage.[107,108] These granules are membrane-bound packets of proteolytic enzymes such as myeloperoxidase, lysozyme, cathepsin G, elastase, acid hydrolases and defensins.[109] Defensins are arginine- and cysteine-rich peptides with broad antimicrobial activities.[110] Promyelocytes express CD13 and CD33 antigens but are HLA-DR negative.

Myelocytes

Myelocytes are cells characterized by a variable amount of cytoplasm containing abundant specific granules and a round or oval nucleus with slight indentation, coarse chromatin and lack of distinct nucleoli (see Figure 1-7). At the myelocytic stage, synthesis of primary granules ceases and their number decreases during subsequent divisions.[107] The neutrophilic granules (secondary granules) are smaller and under the electron microscope are more electron lucent than the primary granules. They contain lysozyme and lactoferrin. Myelocytes are HLA-DR negative and CD15 positive, and may express CD13 and CD33 antigens.

Metamyelocytes

Metamyelocytes are recognized by their kidney-shaped or indented nucleus, which contains coarse chromatin but no distinct nucleolus (see Figure 1-7). Metamyelocytes contain abundant cytoplasm loaded with secondary granules. The metamyelocyte, unlike its progenitor cells, is no longer capable of cell division. Metamyelocytes are HLA-DR and CD33 negative but CD15 positive. They may also express CD13 antigen.

Bands and Segmented Neutrophils

Bands or stab forms have not yet acquired the true nuclear lobulation which is characteristic of segmented neutrophils (see Figure 1-7). The nuclei of segmented cells (Segs) or polymorphonuclear leukocytes (PMNs) have two to five distinct lobules connected to each other by filaments. Electron microscopic studies demonstrate that these filamentous connections are extensions of heterochromatin wrapped in nuclear membranes[111] (Figure 1-8). Neutrophils have phagocytic ability and are able to kill and digest bacteria and yeasts by multiple antimicrobial mechanisms, including hydrogen peroxide production, release of lysosomal enzymes and release of defensin molecules. Bands and segmented neutrophils demonstrate alkaline phosphatase activity and express CD10, CD11c, CD15 and CD16 antigens.

The differentiation process from myeloblast to mature neutrophil takes approximately 2 weeks. Neutrophils that are released into the circulation are distributed between pools of granulocytes which adhere to the endothelium of capillaries and a circulating pool of granulocytes which flows freely through the bloodstream. These pools are roughly equal in size and can continuously exchange cells.

Eosinophilic Granulocytes

The stages of maturation of eosinophilic granulocytes are very similar to that of neutrophils except for the structure and content of their primary and specific granules (Figures 1-9 to 1-11). The primary granules in eosinophilic promyelocytes are round, homogeneously electron dense and larger than primary granules in neutrophilic promyelocytes.[107] These granules contain peroxidase, acid phosphatase, aryl sulfatase and other lysosomal enzymes.[112-115] The specific eosinophilic granules (which are considered lysosomal granules) contain a variety of enzymes

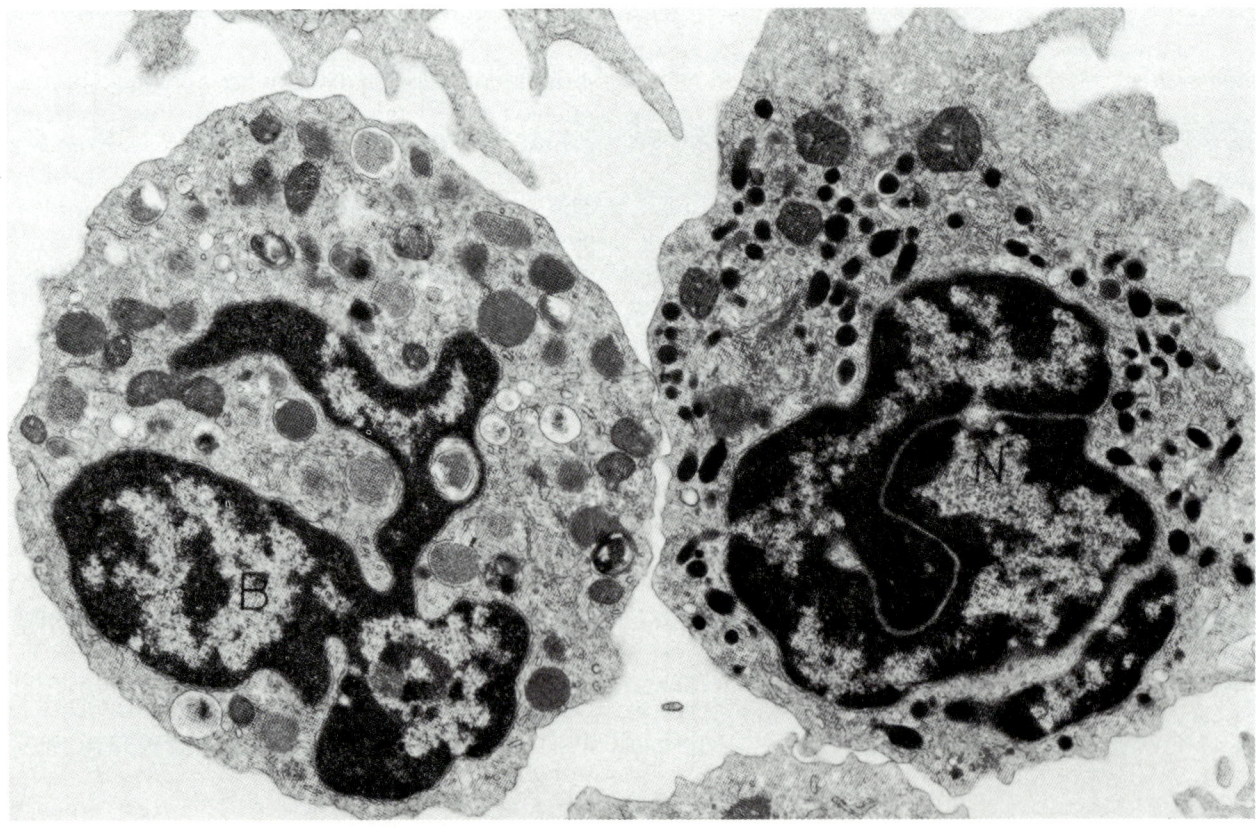

Figure 1-8. Electron microscopic features of a segmented meutrophil (N) and a mature basophil (B) with their typical specific granules. From Dvorak et al: Ultrastructure of eosinophils and basophils stimulated to develop in human cord blood mononuclear cell cultures containing recombinant human interleukin-5 or interleukin-3. *Lab Invest* 61:116, 1989, with permission.

Bone Marrow Structure and Function

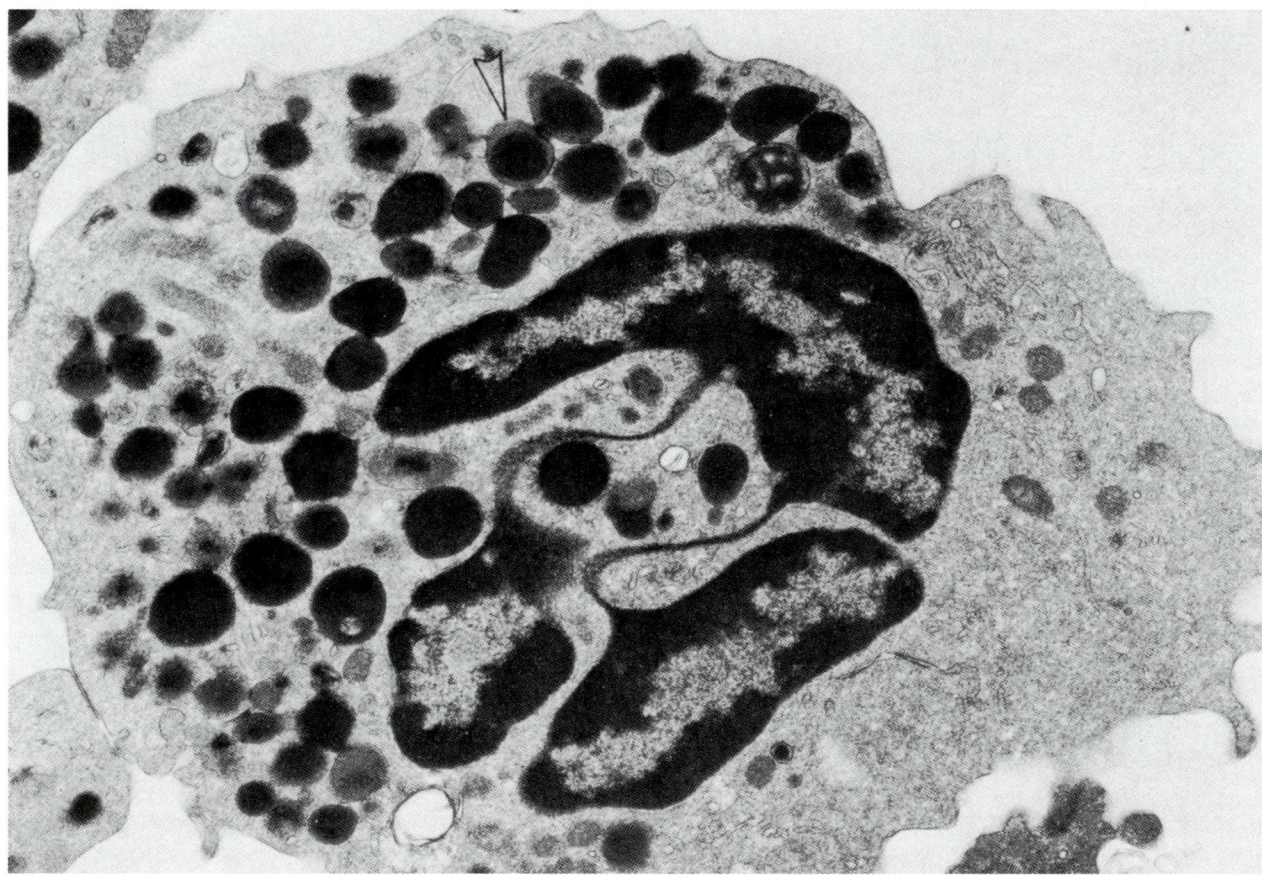

Figure 1-9. Electron microscopic features of a mature eosinophil with numerous specific granules with central crystaloids (arrow), From Dvorak et al: Ultrastructure of eosinophils and basophils stimulated to develop in human cord blood mononuclear cell cultures containing recombinant human interleukin-5 or interleukin-3. *Lab Invest* 61:116, 1989, with permission.

such as myeloperoxidase, acid phosphatase, phospholipase, ribonuclease and cathepsin.[112] Eosinophilic granules are oval or round, membrane-bound structures with a central bar that differs in electron density from the surrounding matrix (see Figures 1-9 and 1-10). The bar, which is also referred to as a "core," "internum" or "crystalloid," is composed of a basic protein with a high arginine content known as "eosinophilic major basic protein."[115] Eosinophils have the ability to phagocytose particles such as immune complexes, and appear to play an important role in anaphylactic and allergic reactions. The eosinophilic basic protein is toxic to certain parasites and normal host cells. Mature eosinophils usually have bilobed nuclei and are loaded with specific granules which are larger than the neutrophilic granules and stain orange to deep red by Wright's and H&E stains (see Figure 1-11).

Basophils and Mast Cells

Basophils and mast cells are characterized by their basophilic granules and their closely related structural and functional properties (Figures 1-9, 1-11 and 1-12). The similarities between basophils and mast cells have raised speculations that these two cells are derived from the same committed stem cell and that the mast cell represents the tissue form of the basophil.[116,117] However, basophils and mast cells have numerous differences. Mast cells are larger and have more abundant cytoplasm than do basophils. The mast cell nucleus is not segmented, and its nuclear chromatin is less condensed than that of the segmented nucleus of basophils. Aggregates of cytoplasmic glycogen are present in basophils but absent in mast cells. Mast cell cytoplasmic granules

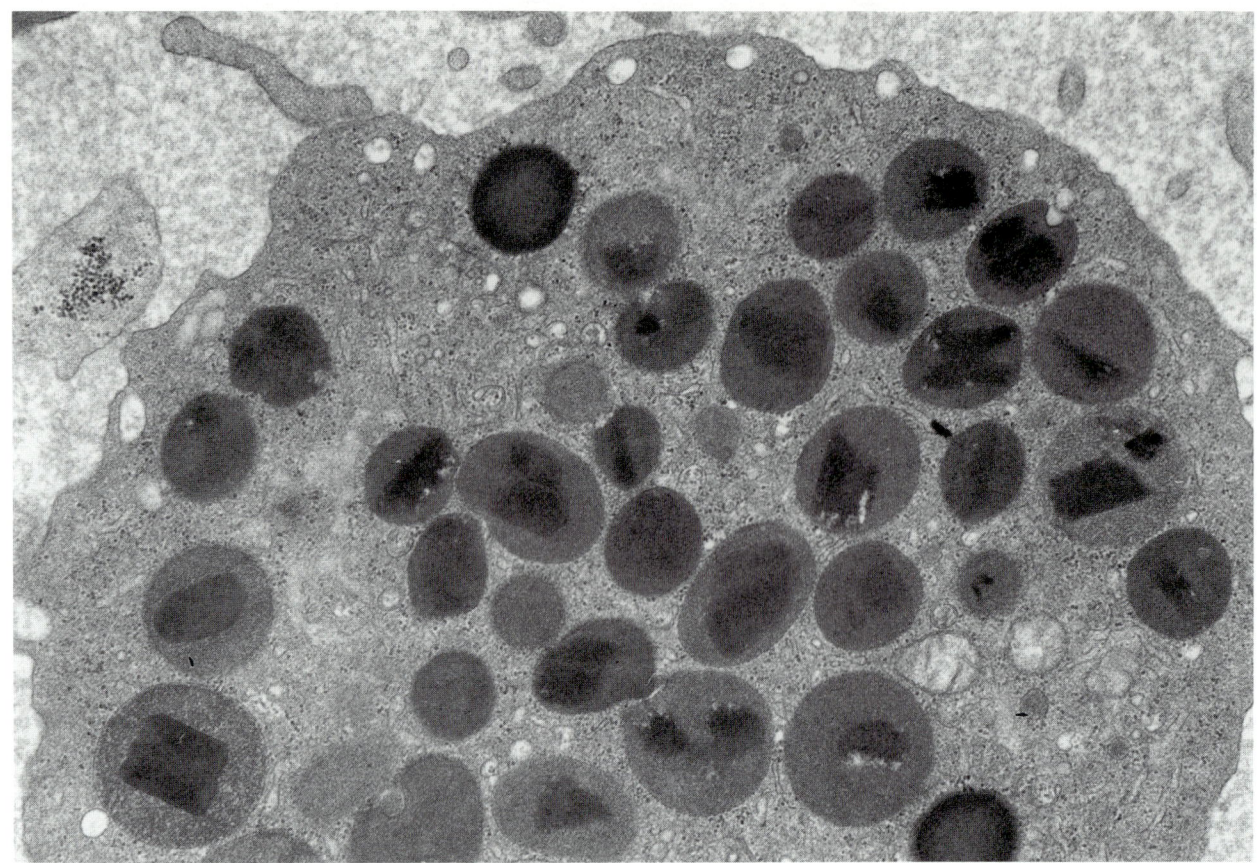

Figure 1-10. Electron microscopic features of specific granules in a mature eosinophil. The majority of granules contain central crystalloids.

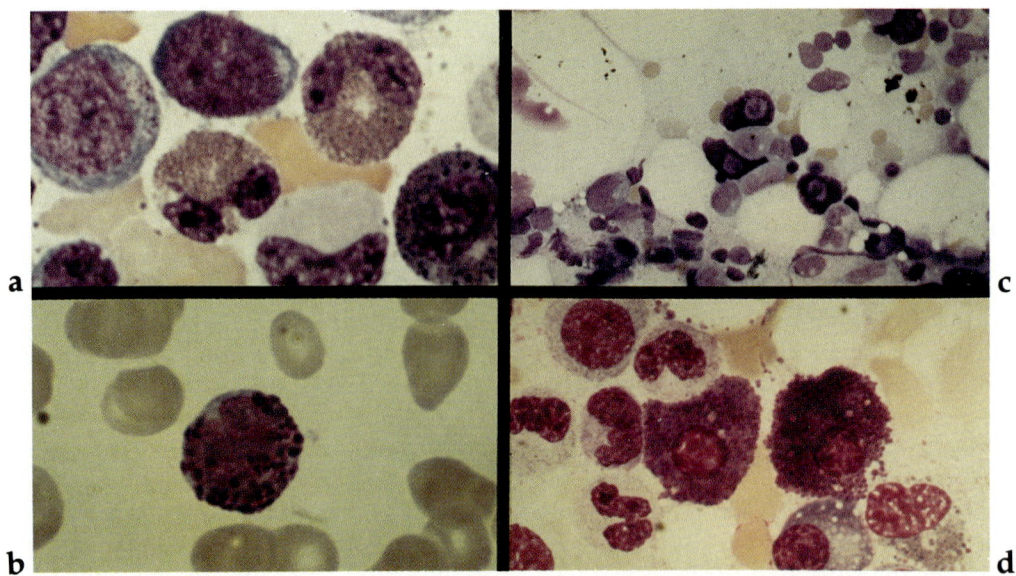

Figure 1-11. Bone marrow smears demonstrating eosinophils (a), a basophil (b) and several mast cells (c, d).

Bone Marrow Structure and Function

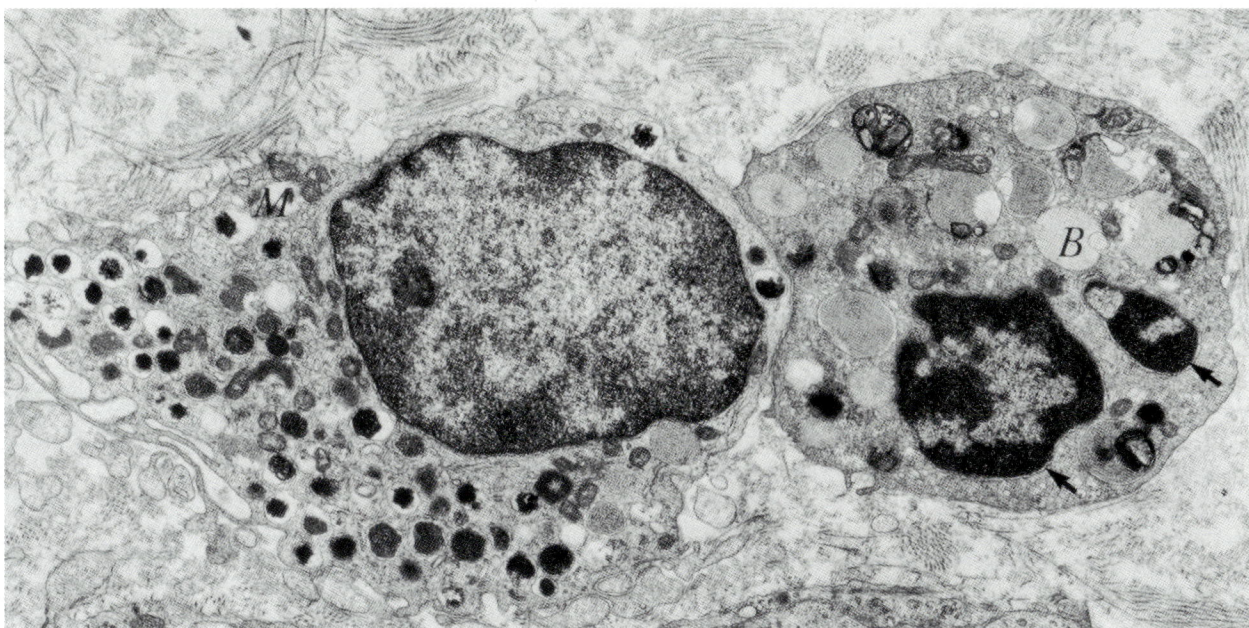

Figure 1-12. Electron microscopic features of a basophil (B) and a mast cell (M). The mast cell granules are smaller, more numerous, and more variable in shape and content than those of the basophil. From Galli SJ: New insights into the riddle of the mast cells: Microenvironmental regulation of mast cell development and phenotypic heterogeneity. *Lab Invest* 62:1, 1990, with permission.

are smaller, more numerous, more variable in appearance and less water-extractable than basophil cytoplasmic granules.[107,118,119] Mast cell granules contain histamine, heparin, serotonin, hydrolytic enzymes and eosinophil chemotactic factor of anaphylaxis (ECF-A). Basophils lack serotonin, protease, acid and alkaline phosphatase but, unlike mast cells, do contain peroxidase.[107,118] Granule-granule fusion during degranulation is rare in basophils but common in mast cells.[119] Normally, mast cells reside and mature in connective tissues and serosal cavities, where they show a diverse morphology. Basophils mature in the bone marrow and remain in peripheral blood until immunologic or inflammatory signals cause them to leave the circulation and enter the tissues. Mast cells have a longer life span than basophils.[119] Mast cells and basophils are primarily involved in allergic and anaphylactic reactions by releasing the contents of their granules into the environment (degranulation). This process is mediated in various ways, including interaction of the surface IgE with antigens and anti-IgE antibodies.[107,120,121]

The Monocyte-Macrophage Lineage

Monocytes and macrophages are derived from a progenitor cell, the CFU-GM, which also serves as the progenitor for granulocytes. Like other hematopoietic cell lineages, monocytes pass through a maturation process which starts at a blast stage (monoblast), passes through promonocyte stage and subsequently ends up as monocytes, and later as macrophages and sometimes as multinucleated giant cells. Monoblasts are morphologically similar to myeloblasts, except that their nuclear shape may be cleft or slightly lobulated. Promonocytes are larger than monoblasts, contain a few azurophilic (lysosomal) granules and have a rounded, oval or lobulated nucleus with one or more prominent nucleoli. Monocytes have abundant grayish-blue cytoplasm with small azurophilic granules and often one or several intracytoplasmic vacuoles (Figure 1-13). The nucleus is usually eccentrically placed and is folded or kidney-shaped, with a fine, lacy chromatin pattern. The lysosomal granules

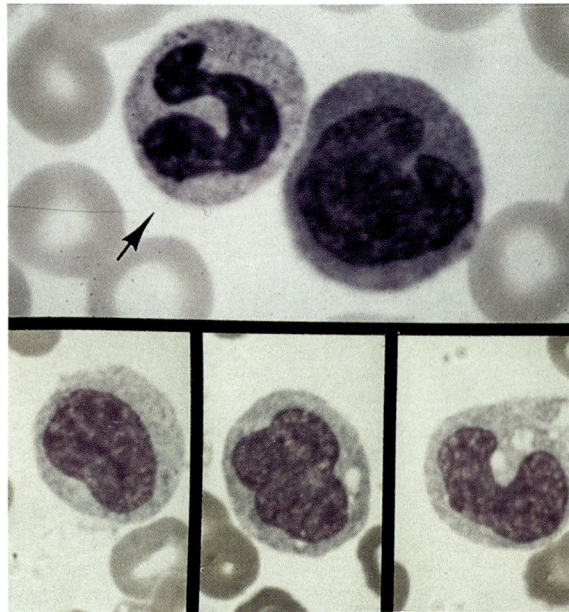

Figure 1-13. Peripheral blood smears demonstrating a neutrophilic band (arrow) and several monocytes.

contain a variety of hydrolytic enzymes including acid phosphatase, esterases, lysozyme, and galactosidases.

In addition to the proteolytic enzymes, monocytes secrete a large number of bioactive products which play an important role in inflammatory, proliferative and immune responses.[122,123] These products include complement components, binding proteins (transferrin, transcobalamin II, fibronectin), growth factors (GM-CSF, G-CSF, M-CSF, IL-1), antiproliferating factors (interferons, TNF) and arachidonate metabolites (e.g., prostaglandin E2, thromboxane). Monocytes express HLA-DR, CD13, CD14, CD15, CD11b (C3 receptor) and CD11c (integrin) antigens.

The process by which monocytes are released from bone marrow into the intravascular space is similar to that for granulocytes. In the peripheral blood, monocytes either flow freely through the circulation or adhere to the endothelial cells of the capillaries and small venules.[4,124] They migrate out of the circulation into the various tissues after 16 to 76 hours and transform into macrophages or tissue histiocytes (resident macrophages) (Figure 1-14). Thus, the mononuclear phagocytic (reticuloendothelial) system in man, includes hepatic Kupffer cells, pulmonary alveolar macrophages, soft tissue histiocytes, serous

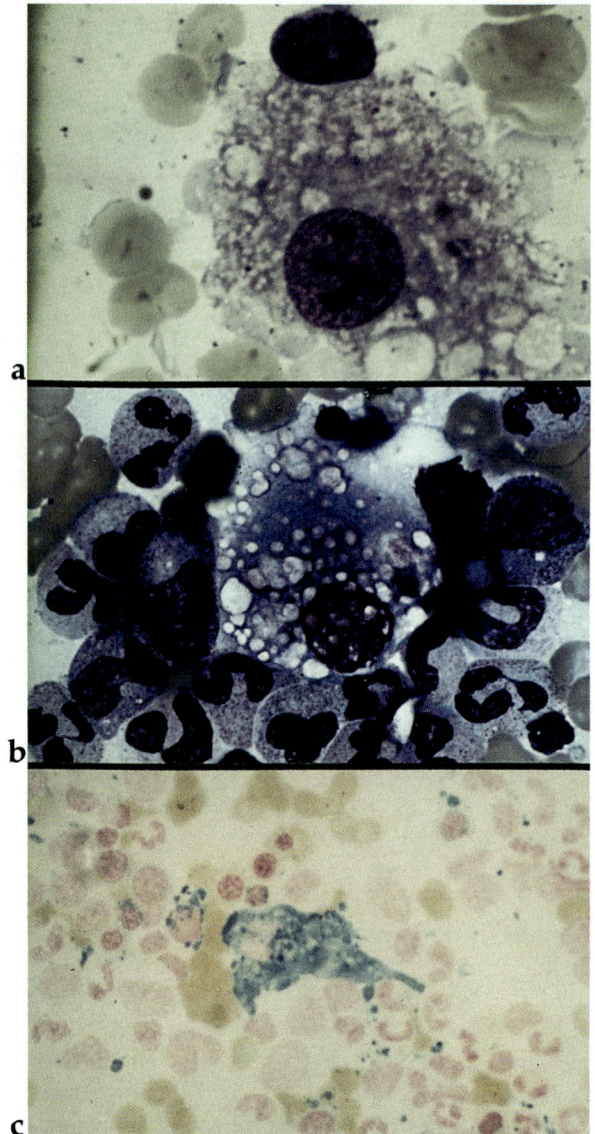

Figure 1-14. Bone marrow smears demonstrating vacuolated macrophages (a, b) and a hemosiderin-loaded macrophage stained with prussian blue (c).

cavity macrophages, central nervous system microglial cells and osteoclasts.[122-124] This system is involved in the removal of damaged and senescent cells, microorganisms and foreign materials and the storage of iron. It also plays an important role in antigen presentation and cell–cell interactions in the immune system, and is involved in the production and release of a large number of mediators which play an important role in inflammatory and immune responses.

Bone Marrow Structure and Function

Tissue histiocytes are less phagocytic and have fewer lysosomal granules than macrophages; their primary function is antigen presentation to lymphocytes. Langerhans cells in skin and interdigitating and dendritic reticulum cells in lymph nodes, which are characterized by expressing CD1 antigen and S-100 protein, are considered a subtype of tissue histiocytes.[125–129]

Iron is stored in bone marrow macrophages as ferritin (soluble in aqueous tissue extracts) and, more abundantly, as hemosiderin (insoluble aggregates).[130,131] Hemosiderin appears as dark blue granules by Prussian blue stain (potassium ferrocyanide) and is assumed to be derived from ferritin or its degraded forms (see Figure 1-14). The stored iron comes almost exclusively from the phagocytosis of senescent or defective erythrocytes. In normal conditions, approximately two-thirds of the phagocytosed iron is rapidly (within 30-60 minutes) recycled to plasma transferrin, and the remaining one-third enters the storage pool.[130] The recycling of iron to plasma transferrin requires ascorbic acid.[132,133]

Erythroid Precursors

The earliest morphologically identifiable erythroid cell is the erythroblast (rubriblast, pronormoblast), which is derived from the CFU-E. The erythroblast has a diameter of 15–30 μm, with a high nuclear/cytoplasmic ratio, a deep blue cytoplasm with a perinuclear pale area (representing the Golgi system) and no cytoplasmic granules (Figure 1-15). The nuclear chromatin is fine, and one or two prominent nuclei are present. The erythroblast divides into two basophilic erythroblasts (basophilic normoblasts, prorubricytes) which are smaller (10–18 μm) and have a deep blue cytoplasm. The nuclear chromatin of the

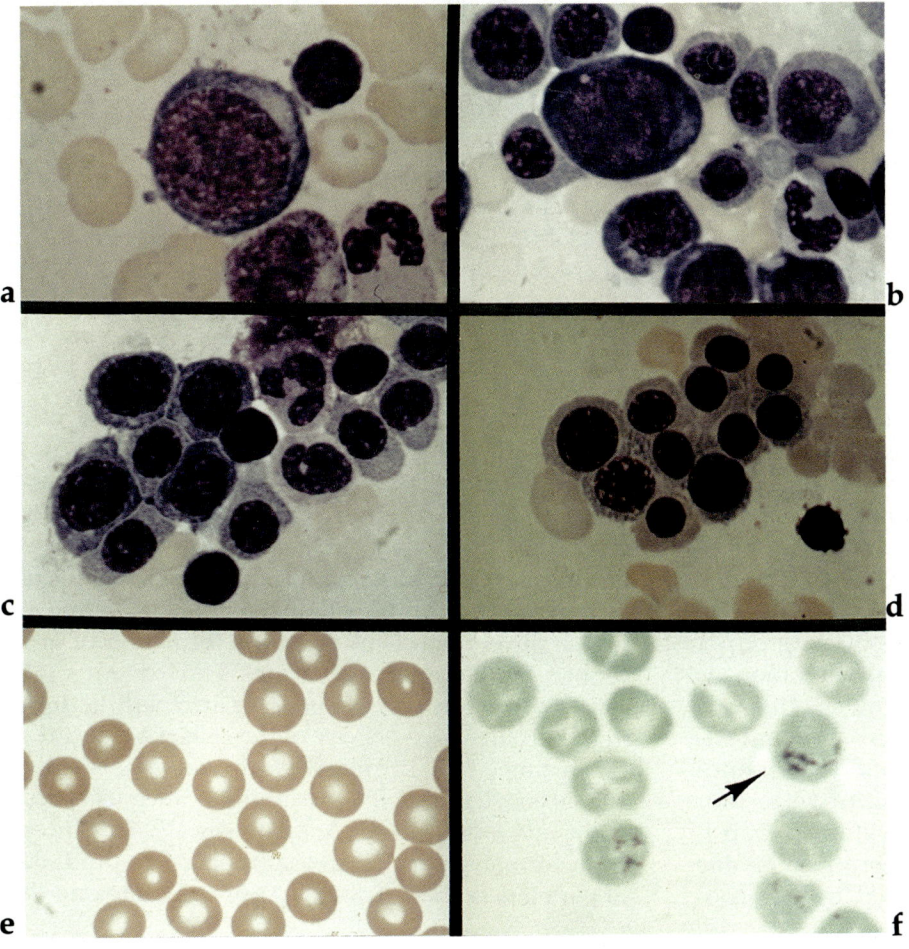

Figure 1-15. Bone marrow (a-d) and peripheral blood (e,f) smears demonstrating the stages of differentiation from rubriblast to erythrocyte. Reticulocytes are demonstrated in (f) (arrow); methylene blue staining.

basophilic erythroblast is not as fine as that of the pronormoblast, and its nucleoli are not distinct. The basophilic erythroblast undergoes three cell divisions and continues maturation, forming polychromatophilic erythroblasts (rubricytes) (see Figure 1-15). Rubricytes are unable to undergo further cell division, though maturation continues, leading to the formation of orthochromic erythroblasts (metarubricytes) and then reticulocytes (see Figure 1-15). As this maturation process proceeds, the erythroid cells become smaller, the nuclear chromatin gets denser, and the nucleus becomes pyknotic and is eventually extruded from the cell via the red cell cytoskeletal system.[134] The early non-nucleated erythroid cells (reticulocytes) still contain a significant number of ribosomes and appear grayish-red with Romanowsky stains. The ribosomes present in these cells show a reticular pattern when stained with a supravital stain such as methylene blue. It takes 3–5 days for the pronormoblast to develop into the reticulocyte. Reticulocytes are released into the circulation after 1–2 days. Reticulocytes gradually lose their ribosomes (over 1–2 days) and become mature red blood cells. Along with this maturation process, erythroid precursors express a number of proteins and glycoproteins including transferrin (TF) receptor, glycoprotein (GP) IV, carbonic anhidrase, blood group antigens, glycophorin A and C, spectrin, band 3 and hemoglobin. TF receptor and GP IV disappear during the maturation of reticulocytes.

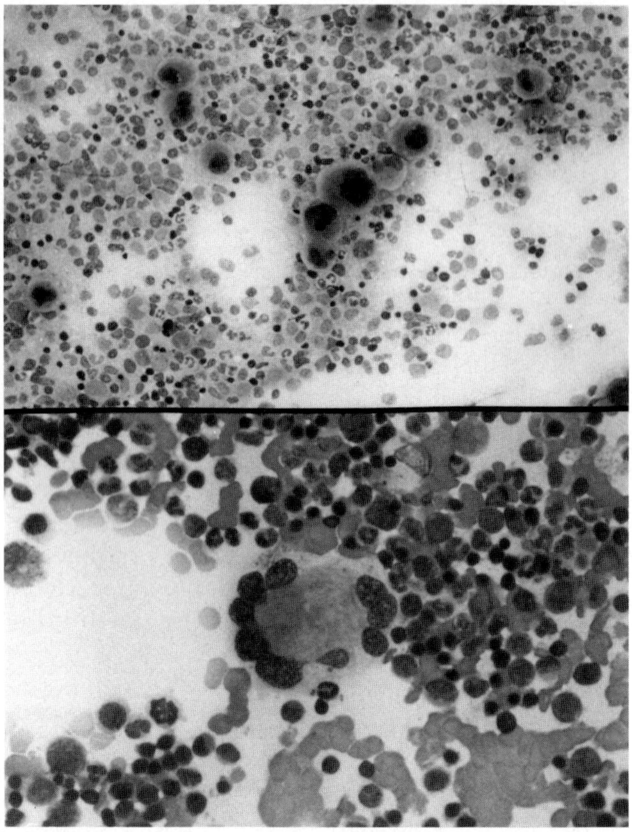

Figure 1-16. Magakaryocytes are the largest bone marrow cells and demonstrate various degrees of nuclear lobulation (a). A megakaryocyte with a marked nuclear lobulation is shown in (b).

Platelet Precursors

Megakaryocytes are the largest hematopoietic elements in the bone marrow. They are highly pleomorphic with respect to both their morphology and size (which may range from 15 to > 80 μm in diameter) (Figures 1-16 and 1-17).

Megakaryocytes are derived from the CFU-megakaryocyte (CFU-Meg). The progeny of the CFU-Meg is the megakaryoblast (promegakaryoblast, group 1 megakaryocyte). Megakaryoblastic proliferation is regulated by IL-3 and GM-CSF, as well as other factors.[135,136] Megakaryoblasts undergo endomitosis (nuclear division without cytoplasmic division) once or twice and become a larger cell with two to four nuclei referred to as "promegakaryocytes" (group II megakaryocytes). The maturation process of the megakaryocytic series is characterized by the continuation of endomitosis and generation of large cells with lobulated nuclei demonstrating 8, 16 or 32 ploidy. During this process of continuous nuclear division, the cell volume gradually increases, the concentration of ribosomal granules (cytoplasmic basophilia) declines, azurophilic granules increase in number and a complex demarcation membrane system is developed, leading to the formation of group III or granular megakaryocytes[137-140] (Figure 1-18). This maturation process is associated with a decline in the proliferative activity of the cells. Overall, at any given time, 44% of megakaryoblasts, 18% of promegakaryocytes and 2% of granular megakaryocytes show evidence of DNA synthesis.[137] The interval from formation of the megakaryoblast to production of platelets is about 1 week. Approximately one-third

Bone Marrow Structure and Function

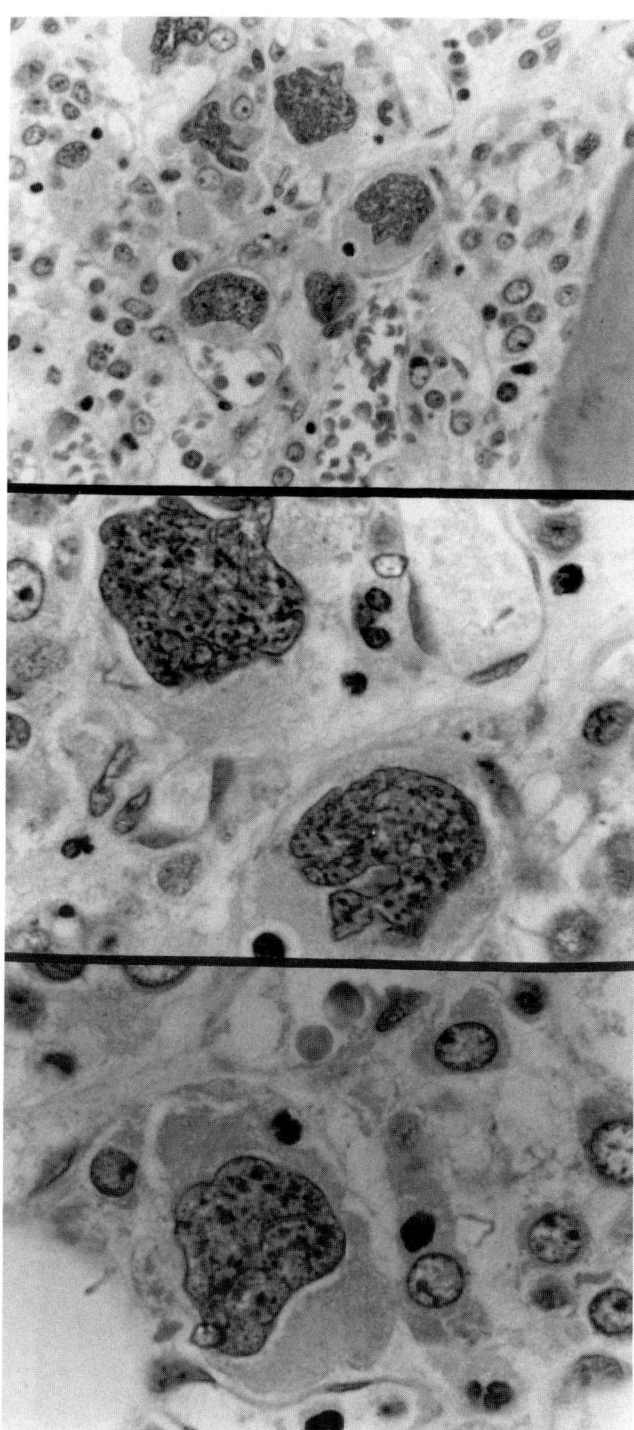

Figure 1-17. A bone marrow biopsy section demonstrating several megakaryocytes in close proximity to the marrow sinusoids.

of the platelets released into the bloodstream are located in the spleen, whereas two-thirds are circulating. Platelets survive for 8–10 days and play an important role in blood coagulation.

The granular megakaryocytes are the platelet-producing cells, capable of passing through sinus endothelial cells and releasing platelets into the circulation. Granular megakaryocytes have a complex cytoplasmic structure divided into three ill-defined zones: perinuclear, intermediate and marginal.[137,140-145] Most of the cytoplasmic organelles including ribosomes, rough endoplasmic reticulum, centrioles, mitochondria and the Golgi system are found in the perinuclear region, suggesting that this region is the primary site of biosynthetic activity in the megakaryocyte.[137, 142] The demarcation membranes, structures unique to the megakaryocytes, develop in the intermediate zone (see Figure 1-18). Whether the demarcation membranes develop from the Golgi membranes or from the plasma membrane of megakaryocytes remains controversial,[137,142] but the formation of these membranes results in the demarcation of platelet fields. The cytoplasm in the intermediate zone contains platelet granules, mitochondria, microfilaments and microtubules, and glycogen. In addition to the above-mentioned zones, some megakaryocytes show a thin (1–2 μm) marginal zone which contains few or no granules and consists primarily of actin-containing microfilaments.

One of the frequent morphologic observations in megakaryocytes is the phenomenon of "emperipolesis," which is the temporary presence of one cell within the cytoplasm of another. Hematopoietic as well as nonhematopoietic cells (i.e., metastatic tumors) may be found inside the cytoplasm of megakaryocytes (Figure 1-19). It has been suggested that some hematopoietic cells may reach the circulation by emperipolesis via the processes of megakaryocytic cytoplasm that protrude into the adjacent bone marrow sinuses.[137]

Platelets are the end products of the megakaryocytic lineage. They are cytoplasmic fragments measuring 2–4 μm in diameter, staining pale blue with fine azurophilic granules. Ultrastructural studies demonstrate four types of granules: (1) alpha granules which contain platelet factor 4, factor VIII-related antigen, beta-thromboglobulin, platelet-derived growth factor, albumin, fibronectin, fibrinogen and thrombospondin; (2) delta granules (dense granules) containing serotonin, calcium, pyrophosphate, and ADP and ATP storage pools; (3) gamma (lysosomal)

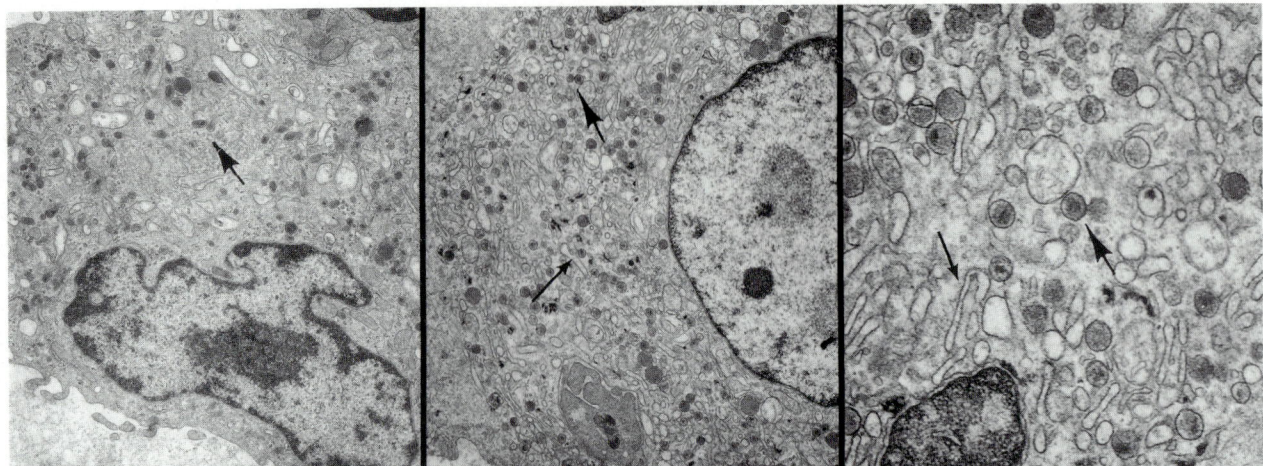

Figure 1-18. Electron microscopic features of granular megakaryocytes. Demarcation membranes (short-headed arrows) and numerous granules (long-headed arrows) are present.

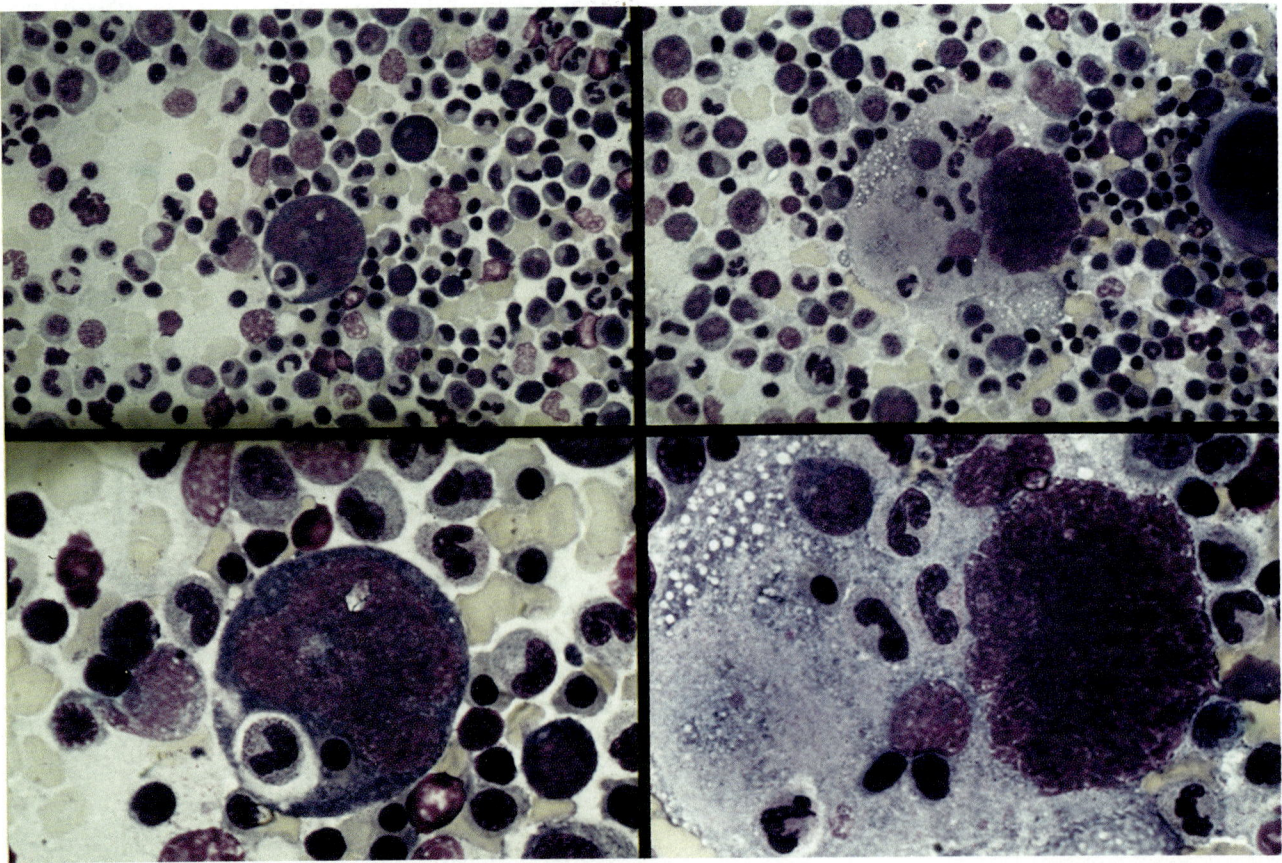

Figure 1-19. Megakaryocytes demonstrating emperipolesis.

Bone Marrow Structure and Function

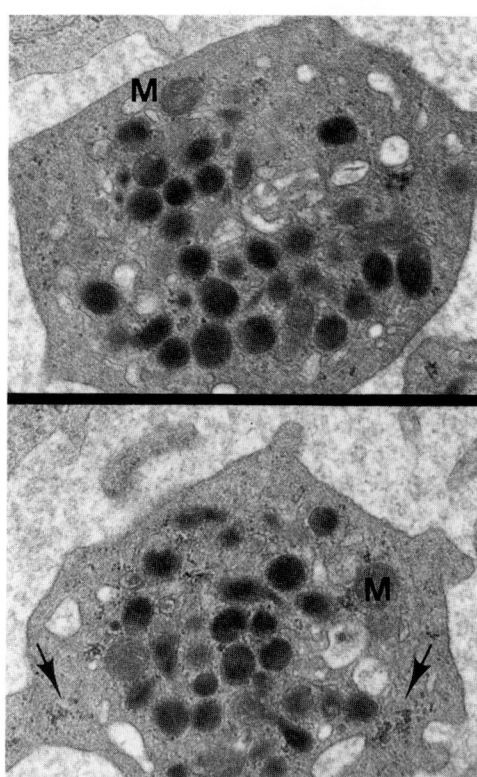

Figure 1-20. Platelets demonstrating numerous granules, scattered mitochondia (M) and glycogen particles (arrow).

granules which contain acid phosphatase, beta-glucuronidase and aryl sulfatase; and (4) peroxisomes containing catalase.[146,147] In addition to these granules, platelets contain mitochondria and glycogen particles (Figure 1-20). Two membrane systems have been demonstrated in platelets: a surface-connected canalicular system and a dense tubular system. Granular megakaryocytes and platelets react with antibodies against CD41, CD42, CD61, von Willebrand factor, platelet factor 4 and fibrinogen (see Figure 10-1, Chapter 10).[135]

Lymphocytes and Plasma Cells

Lymphocytes, similar to the other hematopoietic cells, are derived from the uncommitted pluripotential stem cell (CFU-S). The earliest morphologically identifiable cell in this lineage is the lymphoblast. Lymphoblasts measure 10–15μm in diameter, have a high nuclear/cytoplasmic ratio with a narrow rim of nongranular deep blue cytoplasm, and a round to oval nucleus with finely dispersed chromatin and one or two nucleoli (Figure 1-21). The morphologic stages associated with the transition from lymphoblast to lymphocyte are not well defined. The term "prolymphocyte" is often used to describe lymphoid cells which are less mature than lymphocytes and more mature than lymphoblasts. Prolymphocytes have more cytoplasm and a larger nucleus than lymphocytes, and display a coarse chromatin and often a prominent nucleolus (see Figure 1-21). Lymphid maturation results in the formation of T lymphocytes (thymus derived) and B lymphocytes (bone marrow derived) in man. The functional and immunophenotypic characteristics of both B and T cells during their maturation process have been extensively studied (Tables 1-1 and 1-2).[148-151] Both B and T cells can undergo cell division when they are exposed to mitogens and/or antigens. These transformed or activated lymphocytes are usually large (15–25 μm), with abundant cytoplasm and a highly polymorphic nuclear morphology. These cells may have fine to coarse chromatin and indistinct to prominent nucleoli. B and T lymphocytes and their precursors are morphologically indistinguishable from each other, though their immunophenotypic characteristics are well defined (Figure 1- 22) (Tables 1-1 and 1-2). A small population of the lymphocytes in the bone marrow and peripheral blood have NK activities (i.e., are able to kill target cells without major histocompatibility complex restriction).[152] NK cells are often large, with abundant cytoplasm and cytoplasmic azurophilic granules (large granular lymphocytes)[153] (see Figure 1-21). NK cells express CD11b, CD16, CD56 and CD57 and include a subtype of CD8+ lymphocytes.

Plasma cells are the end product of B lymphocytes and are characterized by abundant deep blue cytoplasm, a pale perinuclear zone, and an eccentric nucleus (see Figure 1-21). The nucleus has coarse chromatin, often with a cartwheel appearance in tissue sections. Plasma cells contain several small, rounded inclusions (Mott or morular cells). They may also contain large eosinophilic cytoplasmic (Russell bodies) or nuclear (Dutcher bodies) inclusions (see Figure 1-21). Flame cells are plasma cells whose cytoplasm is partially or totally eosinophilic.

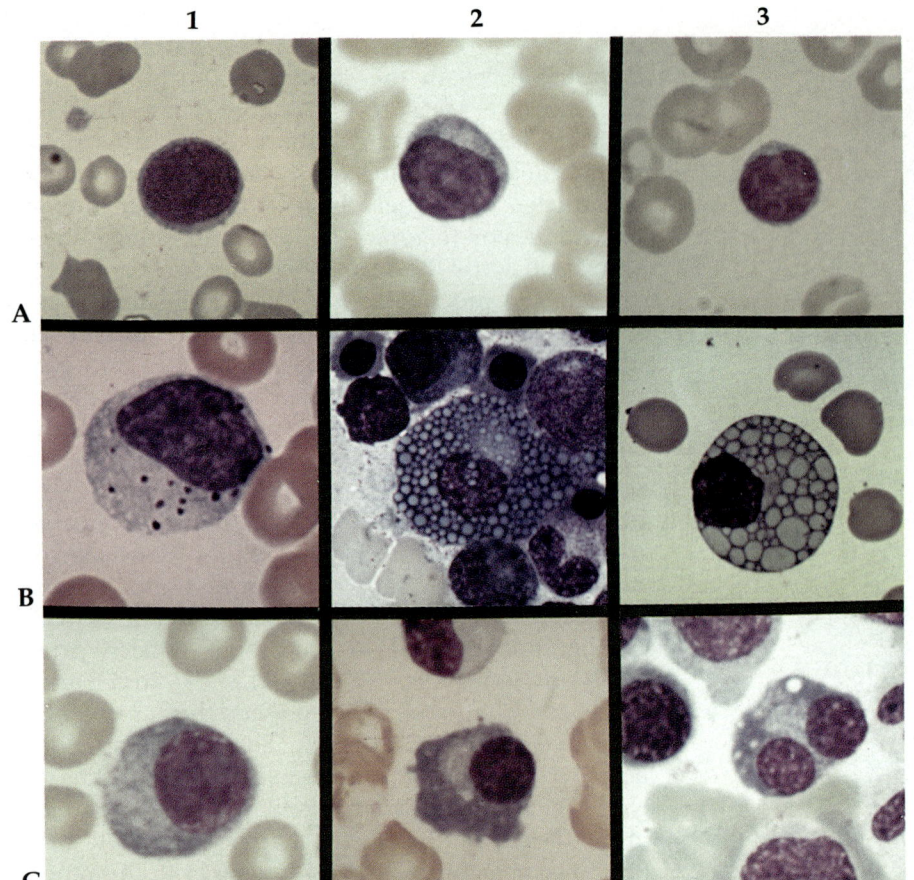

Figure 1-21. (A1) lymphoblast, (A2) prolymphocyte, (A3) lymphocyte, (B1) large granular lymphocyte, (B2) and (B3) vacuolated plasma cell (C1), immature plasma cell, (C2) mature plasma cell, and (C3) binucleated plasma cell.

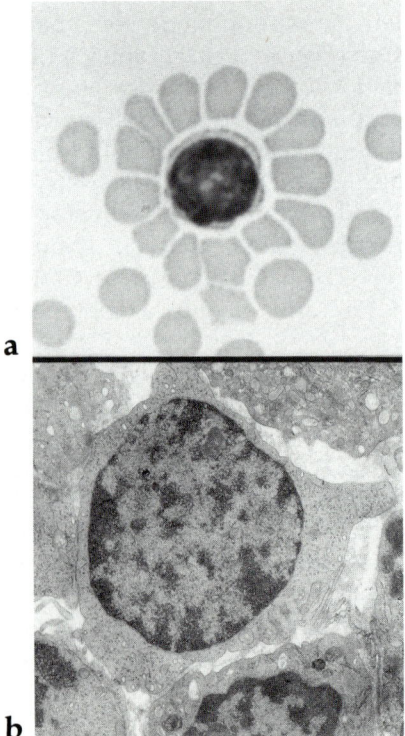

Figure 1-22. A T lymphocyte demonstrating sheep erythrocyte rosetting (a) and electron microscopy of a mature lymphocyte showing prominent heterochromatin, abundant polyribosomes and scattered mitochondria (b).

Table 1-1 Characteristics of B Lymphocytes*

Cell Type	Pluripotent Stem Cell	Committed Progenitor	Pre-B Cell	Immature B Lymphocyte	Mature B Lymphocyte	Plasma Cell
Antigen Ig	Germ-Line Ig Genes	Rearranged Ig Genes	CIg⁺† SMIg⁻	SMIg⁺	SMIg⁺⁺	CIg⁺⁺⁺
HLA-DR		═══	═══	═══	═══	
PI 153/3		═══	═══	═══	═══	
CD9		═══	═══	═══	═══	
CD19		═══	═══	═══	═══	
CD24		═══	═══	═══	═══	
CD10		═══	═══			
HL25		═══	═══	═══		
CD20		═══	═══	═══	═══	
CD21			═══	═══	═══	
FMC1				═══	═══	
41H.16				═══	═══	
L26				═══	═══	
L27					═══	
FMC7				═══		
L22			═══	═══	═══	
L23			═══	═══	═══	
L24			═══	═══	═══	
CD38						═══
PCA1						═══
PC1						═══

* Adapted from Zola H., Differentiation and maturation of human B lymphocytes: A review. *Pathology* 17:365, 1985.
† CIg: cytoplasmic Ig; SMIg, surface membrane Ig.

Table 1-2 Cell Surface Antigen Expressions in the T-Cell Lineage

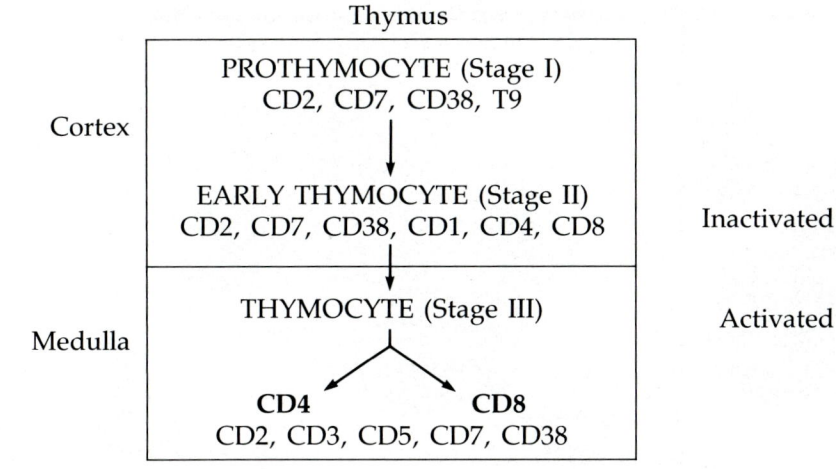

	Thymus		Peripheral Blood	
			Inducer	Suppressor
Cortex	PROTHYMOCYTE (Stage I) CD2, CD7, CD38, T9 ↓ EARLY THYMOCYTE (Stage II) CD2, CD7, CD38, CD1, CD4, CD8	Inactivated	**CD4**, CD2, CD3, CD5, CD7	**CD8**, CD2, CD3, CD5, CD7
Medulla	↓ THYMOCYTE (Stage III) ↙ ↘ **CD4** **CD8** CD2, CD3, CD5, CD7, CD38	Activated	**CD4**, CD2, CD3, CD5, CD7, CD25, HLA-DR	**CD8**, CD2, CD3, CD5, CD7, CD25, HLA-DR

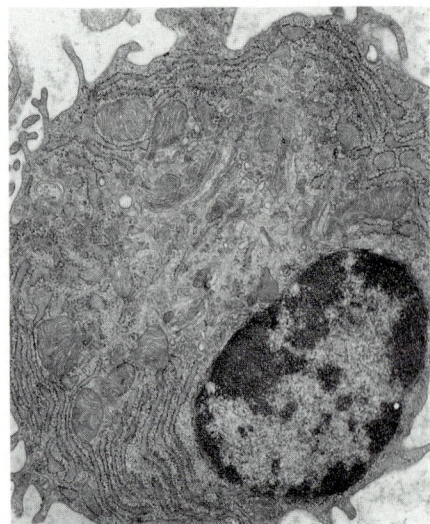

Figure 1-23. Electron microscopy of a plasma cell demonstrating an eccentric nucleus, abundant rough endoplasmic reticulum, scattered mitochondria and a perinuclear Golgi system.

Ultrastructurally, plasma cells are characterized by a well-developed Golgi system and abundant rough endoplasmic reticulum, which are necessary for the large-scale production of immunoglobulins. A moderate number of mitochondria and occasional lysosomal granules are also present (Figure 1-23).

Osteoblasts and Osteoclasts

In bone marrow biopsy sections, osteoblasts and osteoclasts are located along the bone trabeculae. Osteoblasts are involved in osteoid deposition and new bone formation. They are elongated mononuclear

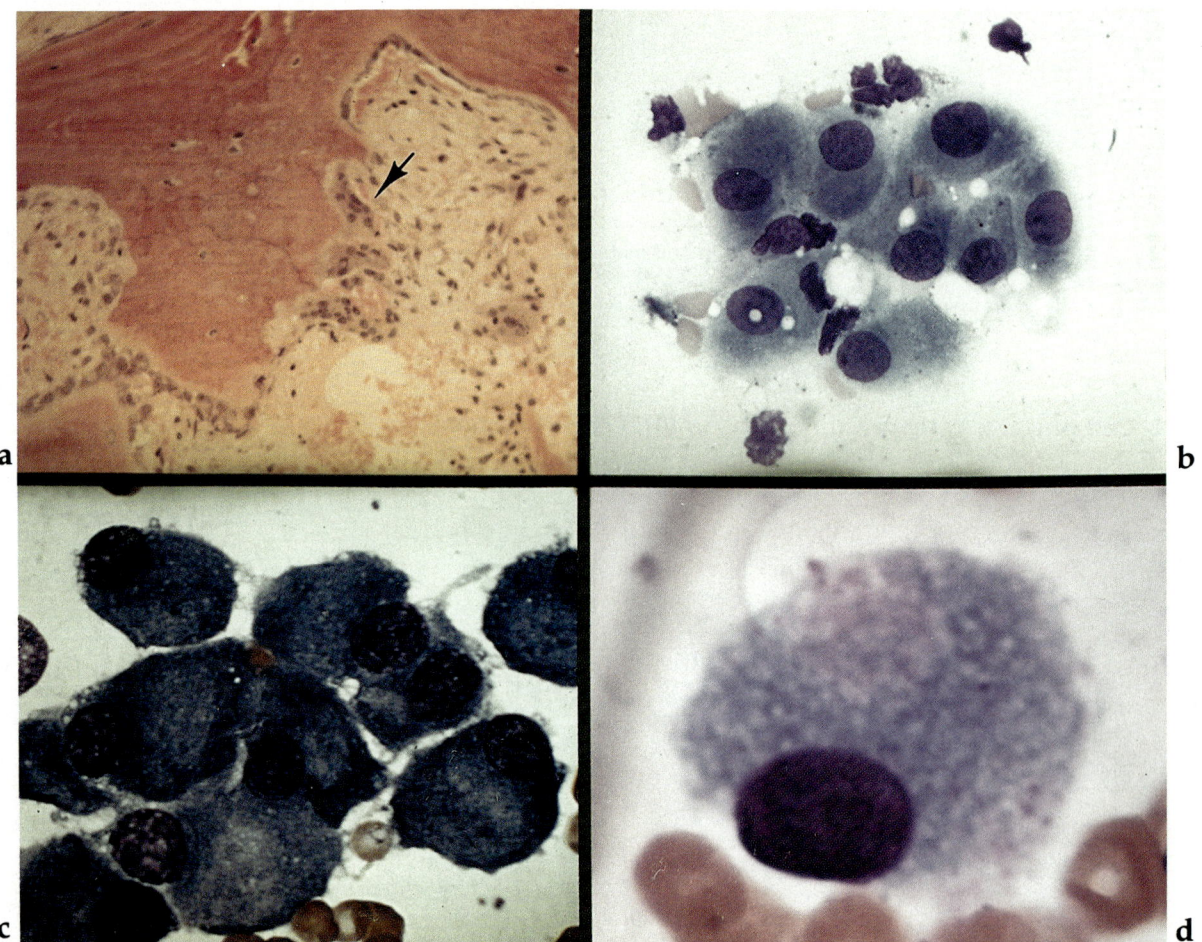

Figure 1-24. Osteoblasts are demonstrated in a biopsy section at the margins of the bone trabeculae (arrow) (a) and in bone marrow smears (b, c, d).

Bone Marrow Structure and Function

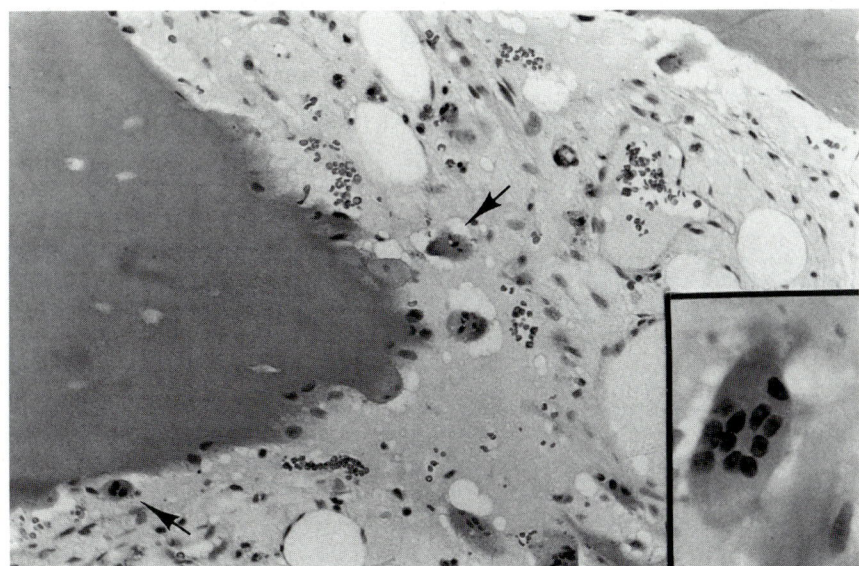

Figure 1-25. A bone marrow biopsy section demonstrating several osteoclasts (arrow and insert).

cells with a variable amount of cytoplasm and an eccentric nucleus (Figure 1-24). In bone marrow smears, osteoblasts often appear as a small cluster of oval or elongated cells that contain a single eccentric nucleus and one or more nucleoli. Osteoblasts have some resemblance to plasma cells, but they are larger than plasma cells, their Golgi system is not as close to the nucleus and their nuclear chromatin is finer than that of the plasma cell (see Figure 1-24).

Osteoclasts are multinucleated giant cells, derived from the monocytic lineage, that are involved in bone resorption and remodeling. Their abundant cytoplasm contains numerous azurophilic granules (Figures 1-25 and 1-26). They are frequently found in bone marrow specimens from patients with Paget's disease or hyperparathyroidism or from pediatric patients. Osteoclasts bear some resemblance to megakaryocytes. However, unlike megakaryocytes, the multiple nuclei present in each cell are uniform in size and separate from each other.

Adipocytes

Adipocytes (lipocytes, fat cells) are the most prominent component of the bone marrow stroma. These are large cells with fat-laden cytoplasm and a small,

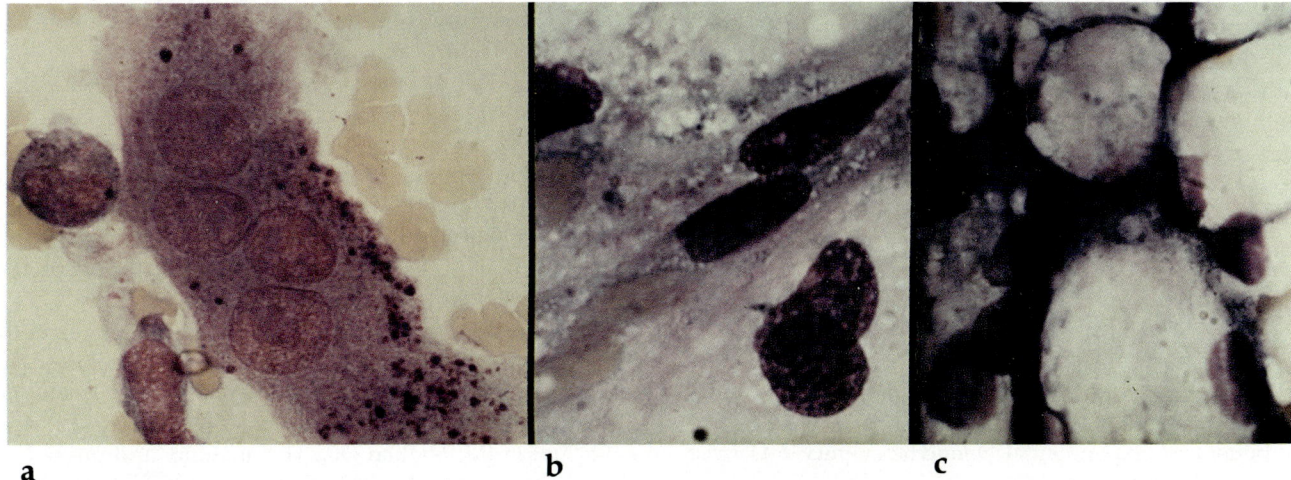

Figure 1-26. Marrow smears showing an osteoclast (a), endothelial cells (b) and adipocytes (c).

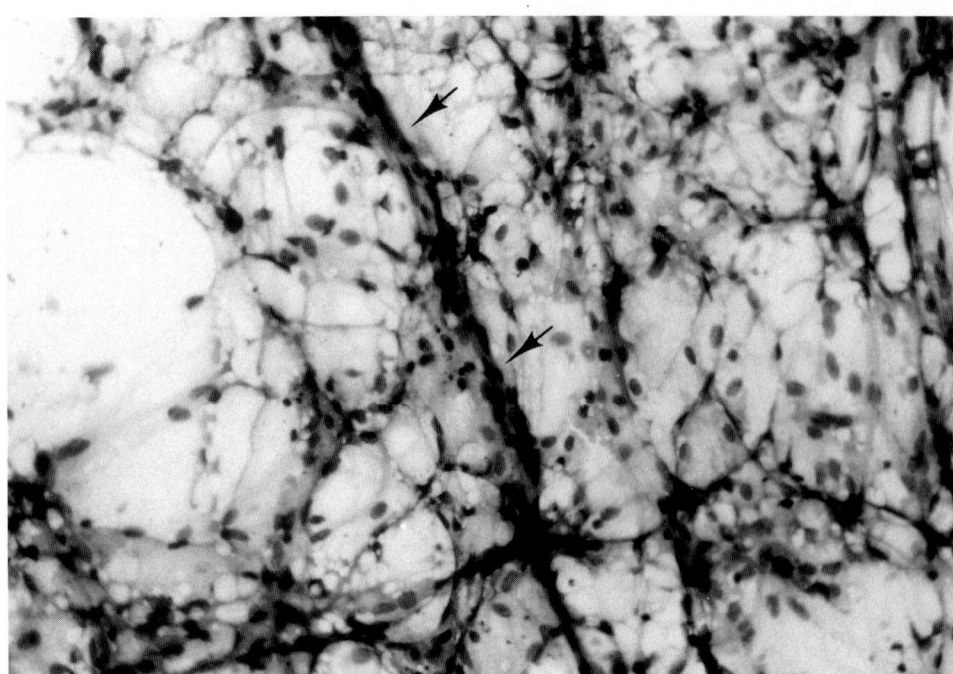

Figure 1-27. Bone marrow smear demonstrating numerous adipocytes and a collapsed capillary (arrow).

pyknotic nucleus often eccentrically located (Figures 1-26 and 1-27). Bone marrow fatty tissue can be rapidly replaced by hematopoietic tissue when there is a need for more blood cells.

Fibroblast-Like Cells and Endothelial Cells

Fibroblast-like cells (reticulum cells) support the wall of the bone marrow sinuses and make up the skeletal framework that supports the hematopoietic cells in the marrow. These cells are usually large (15–30 µm) and elongated or polygonal, with pale blue cytoplasm and round, oval or folded nuclei. Their nuclear chromatin is fine, and one or more nucleoli may be seen. Their cytoplasm may contain a variable number of azurophilic or eosinophilic granules. Endothelial cells appear very similar to the fibroblast-like cells on Wright's-stained marrow smears (see Figure 1-26).

References

1. Weiss L: The structure of bone marrow; functional interrelationships of vascular and hematopoietic components in experimental hemolytic anemia. *J Morphol* 117:467, 1965.
2. De Bruyn PPH: Structural substrates of bone marrow function. *Semin Hematol* 18:179, 1981.
3. Politis C, Karamerou A, Block M: Pathophysiologic aspects of the bone/marrow/fat relationship. *Lab Management* 21:40, 1983.
4. Gulati GL, Ashton JK, Hyun BH: Structure and function of the bone marrow and hematopoiesis. *Hematol Oncol Clin North Am* 2:495, 1988.
5. DeBruyn PPH, Breen PC, Thomas TB: The microcirculation of the bone marrow. *Anat Rec* 168:55, 1970.
6. Doan CA: The circulation of the bone marrow. *Carnegie Inst Wash Contrib Embryol* 14:27, 1922.
7. Hartsock R, Smith EB, Petty CS: Normal variations with aging at the amount of hematopoietic tissue in bone marrow from the anterior iliac crest. *Am J Clin Pathol* 43:326, 1965.
8. Custer RP: *An Atlas of the Blood and Bone Marrow*, ed 2, Philadelphia, WB Saunders, 1974, p 33.
9. Rozman C, Feliu E, Berga L, et al: Age-related variations of fat tissue fraction in normal human bone marrow depend both on size and number of adipocytes; a stereological study. *Exp Hematol* 17:34, 1989.
10. Chertkov JL: Early hematopoietic and stromal precursor cells. *Int Rev Cytol* 102:271, 1986.
11. Dexter TM, Moore M: Growth and development in the hematopoietic system; the role of lymphokines and their possible therapeutic potential in disease and malignancy. *Carcinogenesis* 7:509, 1986.
12. Lipton JM, Nathan DG: The anatomy and physiology of hematopoiesis, in Nathan DG, Oski FE (eds), *Hema-*

topoietic Stem Cell, ed 3. New York, Marcel Dekker, 1985, p 145.
13. Takashina J: Hemopoiesis in the human yolk sack. J Anat 151:125, 1987.
14. Nelson DA, Davey FR: Hematopoiesis, in Henry JB (ed), Clinical Diagnosis and Management by Laboratory Methods. Philadelphia, WB Saunders, 1984, p 626.
15. Erslev AJ, Weiss L: Structure and function of the marrow, in Williams WJ, Beutler E, Erslev AJ, et al (eds), Hematology, ed 3. New York, McGraw-Hill, 1983, p 75.
16. Albelda SM, Buck CA: Integrins and other adhesion molecules. FASEB J 4:2868, 1990.
17. Tavassoli M, Hardy CL: Molecular basis of homing of intravenously transplanted stem cells to the marrow. Blood 76:1059, 1990.
18. Roberts R, Gallagher J, Spooner E, et al: Heparan sulfate-bound growth factors: A mechanism for stromal cell-mediated hematopoiesis. Nature 332:376, 1988.
19. Dexter TM: Heparan sulphate bound growth factors; a mechanism for stromal cell mediated hemopoiesis. Nature 332:376, 1988.
20. Gordon MY, Riley GP, Watt SM, et al: Compartmentalization of a hematopoietic growth factor (GM-CSF) by glycosaminoglycans in the bone marrow microenvironment. Nature 326:403, 1987.
21. Zipori D: Modulation of hemopoiesis by novel stromal cell factors. Leukemia 2 (suppl 12):9S, 1988.
22. Zipori D, Lee F: Introduction of interleukin-3 gene into stromal cells from the bone marrow alters hemopoietic differentiation but does not modify stem cell renewal. Blood 71:586, 1988.
23. Campbell AD: Haemonectin, a bone marrow adhesion protein specific for cells of granulocyte lineage. Nature 329:744, 1987.
24. De Bruyn PPH, Michelson S, Thomas TB: The migration of blood cells of the bone marrow through the sinusoidal wall. J Morphol 133:417, 1971.
25. Campbell F: Ultrastructural studies of transmural migration of blood cells in the bone marrow of rats, mice and guinea pigs. Am J Anat 135:521, 1972.
26. Muto M: A scanning and transmission electron microscopic study on rat bone marrow sinuses and transmural migration of blood cells. Arch Histol Jpn 39:51, 1976.
27. Becker RP, De Bruyn PPH: The transmural passage of blood cells into myeloid sinusoids and the entry of platelets into the sinusoidal circulation; a scanning electron microscopic investigation. Am J Anat 145:183, 1976.
28. Huyn BH, Gulati GL, Ashton JK: Color Atlas of Clinical Hematology. New York, Igaku-Shoin, 1986, p 4.
29. Jandl JH: Blood: Textbook of Hematology. Boston, Little, Brown, 1987, p 1.
30. Kushner JA: Hematopoietic stem cell proliferation. Lab Med 12:279, 1981.
31. Yoffey JM: Stem cell kinetics: Correlation of in vivo and in vitro data. Exp Hematol 15:110, 1987.
32. Ogawa M, Porter PN, Nakahata T: Renewal and commitment to differentiation of hemopoietic stem cells. Blood 61:823, 1983.
33. Till JE, McCulloch EA: A direct measurement of the radiation sensitivity of normal mouse bone marrow cells. Radiat Res 14:213, 1961.
34. Siminovitch L, Till JE, McCulloch EA: Decline in colony-forming ability of marrow cells subjected to serial transplantation into irradiated mice. J Cell Comp Physiol 64:23, 1964.
35. Reviewed in Schofield R: The relationship between spleen colony-forming cells and the haematopoietic stem cell. Blood Cells 4:7, 1978.
36. Hodgson GS, Bradley TR: Properties of haematopoietic stem cells surviving 5-flurouracil treatment: Evidence for a pre-CFU-S cell? Nature 281:381, 1979.
37. Van Zant G: Studies of hematopoietic stem cells spared by 5-fluorouracil. J Exp Med 159:679, 1984.
38. Bradley TR, Metcalf D: The growth of mouse bone marrow cells in vitro. Aust J Exp Biol Med Sci 44:287, 1966.
39. Pluznik DH, Sachs L: The cloning of normal "mast" cells in tissue culture. J Cell Comp Physiol 66:319, 1965.
40. Nakahata T, Ogawa M: Identification in culture of a class of hematopoietic colony-forming units with extensive capability to self-renew and generate multipotential colonies. Proc Natl Acad Sci USA 79:3843, 1982.
41. Spangrude GJ, Heimfled S, Weissman IL: Purification and characterization of mouse hematopoietic stem cells. Science 241:58, 1988.
42. Civin CI, Strauss LC, Brovall C, et al: Antigenic analysis of hematopoiesis III. A hematopoietic progenitor cell surface antigen defined by a monoclonal antibody raised against KG-1a cells. J Immunol 133:157, 1984.
43. Beschorner WE, Civin CI, Strauss LC: Localization of human hematopoietic progenitor cells in tissue with anti-MY-10 monoclonal antibody. Am J Pathol 119:1, 1985.
44. Ikebuchi K, Wong GG, Clark SC, et al: Interleukin 6 enhancement of interleukin 3-dependent proliferation of multipotential hematopoietic progenitors. Proc Natl Acad Sci USA 84:9035, 1987.
45. Ikebuchi K, Ihle JN, Hirai Y, et al: Synergistic factors for stem cell proliferation: Further studies of target stem cells and the mechanism of stimulation by interleukin-1, interleukin-6, and granulocyte colony-stimulating factor. Blood 72:2007, 1988.
46. Leary AG, Ikebuchi K, Hiari Y, et al: Synergism between interleukin-6 and interleukin-3 in supporting proliferation of human hematopoietic stem cells: Comparison with interleukin-1α. Blood 71:1759, 1988.

47. Ikebuchi K, Clark SC, Ihle JN, et al: Granulocyte colony-stimulating factor enhances interleukin-3-dependent proliferation of multipotential hematopoietic progenitors. *Proc Natl Acad Sci USA* 85:3445, 1988.
48. Leary AG, Yang YC, Clark S, et al: Recombinant gibbon interleukin 3 supports formation of human multilineage colonies and blast cell colonies in culture: Comparison with recombinant human granulocyte-macrophage colony-stimulating factor. *Blood* 70:1343, 1987.
49. Messner HA, Yamasaki K, Jamal N, et al: Growth of human hematopoietic colonies in response to recombinant gibbon interleukin-3: Comparison with human recombinant granulocyte-macrophage colony-stimulating factor. *Proc Natl Acad Sci USA* 84:6765, 1987.
50. Golde DW: Overview of myeloid growth factors. *Semin Hematol* 27 (Suppl 3):1, 1990.
51. Morytyn G, Burgess AW: Hematopoietic growth factors: A review. *Cancer Res* 48:5624, 1988.
52. Sieff C: Hematopoietic growth factors. *J Clin Invest* 79:1549, 1987.
53. Metcalf D: The molecular biology and functions of the granulocyte-macrophage colony-stimulating factors. *Blood* 67:257, 1986.
54. Storber W, James SP: The interleukins. *Pediatr Res* 24:549, 1988.
55. Champlin R, Nimer SD, Ireland P, et al: Treatment of refractory aplastic anemia with recombinant human granulocyte-macrophage colony-stimulating factor. *Blood* 73:694, 1989.
56. Ganser A, Voelkers B, Greher J, et al: Recombinant human granulocyte-macrophage colony-stimulating factor in patients with myelodysplastic syndromes—A phase I/II trial. *Blood* 73:31, 1989.
57. Warren MK, Ralph P: Macrophage growth factor CSF-1 stimulates human monocyte production of interferon, tumor necrosis factor, and colony-stimulating activity. *J Immunol* 137:2281, 1986.
58. Ikebuchi K, Wong GG, Clark SC, et al: Interleukin 6 enhancement of interleukin 3-dependent proliferation of multipotential hematopoietic progenitors. *Proc Natl Acad Sci USA* 84:9035, 1987.
59. Ikebuchi K, Clark SC, Ihle JN, et al: Granulocyte colony-stimulating factor enhances interleukin-3 dependent proliferation of multipotential hematopoietic progenitors. *Proc Natl Acad Sci USA* 85:3445, 1988.
60. Leary AG, Ikebuchi K, Hirari Y, et al: Synergism between interleukin-6 and interleukin-3 in supporting proliferation of human hematopoietic stem cells. Comparison with interleukin-1α. *Blood* 71:1759, 1988.
61. Velenga E, Young DC, Wagner K, et al: The effects of GM-CSF and G-CSF in promoting growth of colonogenic cells in acute myeloblastic leukemia. *Blood* 69:1771, 1987.
62. Delwel R, Dorssers L, Touw I, et al: Human recombinant multilineage colony stimulating factor (interleukin-3): Stimulator of acute myelocytic leukemia progenitor cells in vitro. *Blood* 70:333, 1987.
63. Heubner K, Isobe M, Croce CM, et asl: The human gene encoding GM-CSF is at 5q21–q32, the chromosome region deleted in 5q-anomaly. *Science* 230:1282, 1985.
64. Chan JY, Slamon DJ, Nimer SD, et al: Regulation of expression of human granulocyte-macrophage colony-stimulating factor (GM-CSF). *Proc Natl Acad Sci USA* 83:8669, 1986.
65. Thorens B, Mermod JJ, Vassalli P: Phagocytosis and inflammatory stimuli induce GM-CSF mRNA in macrophages through posttranscriptional regulation. *Cell* 48:671, 1987.
66. Broudy VC, Zuckerman KS, Jermalani S, et al: Monocytes stimulate fibroblastoid bone marrow stromal cells to produce multi-lineage hematopoietic growth factors. *Blood* 68:530, 1986.
67. Strife A, Lambek C, Wisniewski D, et al: Activities of four purified growth factors on highly enriched human hematopoietic progenitor cells. *Blood* 69:1508, 1987.
68. Tomonaga M, Golde DW, Gasson JC: Biosynthetic (recombinant) human granulocyte-macrophage colony-stimulating factor: Effects on normal bone marrow and leukemia cell lines. *Blood* 67:31, 1986.
69. Sieff CA, Emerson SG, Donahue RE, et al: Human recombinant granulocyte-macrophage colony-stimulating factor: A multilineage hematopoietin. *Science* 230:1171, 1985.
70. Groopman JE, Mitsuyasu RT, Deleo MJ, et al: Effect of recombinant human granulocyte-macrophage colony-stimulating factor on myelopoiesis in the acquired immunodeficiency syndrome. *N Engl J Med* 317:593, 1987.
71. Antman KS, Griffin JD, Elias A, et al: Effects of recombinant human granulocyte-macrophage colony-stimulating factor on chemotherapy-induced myelosuppression. *N Engl J Med* 319:593, 1988.
72. Naeim F, Champlin R, Nimer S: Bone marrow changes in patients with refractory aplastic anemia treated by recombinant GM-CSF. *Hematol Pathol* 4:79, 1990.
73. Simmers RN, Webber LM, Shannon MF, et al: Localization of the G-CSF gene on chromosome 17 proximal to the breakpoint in the t(15, 17) in acute promyelocytic leukemia. *Blood* 70:330, 1987.
74. Nagata S, Tsuchiya M, Asano S, et al: Molecular cloning and expression of cDNA from human granulocyte-colony stimulating factor. *Nature* 319:415, 1986.
75. Glaspy JA, Baldwin GC, Robertson PA, et al: Therapy for neutropenia in hairy cell leukemia with recombinant human granulocyte colony-stimulating factor. *Ann Intern Med* 109:789, 1988.

76. Jakubowski AA, Souza L, Kelly F, et al: Effects of human granulocyte colony-stimulating factor in a patient with idiopathic neutropenia. *N Engl J Med* 320:38, 1989.
77. Kobayashi Y, Okabe T, Ozawa K, et al: Treatment of myelodysplastic syndromes with recombinant human granulocyte colony-stimulating factor: A preliminary report. *Am J Med* 86:178, 1989.
78. Hammond WP, Price TH, Souza LM, et al: Treatment of cyclic neutropenia with granulocyte colony-stimulating factor. *N Engl J Med* 320:1306, 1989.
79. Morstyn G, Souza L, Keech J, et al: Effects of granulocyte colony stimulating factor on neutropenia induced by cytotoxic chemotherapy. *Lancet* 1:667, 1988.
80. Wong GG, Temple PA, Leary AC, et al: Human CSF-1: Molecular cloning and expression of a 4 kb cDNA encoding the hematopoietin and determination of the complete amino acid sequence of the human urinary protein. *Science* 235:1504, 1987.
81. Morris SW, Valentine MB, Shapiro DN, et al. Reassignment of the human CSF1 gene to chromosome 1p13-p21. *Blood* 78:2013, 1991.
82. Fibbe WE, Van Damme J, Billiau A, et al: Human fibroblasts produce granulocyte-CSF, macrophage-CSF, and granulocyte-macrophage-CSF following stimulation by interleukin-1 and poly(rI), poy (rC). *Blood* 72:860, 1988.
83. Horiguchi J, Warren MK, Kufe D: Expression of the macrophage specific colony stimulating factor in human monocytes treated with granulocyte-macrophage colony-stimulating factor. *Blood* 69:1259, 1987.
84. Masaoka T, Motoyoshi K, Takaku F, et al: Administration of human urinary colony stimulating factor after bone marrow transplantation. *Bone Marrow Trans* 3:121, 1988.
85. Spivak JL, Smith RRL, Ihle JN: Interleukin-3 promotes the in vitro proliferation of murine pluripotent hematopoietic stem cells. *J Clin Invest* 76:1613, 1985.
86. Le Beau MM, Epstein ND, O'Brien SJ, et al: The interleukin 3 gene is located on human chromosome 5 and is deleted in myeloid leukemias with deletion of 5q. *Proc Natl Acad Sci USA* 84:5913, 1987.
87. Saeland S, Caux C, Favre C, et al: Effects of recombinant human interleukin-3 on CD34-enriched normal hematopoietic progenitors and on myeloblastic leukemia cells. *Blood* 72:1580, 1988.
88. Ganser A, Lindeman A, Ottman OG, et al: Effects of recombinant human IL-3 in vivo—a phase I study, abstracted. *Exp Hematol* 17:484, 1989.
89. Law ML, Cai GY, Lin FK, et al: Chromosomal assignment of the human erythropoietin gene and its DNA polymorphism. *Proc Natl Acad Sci USA* 83:6920, 1986.
90. Koury ST, Bondurant MC, Koury MJ: Localization of erythropoietin synthesizing cells in murine kidneys by in situ hybridization. *Blood* 71:524, 1988.
91. Zanjani ED, Poster J, Burlington H, et al: Liver as the primary site of erythropoietin formation in fetus. *J Lab Clin Med* 89:640, 1977.
92. Migliaccio G, Migliaccio AR, Visser JWM: Synergism between erythropoietin and interleukin-3 in the induction of hematopoietic stem cell proliferation and erythroid burst colony formation. *Blood* 72:944, 1988.
93. Eschbach JW, Kelly MR, Haley NR, et al: Treatment of the anemia of progressive renal failure with recombinant human erythropoietin. *N Engl J Med* 321:158, 1989.
94. Dinarello CA: Biology of interleukin-1. *FASEB J* 2:108, 1988.
95. March CJ, Mosley B, Larsen A, et al: Cloning sequence and expression of two distinct human interleukin-1 complementary DNAs. *Nature* 315:641, 1985.
96. Zsebo KM, Wypych J, McNiece IK, et al: Identification, purification, and biological characterization of hematopoietic stem cell factor from buffalo rat liver-conditioned medium. *Cell* 63:195, 1990.
97. Copeland NG, Gilbert DJ, Cho BC, et al: Mast cell growth factor maps near the steel locus on mouse chromosome 10 and is deleted in a number of steel alleles. *Cell* 63:175, 1990.
98. Paul SR, Bennet F, Calvetti JA, et al: Molecular cloning of a cDNA encoding interleukin-11, a novel stromal cell-derived lymphopoietic and hematopoietic cytokine. *Proc Natl Acad Sci USA* 87:7512, 1990.
99. Malkovsky M, Loveland B, North M, et al: Recombinant interleukin-2 directly augments the cytotoxicity of human monocytes. *Nature* 325:262, 1987.
100. Paul WE: Interleukin 4/B cell stimulatory factor 1: One lymphokine, many functions. *J Fed Am Soc Exp Biol* 1:456, 1987.
101. Zlotnik A, Fischer M, Roehm N, et al: Evidence for effects of interleukin 4 (B cell stimulatory factor 1) on macrophages: Enhancement of antigen presenting ability of bone marrow-derived macrophages. *J Immunol* 138:4279, 1987.
102. Essner R, Rhoades K, McBride TW, et al: IL-4 down-regulates IL-1 and TNF gene expression in human monocytes. *J Immunol* 142:3857, 1989.
103. Lopez AF, Sanderson CJ, Gamble JR, et al: Recombinant human interleukin 5 is a selective activator of human eosinophil function. *J Exp Med* 167:219, 1988.
104. Namen AE, Lupton S, Hjerrild K, et al: Stimulation of B-cell progenitors by cloned murine interleukin-7. *Nature* 333:571, 1988.
105. Chazen GD, Pereira GMB, LeGros G, et al: Interleukin 7 is a T-cell growth factor. *Proc Natl Acad Sci USA* 86:5923, 1989.
106. Hansson M: Growth and differentiation factors for B and T cells. *Leukemia Res* 14:705, 1990.
107. Zuker-Franklin D, Greaves MF, Grossi CE, et al: *Atlas of Blood Cells*. Philadelphia, Lee and Febiger, 1981.

108. Bainton DF, Ullyot JL, Farquhar MG: The development of neutrophilic polymorphonuclear leukocytes in human bone marrow. *J Exp Med* 134:907, 1971.
109. Bainton DF, Farquhar MG: Origin of granules in polymorphonuclear leukocytes: Two types derived from opposite faces of the Golgi complex of developing granulocytes. *J Cell Biol* 28:277, 1966.
110. Lehrer RI, Ganz T, Selsted ME, et al: Neutrophils and host defense. *Ann Intern Med* 109:127, 1988.
111. Zucker-Franklin D: Electron microscopic studies of human granulocytes: Structural variations related to function. *Semin Hematol* 5:109, 1968.
112. Archer GT, Hirch JG: Isolation of granules from eosinophil leukocytes and study of their enzyme content. *J Exp Med* 118:277, 1963.
113. Bainton DF, Farquhar MG: Segregation and packaging of granule enzymes in eosinophilic leukocytes. *J Cell Biol* 45:54, 1970.
114. Hardin JH, Spicer SS: An ultrastructural study of human eosinophil granules: Maturational shapes and pyroantimonate reactive cation. *Am J Anat* 128:283, 1970.
115. Olsson I, Venge P, Spitznagel JK, et al: Arginine-rich cationic proteins of human eosinophil granules. *Lab Invest* 36:493, 1977.
116. Zucker-Franklin D: Ultrastructural evidence for the common origin of human mast cells and basophils. *Blood* 56:534, 1980.
117a. Dvorak AM, Dvorak HF, Galli SJ: Ultrastructural criteria for identification of mast cells and basophils in humans, guinea pigs, and mice. *Am Rev Respir Dis* 128:S49, 1983.
117b. Dvorak AM, Saito H, Estrella P, et al: Ultrastructure of eosinophils and basophils stimulated to develop in human cord blood mononuclear cell cultures containing recombinant human interleukin-5 or interleukin-3. *Lab Invest* 61:116, 1989.
118. Wickramasinghe SN: *Blood and Bone Marrow.* London, Churchill Livingstone, 1986.
119. Galli SJ: New insights into the riddle of the mast cells: Microenvironmental regulation of mast cell development and phenotypic heterogeneity. *Lab Invest* 62:1, 1990.
120. Ryan GB, Majno G: *Inflammation.* Kalamazoo, Mich, Upjohn, 1977.
121. Beaven MA, Cunha-Melo JR: Membrane phosphoinositide-activated signals in mast cells and basophils. *Prog Allergy* 42:123, 1988.
122. Nathan CF, Murray HW, Cohn ZA: The macrophage as an effector cell. *N Engl J Med* 303:622, 1980.
123. Lasser A: The mononuclear phagocytic system: A review. *Human Pathol* 14:108, 1983.
124. van Furth RL: Origin and turnover of monocytes and macrophages. *Curr Top Pathol* 79:125, 1989.
125. Birbeck MS, Breathnach AS, Eversall JD: An electron microscope study of basal melanocytes and high-level clear cells (Langerhans cells) in vitiligo. *J Invest Dermatol* 37:51, 1961.
126. Murphy GF, Bhan AK, Sato S, et al: A new immunologic marker for human Langerhans cells. *N Eng J Med* 304:791, 1981.
127. Naeim F, Hoon DS, Cheng L, et al: Reactivity of neoplastic cells of hairy cell leukemia with antisera to S-100 protein. *Am J Clin Pathol* 88:86, 1987.
128. Gonzalez CL, Jaffe ES: The histiocytosis: Clinical presentation and differential diagnosis. *Oncology* 4:47, 1990.
129. Takahashi K, Tokiashi I, Ohtsuki Y, et al: Immunohistochemical localization and distribution of S-100 protein in the human lymphoreticular system. *Am J Pathol* 116:497, 1984.
130. Brittenham GM, Danish EH, Hariss JW: Assessment of bone marrow and body iron stores: Old techniques and new technologies: *Semin Hematol* 18:194, 1981.
131. Hershko C: Storage iron regulation. *Prog Hematol* 10:105, 1977.
132. Fillet G, Cook JD, Finch CA: Storage iron kinetics. VII. A biologic model for reticuloendothelial iron transport. *J Clin Invest* 53:1527, 1974.
133. Lipschitz DA, Bothwell TH, Seftel HC, et al: The role of ascorbic acid in the metabolism of storage iron. *Br J Haematol* 20:155, 1971.
134. Lazarides E: From genesis to structural morphogenesis: The genesis and epigenesis of a red blood cell. *Cell* 51:345, 1987.
135. Vainchenker W, Kieffer N: Human megakaryocytopoiesis: In vitro regulation and characterization of megakaryocytic precursor cells by differentiation markers. *Blood Rev* 2:102, 1988.
136. Hegyi E, Navarro S, Debili N, et al: Regulation of human megakaryocytopoiesis: Analysis of proliferation, ploidy and maturation in liquid cultures. *Int J Cell Cloning* 8:236, 199.
137. Wickramasighe SN: Normal hematopoiesis: Cellular composition and normal bone marrow. In Wickramasinghe SN (ed), *Blood and Bone Marrow*, ed 3. London, Churchill Livingstone, 1986, p 57.
138. Odell TT Jr, Jackson TW, Friday TJ: Megakaryocytopoiesis in the rat with special reference to polyploidy. *Blood* 35:775, 1970.
139. Burkhardt R: Bone marrow in megakaryocytic disorders. *Hematol Oncol North Am* 2:695, 1988.
140. Huffman R, Straneva J, Yank HH, et al: New insights into the regulation of megakaryocytopoiesis. *Blood Cells* 13:75, 1987.

141. Zucker-Franklin D: Megakaryocytes and platelets, in Zucker-Franklin D, Greaves MF, Grossi CE, et al (eds), *Atlas of Blood Cells: Function and Pathology*. Philadelphia, Lea and Febiger, 1981, p 557.
142. Zucker-Franklin D, Petursson S: Thrombocytopoiesis—analysis by membrane tracer and freeze-fracture studies on fresh human and cultured mouse megakaryocytes. *J Cell Biol* 99:390, 1984.
143. Paulus JM, Bury J, Grosdent JC: Control of platelet territory development in megakaryocytes. *Blood Cells* 5:59, 1979.
144. Becker RP, de Bruyn PPH: The transmural passage of blood cells into myeloid sinusoids and entry of platelets into the sinusoidal circulation: A scanning electron microscopic investigation. *Am J Anat* 145:183, 1976.
145. Lichtman MA, Chamberlain KK, Simon W, et al: Parasinusoidal location of megakaryocytes in marrow: A determinant of platelet release. *Am J Hematol* 4:303, 1978.
146. Zucker-Franklin D: Platelet morphology and function, in Williams WJ, Beutler E, Erslev AJ, et al (eds), *Hematology*, ed 4. New York, McGraw-Hill, 1990 p 1172.
147. Rao KA, Holmsen H: Congenital disorders of platelet function. *Semin Hematol* 23:102, 1986.
148. Zola H: Differentiation and maturation of human B lymphocytes: A review. *Pathology* 17:365, 1985.
149. Mechanisms that regulate immunoglobulin gene expression. *Annu Rev Immunol* 3:159, 1985.
150. Inglis JR: *T Lymphocytes Today*. Amsterdam, Elsevier, 1983.
151. Minden MD, Mak TW: The structure of the T cell antigen receptor genes in normal and malignant T cells. *Blood* 68:327, 1986.
152. Hercend T, Schmidt RE: Characteristics and uses of natural killer cells. *Immunolgy Today* 9:291, 1988.
153. Timonen T, Ortaldo JR, Herbermen RB: Characteristics of human large granular lymphocytes and relationship to natural killer and K cells. *J Exp Med* 153:569, 1981.

2 BONE MARROW EXAMINATION: SPECIAL PROCEDURES

SAMPLE PREPARATION

Bone marrow examination is a common practice in medicine. It is not only the primary source of information for hematologic disorders but has become an important component of patient evaluation, particularly in those who are receiving chemotherapy or radiation therapy for malignant diseases and those who are suspected of having disseminated infections.

The procedure for bone marrow aspiration or biopsy is accompanied by some discomfort and pain, which are not severe in most instances. Complications of bone marrow aspiration or biopsy are uncommon and are usually not severe. Hemorrhage, and occasionally infection, at the site of aspiration/biopsy are the anticipated complications. However, perforation of iliac bone with retroperitoneal hemorrhage in patients with osteoporosis and cardiac tamponade due to perforation of the lower plate of the sternum may happen because of inexperience or carelessness.[1,2] Bone marrow aspiration/biopsy is contraindicated in severe coagulation deficiencies.

The most frequent area used for bone marrow aspiration and/or biopsy at any age is the posterior iliac crest. The anterior iliac crest is chosen in infants and children or in adults when the posterior iliac crest is not accessible (e.g., in a patient with obesity or in a cast). The sternum is used only for bone marrow aspiration in adults. This area should not be used in infants and children. The tibia is used for aspiration only in infants, preferably those below 18 months of age.[1]

Bone marrow samples are obtained by the use of Jamshidi or other appropriate needles and are prepared in various ways, including smears, sections and touch preparations.

Bone Marrow Smears

Smears are made from the marrow aspirates. A small amount of the aspirated marrow (about 0.2 ml) is used to make several thin smears. Marrow smears are primarily used for differential counts and assessment of the myeloid:erythroid ratio. They are the most suitable preparations for studying cellular details and the maturation process of the hematopoietic cells and for characterizing the abnormal cells (Figures 2-1 and 2-2). For the differential count, 200 nucleated cells in randomly selected high-power light microscopic field are usually counted (Table 2-1).

Marrow smears are also useful in the evolution of iron store and are the primary source of special cytochemical stains.

Bone Marrow Sections

Bone marrow sections are useful sources for the estimation of bone marrow cellularity and for identification of pathologic processes such as fibrosis, granulomatosis, amyloidosis, metastatic lesions and primary malignancies.[1,3-6] Bone marrow sections are of two types: (1) marrow particle sections and (2) biopsy sections.

Marrow particle sections

Marrow particle sections are prepared from aspirated bone marrow. The most simple and practical method is to let the aspirated marrow clot and fix it in a proper fixative (e.g., formaldehyde, B5, Zenker's). The fixed clot is then prepared for paraffin sections

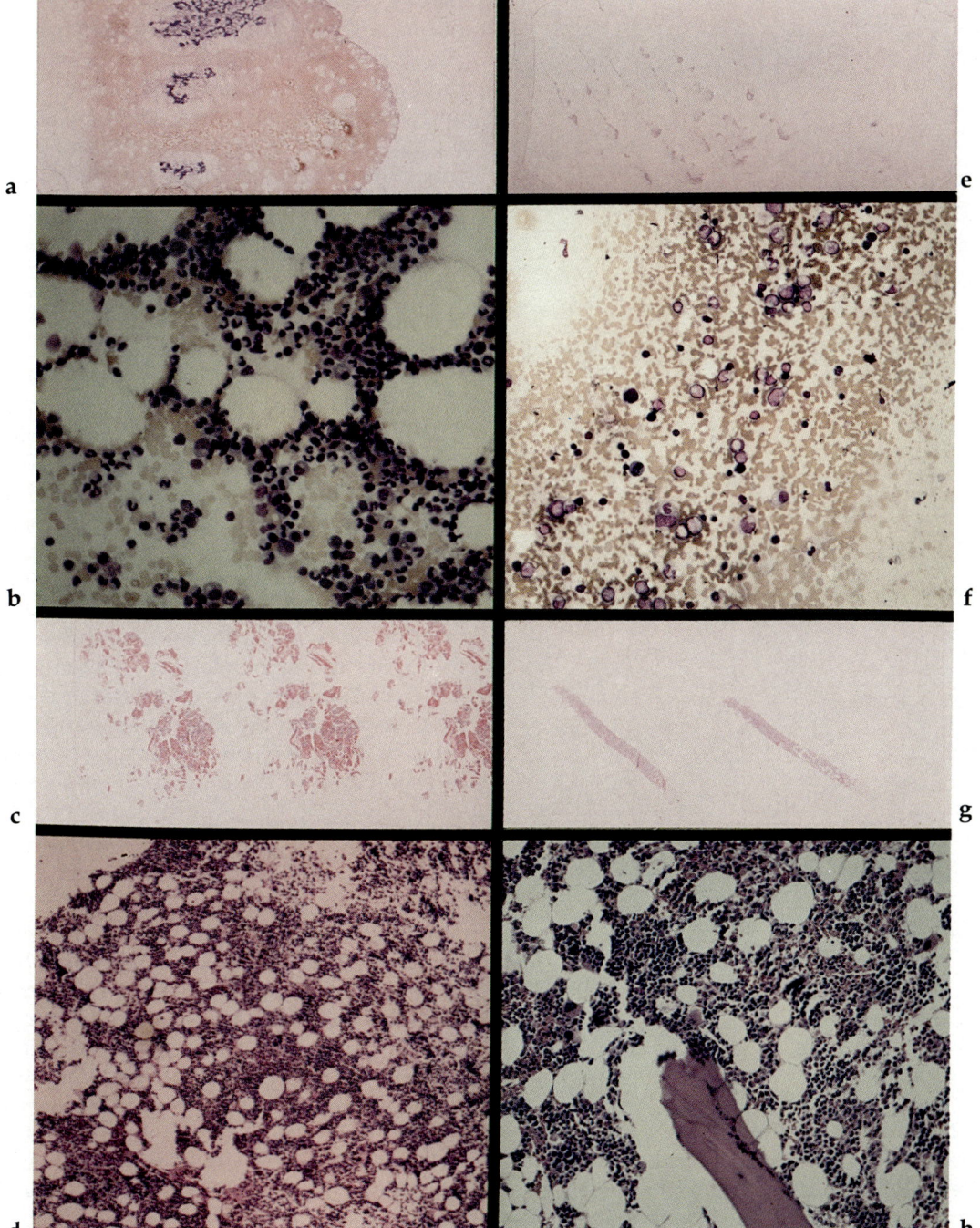

Figure 2-1. Representative examples of glass slide preparations of bone marrow and the corresponding microscopic features: smear (a, b), clot section (c, d), touch preparation (e, f), and biopsy section (g, h).

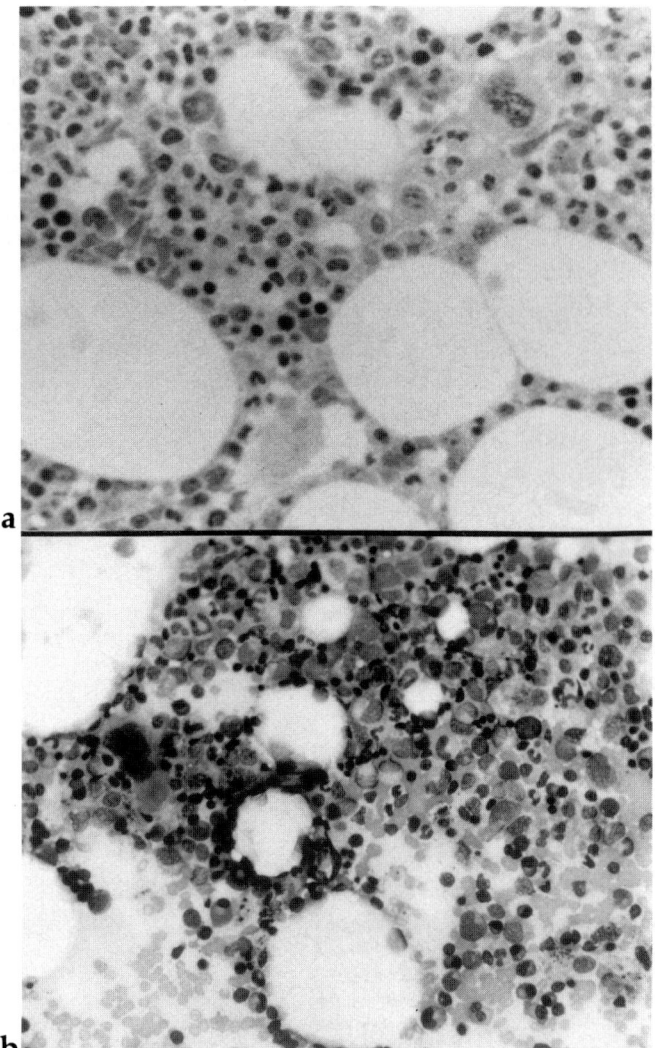

Figure 2-2. A marrow clot section (a) and a marrow smear (b) demonstrating hematopoietic cells in various stages of differentiation.

(see Figures 2-1 and 2-2). Because of the excess blood clot in this preparation and the technical difficulty of cutting reasonably thin sections, a number of laboratories add heparin to the aspirated bone marrow to prevent clot formation and then pass the marrow particles through a fine filter paper. The particles remaining on the paper are fixed promptly and prepared for paraffin sections and staining.

Biopsy sections

Biopsy sections are prepared in two different ways. The traditional method is fixation, decalcification and paraffin embedding of the biopsy cores prior to sectioning. This standard procedure has a number of disadvantages, including decalcification artifact, degradation of certain proteins, loss of cellular details and inability to produce semithin sections (0.5 to 3 μm). However, when all marrow preparations (e.g., smears, biopsy cores) are available for examination, high-quality, paraffin-embedded sections will provide adequate information (see Figure 2-1). To avoid the unwanted effects of decalcification and paraffin embedding, plastic embedding has been recommended. In this procedure, instead of paraffin, biopsy cores are embedded in glycol methacrylate without going through the decalcification process. The advantages of plastic embedding are the ability to cut thinner sections, well-preserved cellular details, better preservation of proteins and maintenance of the chemical composition of bone.[9,10] The disadvantages are the extra cost, longer processing and sectioning time and difficulty in achieving high-quality staining.[9] Plastic embedding is strongly recommended for the laboratories that handle only bone marrow biopsy specimens. One difficulty is that pathologists and hematologists are often accustomed to either paraffin- or plastic-embedded sections. Therefore, disparity in the morphology and staining properties of these two procedures may create problems in interpretation of the bone marrow lesions.

Touch Preparations

Touch preparations are made by gently pressing (touching) the glass slides over the bone marrow biopsy specimens (see Figure 2-1). They are the least desirable preparations for morphologic examination because they show significant artifactual changes. However, they are useful, particularly when bone marrow aspiration fails to yield marrow tissue ("dry tap"). Dry tap may occur when the bone marrow is involved with fibrosis, metastatic tumor, or a granulomatous process, and sometimes in pernicious anemia or leukemia.

Bone marrow smears and touch preparations are usually stained with Wright's and/or Giemsa stains (Romanovsky's method), and biopsy and clot sections are most often stained with hematoxylin and eosin (H&E) stain (Maximov's method). With Wright's stain, red blood cells are pink, the nuclei of the bone marrow cells are purplish blue, eosinophilic granules are red-orange and basophilic granules are dark blue. With Maximov's stain, red blood cells and

Bone Marrow Examination: Special Procedures

Table 2-1 Bone Marrow Differential Counts in Healthy Persons*

Cell type	Age		
	0 month	18 months	Adult
Myeloblast	—	—	1.5 (0.3–5.0)
Promyelocyte	0.8 ± 0.9	0.6 ± 0.7	3.5 (1.0–8.0)
Neutrophilic series			
Myelocyte	4.0 ± 3.0	2.5 ± 1.4	10.0 (5.0–19.0)
Metamyelocyte	19.0 ± 5.0	12.5 ± 4.0	26.0 (13.0–32.5)
Band	29.0 ± 7.5	14.0 ± 5.5	16.0 (12.0–30.0)
Segmented	7.5 ± 4.5	6.5 ± 4.0	15.0 (7.0–30.0)
Eosinophilic series	2.7 ± 1.0	2.7 ± 2.0	2.0 (0.5–6.0)
Basophilic series	0.1 ± 0.2	0.1 ± 0.1	0.8 (0.0–1.0)
Monocytic series	0.8 ± 0.8	2.0 ± 1.5	2.0 (0.0–4.0)
Proerythroblast	0.02 ± 0.06	0.1 ± 0.1	0.5 (0.2–2.0)
Erythroblast			
Basophilic	0.2 ± 0.2	0.5 ± 0.3	2.5 (1.5–6.0)
Polychromic	13.0 ± 7.0	7.0 ± 3.5	11.0 (5.0–25.0)
Orthochromic	0.1 ± 0.1	0.5 ± 0.5	5.0 (2.0–20.0)
Megakaryocyte	0.05 ± 0.1	0.05 ± 0.1	0.3 (0.04–2.0)
Lymphocyte	14.5 ± 6.0	43.5 ± 9.0	10.0 (3.0–20.0)
Plasma cell	0.0 ± 0.02	0.05 ± 0.08	0.5 (0.0–2.0)
M:E ratio	4.4:1	4.8:1	3–3.5:1

* Modified from Williams WJ, Nelson DA: Examination of the bone marrow, in Williams WJ, Beutler E. Erslev AJ, et al (eds), *Hematology*. ed 4. New York, McGraw-Hill, 1990, p 24, and Naeim F: Some technical aspects in hematology, in Figueroa WG (ed), Hematology. New York, Wiley, 1981, p 384.

eosinophilic granules appear pink, granules in basophils stain purple and nuclei appear dark blue.

All bone marrow preparations should be examined together and should be interpreted in view of the peripheral blood and all available clinical and laboratory findings.[7,8]

In addition to routine tissue processing and staining procedures, a number of special procedures and advanced techniques are available for further characterization of hematologic disorders. These special procedures are briefly discussed here.

SPECIAL STAINS

The application of cytochemical stains for the evaluation of cellular components such as nucleoproteins, proteins, carbohydrates, lipids and enzymes is a common practice in hematopathology. It provides valuable information regarding the lineage and differentiation of the hematopoietic cells and plays an important role in the evaluation of hematologic disorders, especially in the differential diagnosis and classification of hematologic malignancies (Table 2-2). The most commonly used cytochemical stains are discussed below.

Prussian Blue Reaction (Iron Stain)

Prussian blue is a stain developed by the production of ferric ferrocyanide when an acidified solution of ferrocyanide reacts with ferric ions. This stain is widely used for assessment of the marrow iron store. Hemosiderin is stored in the mononuclear phagocytic system and with Prussian blue stain appears as irregular small and large blue cytoplasmic granules (Figure 2-3). The presence of iron granules in sideroblasts (iron-containing normoblasts) and siderocytes (iron-containing red blood cells) is also demonstrated with the use of Prussian blue staining. In

Table 2-2 Cytochemical Reactions in Leukemias

Stain	Nonlymphoid Leukemias				Lymphoid Leukemias	
	Myeloblasts/Promyelocytes	Monoblasts	Erythroblasts	Megakaryoblasts	HCL	Others
PAS*	−	±	+	±	−	+
Sudan black	+	±	−	−	−	−
Peroxidase	+	+	−	−	−	−
Esterases†						
Nonspec.	−	+	+	+	±	±
Naph. AS-D	+	+	+	+	−	−
Chloroac.	+	±	±	±	−	−
TRAP‡	−	−	−	−	+	−

* Coarse cytoplasmic granules.
† Nonspec. = nonspecific esterase stain; fluoride sensitive in monoblastic (M4, M5) and megakaryoblastic (M7) leukemias.
Naph. AS-D = naphthol AS-D.
Chloroac. = Chloroacetate esterase
Esterases may show focal cytoplasmic positivity in lymphoid cells, especially T cells.
‡ Tartrate-resistant acid phosphatase.

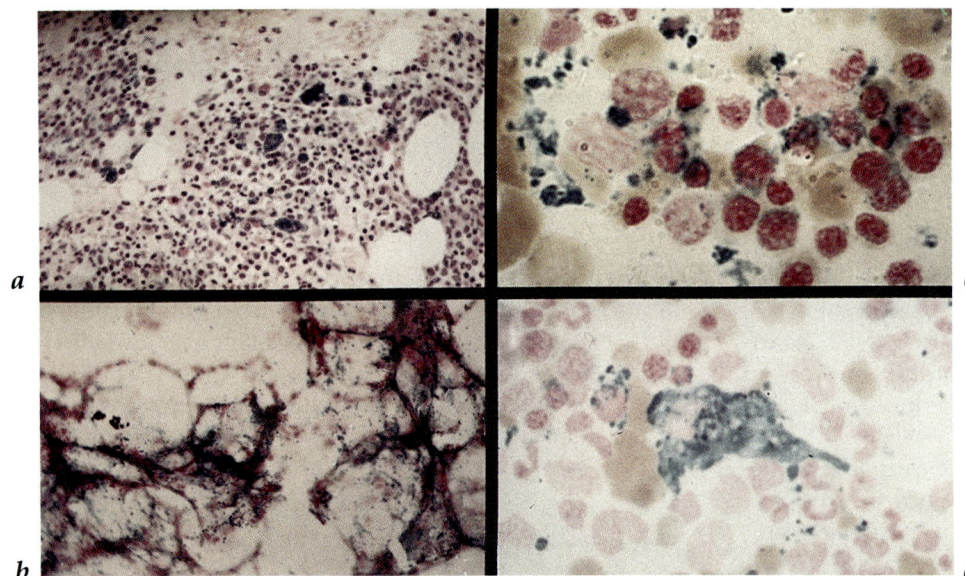

Figure 2-3. Iron stain on the marrow clot section (a) and smear (b, c, d) of a patient with refractory anemia. The blue stain represents hemosiderin. Several ringed sideroblasts are present (c), and a hemosiderin-loaded macrophage is demonstrated (d).

refractory anemias, iron may be retained in the mitochondria of the normoblasts. The result is a perinuclear ring of blue granules caused by an iron stain. These cells are called "ringed sideroblasts" (see Figure 2-3). Increased marrow hemosiderin is observed in hemochromatosis, hemolytic anemias, recurrent blood transfusions and ineffective eythropoiesis. Stainable iron is absent or markedly decreased in iron deficiency anemia.

Periodic Acid-Schiff (PAS) Reaction

Periodic acid oxidizes the 1-2 glycol group or its amino or alkylamino derivatives.[11] The outcome is the production of aldehydes that react with Schiff's reagent to produce a purple color.[11,12] A positive reaction may be found in a variety of naturally occurring carbohydrates such as monosaccharides, poly-

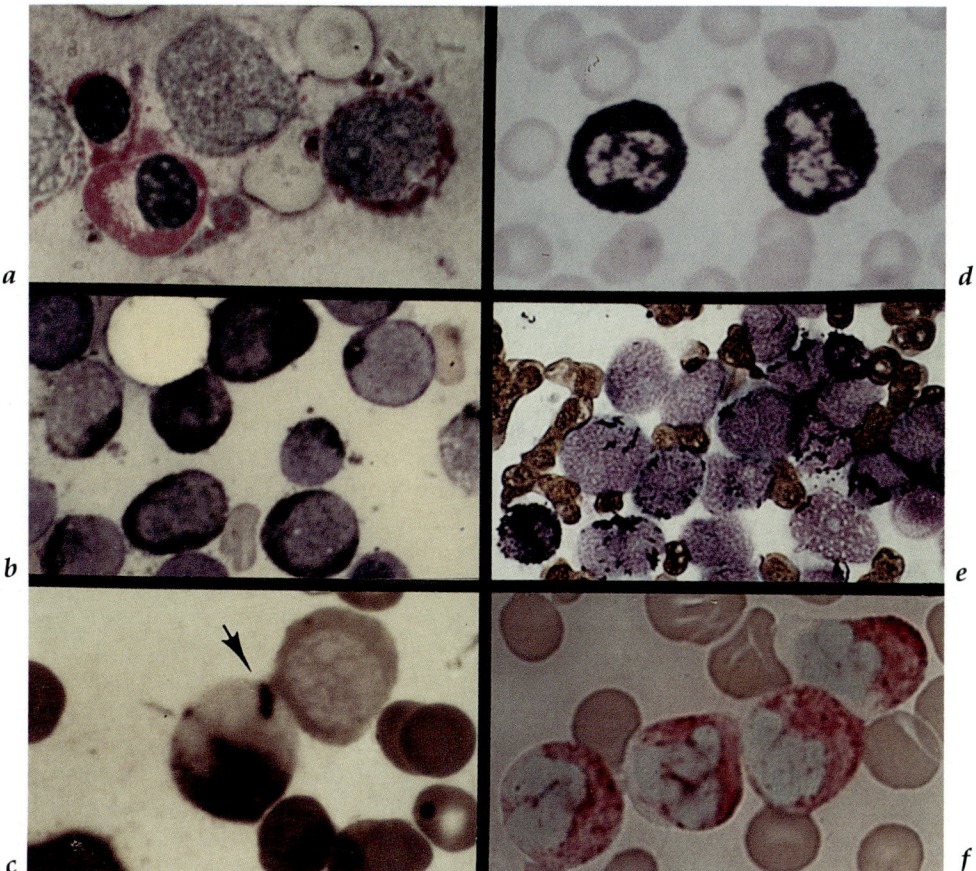

Figure 2-4. (a) A PAS stain demonstrating coarse, positive granules in a lymphoblast and diffuse cytoplasmic staining in two nucleated red blood cells; (b, c) several myeloblasts positive for myeloperoxidase, one demonstrating an Auer rod (c, arrow); (d, e) Sudan black B-positive, segmented neutrophils and immature myeloid cells; (f) chloroacetate esterase staining in segmented neutrophils.

saccharides, glycoproteins, mucoprotein conjugates and cerebrosides.[12]

The positive PAS reaction in hematopoietic cells is primarily due to the presence of cytoplasmic glycogen. In normal conditions, erythroid precursors do not show any detectable PAS reaction. Granulocytic cells show diffuse, fine, PAS-positive granules. This reaction is stronger in more mature cells. The eosinophilic- and basophilic-specific granules are usually PAS negative, although the cytoplasm of eosinophils and basophils displays a diffusely positive reaction.[11,13,14] Monocytes usually demonstrate a light, diffuse cytoplasmic PAS positivity with scattered coarse, positive granules. Lymphocytes often show a small number of coarse, PAS-positive granules in both B- and T-cell subtypes. Megakaryocytes show diffuse positivity as well as blocks of cytoplasmic positivity. Platelets often demonstrate diffuse, light PAS staining in their periphery and dense, clumped staining in their center.

In acute lymphoblastic leukemia, blast cells often show numerous perinuclear coarse, PAS-positive granules which may vary in size and intensity (Figure 2-4). Blast cells in the majority of acute myelogenous leukemias, especially M1 to M3 of the FAB classification (Chapter 6), usually display a light, diffuse, finely granular, PAS-positive reaction. Acute myelomonocytic and monocytic leukemias (M4 and M5) may show various patterns of PAS reactivity ranging from a light, diffuse reaction to the presence of strong, coarse, PAS-positive granules or a combination of both. In acute myelogenous leukemias which show increased numbers of atypical eosinophils, such as those associated with an inversion of chromosome 16 (M4) or 8;21 translocation (M2), eosinophilic granules may show PAS reactivity.[15-17] Dysplastic eythroid precursors and immature erythroid cells in refractory anemias and erythroleukemia (M6) often show coarse, PAS-positive granules. Blast cells in megakaryoblastic leukemia (M7) may also show coarse, PAS-positive granules. PAS stain is also used for the detection of fungal infections.

Sudan Black B

Sudan black B is a lipophilic dye that, through uncertain mechanisms, stains granulocytic and monocytic elements. Its reactivity appears to correlate with the presence of peroxidase-containing granules in these cells.[11] The intensity of the Sudan black B stain increases with the maturity of the granulocytic cells; myeloblasts are either negative or show a small number of perinuclear positive granules; promyelocytes show a larger number of Sudan black B-positive granules; and neutrophilic myelocytes, metamyelocytes and segmented cells are strongly Sudan black B positive[18] (see Figure 2-4). Similarly, eosinophils show increasing Sudan black positivity with progressive maturation. On the other hand, Sudan black staining is stronger in immature basophils than in the mature forms.[11]

Sudan black B is either negative or weakly positive in the monocytic lineage. The positive cells show scattered, fine or moderately coarse cytoplasmic granules which are mostly perinuclear. Erythroid precursors, as well as platelets, megakaryocytes and lymphoid cells, are Sudan black negative. Rare megakaryocytes may show a weak background staining with a few cytoplasmic Sudan black-positive granules. Occasionally, lymphocytes may also show a few perinuclear positive granules, especially when a counterstain is not used.[11]

Sudan black B is an excellent stain for confirming the diagnosis of myelogenous and myelomonocytic leukemias. However, rare cases of acute lymphoblastic leukemia have been reported as being Sudan black B positive.[19-21] In such cases, Sudan black B-positive granules in blast cells are often coarse, globular, and few in number.

Peroxidase

Myeloperoxidase is a lysosomal enzyme present in the granulocytic and monocytic cells (see Figure 2-4). Several peroxidase isoenzymes have been identified.[22-25] Two distinct peroxidase activities have been demonstrated in primary and secondary granules[26,27]; after the myelocyte stage, because of a progressive increase in tertiary granules and a decrease in primary and secondary granules, myeloperoxidase activity declines. Several monoclonal antibodies have been raised against myeloperoxidase and its subunits.[28,29] These antibodies are helpful in the detection of myeloperoxidase molecules in blast cells in myelogenous leukemias. It has been suggested that the gene for human myeloperoxidase is located on chromosome 17, in close proximity to the translocation breakpoint observed in acute progranulocytic leukemia.[30,31]

Peroxidase activity is detected in neutrophilic and eosinophilic lineages in all stages of differentiation. The peroxidase staining is stronger in immature basophils and gradually decreases by maturation; fully mature basophils are peroxidase negative.[32] Monocytes often show scattered peroxidase-positive granules. Erythroid precursors and lymphocytes are myeloperoxidase negative.

Platelets and megakaryocytes contain a peroxidase isoenzyme located in the dense tubular system.[33] Platelet peroxidase (PPO) has been detected at the electron microscopic level, and has been found not only in platelets and megakaryocytes but also in early erythroid blast cells.[34,35] A method which allows the detection of PPO at the light microscopic level has been developed by Khalaf and Hayhoe.[36] With this technique, in addition to platelets and megakaryocytes, myeloblasts and cells in certain lymphoid malignancies (i.e., hairy cell leukemia, large cell follicular lymphoma and plasma cell leukemia) may demonstrate PPO positivity.[1]

Esterases

Three major esterase reactions are used in hematology: alpha-naphthyl butyrate (or acetate) esterase, naphthol AS-D acetate esterase and naphthol AS-D chloroacetate esterase. Esterase cytochemistry has been traditionally used to distinguish cells of granulocytic and monocytic origin. However, other hematopoietic cells, such as lymphocytes and megakaryocytes, also demonstrate esterase activity.

Alpha-Naphthyl Butyrate (or Acetate) Esterase

This esterase, which is also known as "nonspecific esterase," is strongly positive in cells of monocytic lineage and usually negative in cells of the gran-

Bone Marrow Examination: Special Procedures

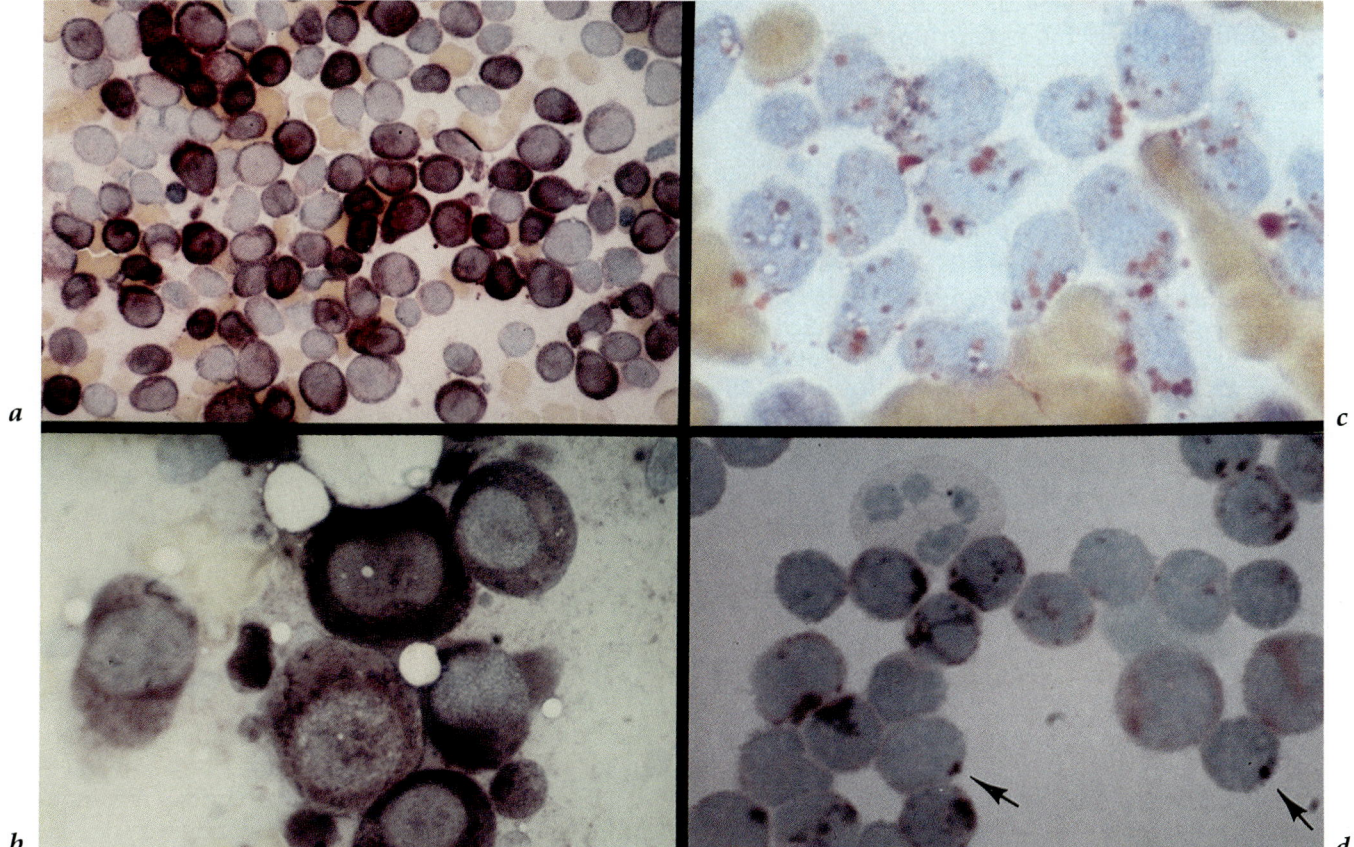

Figure 2-5. A marrow smear demonstrating numerous blasts positive for nonspecific esterase acivity (a, b); marrow smear of a patient with Burkitt's lymphoma showing positive reaction with Oil Red O (c); a peripheral blood smear stained for beta-glucuronidase (d): monocytes show diffuse cytoplasmic staining, and lymphocytes demonstrate focal staining (arrow).

ulocytic series (Figure 2-5). Occasional granulocytic cells may show a few scattered positive granules. Nonspecific esterase staining is helpful in the diagnosis of monocytic and histiocytic lesions. However, it has been reported to be positive in the leukemic cells of some patients with promyelocytic leukemia.[37] Normal erythroid precursors are either negative or weakly positive, while megaloblasts and blast cells in erythroleukemia are often positive. Alpha-naphthyl esterase activity is fluoride sensitive in monocytes, platelets and megakaryocytes, and the acetate derivative reacts more strongly with platelets and megakaryoctytes than the butyrate derivative. Lymphocytes, especially T cells, may show a few dotlike, positive granules at pH 5.8 with prolonged incubation.[38-40]

Naphthtol AS-D Acetate Esterase

Activity of this enzyme is demonstrated in granulocytic cells of various stages of differentiation but is strongest in promyelocytes and myelocytes. This activity is not inhibited by sodium fluoride. Cells of monocytic lineage are strongly positive with this enzyme, but the enzyme's activity is inhibited by sodium fluoride. Erythroid precursors show some positivity, which decreases with increasing maturity. Platelets and megakaryocytes also demonstrate naphthol AS-D acetate esterase activity which is fluoride sensitive. Lymphocytes, especially T cells, may demonstrate a few dot-like, positive granules.

Naphthol AS-D Chloroacetate

This enzyme is primarily demonstrated in granulocytic series (see Figure 2-4). Auer rods are positive. Other hematopoietic cells are essentially negative, though some monocytes and megakaryocytes and/or their leukemic counterparts may show a weak reaction. Pronormoblasts in erythroleukemia may also show chloroacetate positivity.[11]

Alkaline Phosphatase

The determination of alkaline phosphatase activity in neutrophilic granulocytes has a significant clinical application. The cytochemical determination of alkaline phosphatase is based on the formation of a colored precipitate, the intensity of which is subjectively graded from 0 to 4. The score of the leukocyte (or, more accurately, neutrophil) alkaline phosphatase in a given smear is the sum of the staining scores of 100 neutrophilic leukocytes (Figure 2-6). The leukocyte alkaline phosphatase (LAP) score for healthy controls ranges from 15 to 75 in our laboratory, but this range may vary in different laboratories.[41,42] Miller et al. demonstrated two LAP isoenzymes, slow and fast, by polyacrylamide gel electrophoresis.[43,44] The slow LAP isoenzyme is the predominant one and accounts for 90% or more of the LAP in granulocytes. Alkaline phosphatase activity is essentially confined to the neutrophilic segmented cells, stabs and, to a lesser degree, metamyelocytes. Eosinophils, basophils, and monocytic, erythroid, megakaryocytic and lymphoid series all are LAP negative in normal conditions. Bone marrow stromal cells may demonstrate strong enzyme activity.

High LAP scores are found in pregnancy, in patients receiving corticosteroids, in a variety of stress situations and in women taking oral contraceptives.[45-47] LAP scores are also high in healthy newborns. In pathologic conditions, elevated LAP scores are noted in leukemoid reaction, polycythemia vera, and Down's syndrome,[42-48,49] as well as in some cases of myelofibrosis, aplastic anemia, multiple myeloma, Hodgkin's disease, and lymphoid leukemias including acute lymphoblastic leukemia (ALL), chronic lymphocytic leukemia (CLL) and hairy cell leukemia.[42,50-52] Rare cases of chronic myelogenous leukemia (CML) have also demonstrated increased LAP activity.[53,54] Elevated LAP activity may be associated with blast transformation in CML,[55] which, according to Miller et al., is due to increased levels of both slow and fast LAPs.[44]

The LAP score is low in CML, paroxysmal nocturnal hemoglobinuria, congenital hypophosphatasia, the active phase of infectious mononucleosis and sideroblastic anemia.[56-58]

Acid Phosphatase

Acid phosphatase activity has been demonstrated in all hematopoietic cells (see Figure 2-6). Several isoenzymes have been identified by various techniques, and a specific combination of isoenzymes has been demonstrated in each hematopoietic cell type.[59-65] For example, Li et al. identified seven isoenzymes of acid phosphatase in leukocyte extracts by acrylamide gel electrophoresis, designated as 0, 1, 2, 3, 3b, 4 and 5.[60,61] The predominant isoenzymes in neutrophils were 1, 2 and 4, in monocytes 1 and 4, in lymphocytes and platelets 3, in Gaucher cells 0, and in cells of hairy cell leukemia 5. Isoenzyme 5 is a tartrate-resistant acid phosphatase (TRAP) and is the most helpful diagnostic marker for hairy cell leukemia.[66,67] However, TRAP positivity has also been reported in a variety of other lymphoproliferative disorders.[68-70]

Other Special Stains

Several other cytochemical stains have been used in hematology, such as Oil Red O, methyl green pyronine (MGP), dehydrogenases, dipeptidyl aminopeptidase (DAP), β-glucuronidase (β-G), trichrome, reticulin, and supravital stains (see Figure 2-5). Reactivity of these stains with hematopoietic cells is summarized as follows:

Bone Marrow Examination: Special Procedures

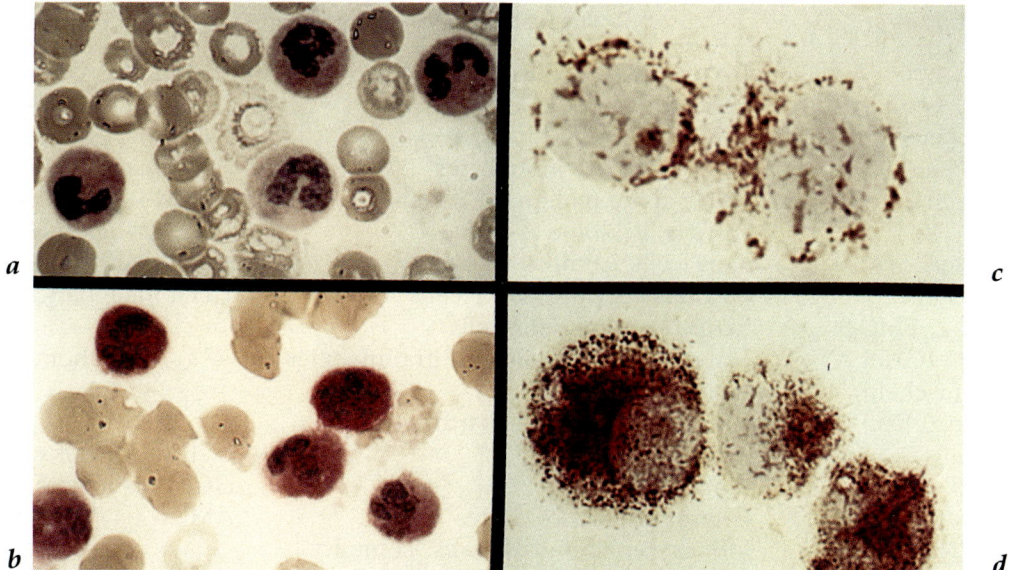

Figure 2-6. Periphereal blood smears (a, b) showing weak to strong LAP activity. Bone marrow smears (c,d) stained for acid phosphatase demonstrating positive monocytes (c) and macrophages (d).

Stain	Predominant Reactivity
Oil Red O	Lymphoid cells, ALL, Burkitt's lymphoma
MGP	Blast cells, plasma cells
Dehydrogenases	Early hematopoietic cells, lymphocytes
DAP	Early and late hematopoietic cells
β-G	Coarse granules in lymphocytes
Lysozyme	Monocytes and histiocytes
Reticulin	Reticulin (fine-collagen) fibers
Trichrome	Coarse-collagen fibers
Supravital	Reticulocytes, red cells with unstable hemoglobin (Heinz bodies).

MONOCLONAL ANTIBODIES

The immunophenotypic studies of the cellular elements in hematopoietic tissues are of great value in evaluation of the differentiation process in normal hematopoietic precursor cells, as well as in the further characterization of hematologic malignancies.

The availability of a large number of monoclonal and highly specific polyclonal antibodies has improved the identification and classification of the lymphoid and nonlymphoid subsets significantly. Monoclonal antibodies have been classified based on their reactivity with the lineage and/or differentiation-associated antigens and have been given a common cluster designation (CD) (Table 2-3). It should be emphasized that virtually none of the currently available monoclonal antibodies are tumor specific; they react with nonneoplastic hematopoietic cells as well. Several of the CD antigens have been shown to represent surface adhesion molecules (integrins).[71] A large number of the antibodies are also not lineage specific, and react with various types of hematopoietic and nonhematopoietic cells.[72,73] Therefore, the results of immunophenotypic studies should always be incorporated with other available data such as clinical findings, histopathologic observations, cytochemical stains, cytogenetic studies, DNA content analysis, and the results of DNA or RNA hybridization techniques.

Various methods are available for screening and evaluating reactivities of monoclonal and highly specific polyclonal antibodies against the hematopoietic cells. The most popular ones are immunoenzyme, immunofluorescent and immunogold techniques.

Table 2-3 Monoclonal Antibodies Frequently Used for Diagnosis and Classification of Tumors of the Hematopoietic System

Name	Prototype	Distribution	Practical Use
CD1	OKT6, Leu6	Thymocytes, dendritic cells	Langerhans cell histiocytosis
CD2	OKT11, Leu5	E-rosetting T cells	T-cell malignancies
CD3	OKT3, Leu4,	PanT, linked to Ag receptor	T-cell malignancies
CD4	OKT4, Leu3	Helper T cells, monocytes	T-cell malignancies
CD5	T101, Leu1, Sc-1	PanT, some malignant B cells	T- and B-cell malignancies
CD6	OKT17, 12.1	PanT cells, some B cells	T-cell malignancies
CD7	3A1, Leu9, 4A	PanT cells, some AML cells	T-cell malignancies
CD8	OKT8, Leu2	Cytotoxic/suppressor T cells	T-cell malignancies/LGL leukemia
CD9	BA-2, J-2, FMC-8	Early hematopoietic cells	
CD10	BA-3, J5 (CALLA)	Some B cells, T cells and granulocytes	ALLs, lymphomas
CD11a	LFA-1 (α-chain)	Leukocytes	
CD11b	Leu15 (C3 Rec)	Granulomonocytes, dendritic cells, NK cells	LGL (NK) leukemia
CD11C	Leu M5, S-HCL-3	Monocytes, hairy cells	HCL, histiocytic tumors
CD13	MY7, MCS2	Granulocytes/monocytes	AMLs
CD14	MY4, LeuM3, Mo2	Monocytes, dendritic cells, some B cells	AML (M4 and 5)
CD15	LeuM1, My1	Monocytes, granulocytes, R-S cells	AMLs, Hodgkin's disease
CD16	Leu11, 3G8	NK cells, some granulocytes, monocytes	LGL leukemia
CD17	T5A7, G-035	Granulocytes, monocytes, thymocytes	
CD18	LFA-1 (beta-chain)	Leukocytes	
CD19	Leu12, B4	Early B cells, B-specific	Lymphoid malignancies
CD20	Leu16, B1	Pan B, B-specific	Lymphoid malignancies
CD21	HB5, B2 (C3d Rec)	Mature B cells, dendritic cells	Lymphoid malignancies
CD22	Leu14, SHCL-1	Pan B, B specific	Lymphoid malignancies
CD23	Blast-2, PL-13	Activated B cells, dendritic cells	Lymphoid malignancies
CD24	BA-1, HB6	B cells, granulocytes, monocytes	Lymphoid malignancies
CD25	Anti-TAC, Tu69	Activated T and B cells, HCL cells	T-cell tumors, HCL
CD30	Ki-1, Ber-H2	Activated T and B cells, R-S cells	Lymphoma, Hodgkin's disease
CD33	MY9, L4F3	Early myeloid cells	AMLs
CD34	MY10, HPCA-1	Stem cells	Acute leukemias
CD38	OK10, HB-7, Leu17	Activated T cells, plasma cells	Multiple myeloma
CD41	gp IIb	Platelets	AML (M7)
CD42b	gp 1bα	Platelets	AML (M7)
CD45	CLA, HLe-1, T200	Leukocytes	Lymphomas
CD45R	Leu18, MY11	Suppressor T cells, B cells, myeloid cells	
CD56	Leu19	NK cells, some T cells	LGL leukemia
CD57	Leu7	NK cells, some T cells	LGL leukemia
CD58	LFA-3	Leukocytes, other cells	
CD61	gp IIIa	Platelets	AML (M7)
CD68	KP1, EBM11	Macrophages/histiocytes	Histiocytic lesions
CD70	KI-24	Activated B and T cells, R-S cells	Lymphoid malignancies
CD71	Transferrin rec.	Activated lymphocytes, monocytes	
CD72	S-HCL-2	Pan B cells	Lymphoid malignancies
CDW75	LN-1	Mature B cells, some T cells	Lymphoid malignancies
None	Ig (L, K, G, M...)	B cells	Lymphomas, B-ALL
None	PCA-1	Plasma cells, HCL cells	Multiple myeloma
None	Glycophorin A	Erythroid precursor cells	AML (M6)
None	HLA-DR	B cells, monocytes, blasts, activated T cells	Lymphoid malignancies

Bone Marrow Examination: Special Procedures

Immunoenzyme Staining

This is a technique in which enzyme (usually peroxidase or alkaline phosphatase)-conjugated antibodies are used for the demonstration of antigens in tissue sections, smears and cytospin preparations. This technique provides information regarding the pattern, intensity and location of the antibody–antigen interactions in the tissues and cells (Figures 2-7 and 2-8). The stain is permanent; thus, slides can be kept on file for a long period of time. However, there are a number of pitfalls including background staining, limited sensitivity of the technique, and difficulty of accurately enumerating the positive cells in the tissue sections. In addition, tissue fixation and processing (e.g., paraffin embedding, decalcification, heat, organic solvents) may cause protein degradation and alteration in the antigenicity of the cellular components, especially membrane integral proteins. However, certain monoclonal antibodies appear to work reasonably well on formalin-fixed, paraffin-embedded tissues, and their number is continuously increasing[74,75a,75b] (see Figures 2-7 and 2-8). The antibodies recommended for formalin-fixed paraffin-embedded tissues include T cell markers such as UCHL 1, L60, MT1, MT2 and βF1, B cell markers such as L26, LN1, LN2, MB1, MB2 and F8-11-13, and monocyte markers such as Leu M1 and Mac 387. Overall, fresh or fresh-frozen (-70 C) tissues are the most suitable samples for immunoenzyme staining.

Immunofluorescent Staining

Immunofluorescent staining is based on the application of fluorescent-conjugated antibodies on tissue and/or cell preparations. The stained tissues/cells are analyzed by either a flow cytometer or a fluorescent microscope.

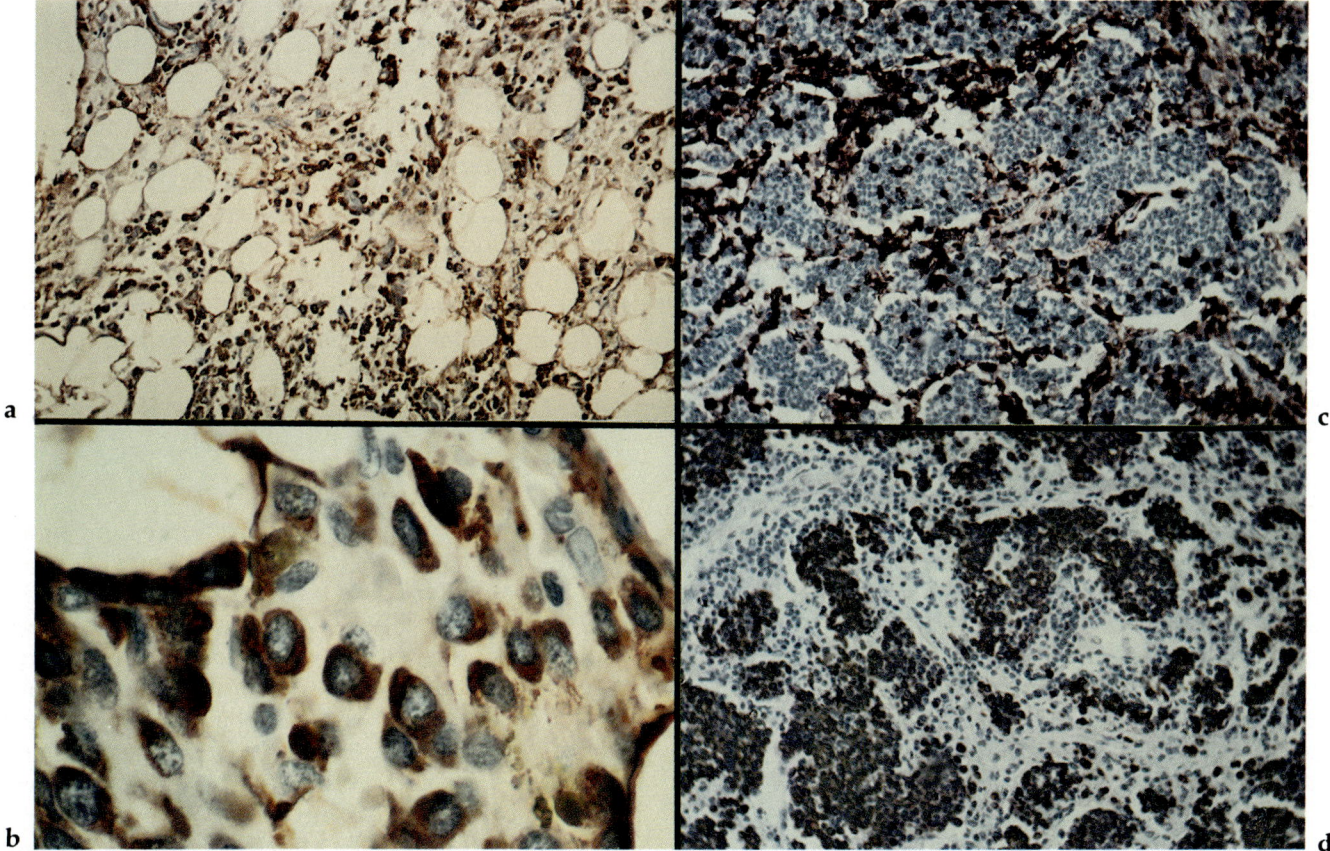

Figure 2-7. Immunoperoxidase staining in marrow biopsy sections. Cytoplasmic Ig kappa positivity is demonstrated in the majority of plasma cells in a patient with multiple myeloma (a, b); the biopsy specimen was formalin-fixed and paraffin-embedded. A bone marrow lymphoid infiltrate demonstrating CD3$^+$ cells (c) surrounding aggregates of CD20$^+$ cells (d) in a patient with B-cell lymphoma (frozen tissue).

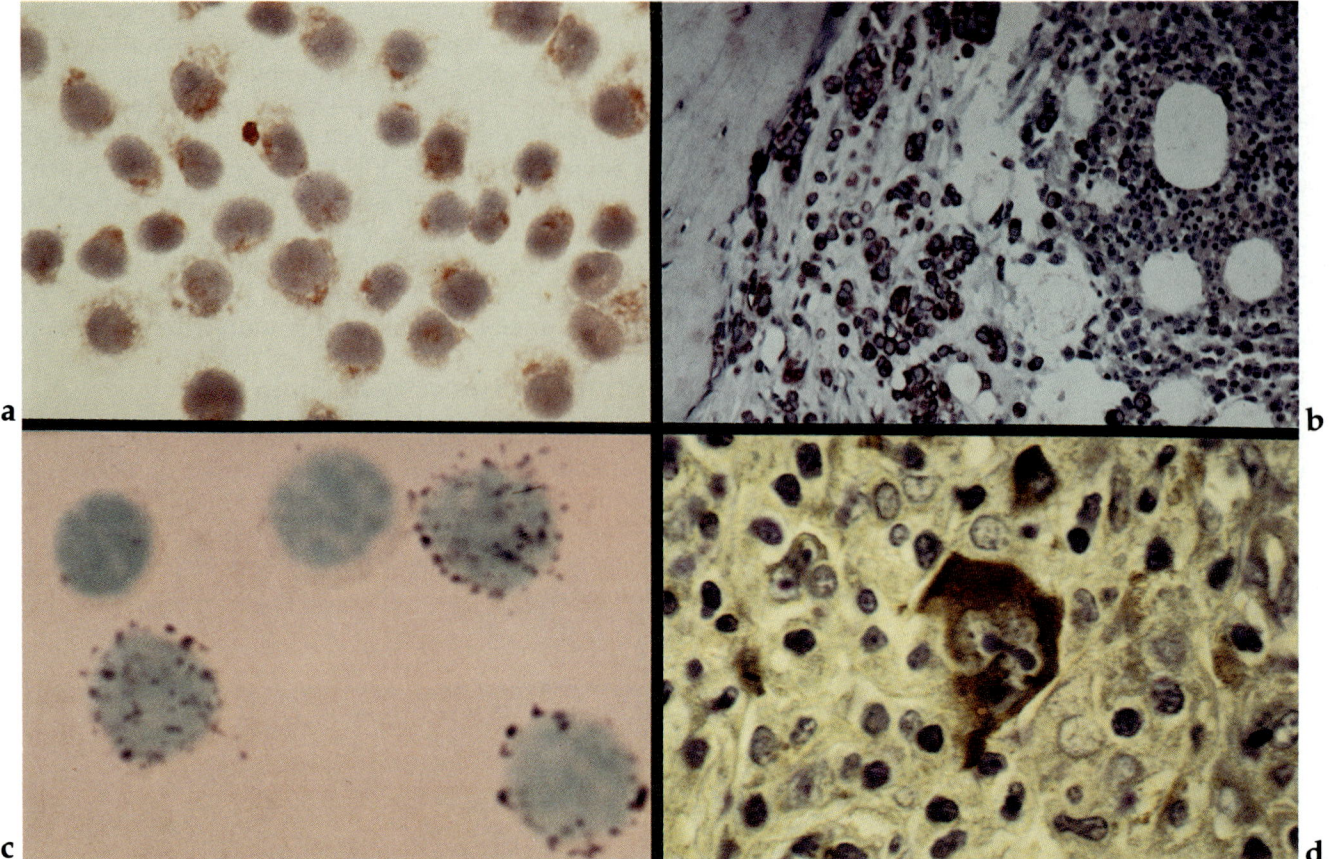

Figure 2-8. Parts (a), (b) and (d) demonstrate immunoperoxidase staining: (a) mononuclear preparation from peripheral blood of a patient with hairy cell leukemia showing S-100 positivity; (b) bone marrow biopsy section demonstrating metastatic carcinoma with tumor cells stained for cytokeratin; (d) bone marrow biopsy section showing Hodgkin's disease, with a Reed-Sternberg cell expressing CD15 (Leu M1) antigen. (c) Immunogold technique demonstrating surface Ig expression in peripheral blood mononuclear cells of a patient with chronic lymphocytic leukemia.

Flow Cytometry

Most of the currently available flow cytometers are equipped to analyze simultaneously at least four or five parameters: two or three fluorescent and two nonfluorescent signals. These signals are generated by cells hitting a laser beam while passing through a flow sheath (Figure 2-9). One of the nonfluorescent signals (forward scatter) represents cell volume, and the other (side scatter) reflects cellular texture and granularity. The two most popular fluorochromes currently used for analyzing monoclonal antibodies are fluorescein isothiocyanide (FITC) and phycoerythrin (PE). Additional fluorochromes, such as DuoChrome complex (phycoerythrin-Texas red) or PerCP (peridinin chlorophyll protein reagent), have recently been introduced as a third fluorescent signal for single-laser flow cytometers. The newly developed programs for computing the data generated by flow cytometers offer numerous analytical approaches including dot plots, contour graphs, a variety of histograms and statistical analysis. It is also possible to gate one or several subgroups of cells and analyze them. Some flow cytometers have sorting facilities and are able to isolate the gated cells physically from the sample with over 95% purity. Most flow cytometers are able to analyze particles as small as 0.5 μm and to detect cell membrane receptors with a density of about 2000 molecules per cell.

Flow cytometry has been applied to many different areas in hematology including leukocyte differen-

Bone Marrow Examination: Special Procedures

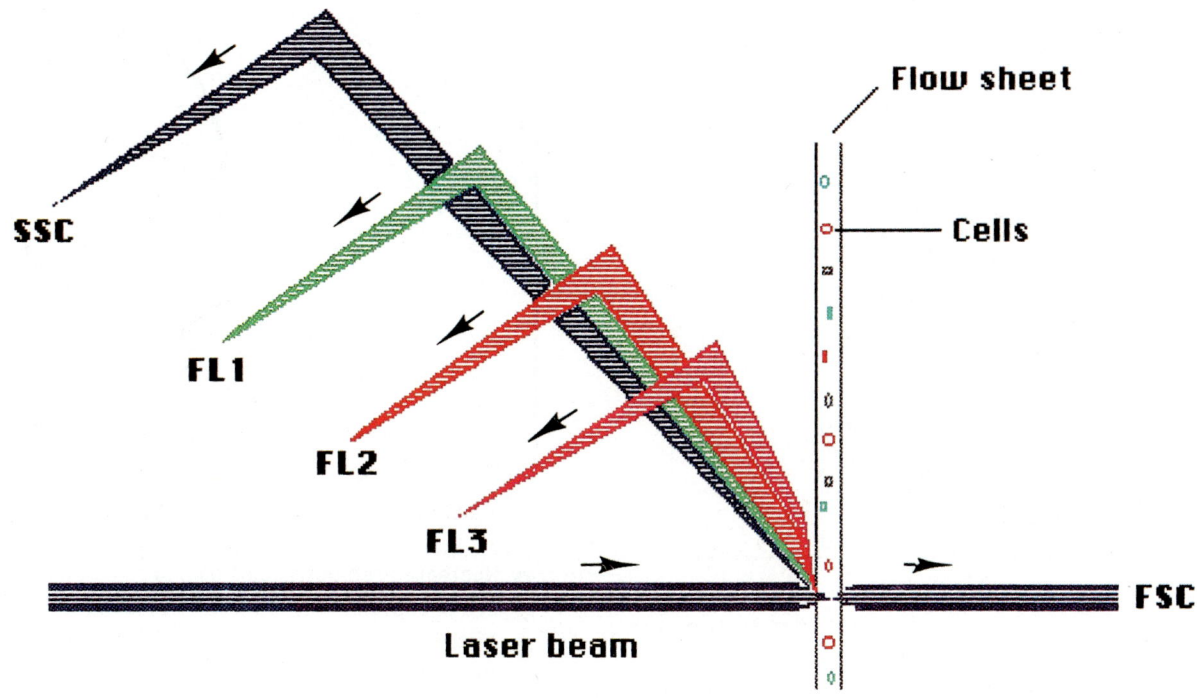

Figure 2-9. A simplified diagram of a flow cytometer:
  FSC: forward scatter
  SSC: side scatter
  FL1: fluorochrome 1, green (fluorescein isothiocyanate)
  FL2: fluorochrome 2, orange (phycoerythrin)
  FL3: fluorochrome 3, red; a recently introduced fluorochrome, such as PerCP, for three color analysis.

tial count, reticulocyte enumeration, detection of antibody-coated red blood cells and platelets, immunophenotypic studies in patients with immune deficiencies and leukemias, monocyte and granulocyte functional assays, and DNA content analysis.[76-85]

For bone marrow flow cytometry, marrow aspirates are cleared from tissue particles by filtration and are depleted from red blood cells, platelets and granulocytes by gradient centrifugation or from erythrocytes by a red blood cell lysing process. The marrow cells are properly stained with fluorescent-conjugated antibodies and analyzed by a flow cytometer. One approach for the analysis of the flow cytometry data is to divide the bone marrow cells into three major clusters based on their size (forward scatter) and granularity (side scatter) (Figure 2-10). These three clusters represent (1) the nongranular small cell population (lymphocyte-enriched), (2) the nongranular or slightly granular large cell population (monocyte/blast-enriched) and (3) the intensely granular cell population (granulocyte precursor-enriched). Although these three clusters are easily distinguishable in normal marrow, they have ill-defined boundaries and merge into each other (Figure 2-11). The lymphocyte-enriched cluster is the most informative cluster in immunodeficiency syndromes and in lymphoproliferative disorders of the small cell type such as chronic lymphocytic leukemia and low-grade lymphomas (Figure 2-12). The large cell nongranular or slightly granular cluster is the primary source of analysis in acute leukemias, histiocytic lesions, NK proliferative disorders and intermediate and high-grade lymphomas. In the interpretation of results generated by this cluster, one should be aware of the nonspecific binding of the monocytes to the free fluorescent stain or fluorescent conjugated antibodies. Some antibodies, particularly those against Ig kappa and lambda light chains, may bind to a variety of non-B cells such as monocytes, NK cells and CD8+ T cells. Analysis of the granulocyte-enriched cluster may provide useful information in conditions such as promyelocytic leukemia and certain storage disorders (mucopolysacharidosis).

Another approach in analyzing flow cytometry data is to gate and study the cells of interest based on their immunophenotypic expression. For example,

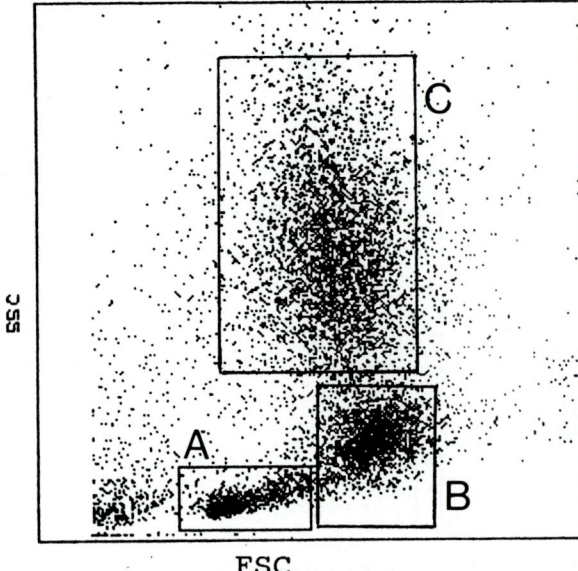

Figure 2-10. A dot plot forward scatter (FSC) and side scatter (SSC) analysis of bone marrow cells. Gate A represents a lymphocyte-enriched population. Other cells such as microblasts and nucleated red blood cells may be also present in this gate. Gate B represents a large nongranular to slightly granular cell population. Blast cells and monocytes are detected mainly in this area. Other cells such as large lymphocytes and promyelocytes may also be present in this cluster. Gate C represents a granulocyte-enriched population.

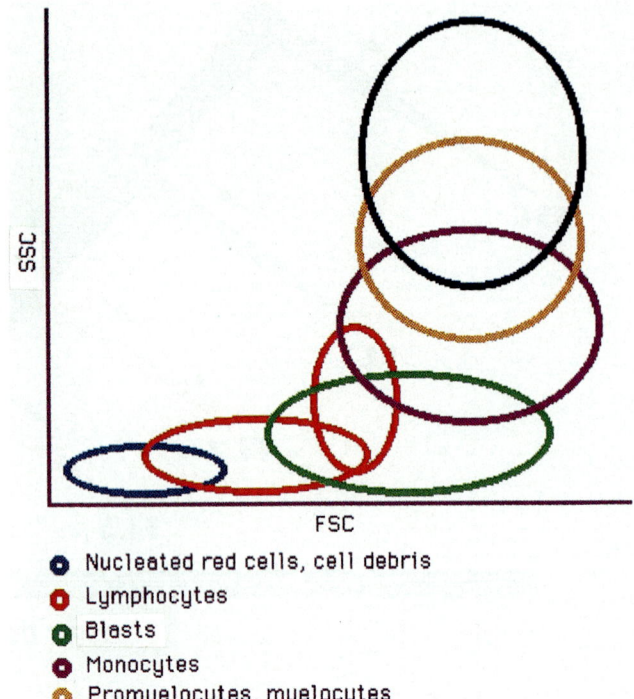

- Nucleated red cells, cell debris
- Lymphocytes
- Blasts
- Monocytes
- Promyelocytes, myelocytes
- Stabs, segmented cells

Figure 2-11. A diagram of FSC/SSC flow analysis of bone marrow cells demonstrating overlapping cell clusters.

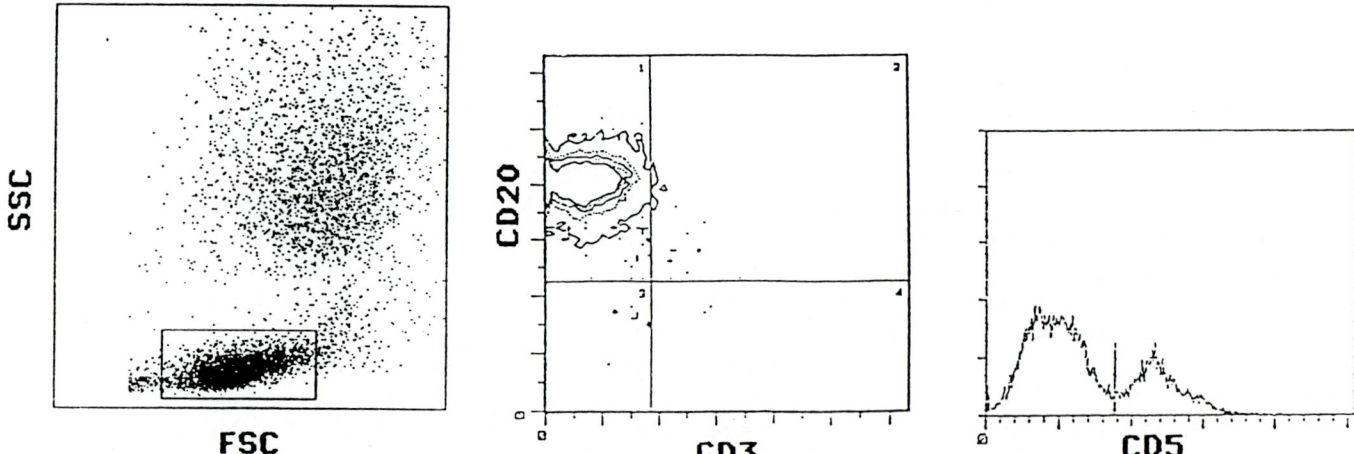

Figure 2-12. Flow analysis of bone marrow cells in a patient with chronic lymphocytic leukemia (CLL). Lymphocytes are gated in an FSC/SSC dot plot (left), and their surface expression for CD20, CD3 and CD5 is analyzed by a contour graph (middle) and a single histogram (right), respectively. CLL cells are CD20 and CD5 positive and CD3 negative. From Naeim et al: Recent advances in diagnosis and classification of leukemias and lymphomas. *Disease Marker* 8:231, 1990, with permission.

Bone Marrow Examination: Special Procedures

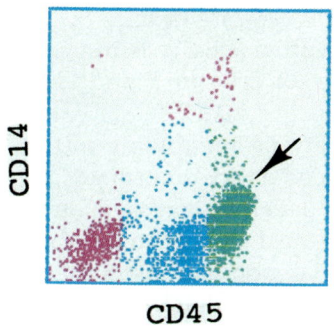 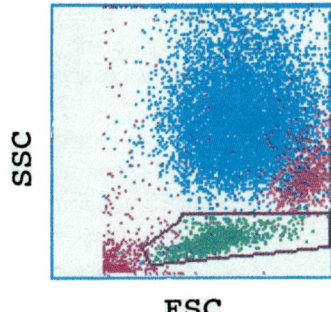

Figure 2-13. Some of the recent software packages offer multicolor programs. For example, in this figure, a program called Simulset (Becton Dickinson) identifies lymphocytes by double staining cells with anti-CD14 and CD45 antibodies (green cluster shown with arrow, left dot plot) and then gates the same color in the FSC/SSC dot plot (right). The gated cells are used for further phenotypic analysis. Granulocytes and monocytes are represented in blue and orange, respectively; red represents erythrocytic cells and cell debris.

for lymphoproliferative disorders, marrow cells are stained with a battery of relevant monoclonal antibodies, including double staining with DC14 and CD45. Lymphoid cells are strongly CD45$^+$ and CD14$^-$, granulocytes are weakly CD45$^+$ and CD14$^-$, and monocytes are CD45$^+$ and CD14$^+$. Thus it is possible to gate the lymphoid (strongly CD45$^+$ CD14$^-$) cluster and analyze the gated cells (Figure 2-13).

Fluorescent Microscopy

Fluorescent microscopy is another way of examining the phenotypic expressions of monoclonal antibodies. Although fluorescent microscopy is not as sensitive and fast as flow cytometry, it provides an opportunity to evaluate tissue and cell morphology and to determine which cell type or cellular component is staining (Figure 2-14). It is highly recommended that flow cytometry laboratories also have access to a fluorescent microscope.

Immunogold Technique

This is a nonfluorescein technique based on the use of colloidal gold particles. The gold particles, which are usually coated with primary or secondary antibodies, stick to the antigenic properties of the cells such as cell membrane receptors and, based on their size, appear as yellow-brown to dark brown granules (see Figure 2-8). Since the colloidal gold particles are electron-dense, the technique is often used in immunoelectron microscopy.

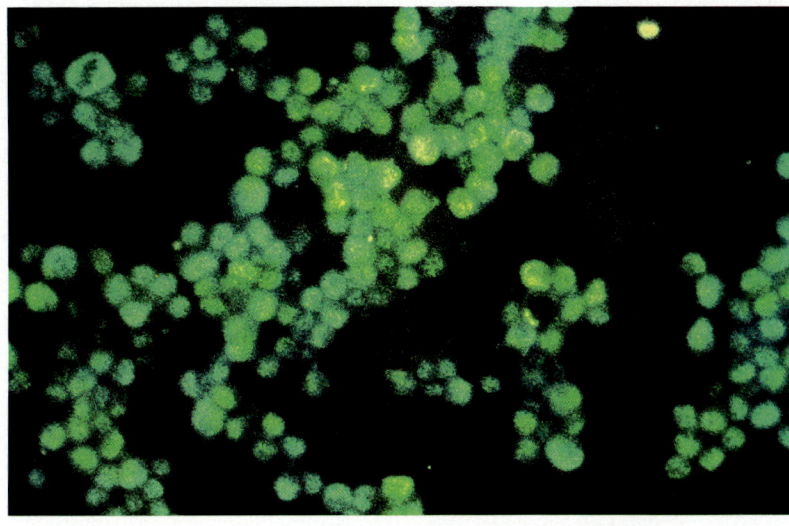

Figure 2-14. A bone marrow smear from a patient with acute leukemia demonstrating TdT-positive cells under a fluorescent microscope. From Schumacher HS: *Acute Leukemia: Approach to Diagnosis.* New York, Igaku-Shoin, 1990, with permission.

DNA CONTENT AND CELL CYCLE ANALYSIS

DNA content assays provide information regarding the proliferation state and ploidy of the cells. Currently, there are two common methods of measuring DNA content in pathology laboratories. One is static cytophotometry or image analysis, a microscope-based system in which tissue sections, smears or cytospin preparations are stained with a DNA fluorescent dye, and the intensity of the stain in selected cells (approximately 100–200 cells are examined) is measured by absorption fluorometry. The other method is flow cytometry. Flow cytometry, as discussed, is an efficient and rapid technique in which a large number of cells (20,000 to 30,000) can be studied in a few minutes. In DNA flow cytometry a variety of DNA dyes such as propidium iodide, acridine orange, diamidine phenylindole, ethidium bromide or mithramycin are incorporated into nuclei, and their fluorescence upon laser excitation is measured and analyzed. Propidium iodide is the most commonly used dye.

Flow cytometry provides information regarding the proliferation status (percentage of cells in G_0/G_1, S and G_2/M phases) and DNA ploidy of the cells in a sample (Figure 2-15). For cell cycle analysis by flow cytometry, several computer programs are available. These programs, by utilizing mathematical models, calculate the percentage of cells in G_0/G_1, S, and G_2/M phases. High proliferative activity is indicated by an increased percentage of cells in S and G_2/M phases.

DNA content abnormality or aneuploidy in flow cytometry is usually identified as an abnormal G_0/G_1 peak. This abnormality is usually expressed as the DNA index—the ratio of the DNA content of the G_0/G_1 cells in the abnormal population to that of the G_0/G_1 of a normal diploid population. The DNA index of diploid, hyperdiploid and hypodiploid cells is 1.00, >1.00 and <1.00, respectively (Figure 2-16). Tetraploid cells have a DNA index of 2.00. Currently

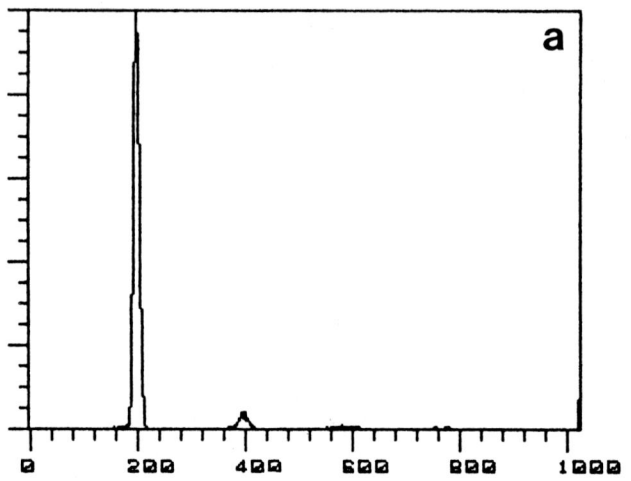

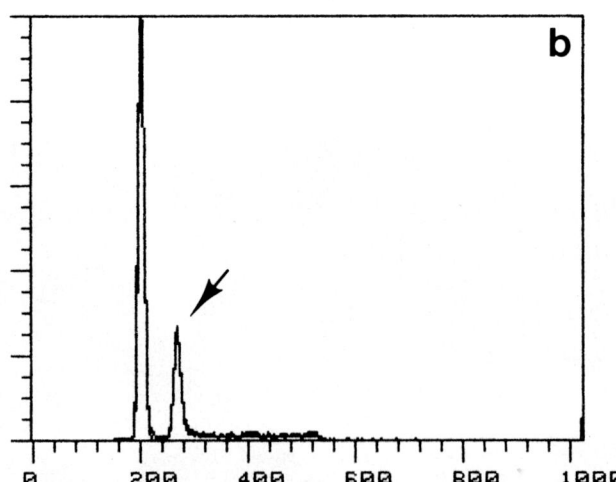

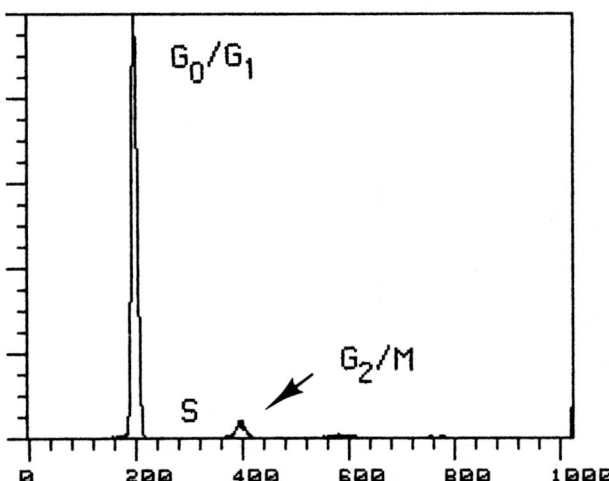

Figure 2-15. A DNA histogram from peripheral blood lymphocytes demonstrating G_0/G_1, S and G_2/M phases of the cell cycle. Most cells are in the G_0/G_1 phase.

Figure 2-16. DNA histograms of normal peripheral blood lymphocytes (a) and cells from a T-cell lymphoma (b). Lymphoma cells demonstrate a hyperdiploid aneuploid peak (arrow) with a DNA index of 1.3.

available flow cytometers are able to distinguish two clonal populations when there is at least a 4% difference in DNA content between them.[81,86]

Several studies have demonstrated a strong correlation between DNA content and disease prognosis in a variety of hematologic disorders.[87-100] Aggressive lymphomas are frequently associated with high proliferative activity (Figure 2-17). Aneuploid lymphomas are usually of the T-cell type and appear to have shorter survival than diploid tumors.[93-100] Several studies have also demonstrated an association between aneuploidy and advanced-stage, shorter-remission duration and reduced survival in patients with multiple myeloma.[101-103] In a series of 123 patients with AML, those who demonstrated aneuploidy (41%) had longer remissions.[82] It has been reported that patients with myelodysplastic syndrome who demonstrate DNA hypodiploidy have a higher level of marrow blasts and shorter survival than those with DNA diploidy or hyperdiploid aneuploidy.[88] Hyperdiploid aneuploidy in childhood ALL has been reported in association with improved survival.[89-91] However, a report on childhood ALL by Pui et al. suggests an association between hypodiploidy and a poor prognosis.[92] DNA content analysis in association with cell marker studies may help to detect minimal residual tumors or early relapses in patients who have been treated for aneuploid hematologic malignancies.

DNA HYBRIDIZATION TECHNIQUES

Principle and Methodology

Recent advances in molecular biology techniques have added new dimensions to the diagnosis of hematologic disorders. These techniques provide an opportunity to explore the structure of the human genome and gene expression.

In molecular pathology, unique segments of nucleic acid sequences (DNA probes) are used to demonstrate the presence of a complementary sequence of either DNA or RNA in the pathologic samples.

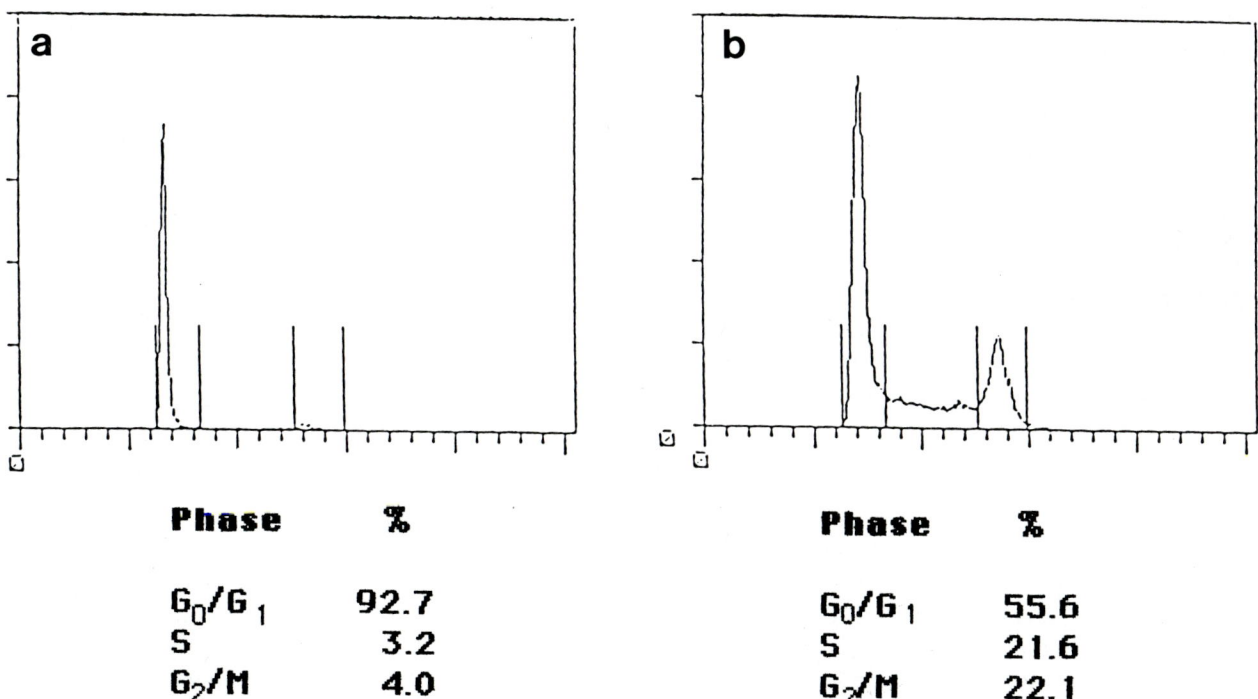

Figure 2-17. The left histogram (a) demonstrates the cell cycle of chronic lymphocytic leukemia cells; the majority of the cells are in the G_0/G_1 phase. The right histogram (b) (large cell lymphoma) demonstrates a high proportion of cells in the S and G_2/M phases. From Naeim et al: Recent advances in diagnosis and classification of leukemias and lymphomas. *Disease Marker* 8:231, 1990, with permission.

Since the complementary target is composed of hundreds or thousands of nucleotide bases, the reaction of a single strand of DNA with its complementary target (DNA hybridization) is the tightest and most specific intermolecular interaction between two biological macromolecules known in nature.[104] Several hybridization techniques are used; they will now be briefly discussed.

Southern Blot Technique

The DNA probes are labeled with a radioactive or nonradioactive signal moiety and thus can be detected after hybridization. The DNA probe is used as a template for second-strand synthesis of DNA with radiolabeled nucleotides in a DNA polymerase reaction. The radioactive-labeled copy of the DNA probe is then detected by autoradiography after hybridization. In nonradioactive DNA labeling procedures, nucleotides are conjugated with biotin or other protein binders such as digoxigenin. Biotin binds specifically to the protein avidin with a very high affinity. Avidin is a polyvalant protein which can be linked to chromogenic enzymes, fluorescein compounds or electron-dense particles. DNA can be labeled by direct incorporation of biotinylated nucleotide derivatives using DNA polymerase reaction techniques. The disadvantages of radioactive labeled DNA probes over nonradioactive labeled ones are radiation hazard and the requirement of special procedures for disposal of the radioactive contaminated wastes; the short shelf life of radioactive probes; and the elongated autoradiography step, which may extend to several days or even weeks. However, in practice, methods using radiolabeled probes have a sensitivity 5- to 10-fold more than the sensitivity of those using non-radioactive probes.[104]

The labeled probes are hybridized to the extracted cellular DNA. Prior to hybridization, the extracted DNA is digested with one or more restriction endonucleases to create discrete length fragments, which are then separated on the basis of size by agarose gel electrophoresis and transferred to a nitrocellulose or nylon filter by buffer transfer through capillary action, or by electrophoretic current or by application of a vacuum. The fragments bound to the filter represent the exact replica of the DNA pattern within the gel. The blotted filter is then immersed in a solution containing the labeled DNA probe for hybridization.[105]

Northern Blot

Northern blot is a technique basically similar to Southern blot, except that it is used to transfer RNA from a gel to a blot instead of DNA.[106]

Dot Blot

Dot blot is a simpler technique which is able to detect the hybridizable sequences in the target samples but does not provide information regarding the size of the hybridized fragment. With this technique, extracted DNA or RNA from the target specimen is spotted onto the filter without the prior electrophoresis and transfer steps.

Polymerase Chain Reaction (PCR)

The recent advancement in recombinant technology is the development of a method for amplification of target DNA.[107] In this method, complementary oligonucleotide primers from either end of the target DNA are added to the sample along with a heat-resistant DNA polymerase. If the target sequence is present, the primers hybridize to it and provide a starting point for polymerase to initiate the synthesis of second-strand DNA. Then the newly synthesized double-stranded DNA is denatured by heating and is exposed again to polymerase at a lower temperature. After completion of 10 to 20 such cycles, which may take about 1 to 2 hours, the specific target sequence is amplified up to half a million to 1 million-fold (Figure 2-18). This powerful and highly sensitive technique is able to detect a specific DNA sequence in a single cell. However, because of its hypersensitivity, PCR may produce high false-positive results.

In Situ Hybridization

In situ hybridization is a technique in which DNA probes are directly applied to the tissue sections and cytologic or chromosomal preparations on a glass microscope slide. Nucleic acids remain intact in fresh-frozen as well as formalin-fixed, paraffin-embedded tissues. The principle of in situ hybridization is essentially similar to that of the other DNA hybridization techniques, except for deparaffinization and pro-

Bone Marrow Examination: Special Procedures

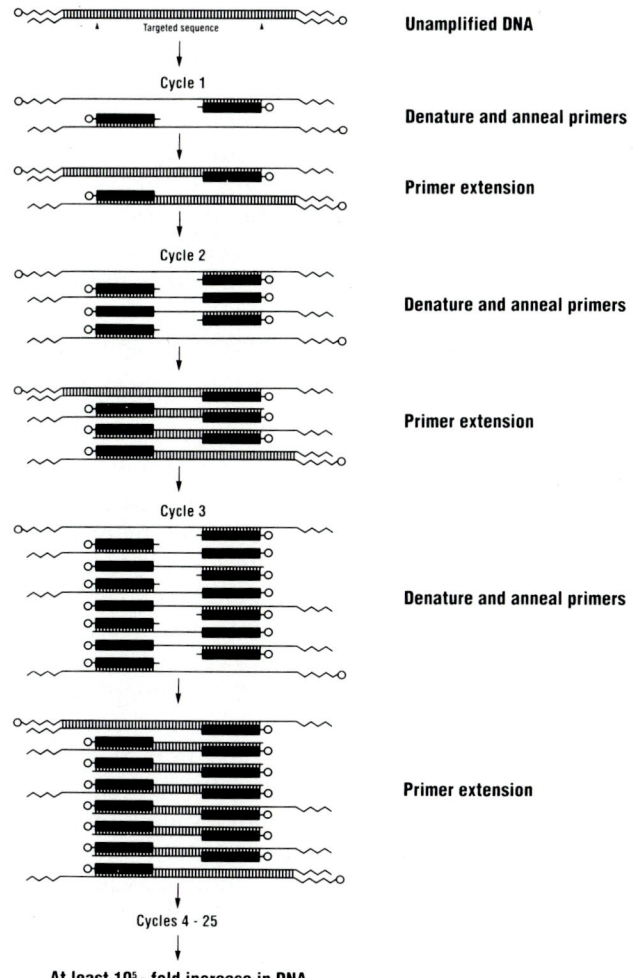

Figure 2-18. Schematic demonstration of the polymerase chain reaction (PCR). From Rose EA: Applications of the polymerase chain reaction to genome analysis. *FASEB J* 5:46, 1991, with permission.

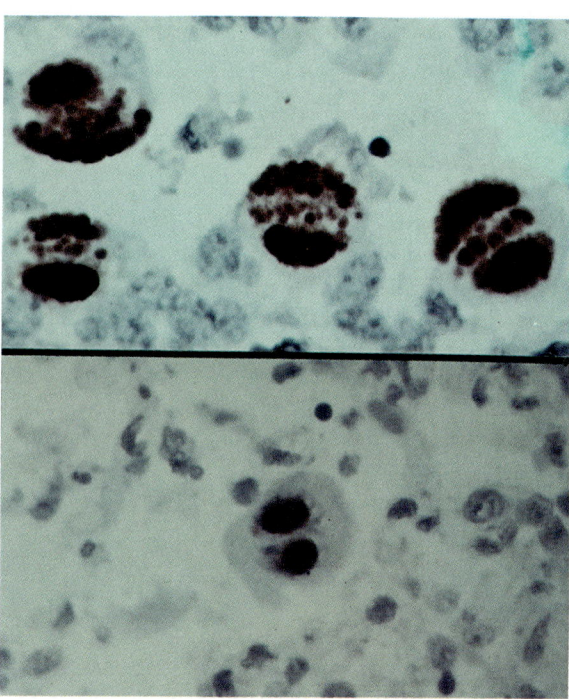

Figure 2-19. Demonstration of nuclear and cytoplasmic cytomegalovirus (CMV) by an in situ hybridization technique using a biotinylated CMV DNA probe.

teolytic digestion of the tissue sections to expose the intracellular nucleic acid targets (Figure 2-19). DNA probes are radioactive-labeled or biotinylated.[108,109]

Molecullar Diagnosis of Hematologic Disorders

DNA hybridization techniques are used in the diagnosis and characterization of a variety of hematologic disorders. They are instrumental in the detection of point mutations, gene or chromosomal deletions, gene rearrangements, chromosomal translocations and oncogene alterations.

Detection of Mutations and Deletions

A number of hematologic disorders result from or are associated with mutation(s) or with partial or complete deletion of certain genes. In such conditions, DNA hybridization techniques play an important role in the establishment of a correct diagnosis and detection of the carriers. Following are some representative examples.

Sickle cell anemia

This is a disorder caused by homozygosity for a nucleotide base pair substitution of adenine (A) to thymine (T) at the second position of the six codon of the beta-globin gene.[110,111] Prenatal diagnosis is performed on cells obtained by amniosynthesis or chorionic villus biopsy. The purified DNA is digested with an enzyme which recognizes a sequence altered by the mutated beta-globulin gene and is hybridized by the diagnostic sickle cell DNA probes by Southern blotting or PCR. A rapid method was recently introduced by Saiki et al. in which nonradioactive, allele-specific oligonucleotide probes and PCR amplification were used.[110]

β-Thalassemia

The molecular diagnosis of β-thalassemia is difficult and complicated because of the disease diversity due to multiple mutations. Over 50 known alleles account for this disease.[112] However, since different mutant alleles are observed in specific ethnic groups, it is possible to use a limited number (up to six) of allele-specific probes to detect up to 90% of the mutations in an ethnic population.[112] The recommended technique for the detection of the β-thalassemia mutations is PCR.[112,113]

Hemophilia A

This is the most common inherited disease of blood coagulation, which is caused by a deficiency or abnormality of factor VIII clotting factor as an X-linked trait. This disorder is associated with a large number of mutant alleles, which makes the diagnosis with allele-specific oligonucleotide probes even more difficult than that of β-thalassemia. However, prenatal diagnosis and carrier detection of hemophilia A has been recommended by several authors using probes consisting of intragenic polymorphic sequences of factor VIII gene by Southern blot and PCR techniques.[114-116] A rapid, nonradioactive PCR technique has been introduced by Kogan and associates for the carrier detection and prenatal diagnosis of hemophilia A.[116]

Von Willebrand disease

This disease is characterized by undetectable or trace quantities of von Willebrand factor (vWF) in plasma and tissues. Homozygous and heterozygous deletions of vWF gene can be detected by Southern blot and dot blot analysis, using vWF cDNA probes.[117,118]

Gene Rearrangements and Translocations

DNA restriction fragment sizes change whenever a translocation, inversion or gene rearrangement occurs in the area detected by a particular DNA probe. This concept has clinical applications in several diagnostic areas in hematopathology, including distinction of clonal from polyclonal lymphoproliferations, determination of the B- or T-cell identity of lymphoid malignancies, detection of rearrangements associated with chromosome translocations in lymphomas and leukemias, search for minimal residual disease during clinical remission or early relapse, and establishment of the relationship between a relapsing malignancy and the original clonal population.[104]

Diagnosis of lymphoid malignancies

The maturation process in the lymphoid system is associated with somatic gene rearrangements of immunoglobulin (Ig) heavy and light chain genes in B cells and T-cell receptor (TCR) genes in T cells.[119-125] Gene rearrangements are random and, therefore, the structure of the rearranged genes varies from one cell to another. Clonal expansion of the neoplastic cell results in identical rearrangements for all cells of the clone. By Southern blot analysis, it is possible to identify a clonal population and to distinguish this population from any other clonal populations or from a nonclonal population of lymphocytes (Figure 2-20). This technique is able to detect monoclonality when clonal cells account for at least 1–5% of the cell population.[126]

T-cell neoplasms display a very diverse morphology which may mimic reactive lymphadenopathy or Hodgkin's disease. The currently available T-specific monoclonal antibodies are helpful in the establishment of T-cell lymphoproliferative disorders, but they often do not detect monoclonality in such lesions. Thus, TCR gene rearrangement studies are the most definitive nonmorphologic approach for the diagnosis of T-cell malignancies. The TCR-β gene is the most informative probe, though its rearrangement has been reported in other hematopoietic malignancies[127,128] (Figures 2-21 and 2-22).

The use of B-specific antibodies, especially antibodies against Ig light chains, has significantly improved the ability of pathologists to diagnose B-cell lymphomas. However, a small percentage of tumors still remain equivocal after extensive morphologic and immunophenotypic studies. In such cases, Ig gene rearrangement studies may solve the problem and establish the diagnosis of malignancy. The most common Ig probes used for the diagnosis of B-cell

Bone Marrow Examination: Special Procedures

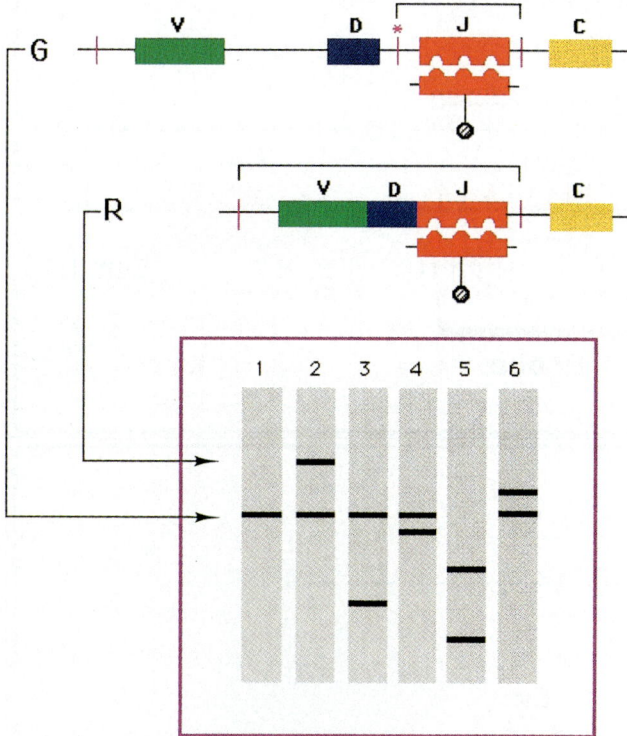

Figure 2-20. Schematic showing the organization of DNA gene complexes that undergo somatic rearrangements prior to expression. The top line (G) represents the genomic DNA prior to rearrangement. The second line (R) represents the rearranged DNA. V, D, J and C depict clusters of gene segments coding for variable, diversity, joining and constant portions, respectively, of T-cell receptors or Ig molecules. In this example, a labeled DNA probe for the joining region hybridizes with complementery DNA sequences on the Southern blot containing DNA from six samples. In the rearranged DNA, some of the restriction endonuclease sites are lost (asterisk). This loss may result in a larger DNA fragment, as shown here in line R and lanes 2 and 6, or, alternatively, a shorter DNA fragment (lanes 3, 4 and 5). The genomic pattern is usually retained in the cell's other chromosome, as seen in lanes 2, 3, 5 and 6. Alternatively, lane 4 represents a cell in which both chromosomes have rearranged their DNA and a genomic fragment is absent. No rearranged DNA band is demonstrated in lane 1.

malignancies are the joining segment of Ig heavy chain and the constant regions of the kappa and lambda light chains[124,126] (Figures 2-22 to 2-24).

Approximately 85% of follicular lymphomas and 30% of high-grade lymphomas demonstrate a t(14;18)(q32;q21) translocation which involves the *bcl-2* gene and occurs within two very short breakpoint regions at the 3' untranslated region of the *bcl-2* gene[129-132a,132b] (Figure 2-25). These two breakpoint regions are designated the "major breakpoint region (mbr)" and the "minor cluster region (mcr)," and contain, respectively, 60% and 25% of the t(14;18) translocations. Occasionally the breakpoint may occur 5' to the *bcl-2* gene. The *bcl-2* gene encodes a 25-kD membrane bound protein which is expressed at high levels in B-cell non-Hodgkin's lymphomas, particularly of the follicular type.[133]

Some of the diffuse lymphomas, including the small lymphocytic and large lymphocytic subtypes, are associated with t(11;14)(q13;q32) chromosome translocation.[134,135] With this translocation the *bcl-1* gene, normally located in chromosome segment 11q13, translocates to the heavy chain locus on chromosome 14q32.

Diagnosis of chronic myelogenous leukemia (CML)

The t(9;22) in CML is associated with the translocation of the *c-abl* gene from the long arm of chromosome 9(q34) to the long arm of chromosome 22(q11).[136-138] The translocated chromosome 22 is called the "Philadelphia chromosome (Ph^1)." The translocation breakpoint on chromosome 22 occurs in a small region called the "breakpoint cluster region (bcr)," leading to a *bcr-abl* fusion gene.[119-121] Thus, detection of the 8.5-kb fusion transcript and/or the 210-kD fusion protein is a pathognomonic feature of CML (Figure 2-26). This event is also detected in approximately half of the adult Ph^1+ ALLs. However, in the other half of the adult Ph^1+ ALLs and in almost all childhood Ph^1+ ALLs, the *bcr* fusion site is different, leading to a 7.0-kb fusion transcript and a 190-kD fusion protein.[139]

Detection of Donor and Recipient Origin of the Marrow in Bone Marrow Transplantation Patients

Recent advances in DNA "fingerprinting" have made it possible to distinguish donor cells from recipient

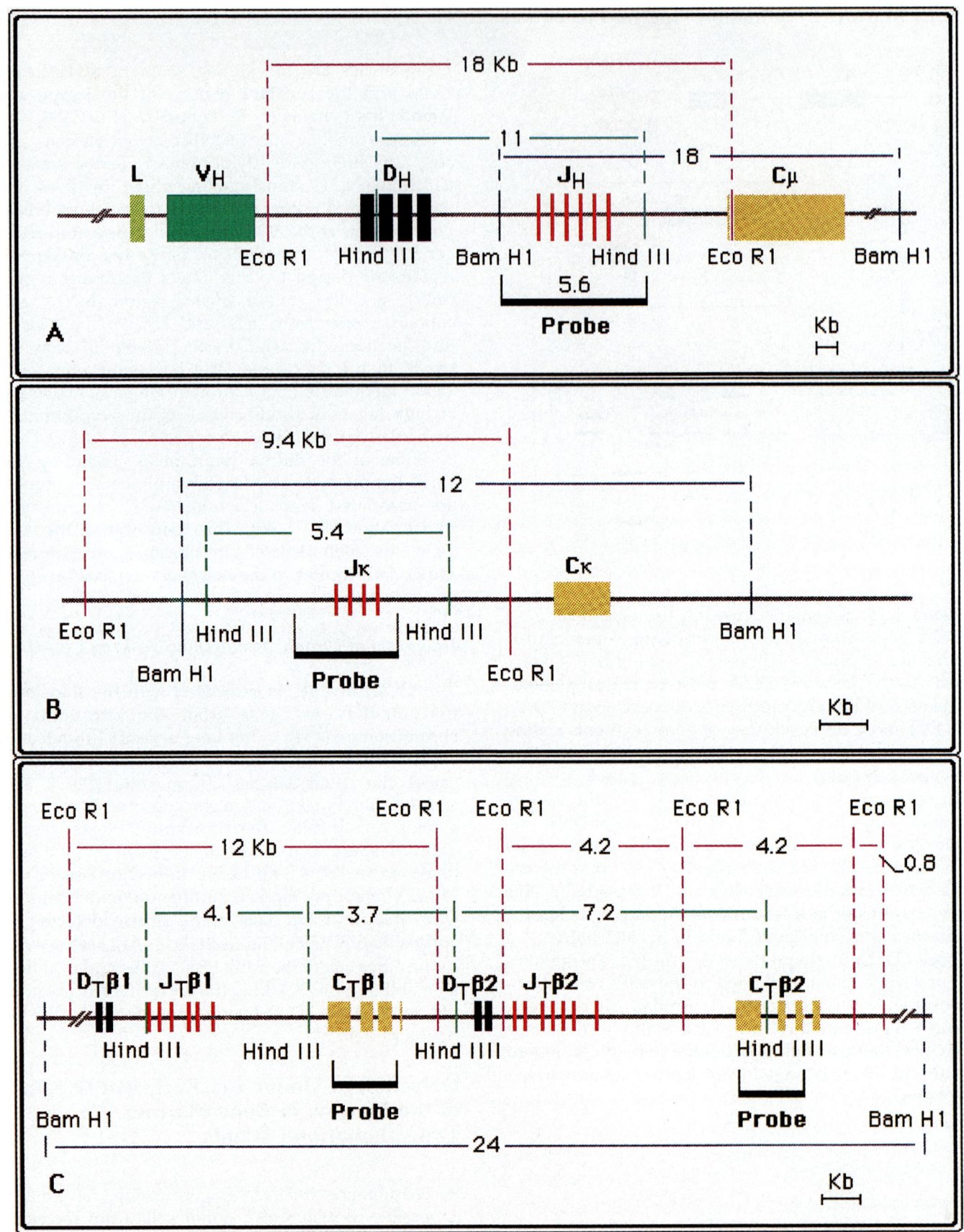

Figure 2-21. Genomic restriction maps of the Ig heavy chain gene (A), the Ig kappa chain gene (B), and the T-cell receptor beta chain gene (C) demonstrating regions which are commonly used as probes for gene rearrangement studies.

Bone Marrow Examination: Special Procedures

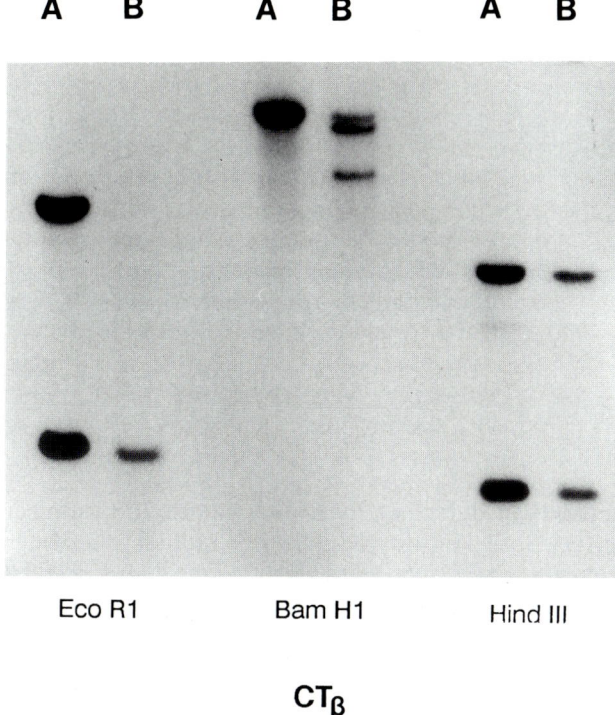

CT$_\beta$

Figure 2-22. Southern blot analysis for T-cell receptor gene rearrangements. The DNA probe is from the constant region of the T-cell receptor beta chain (CTβ). Three restriction enzymes are used. Sample A (control) represents germline bands. Sample B demonstrates rearranged bands with enzymes Eco R1 (loss of a band) and enzyme Bam H1 (two additional bands).

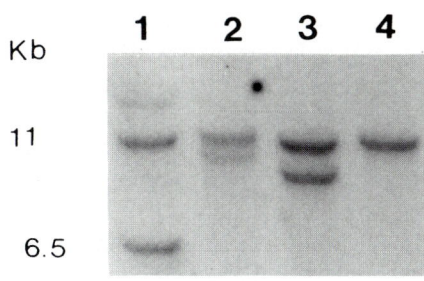

J$_H$

Figure 2-23. Southern blot analysis for Ig gene rearrangements. The DNA probe is from the joint region of Ig heavy chain (JH) and the restriction enzyme is Hid III. Lanes 1, 2 and 3 demonstrate rearranged bands. Lane 4 (control) represents germline DNA.

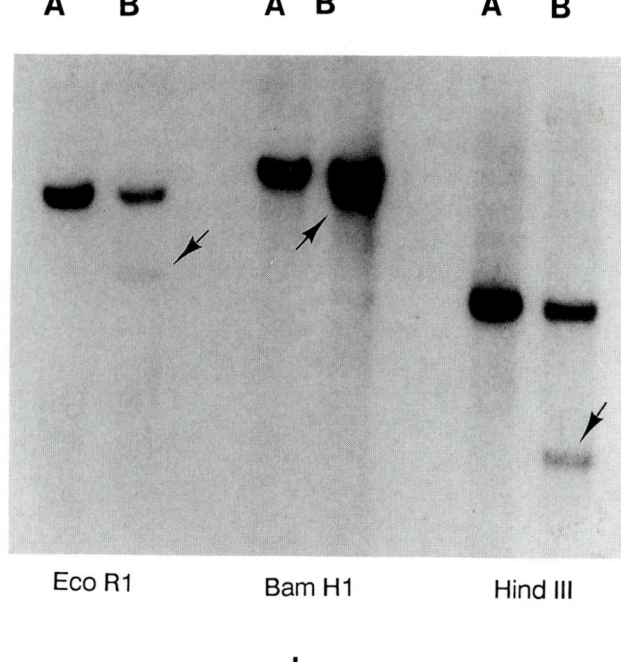

J$_\kappa$

Figure 2-24. Southern blot analysis for Ig gene rearrangements. The DNA probe is from the joint region of the Ig kappa light chain (Jκ). Three restriction enzymes are used. Sample A (control) shows germline bands. Sample B demonstrates rearranged bands (arrows).

cells unless the donor and recipient are identical. The principle of DNA fingerprinting or restriction-fragment length polymorphism (RFLP) is based on comparing the DNA polymorphisms of the donor and the recipient. Certain areas of the human genome vary so greatly between people that they have been designated "hypervariable regions." DNA probes derived from these regions reveal many variations in restriction fragment sizes on Southern blot analysis. The resulting patterns are so complex that essentially no two persons, except for identical twins, will demonstrate the same pattern[104,140] (see Chapter 11).

Detection of Microorganisms

Invasion of human tissue by microorganisms involves the presence of a foreign species of DNA which can readily be distinguished from the endogenous human genomic sequences by the use of a specific DNA probe. In situ hybridization and PCR are effective

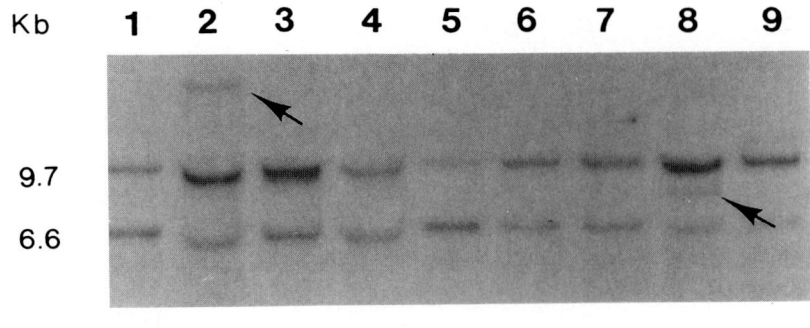

Figure 2-25. Southern blot analysis of DNA samples obtained from lymph nodes of nine patients suspected of having lymphoma. Patients 2 and 8 show rearranged bands when a *bcl-2* DNA probe is used (arrows.) From Grody W, Gatti, RA, Naeim, F: Diagnostic molecular pathology. Modern pathol 2:553, 1989, with permission.

methods of detecting infectious agents in tissue sections. Both biotinylated and radioactive-labeled probes are available and in use for viral and nonviral infectious agents[96,141,142] (see Figure 2-19).

ONCOGENES

Cellular oncogenes (c-oncogenes) are genomic structures homologous to various viral oncogenes (v-oncogenes) identified in acute transforming retroviruses.[143,144] In normal cells, c-oncogenes are involved in the regulation of cell growth and differentiation.[145,146] In most retrovirus-induced tumors in experimental animals, expression of the v-oncogene is responsible for neoplastic transformation. In a number of human neoplasms, such as hematologic malignancies, activation of c-oncogenes is altered. This alteration may be caused by point mutation, deletion, amplification, chromosomal rearrangements, promoter insertion or other mechanisms.[147] Although there is no direct evidence of an etiologic role for proto-oncogenes in hematologic malignancies, recent investigations suggest that cancer results from activation of several c-oncogenes, along with the loss of suppressor genes.[148] Several cellular oncogenes implicated in human hematologic malignancies are presented in Table 2-4.

Change in oncogene activation may be detected at DNA, RNA or protein levels. For example, DNA alteration of *c-myc* in Burkitt's lymphoma, *c-abl* in CML, *bcl-1*, *bcl-2* and *bcl-3* in B-cell lymphomas, and *tcl-1*, *tcl-2* and *tcl-3* in T-cell malignancies are all the result of chromosomal translocations involving these oncogenes. Abnormalities in the *c-ras* family, fre-

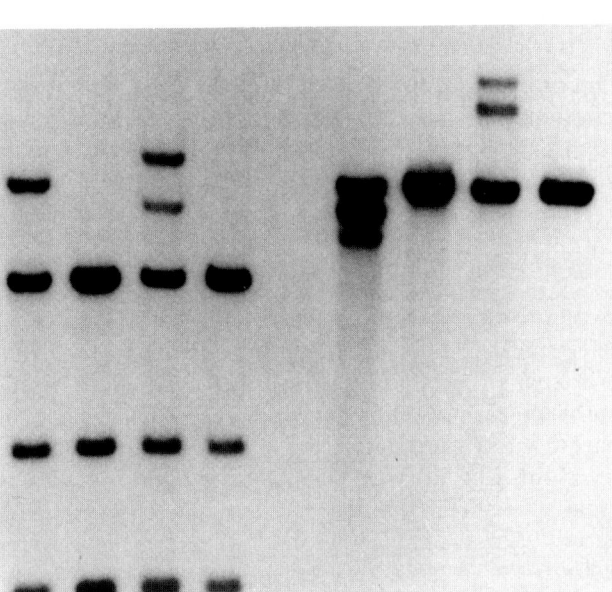

Figure 2-26. Southern blot analysis for the detection of t(9;22) using a *bcr* DNA probe. Enzymes Bgl II and XbaI are used. The positive control (+) and sample A demonstrate rearranged bands with both enzymes. DNA bands in sample B and negative (−) control are identical, indicating no *bcr* rearrangement.

Table 2-4 Oncogenes Implicated in the Pathogenesis of Human Leukemias*

c-Oncogene	Chromosome Location	Related Protein/Site
c-myc	8q24.1	DNA binding/nucleus
c-myb	6q23	?/nuclear
c-abl	9q34.1	Tyrosine Kin.[1]/cytoplasm
N-ras	1p11-13	GTpase/cytoplasm
Ha-ras	11p14-15	GTpase/cytoplasm
Ki-Ras	12p12	GTpase/cytoplasm
c-fes	15q24-26	Tyrosine Kin./cytoplasm
c-fos	14q21-22	?/nucleus
c-fms	5q34	CSF1 receptor/cytoplasm
c-src	1p36/20p13	Tyrosine Kin./cytoplasm
c-sis	22q11-21	PDGF[2]/cytoplasm
c-erb A	17q21	? Carbonic anhydrase/?
c-erb B1	7p	EGF[3] receptor/cytoplasm
c-erb B2	17q21	EGF receptor/cytoplasm
c-mos	8q22	Serine kinase/cytoplasm
Blym 1	1p32	?Transferrin/nucleus
p53 gene	17p13	?/nucleus
bcl-1	11q13	?/?
bcl-2	18q21	?/?
tcl-1	14q32.1	?/?

* Modified from Butturini et al; Oncogenes in human leukemias. *Cancer Invest* 6:305, 1988.
[1]—Kinase.
[2]—Platelet-derived growth factor.
[3]—Epithelial growth factor.

quently observed in AML, are often secondary to point mutations.[149-152] Recent studies have demonstrated a strong association between *ras* mutation and myelodysplastic syndrome (MSD). A high incidence of mutation was found mainly in the *N-ras* oncogene among patients who have chronic myelomonocytic leukemia, a variant of MDS.[154] The majority of MDS patients with a *ras* mutation developed acute leukemia, mostly myelomonocytic. Such findings suggest that a *ras* mutation tends to influence hematopoietic cell differentiation preferentially toward the myelomonocytic cell lineage. In fact, among patients with AML, a *ras* mutation has been reported in those who have myelomonocytic (AML-M4) or monocytic (AML-M5) disease.[154-156]

Qualitative and quantitative changes in mRNA oncogenes have been reported in hematologic malignancies. These changes are detected by a variety of techniques such as Northern or dot blot analysis, PCR, or less frequently, by in situ hybridization techniques. Elevated levels of *c-myc*, *c-myb* and *c-fos* have been demonstrated in most human leukemias.[157-159] *c-sis* mRNA expression is reported in patients with CML in accelerated phase or blast transformation,[159] and elevated *c-fos* mRNA levels are detected in myelomonocytic (M4) and monocytic (M5) leukemias.[158,160] In patients with CML a *c-abl*-related RNA, transcribed from a chimeric gene composed of *bcr* and *c-abl* sequences, has been identified.[136,137]

Several oncogene-encoded proteins have been identified. Some, such as *c-myc* and *c-fos* proteins, are nuclear proteins and are thought to play a role in the regulation of gene expression and/or in splicing out introns in nuclear RNA. The majority of cellular oncogenes encode cytoplasmic proteins. Tyrosine kinase activity has been associated with the expression of a number of cellular oncogenes such as *c-abl*, *c-fes* and *c-src*.[161] The chimeric *bcr/abl* gene present in CML generates a 210-kD protein with tyrosine kinase activity.[162] Similarly, a unique 190-kD *c-abl*-related protein has been found in some patients with Ph+ ALL.[139]

Suppressor Genes ("Anti-Oncogenes")

There is growing evidence supporting the presence of genes which play an important role in the suppression of tumorigenesis.[148,163-166] The retinoblastoma suppressor (Rb) gene and the p53 gene are such examples. The Rb gene is located on chromosome 13 near band q14. Inactivation of the Rb gene due to rearrangements, mutations or deletions may lead to decreased expression of mRNA and protein and subsequently to the development of retinoblastoma, osteosarcoma and megakaryoblastic crisis of CML. Inactivation of the Rb gene has also been demonstrated in a small proportion of human lymphoid neoplasms.[167a] The allelic loss of p53 gene, located on chromosome 17 (p13), is a frequent feature in various human solid tumors. Structural alteration of this gene has also been demonstrated in blast crisis of CML, AML, ALL and Waldenstrom's macroglobulinemia.[167b,167c]

CYTOGENETIC ANALYSIS

Cytogenetic studies in leukemias and lymphomas have provided valuable information regarding the biology of these diseases. With chromosome banding analysis, most human hematologic malignancies have shown chromosomal abnormalities.[168-189] However, this technique has certain limitations such as: (1) it requires cells in metaphase and thus a need for growing bone marrow cells for 1-2 days in culture; (2) interpretation of the results is sometimes difficult because of the small number of recognizable metaphases and/or presence of unidentified chromosome fragments; (3) associated technical problems such as minimal chromosomal spreading, poor banding quality and fuzzy appearance of the chromosome[181b]; and (4) it is time consuming and costly. Availability of chromosome specific DNA probes has provided an opportunity to eliminate some of these limitations by applying in situ hybridization techniques (Figure 2-26). This technique has been applied to cells in interphase as well as metaphase.[181b,182a] Interphase cytogenetics is now being used for both numerical and structural chromosomal aberrations in hematopoietic malignancies.[181b]

Lymphoid Malignancies

Chromosome segments 14q11 and 14q32 are found as a genomic hallmark in approximately two-thirds

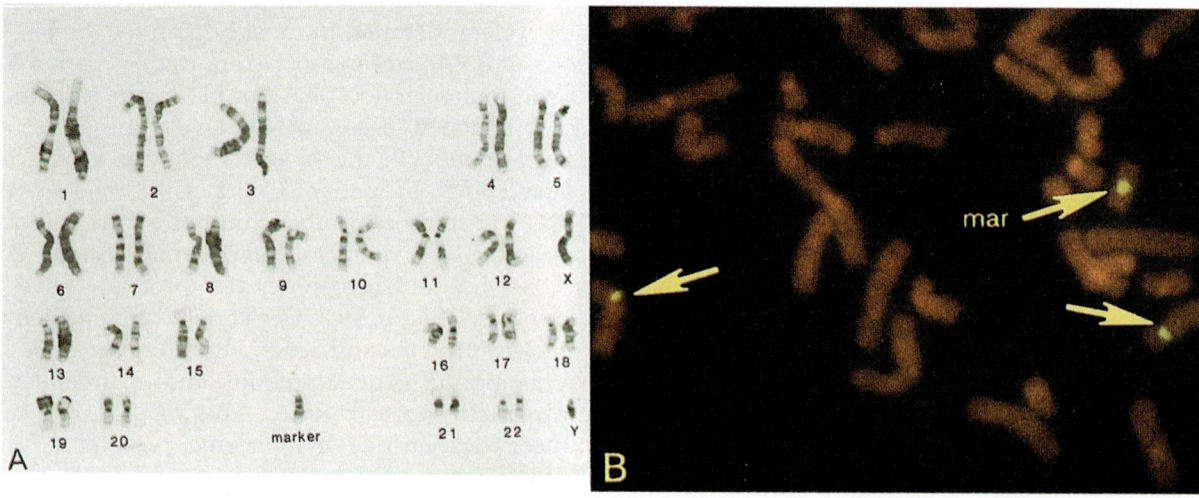

Figure 2-27. Cytogenetic analysis of blast cells in a patient with Acute myelogenous leukemia: (A) karotype demonstrating 46,XY and additional marker chromosome; (B) fluorescent in situ hybridization with the chromosome 12-specific probe showing hybridization of the probe to the two normal 12 chromosomes (unlabeled arrows) and the marker chromosome (mar). With permission, Schad CR, Kraker WJ, Jalal SM, et al. Use of fluorescent in situ hybridization for marker chromosome identification in congenital and neoplastic disorders. *Am J Clin Pathol* 96:203, 1991.

of the patients with non-Hodgkin's lymphoma (NHL)[182] and one-third of those with lymphocytic leukemias.[183] Most of the patients with B-cell malignancies have a characteristic 14q+ chromosome with rearrangement of the IGH genes at band 14q32, while patients with T-cell lymphomas often have a selective rearrangement of the alpha T-cell receptor genes (TCRA) at 14q11[182-188] (Table 2-5, Figure 2-27). The frequent involvement of IGH and TCRA in NHLs and lymphocytic leukemias reflects the fact that these disorders often arise at the pre-B and pre-T stages of cell differentiation, respectively.

Table 2-5 Chromosomes and Genes in Lymphoid Malignancies*

Disease	Chromosome		Rearranged	
	Defect	Breakpoints	Gene	Oncogene
Lymphoma				
Small, noncleaved cell	t(8;14)	8q24.1 and 14q32.3	IGH	c-myc
	t(2;8) or t(8;22)	2p11.2 or 22q11.21	IGK$_1$ or IGL	
Follicular, small, large and mixed cell	t(14;18)	14q32.3 and 18q21.3	IGH	bcl-2
Diffuse, large cell				
	t(3;14)	3p21 and 14q32.3		
	t(3;14)	3q27 and 14q32.3		
	t(8;14)	8q24.1 and 14q32.3	IGH	c-myc
	t(14;18)	14q32.3 and 18q21.3	IGH	bcl-2
	t(11;14)	11q23.3 and 14q32.3	IGH	bcl-3
	t(V;14)†	V and 14q32.3		
Small lymphocytic (CLL)				
	t(2;14)	2p13 and 14q32.3	IGH	
	t(8;14)	8q24.1 and 14q11.2	TRCA	c-myc
	del 11q	11q14.2 and 11q23.3		
	t(11;14)	11q13 and 14q32	IGH	bcl-1
	+12			
	Inv 14 or t(14;14)	14q11.2 and 14q32.1	TCRA	
	t(14;17)	14q32 and 17q23		
	t(14;19)	14q32 and 19q13	IGH	
Acute lymphoblastic leukemia				
	t(1;19)	1q21q23 and 19p13		
L2	t(4;11)	4q21 and 1q23.3		
	t(7;V)	7q34 and V†	TCRB	
L3	t(8;14)	8q24.1 and 14q32.3	IGH	c-myc
	t(8;14)	8q24.1 and 14q11.2	TCRA	c-myc
L1, L2	t(9;22)	9q34.1 and 22q11.21		abl
	t(10;14)	10q24 and 14q11.2	TCRA	
	t(11;14)	11p13 and 14q11.2	TCRA	
	t(11;14)	11p15 and 14q11.2	TCRA	
	t(V;12)	V† and 12p12 or del 12 p12p13		

* Adapted from Yunis JJ; Genes and Chromosomes in the pathogenesis and prognosis of human cancers. *Adv Pathol* 2;143, 1989.
† Variable chromosome.

The vast majority of the patients with Burkitt's lymphoma have a reciprocal translocation t(8;14), with breakpoints at bands 8q24 and 14q32. At the molecular level, the oncogene *c-myc* is rearranged from its normal location at band 8q24 to the joining or switch region of IGH at band 14q32.[184] This rearrangement often results in deregulation of *c-myc* transcription. Approximately 25% of Burkitt's lymphoma patients have a variant chromosomal translocation t(2;8)(p11;q24) or t(8;22)(q24;q11) involving rearrangement of *c-myc* with IGK or IGL, respectively.[184,185]

Among the T-cell lymphomas, the interplay between the oncogene and a cell-differentiation gene in a chromosomal translocation is well illustrated

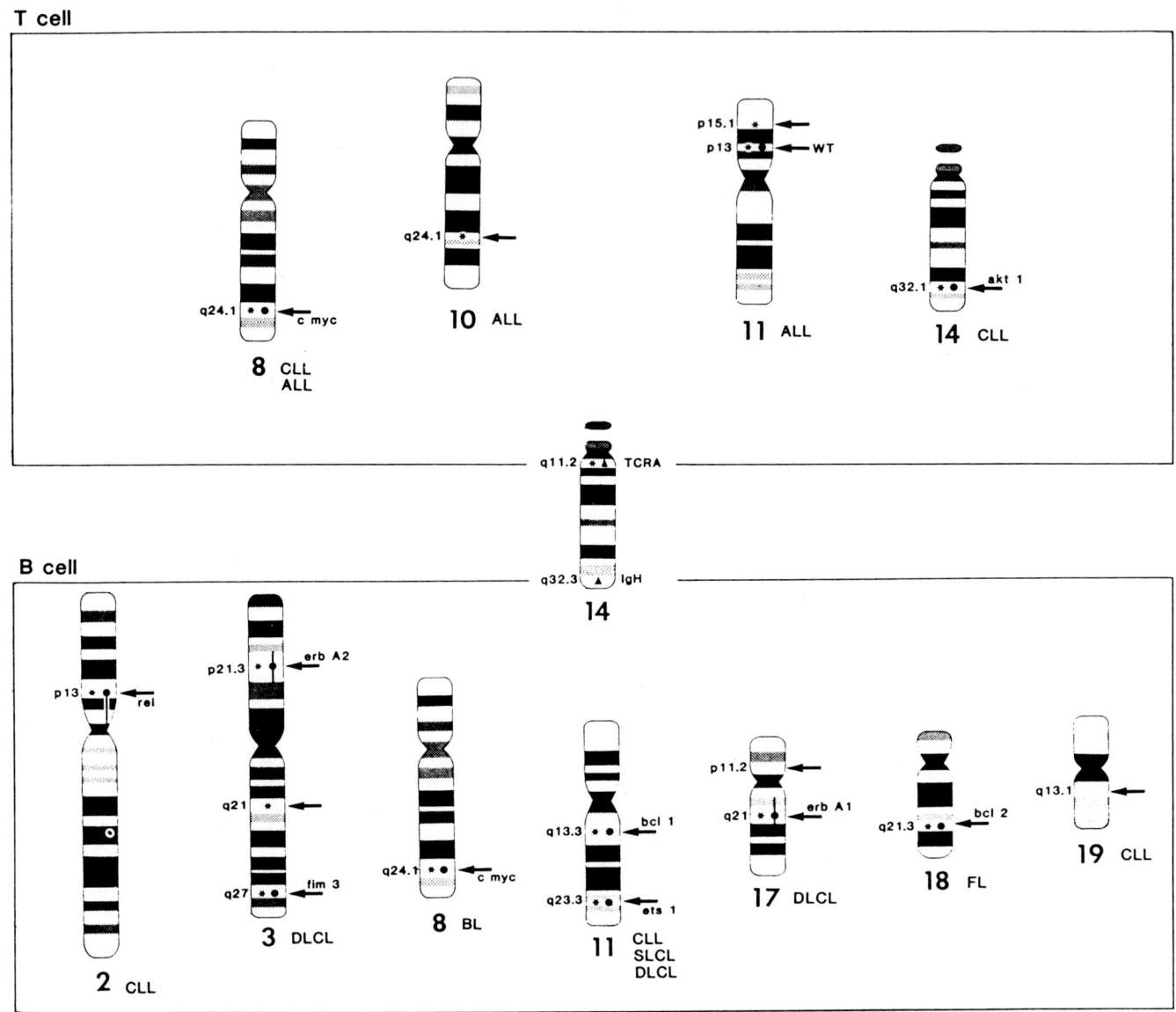

Figure 2-28. Common involvement of T- and B-cell antigen receptors in lymphoid malignancies. Asterisks = fragile sites; dots = oncogenes; triangles = antigen receptors; arrows = recurrent chromosomal break points. From Yumis, JJ, Genes and chromosomes in the pathogenesis and prognosis of human cancers. *Acta Pathol* 2:143, 1989, with permission.

Bone Marrow Examination: Special Procedures

in a subgroup of T-cell lymphoma/leukemia with t(8;14)(q24;q11) in which *c-myc* is rearranged with TCRA[186] (Figure 2-28).

In follicular lymphoma, which represents approximately 40% of NHL, the great majority of patients have t(14;18)(q32;q21), with rearrangement of the putative oncogene *bcl-2* from 18q21 to IGH on chromosome 14q32.[179,181,187,188] The importance of this genomic abnormality to the disease process is denoted by the finding of *bcl-2* rearrangement in patients with not only follicular small-cleaved cell (FSC) but also follicular mixed cell (FMC) and follicular large-cell disease (FLC)[181,187] (Figures 2-28 and 2-29). Patients who do not have a t(14;18)/*bcl-2* rearrangement show a better response to therapy and longer median survival than patients with a t(14;18)/*bcl-2* rearrangement.[181,187]

Approximately one-third of patients with ALL have a chromosomal translocation. Of these, about 5% are diagnosed as having ALL-L3 (Burkitt's type), according to the FAB classification, and generally have a 14q+ chromosome representing a t(8;14) translocation (see Table 2-5). Of the remaining patients, approximately 30% have a chromosome translocation not involving IGH, while others have extra chromosomes, recurrent deletions or normal chromosomes.

As discussed, in some ALL patients with a t(9;22), *abl* and *bcr* are arranged, producing a p210 protein. In others, the breakpoint occurs close to but not in the *bcr* gene, and the product is a p190 protein. Several other cytogenetic abnormalities have been defined for ALL.[189-191]

Myeloid Malignancies

A t(9;22) translocation is observed in approximately 90 to 95% of adults diagnosed with CML, and the

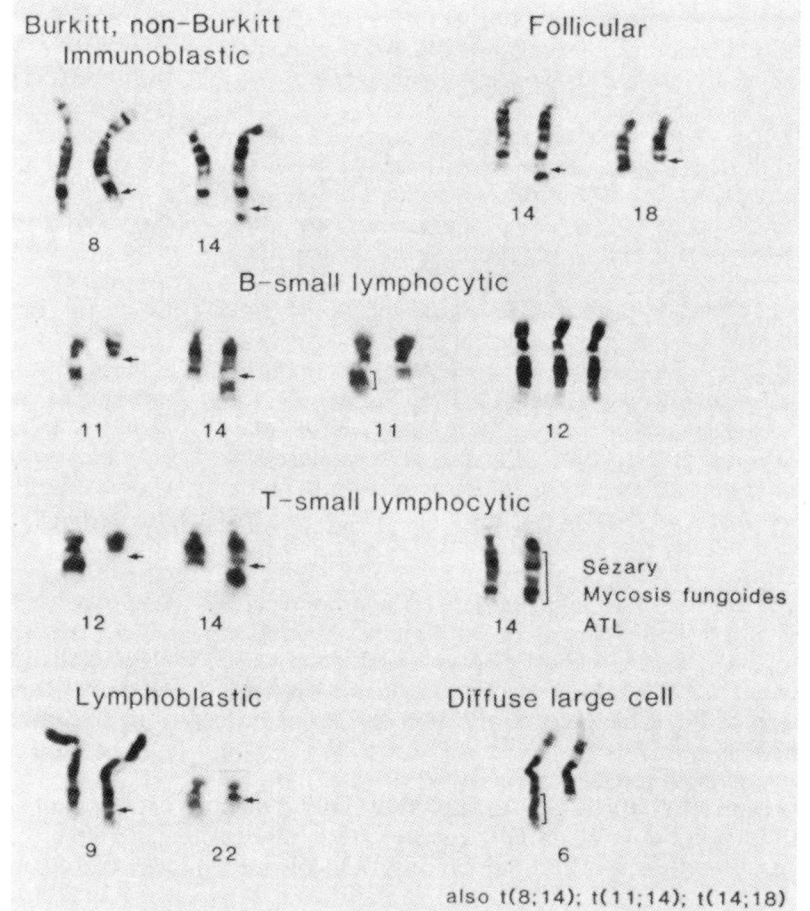

Figure 2-29. Selected G-banded chromosomes depicting specific chromosome defects preferentially found in various histologic subtypes of non-Hodgkin's lymphoma. Yunis JJ: Chromosomal rearrangements, genes and fragile sites in cancer: Clinical and biologic implications, in De Vita V, et al (eds), Important Advances in Oncology. Philadelphia, JB Lippincott, 1986, p 93, with permission.

defect is found throughout the evolution of the disease. As discussed before, this translocation is associated with rearrangement of the *c-abl* and formation of an *abl-bcr* segment, producing a hybrid mRNA and protein found only in the leukemic cells.[191-195]

The presence of t(9;22) and, more recently, *bcr* rearrangement in patients with the diagnosis of CML is important as a prognostically favorable indicator because these patients have a median survival of 42 months, whereas the remaining 5 to 10% of CML patients who do not have such a defect survive for an average of only 15 months[196] (Figure 2-30).

Approximately 80% of CML patients in blast crisis show additional cytogenetic abnormalities such as a second Ph chromosome, an isochromosome 17q, trisomy 8, trisomy 1, or trisomy 17.[178,197] A t(1;17) translocation has also been observed.[198]

Unlike CML, which basically represents a homogeneous disorder, de novo AML is quite heterogeneous and includes at least 10 different types of recurrent chromosomal abnormalities (Table 2-6). Patients with an inv(16), t(8;21) and t(15;17), as well as those with normal chromosomes, have a relatively better prognosis than those with t(9;11).

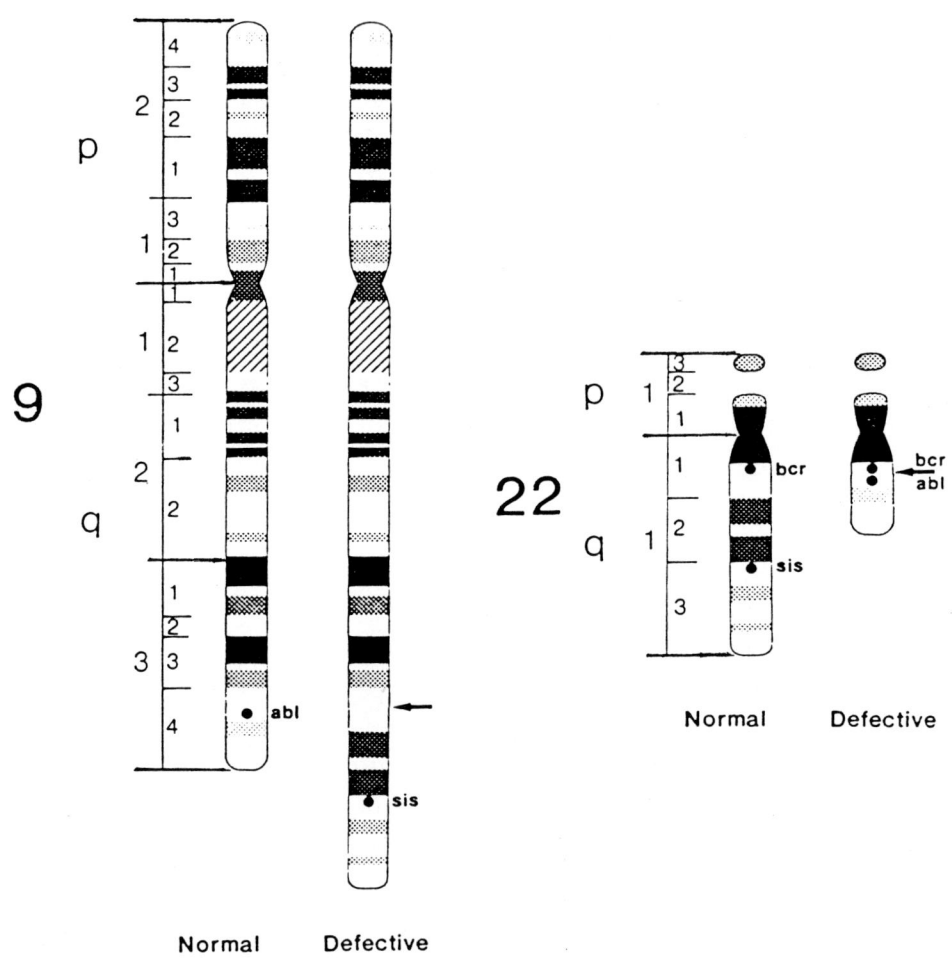

Figure 2-30. Schematic demonstration of t(9;22) translocation in chronic myelogenous leukemia and formation of an *abl-bcr* hybrid. Adapted from Yunis JJ, Chromosomal rearrangements, genes and fragile sites in cancer: Clinical and biologic implications, in De Vita V, et al (eds), Important Advances in Oncology. Philadelphia, JB Lippincott, 1986, p 93.

Bone Marrow Examination: Special Procedures

Table 2-6 Consistent Chromosome Defects in Myeloid Leukemia and Myelodysplastic Syndrome*

Disease	Chromosome		Near Breakpoint	
	Defect	Breakpoints	Gene	Oncogene
Leukemia				
CML	t(9;22)	9q34.1 and 22q11.21	bcr‡	abl‡
AML	inv 3	3q21 and 3q26.2		
	t(3;5)	3q21 and 5q31	GM-CSF	
M1, M2	del 5q	5q31 and 5q35		
M2	t(6;9)	6p22.2 and 9q34.1		pim, abl
	del 7p	7p11.2 and 7p22	PDGFA	erb-B1
	t(8;21)	8q22.1 and 21q22.3		mos, ets-2
M1, 2, 4, 5, 6	del 7q	7q31.2 and 7q36		
	+8			
M4, M5	t(9;11)	9p22 and 11q23.3	INF A, B‡	ets-1
M1	t(9;22)	9q34.1 and 22q11.21	bcr‡	abl‡
M3	t(15;17)	15q22 and 17q11.2	MP‡	erb-A1
M2, M4	inv 16	16p13.2 and 16q22	MTI, II‡	
Myelodysplastic syndrome†				
RAEB, RAEB-T	t(1;3)	1p36 and 3q21		
	t(2;11)	2p11.2 and 11q23.3		
RA, RAEB	del 5q	5q31q35		
RAEB	del 7p	7p11.2 and 7p22	PDGFA	erb-B1
RA, RAEB, RAEB-T, CMML	del 7q	7q31.2 and 7q36		
RAEB	+8			
	del 9q	9q13 and 9q22.1		
	del 20q	20q11.3 and 20q13.3		

* Adapted from Yunis JJ: Genes and chromosomes in the pathogenesis and prognosis of human cancers, *Adv Pathol* 2:143, 1989.
† RA: refractory anemia.
  RAEB: refractory anemia with excess blasts.
  RAEB-T: refractory anemia with excess blasts in transformation.
  CMML: chronic myelomoncytic leukemia
‡ Gene/oncogene found rearranged.

ELECTRON MICROSCOPY

Transmission electron microscopy is routinely used to evaluate ultrastructural changes in hematologic disorders. Detection of Auer rods and other abnormal granules in myelogenous leukemia and Birbeck bodies in Langerhans cell histiocytosis are examples (Figure 2-31). Immunoelectron microscopy is used for the detection of specific ultrastructural cellular components by using antibody-coated, electron-dense particles. An example is the demonstration of PPO in megakaryoblastic leukemias. Scanning electron microscopy is also occasionally used in hematopathology when the surface configuration of the cells is of diagnostic value, such as the presence of numerous elongated microvilli in hairy cell leukemia (Figure 2-32). In the following chapters, electron microscopic findings are discussed, along with other morphologic findings in appropriately selected cases.

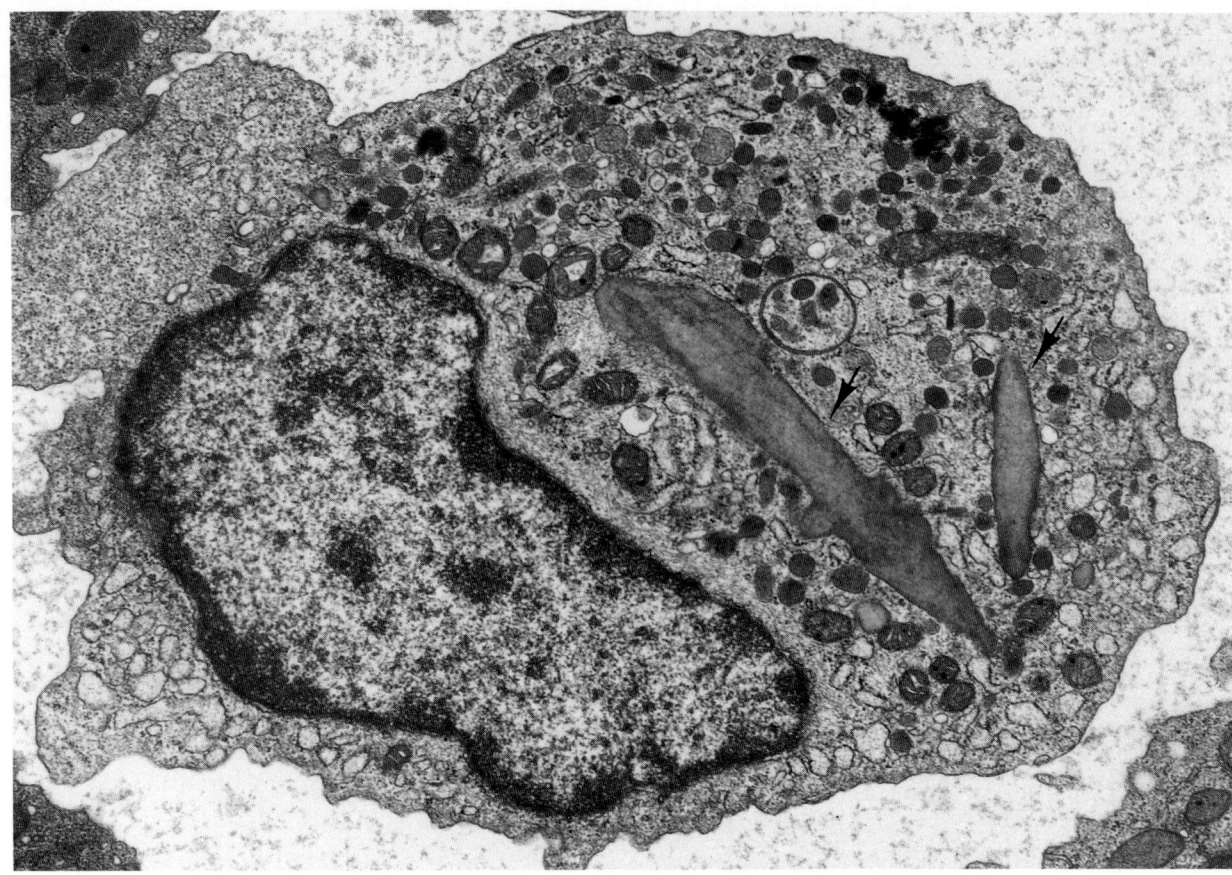

Figure 2-31. An electron microscopic photograph of a promyelocyte with Auer rods (arrow) in a patient with promyelocytic leukemia.

BONE MARROW CULTURE

Improved semisolid and liquid culture procedures have provided a great opportunity for in vitro studies of normal and abnormal hematopoiesis.[199-202] Bone marrow culture is used to investigate the effects of growth factors and regulatory cytokines on hematopoietic cell proliferation and differentiation. It is used for cytogentic analysis, colony assays and detection of stem cell defects, and therapeutic evaluations in disorders such as bone marrow aplasia, myelodysplastic syndromes, myeloproliferative disorders and leukemias. It is also used as one of the purging methods in bone marrow transplantation.[203]

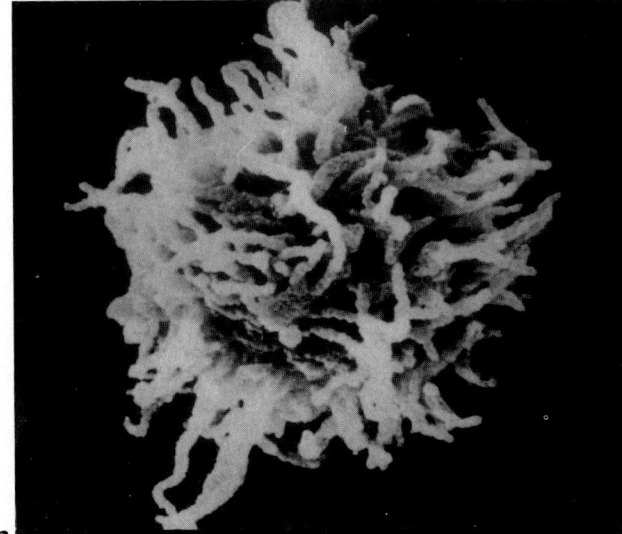
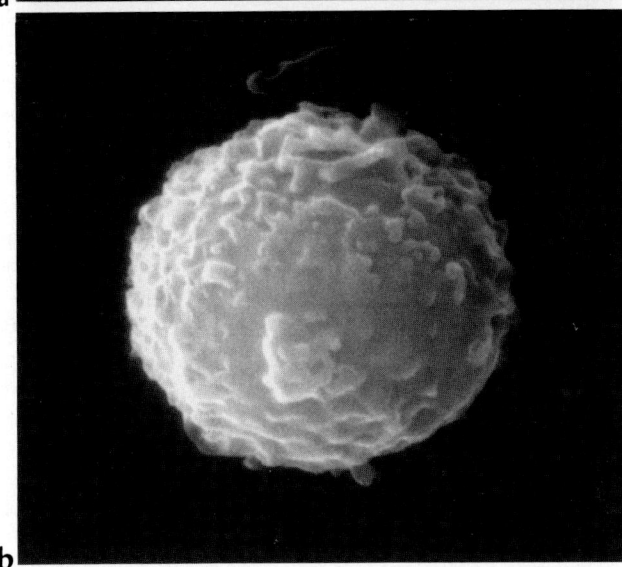

Figure 2-32. Scanning electron microscopic photograph of neoplastic cells: (a) in a patient with hairy cell leukemia; (b) a patient with Sezary syndrome; from Naeim F: Cytoskeletal control of redistribution of surface membrane receptors in hairy cell leukemia. *Am J Clin Pathol* 74:661, 1980, with permission.

References

1. Hyun BH, Gulati GL, Ashton JK: Bone marrow examination: Techniques and interpretation. *Hematol Oncol Clin North Am* 2:513, 1988.
2. Bakir F: Fatal sternal puncture: Report of a case. *Dis Chest* 44:435, 1963.
3. Gulati GL, Ashton JK, Hyun BH: Structure and function of the bone marrow and hematopoiesis. *Hematol Oncol Clin North Am* 2:495, 1988.
4. Beckstead JH: The bone marrow biopsy: A diagnostic strategy. *Arch Pathol Lab Med* 110:175, 1986.
5. Fong TP, Okafor LA, Schnitz TH, et al: An evaluation of cellularity in various types of bone marrow specimens. *Am J Clin Pathol* 72:812, 1979.
6. Gruppo RA, Lampkin BC, Granger S: Bone marrow cellularity determination: Comparison of the biopsy, aspirate and buffy coat. *Blood* 49:29, 1977.
7. Bartl R, Frisch B, Buchenrieder B, et al: Multiparameter studies on 650 bone marrow biopsy cores: Diagnostic value of combined utilization of imprints, cryostat and plastic sections in medical practice. *Bibliotheca haematol* 50:1, 1984.
8. Byrnes RK, Mckenna RW, Sundberg RD: Bone marrow aspiration and trephine biopsy: An approach to a thorough study. *Am J Clin Pathol* 70:753, 1987.
9. Burns WA, Yook CR: Plastic sections and ultrastructural techniques in the evaluation of bone marrow pathology. *Hematol Oncol Clin North Am* 2:525, 1988.
10. Islam A, Frisch B: Plastic embedding in routine histology 1: Preparation of semi-thin sections of undecalcified marrow cores. *Histopathology* 9:1263, 1985.
11. Hayhoe FGJ, Quaglino D: *Hematological Cytochemistry*, ed 2. London, Churchill Livingstone, 1988.
12. Hotchkiss RD: A microchemical reaction resulting in the staining of polysaccharide structures in fixed tissue preparation. *Arch Biochem* 16:131, 1948.
13. Inagaki S: Cytochemical reactions of basophil leukocytes. VII. Periodic acid-Schiff (PAS) reaction. *Acta Hematol Jpn* 31:169, 1968.
14. Kaung DT: Periodic acid-Schiff reaction in human basophilic leukocytes. *Acta Hematol* 42:269, 1969.
15. Bitter MA, Le Beau MM, Larson RA, et al: A morphologic and cytochemical study of acute myelomonocytic leukemia with abnormal marrow eosinophils associated with inv(16)(p13q22). *Am J Clin Pathol* 81:733, 1984.
16. Schmitz N, Godde-Salz E, Gassmann W, et al: Acute myelomonocytic leukemia with involvement of eosinophils and inversion of chromosome 16. *Blut* 48:263, 1984.
17. Swirsky DM, Li YS, Matthews JG, et al: Translocation in acute granulocytic leukemia: Cytological, cytochemical and clinical features. *Br J Haematol* 56:199, 1984.
18. Hayhoe FGJ: The cytochemistry of hematopoiesis, in Britton JC (ed), *Disorders of the Blood*. London, Churchill Livingstone, 1969, p 123.

19. Ho FCS, Chan GTC, Todd D: Non-specificity of Sudan black B in the diagnosis of acute myeloid leukemia. *Br J Haematol* 53:171, 1983.
20. Savage RA, Hoffman GC: Sudan black positivity in non-myeloid leukemia. *Br J Haematol* 54:494, 1983.
21. Stass SA, Pui CH, Melvin S, et al: Sudan black B positive acute lymphoblastic leukemia. *Br J Haematol* 57:413, 1984.
22. Felberg NT, Schultz J: Evidence that myeloperoxidase is composed of isoenzymes. *Arch Biochem Biophys* 148:407, 1972.
23. Lippi U, Cappelletti P: Cytochemical evidence of multiple molecular forms of myeloperoxidase. *Haematologica* 67:807, 1982.
24. Pember S, Shapira R, Kinkade J: Multiple forms of myeloperoxidase from human neutrophilic granulocytes: Evidence for differences in compartmentalization, enzymatic activity, and subunit structure. *Arch Biochem Biophys* 221:391, 1983.
25. Olsson I, Persson AM, Stromberg K, et al: Purification of eosinophil peroxidase and studies of biosynthesis and processing in human bone marrow. *Blood* 66:1143, 1985.
26. Cawley JC, Hayhoe FGJ: *Ultrastructure of Haemic Cells.* London, WB Saunders, 1973.
27. Koeffler HP, Ranyard J, Pertcheck M: Myeloperoxidase: Its structure and expression during myeloid differentiation. *Blood* 65:484, 1985.
28. Morishita Y, Morishima Y, Ogura M, et al: Biochemical characterization of human myeloperoxidase using three monoclonal antibodies. *Br J Haematol* 63:435, 1986.
29. Tetteroo PAT, van der Schoot CE, van dem Borne AEG: New developments in the phenotypic analysis of (im)mature myeloid leukemia: Clinical relevance. *Proc Int Meeting on Genotypic, Phenotypic and Functional Aspects of Haematopoiesis.* Assisi, 1987, p 13A.
30. Chang KS, Schroder W, Siciliano MJ, et al: The localization of the human myeloperoxidase gene is in close proximity to the translocation breakpoint in acute promyelocytic leukemia. *Leukemia* 1:458, 1987.
31. Well SC, Rosner GL, Reid MS, et al: Translocation and rearrangement of myeloperoxidase gene in acute promyelocytic leukemia. *Science* 240:790, 1988.
32. Parwaresch MR: *The Human Blood Basophil.* Berlin, Springer-Verlag, 1976.
33. Breton-Gorius J, Van Haeke D, Pryzwansky KB, et al: Simultaneous detection of membrane markers with monoclonal antibodies and peroxidase activities in leukemia: Ultrastructural analysis using a new method of fixation preserving the platelet peroxidase. *Br J Haematol* 58:447, 1984.
34. Koike T, Nagayama R, Takahashi M, et al: Perinuclear peroxidase activity in erythroblasts. *Br J Haematol* 64:621, 1986.
35. Breton-Gorius J, Villeval JL, Mitjavila MT, et al: Ultrastructural and cytochemical characterization of blasts from early erythroblastic leukemia. *Leukemia* 1:173, 1987.
36. Khalaf MR, Hayhoe FGJ: Cytochemical demonstration of "platelet" peroxidase at light microscope level. *Eur J Haematol* 39:128, 1987.
37. Matsuo T, Jain NC, Bennett JM: Nonspecific esterase of acute promyelocytic leukemia (M3). *Am J Hematol* 29:148, 1988.
38. Ranki A: Nonspecific esterase activity in human lymphocytes. *Clin Immun Immunopathol* 10:47, 1978.
39. Yang K, Bearman RM, Pangalis GA, et al: Acid phosphatase and alpha-naphthyl acetate esterase in neoplastic and nonneoplastic lymphocytes. A statistical analysis. *Am J Clin Pathol* 78:141, 1982.
40. Jaffe ES, Cossman J, Callihan TR: Presence of acid alpha-naphthyl acetate esterase (ANAE) in human B cell lymphomas. *Lab Invest* 42:125, 1980.
41. Kaplow LS: Cytochemistry of leukocyte alkaline phosphatase. Use of complex naphthol AS phosphates in azo-dye coupling techniques. *Am J Clin Pathol* 39:439, 1963.
42. Hayhoe FGJ, Quaglino D: Cytochemical demonstration and measurement of leukocyte alkaline phosphatase activity in normal and pathological states by a modified azo-dye coupling technique. *Br J Haematol* 4:375, 1958.
43. Miller DM, Yang A, Liepman M: Altered isoenzyme patterns of leukocyte alkaline phosphatase in disease states. *Br J Haematol* 57:145, 1984.
44. Miller DM, Yang A, Leipman M: Evidence for two isoenzymes of leukocyte alkaline phosphatase in leukemic leukocytes. *Am J Hematol* 18:159, 1985.
45. Climie ARW, Henrichs WL, Foster IJ: Neutrophil alkaline phosphatase test. A review with findings in pregnancy. *Am J Clin Pathol* 38:95, 1962.
46. Kaplow LS, Beck RE: Leukocyte alkaline phosphatase response to surgical stress. *Surg Gynecol Obstet* 119:97, 1964.
47. Valentine WN, Follette JH, Hardin EB, et al: Studies on leukocyte alkaline phosphatase activity: Relation to stress and pituitary-adrenal activity. *J Lab Clin Med* 44:219, 1954.
48. Koler RD, Seaman AJ, Osgood EE, et al: Myeloproliferative diseases: Diagnostic value of the leukocyte alkaline phosphatase test. *Am J Clin Pathol* 30:295, 1958.
49. Wachstein M: Alkaline phosphatase activity in normal and abnormal human blood and bone marrow cells. *J Lab Clin Med* 31:1, 1946.

50. Lewis SM, Dacie JV: Neutrophil (leukocyte) alkaline phosphatase in paroxysmal nocturnal haemoglobulinuria. *Br J Haematol* 11:549, 1965.
51. Hayhoe FGJ, Neuman Z: Cytology of myeloma cells. *J Clin Pathol* 29:916, 1976.
52. Hayhoe FGJ, Flemans RJ, Burns GF, et al: Leukocyte alkaline phosphatase scores in hairy cell leukemia. *Br J Haematol* 37:158, 1977.
53. Tanzer J, Harel B, Boiron M, et al: Cytochemical and cytogenetic findings in a case of chronic neutrophilic leukemia of mature cell type. *Lancet* 1:387, 1964.
54. Hammouda F, Quaglino D, Hayhoe FGJ: Blast crisis of chronic granulocytic leukemia. Cytochemical, cytogenetic and autoradiographic studies in four cases. *Br Med J* 1:1275, 1964.
55. Rambaldi A, Terao M, Bettoni S, et al: Differences in the expression of alkaline phosphatase mRNA in chronic myelogenous leukemia and paroxysmal nocturnal hemoglobinuria polymorphonuclear leukocytes. *blood* 73:1113, 1989.
56. Burroughs SF, Devine DV, Browne G, et al: The population of paroxysmal nocturnal hemoglobinuria neutrophils deficient in decay-accelerating factor is also deficient in alkaline phosphatase. *Blood* 71:1086, 1988.
57. Macfarlane JD, Poorthuis BJ, van der Kamp JJ, et al: Hypophosphatasia: Biochemical screening of a Dutch kindred and evidence that urinary excretion of inorganic phosphatase is a marker for the disease. *Clin Chem* 34:41, 1988.
58. Cazzalo M, Barosi G, Bobbi PG, et al: Natural history of idiopathic refractory sideroblastic anemia. *Blood* 71:305, 1988.
59. Katayama I, Yang JPS: Reassessment of a cytochemical test for differential diagnosis of leukemic reticuloendotheliosis. *Am J Clin Pathol* 68:268, 1977.
60. Li CY, Yam LT, Lam KW: Acid phosphatase isoenzymes in normal and pathological conditions. *J Histochem Cytochem* 18:473, 1970.
61. Li CY, Yam LT, Lam KW: Studies of acid phosphatase isoenzymes in human leukocytes: Demonstration of isoenzyme cell specificity. *J Histochem Cytochem* 18:901, 1970.
62. Kass L, Munster D: Acid phosphatase in normal human blood cells: Characterization by isoelectric focusing in polyacrylamide gel. *Exp Hematol* 7:272, 1979.
63. Radsun HJ, Parwaresch MR: Isoelectric focusing pattern of acid phosphatase and acid esterase in human blood cells, including thymocytes, T lymphocytes and B lymphocytes. *Exp Hematol* 8:737, 1980.
64. Radsun HJ, Parwaresch MR, Feller AC: Cell-specific polymorphism of acid phosphatase in human blood cells: Their functional and leukemic variants. *Proc Soc Exp Biol Med* 167:394, 1981.
65. Drexler HG, Gaedicke G: Analysis of isoenzyme patterns of acid phosphatase in acute leukemias. *Blut* 47:105, 1983.
66. Li CY, Yam LT, Lam KW: Tartrate resistant acid phosphatase in the reticulum cells of leukemic reticuloendotheliosis. *N Engl J Med* 284:357, 1971.
67. Katayama I, Li CY, Yam LT: Histochemical study of acid phosphatase isoenzyme in leukemic reticuloendotheliosis. *Cancer* 29:157, 1972.
68. Usui T, Konishi H, Sawada H, et al: Existence of tartrate-resistant acid phosphatase activity in differentiated lymphoid leukemic cells. *Am J Hematol* 12:47, 1982.
69. Naeim F, Caspotango VJ, Johnson CE, et al: Sezary syndrome: Tartrate-resistant acid phosphatase in the neoplastic cells. *Am J Clin Pathol* 71:528, 1979.
70. Yam LT, Janckila AJ, Li CY, et al: Cytochemistry of tartrate-resistant acid phosphatase: 15 years experience. *Leukemia* 1:285, 1987.
71. Albelda SM, Buck CA: Integrins and other adhesion molecules. *FASEB J* 4:2868, 1990.
72. Naeim F: Selection of monoclonal antibodies in the diagnosis and classification of leukemias. *Desease Marker* 7:1, 1989.
73. LeBien TW, McCormack RT: The common acute lymphoblastic leukemia antigen (CD10)—emancipation from a functional enigma. *Blood* 73:625, 1989.
74. Ng CS, Chan JK, Hui PK, et al: Monoclonal antibodies reactive with normal and neoplastic T cells in paraffin sections. *Hum Pathol* 19:295, 1988.
75a. Andrade RE, Wick MR, Frizzera G, et al: Immunophenotyping of hematopoietic malignancies in paraffin sections. *Hum Pathol* 19:394, 1988.
75b. Kubic VL, Brunning RD: Immunohistochemical evaluation of neoplasms in bone marrow biopsies using monoclonal antibodies reactive in paraffin-embedded tissue. *Modern Pathol* 2:618, 1989.
76. Ryan DH, Fallon MA, Horan PK: Flow cytometry in the clinical laboratory. *Clin Chim Acta* 171:125, 1988.
77. Neudorf SML, Tucker WLB, Bollum F, et al: Double fluorochrome analysis of human bone marrow lymphoid cells: Studies with terminal transferase and anti-T-cell monoclonal antibodies. *Exp Hematol* 12:69, 1984.
78. Diamond LW, Nathwani BN, Rappaport H: Flow cytometry in the diagnosis and classification of malignant lymphoma and leukemia. *Cancer* 50:1122, 1982.
79. Coon JS, Landay AL, Weinstein RS: Advances in flow cytometry for diagnostic pathology. *Lab Invest* 57:453, 1987.
80. Brylan RC, Benson NA, Nourse VA: Cellular DNA of human neoplastic B-cells measured by flow cytometry. *Cancer Res* 44:5010, 1984.

81. Merkel DE, Dressler LG, McGuire WL: Flow cytometry, cellular DNA content, and prognosis in human malignancies. *J Clin Oncol* 5:1690, 1987.
82. Hiddemann W, Wormann B, Gohde W, et al: DNA aneuploidies in adult patients with acute myeloid leukemia. *Cancer* 57:2146, 1986.
83. Barlogie B, Alexanian R, Dixon D, et al: Prognostic implications of tumor cell DNA content in multiple myeloma. *Blood* 66:338, 1985.
84. Wilson RM, Galvin AM, Robins RA, et al: A flow cytometric method for the measurement of phagocytosis by polymorphonuclear leukocytes. *J Immunol Methods* 76:247, 1985.
85. Bass DA, Parce JW, Dechatelet LI, et al: Flow cytometric studies of oxidative product formation by neutrophils: A graded response to membrane stimulation. *J Immunol* 130:1910, 1983.
86. Vindelov LL, Christensen IJ, Jensen J, et al: Limits of detection of nuclear DNA abnormalities by flow cytometric analysis. *Cytometry* 3:332, 1983.
87. Clark R, Peters S, Hoy T, et al: Prognostic significance of hypodiploid hemopoietic precursors in myelodysplastic syndromes. *N Engl J Med* 314:1472, 1986.
88. Worman B, Hiddemann W, Ritter J, et al: DNA aneuploidy in childhood ALL—incidence and relation to prognostic factors. *Proc Am Assoc Cancer Res* 24:161, 1983.
89. Look AT, Roberson PK, Williams DL, et al: Prognostic importance of blast cell DNA content in childhood acute lymphoblastic leukemia. *Blood* 65:1079, 1985.
90. Smets LA, Slaten RM, Behrendt H, et al: Phenotypic and karyotypic properties of hyperdiploid acute lymphoblastic leukemia of childhood. *Br J Haematol* 61:113, 1985.
91. Smets LA, Homan BJ, Hart A, et al: Prognostic implication of hyperdiploidy as based on DNA flow cytometric measurement in childhood acute lymphocytic leukemia: A multicenter study. *Leukemia* 1:163, 1987.
92. Pui Ch, Williams DL, Raimondi SC, et al: Hypodiploidy is associated with a poor prognosis in childhood acute lymphoblastic leukemia. *Blood* 70:247, 1987.
93. Brylan RC, Diamond LW, Powell ML, et al: Percentage of cells in the S-phase of the cell cycle in human lymphoma determined by flow cytometry. Correlation with labeling index and patient survival. *Cytometry* 1:171, 1980.
94. Shackney SE, Levine AM, Fisher RI, et al: The biology of tumor growth in the non-Hodgkin's lymphomas. *J Clin Invest* 73:1201, 1984.
95. Diamond LW, Brylan RC: Flow analysis of DNA content and cell size in non-Hodgkin's lymphoma. *Cancer Res* 40:703, 1980.
96. Brylan RC, Benson NA, Nourse VA: Cellular DNA of human neoplastic B-cells measured by flow cytometry. *Cancer Res* 44:5010, 1984.
97. Scraffe JH, Crowther D: The pretreatment proliferative activity of non-Hodgkin's lymphoma cells. *Eur J Cancer* 17:99, 1981.
98. McLaughlin P, Osborne BM, Johnston D, et al: Nucleic acid flow cytometry in large cell lymphoma. *Cancer Res* 48:6614, 1988.
99. Egerter DA, Said JW, Epling S, et al: DNA content of T-cell lymphomas. A flow cytometric analysis. *Am J Pathol* 130:326, 1988.
100. Bunn PA, Whang-Peng J, Carney DN, et al: DNA content analysis by flow cytometry and cytogenetic analysis in mycosis fungoides and Sezary syndrome. *J Clin Invest* 65:1440, 1980.
101. Bunn PA, Krasnow S, Makuch RW, et al: Flow cytometric analysis of DNA content of bone marrow cells in patients with plasma cell myeloma: Clinical implications. *Blood* 59:528, 1982.
102. Balogie B, Alexanian R, Gehan EA, et al: Marrow cytometry and prognosis in myeloma. *J Clin Invest* 72:853, 1983.
103. Balogie B, Alexanian R, Dixon D, et al: Prognostic implications of tumor cell DNA and RNA content in multiple myeloma. *Blood* 66:338, 1985.
104. Grody WW, Gatti RA, Naeim F: Diagnostic molecular pathology. *Modern Pathology* 2:553, 1989.
105. Southern EM: Detection of specific sequences among DNA fragments separated by gel electrophoresis. *J Mol Biol* 98:503, 1975.
106. Alwine JC, Kemp DJ, Parker BA, et al: Detection of specific RNAs or specific fragments of DNA by fractionation in gels and transfer to diazobenzyloxymethyl paper. *Methods Enzymol* 68:220, 1979.
107. Saiki RK, Scharf S, Fallona F, et al: Enzymatic amplification of beta-globin genomic sequences and restriction site analysis for diagnosis of sickle cell anemia. *Science* 230:1350, 1985.
108. Bayer EA, Wilchek M: The use of avidin-biotin complex as a tool in molecular biology. *Methods Biochem Anal* 26:1, 1980.
109. Langer PR, Waldrop AA, Ward DC: Enzymatic synthesis of biotin-labeled polynucleotides: Novel nucleic acid affinity probes. *Proc Natl Acad Sci USA* 78:6633, 1981.
110. Saiki RK, Chang CA, Levenson CH, et al: Diagnosis of sickle cell anemia and β-thalassemia with enzymatically amplified DNA and non-radioactive allele-specific oligonucleotide probes. *N Engl J Med* 319:537, 1988.
111. Macityre EA: The use of the polymerase chain reaction in hematology. *Blood Rev* 3:201, 1989.
112. Kazazian HH, Bohem CD: Molecular basis and prenatal diagnosis of β-thalassemia. *Blood* 72:1107, 1988.

113. Wong C, Dowling CE, Saiki RK, et al: Characterization of β-thalassemia mutations using direct genomic sequencing of amplified single copy. *Nature* 330:384, 1987.
114. Gitschier J, Lawn RM, Rotblat F, et al: Antenatal diagnosis and carrier detection of hemophilia A using factor VIII gene probe. *Lancet* 1:1093, 1985.
115. Antonarakis SE, Copeland KL, Carpenter RJ Jr, et al: Prenatal diagnosis of hemophilia A by factor VIII gene analysis. *Lancet* 1:1407, 1985.
116. Kogan SC, Doherty M, Gitschier J: An improved method for prenatal diagnosis of genetic diseases by analysis of amplified DNA sequences. Application to hemophilia A. *N Eng J Med* 317:985, 1987.
117. Shelton-Inloes BB, Chebab FF, Mannucci PM, et al: Gene deletions correlate with the development of alloantibodies in von Willebrand disease. *J Clin Invest* 79:1459, 1987.
118. Ngo KY, Glotz VT, Koziol JA, et al: Homozygous and heterozygous deletion of the von Willebrand factor gene in patients and carriers of severe von Willebrand disease. *Proc Natl Acad Sci USA* 85:2753, 1988.
119. Tonegawa S: Somatic generation of antibody diversity. *Nature* 302:575, 1983.
120. Coleclough C: Chance, necessity and antibody diversity. *Nature* 303:23, 1983.
121. Hood L, Kronenberg M, Hunkapiller T: T-cell antigen receptors and the immunoglobulin supergene family. *Cell* 40:225, 1985.
122. Yoshikai Y, Clark SP, Taylor S, et al: Organization and sequences of the variable, joining and constant region genes of the human T-cell receptor alpha-chain. *Nature* 316:837, 1985.
123. Hayday A, Saito H, Gillies SD, et al: Structure, organization, and somatic rearrangement of T-cell gamma genes. *Cell* 40:259, 1985.
124. Korsmeyer SJ, Waldman TA: Immunoglobin genes; rearrangement and translocation in human malignancy. *J Clin Immunol* 4:1, 1984.
125. Minden MD, Mak TW: The structure of the T cell antigen receptor genes in normal and malignant cells. *Blood* 64:327, 1986.
126. Arnold AJ, Cossman J, Bakhshi A, et al: Immunoglobulin-gene rearrangements as unique clonal markers in human lymphoid neoplasms. *N Engl J Med* 309:1593, 1983.
127. Mack TW: Monoclonality in human T-cell disorders. *Blood Rev* 2:89, 1988.
128. Hoffbrand AV, Leber BF, Browett PJ, et al: Mixed acute leukemias. *Blood Rev* 2:9, 1988.
129. Tsujimoto Y, Finger LR, Yunis JJ, et al: Cloning of the chromosome breakpoint of neoplastic B cells with the t(14;18) translocation. *Science* 226:1097, 1984.
130. Bakhshi A, Jensen JP, Goldman P, et al: Cloning of chromosomal breakpoint of t(14;18) human lymphomas: Clustering around JH on chromosome 14 and near a transcriptional unit on 18. *Cel* 41:899, 1985.
131. Cotter FE: The role of the *bcl-2* gene in lymphoma. *Br J Haematol* 75:449, 1990.
132a. Cleary NL, Smith SD, Sklar J: Cloning and structural analysis of cDNAs for *Bcl-2* and a hybrid *Bcl-2*/immunoglobulin transcript resulting from the t(14;18) translocation. *Cell* 47:19, 1986.
132b. Weiss LM, Warnke RA, Sklar RA, et al: Molecular analysis of the t(14;18) chromosomal translocation in malignant lymphomas. *N Engl J Med* 317:1185, 1987.
133. Ngan BY, Chen-Levy Z, Weiss LM, et al: Expression in non-Hodgkin's lymphoma of the bcl-2 protein associated with the t(14;18) chromosomal translocation. *N Engl J Med* 318:1638, 1988.
134. Tsujimoto Y, Yunis J, Onorato-Showe L, et al: Molecular cloning of the chromosomal breakpoint of B-cell lymphomas and leukemias with t(11;14) chromosome translocation. *Science* 224:1403, 1984.
135. Tsujimoto Y, Cossman J, Gorham J, et al: Clustering of breakpoints on chromosome 11 in human B-cell neoplasms with t(11;14) chromosome translocation. *Nature* 315:340, 1985.
136. De Klein A, Van Kessel GA, Grosveld G, et al: A cellular oncogene is translocated on the Philadelphia chromosome in chronic myelocytic leukemia. *Nature* 300:765, 1982.
137. Groffen J, Stephenson JR, Heisterkamp N, et al: Philadelphia chromosomal breakpoints are clustered within a limited region, bcr, on chromosome 22. *Cell* 36:93, 1984.
138. Stam K, Heisterkamp N, Grosveld G, et al: Evidence of a new chimeric *bcr/c-abl* mRNA in patients with chronic myelocytic leukemia and the Philadelphia chromosome. *N Eng J Med* 313:1429, 1985.
139. Hermans A, Heisterkamp N, von Lindern M, et al: Unique fusion of *bcr* and *c-abl* genes in Philadelphia chromosome positive acute lymphoblastic leukemia. *Cell* 51:33, 1987.
140. Nakamura Y, Leppert M, O'Connell P, et al: Variable number of tandem repeat (VNTR) markers for human gene mapping. *Science* 235:1616, 1987.
141. Grody W, Lewin K, Naeim F: Detection of cytomegalovirus DNA in classic and epidemic Kaposi's sarcoma by in situ hybridization. *Hum Pathol* 19:524, 1987.
142. Tenover FC: Diagnostic deoxyribonucleic acid probes for infectious diseases. *Clin Microbiol Rev* 1:82, 1988.
143. Bishop JM: Cellular oncogenes and retroviruses. *Annu Rev Biochem* 52:301, 1983.
144. Bishop JM: Viruses, genes and cancer: II. Retroviruses and cancer genes. *Cancer* 55:2329, 1985.

145. Muller R: Protooncogenes and differentiation. *Trends Biochem Sci* 11:129, 1986.
146. Hunter T: The epidermal growth factor receptor gene and its product. *Nature* 311:414, 1984.
147. Alitalo K: Amplification of cellular oncogenes in cancer cells. *Med Biol* 62:304, 1984.
148. Srivatsan ES, Benedict WF, Stanbridge EJ: Molecular analysis of the chromosomal control of neoplastic expression in human cell hybrids: Chromosome 11 is implicated in the suppression of tumorigenicity. *Cancer Res* 46:6174, 1986.
149. Bos JL, Takoz D, Marshall CJ, et al: Amino acid substitution at codon 13 of the N-ras oncogene in human acute myelogenous leukemia. *Nature* 45:3262, 1985.
150. Bos JL, Verlaan-de Vries M, van der Erb J, et al: Mutation in N-ras predominate in acute myelogenous leukemia. *Blood* 69:1237, 1987.
151. Hirai H, Tanaka S, Azuma M, et al: Transforming genes in human leukemia cells. *Blood* 66:1371, 1985.
152. Eva A, Tronick SR, Goll RA, et al: Transforming genes of human hemopoietic tumors: Frequent deletion of ras-related oncogenes whose activation appears to be independent of tumor phenotype. *Proc Natl Acad Sci USA* 80:4926, 1983.
153. Mavilio F, Testa U, Sposi NM, et al: Selective expression of c-fos oncogene in acute myelomonocytic leukemias: A molecular marker of terminal differentiation. *Blood* 69:160, 1987.
154. Box JI, Verlaan-de Vires M, van der Eb AJ, et al: Mutations in N-ras predominate in acute myeloid leukemia. *Blood* 69:1237, 1987.
155. Farr CJ, Saiki RK, Erlich HA, et al: Analysis of ras gene mutation in acute myeloid leukemia by polymerase chain reaction and oligonucleotide probes. *Proc Natl Acad Sci USA* 85:1629, 1988.
156. Tokzos D, Farr CJ, Marshall CJ: Ras gene activation in a minor proportion of the blast population in acute myeloid leukemia. *Oncogene* 1:409, 1987.
157. Westin EH, Gallo RC, Arya SK, et al: Differential expression of the amv gene in human hematopoietic cells. *Proc Natl Acad Sci USA* 79:2194, 1982.
158. Romero P, Blick M, Taipaz M, et al: C-sis and c-abl expression in chronic myelogenous leukemia and other hematologic malignancies. *Blood* 67:839, 1986.
159. Preisler HD, Raza A, Larson R, et al: Protooncogene expression and clinical characteristics of acute myelocytic leukemia: A Leukemia intergroup Pilot Study. *Blood* 73:255, 1989.
160. Mavilio F, Testa U, Sposi NM, et al: Selective expression of c-fos oncogene in acute myelomonocytic leukemias: A molecular marker of terminal differentiation. *Blood* 69:160, 1987.
161. Butturini A, Sthivelman E, Canaani E, et al: Oncogenes in human leukemias. *Cancer Invest* 6:305, 1988.
162. Canaani E, Gale RP, Steiner-Salz, D, et al: Altered transcription of an oncogene in chronic myeloid leukemia. *Lancet* 1:593, 1984.
163. Koufos A, Hansen MF, Copeland NG, et al: Loss of heterozygosity in three embryonal tumors suggesting a common pathogenic mechanism. *Nature* 316:330, 1985.
164. Klein G: The approaching era of the tumor suppressor genes. *Science* 238:1539, 1987.
165. Friend SH, Bernards SR, Weinberg RA, et al: A human DNA segment with properties of the gene that predisposes to retinoblastoma and osteosarcoma. *Nature* 323:643, 1986.
166a. Weinberg RA: Finding the anti-oncogene. *Sci Am* 259:44, 1988.
166b. Towatari M, Adachi K, Kato H, et al: Absence of the retinoblastoma gene product in the megakaryoblastic crisis of chronic myelogenous leukemia. *Blood* 78:2178, 1991.
167a. Ginsberg AM, Raffeld M, Cossman J: Inactivation of the retinoblastoma gene in human lymphoid neoplasms. *Blood* 77:833, 1991.
167b. Sugimoto K, Toyoshima H, Sakai R, et al: Mutations of the p53 gene in lymphoid leukemia. *Blood* 77:1153, 1991.
167c. Fenaux P, Jonveaux P, Quiquandon I, et al: P53 gene mutations in acute myeloid leukemia with 17p monosomy. *Blood* 78:1652, 1991.
168. Yunis JJ, Fizzera G, Oken MM, et al: Multiple recurrent genomic defects in follicular lymphoma, a possible model for cancer. *N Engl J Med* 316:79, 1987.
169. Rowley JD: Chromosome abnormalities in leukemia. *J Clin Oncol* 6:194, 1988.
170. Third MIC Cooperative Study Group: Recommendations for a morphologic, immunologic and cytogenetic (MIC) working classification of the primary and therapy related myelodysplastic disorders. *Cancer Genet Cytogenet* 32:1, 1988.
171. Second MIC Cooperative Study Group: Morphologic, immunologic, and cytogenetic (MIC) working classification of acute myeloid leukemias. *Cancer Genet Cytogenet* 30:1, 1988.
172. Berger R, Bernheim A: Cytogenetic studies of Burkitt's lymphoma-leukemia. *Cancer Genet Cytogenet* 7:231, 1982.
173. Le Beau MM: Chromosomal fragile sites and cancer-specific rearrangements. *Blood* 67:849, 1986.
174. Mecucci C, Louwagie A, Thomas J, et al: Cytogenetic studies in T-cell malignancies. *Cancer Genet Cytogenet* 30:63, 1988.
175. Yunis JJ: Genes and chromosomes in human cancer. *Prog Med Virol* 32:58, 1985.
176. Fourth International Workshop on Chromosomes in Leukemia 1982: A prospective study of acute non-

lymphoblastic leukemia. *Cancer Genet Cytogenet* 11:249, 1984.
177. Diez-Martin JL, Dewald GW, Pierre RV: Possible cytogenetic distinction between lymphoid and myeloid blast crisis in chronic granulocytic leukemia. *Am J Hematol* 27:294, 1988.
178. Yunis JJ: Genes and chromosomes in the pathogenesis and prognosis of human cancers. *Adv Pathol* 2:143, 1989.
179. Nowell PC, Croce CM: Chromosome translocations and oncogenes in human lymphoid tumors. *Am J Clin Pathol* 94:229, 1990.
180. Yunis JJ, Lobell M, Arnesen MA, et al: Refined chromosome study helps define prognostic subgroups in most patients with primary myelodysplastic syndrome and acute myelogenous leukemia. *Br J Haematol* 68:189, 1988.
181a. Rowley JD: The biological implications of consistent chromosome rearrangements. *Cancer Res* 44:3159, 1984.
181b. Poddighe PJ, Moesker O, Smeets D, et al: Interphase cytogenetics of hematological cancer: Comparison of classical karyotyping and in situ hybridization using a panel of eleven chromosome specific DNA probes. *Cancer Res* 51:1959, 1991.
182a. Schad CR, Kraker WJ, Jalal SM, et al: Use of fluorescent in situ hybridization for marker chromosome identification in congenital and neoplastic disorders. *Am J Clin Pathol* 96:203, 1991.
182b. Yunis JJ: Chromosomal translocations and gene rearrangements in non-Hodgkin's lymphomas. *Cancer Detect Prevent* 12:291, 1988.
183. Yunis JJ, Brunning RD: Prognostic significance of chromosomal abnormalities in acute leukemias and myelodysplastic syndromes. *Clin Haematol* 15:597, 1986.
184. Leder P, Battey J, Lenoir G, et al: Translocations among antibody genes in human cancer. *Science* 222:765, 1983.
185. Yunis JJ: Chromosomal rearrangements, genes and fragile sites in cancer: Clinical and biologic implications, in De Vita V, Hellman S, Rosenberg S (eds), *Important Advances in Oncology*. Philadelphia, JB Lippincott, 1986, p 93.
186. Gallo RC, Wong-Staal F, Markham PD, et al: Human leukemia viruses: The HTLV "family" and their role in human malignancy and immune deficiency disease. *Prog Cancer Res Ther* 32:183, 1985.
187. Yunis JJ, Mayer MG, Arnesen MA, et al: bcl-2 and other genomic alterations in the prognosis of large-cell lymphoma. *N Engl J Med* 320:1047, 1989.
188. Weiss LM, Warnke RA, Sklar J, et al: Molecular analysis of the t(14;18) chromosome translocation in malignant lymphoma. *N Engl J Med* 317:1185, 1987.
189. Third International Workshop on Chromosomes in Leukemia: Chromosomal abnormalities and their clinical significance in lymphoblastic leukemia. *Cancer Res* 43:868, 1984.
190. Williams DL, Look AT, Melvin SL, et al: New chromosomal translocations correlate with specific immunophenotypes of childhood acute lymphoblastic leukemia. *Cell* 36:101, 1984.
191. Williams DL, Raimondi S, Rivera G, et al: Presence of clonal chromosome abnormalities in virtually all cases of acute lymphoblastic leukemia. *N Engl J Med* 410:640, 1985.
192. Nowell PC, Hungerford DA: A minute chromosome in human granulocytic leukemia. *Science* 132:1497, 1960.
193. Rowley JD: A new consistent chromosomal abnormality in chronic myelogenous leukemia identified by quinacrine fluorescence and Giemsa staining. *Nature* 243:290, 1973.
194. Heisterkamp N, Stam K, Groffen J, et al: Structural organization of the *bcr* gene and its role in the Ph translocation. *Nature* 315:758, 1985.
195. Mes-Masson A-M, Witte ON: Role of the *abl* oncogene in chronic myelogenous leukemia. *Blood* 51:843, 1982.
196. Sandberg AA: The chromosomes, in *Human Cancer and Leukemia*. New York, Elsevier-North Holland, 1980, p
197. Rowley JD: Chromosome changes in acute leukemia. *Br J Haematol* 44:339, 1980.
198. Kerman SL, Miller RB, Heritage DW: Translocation (1;17) in accelerating and blast phases of chronic myelogenous leukemia. *Cancer Genet Cytogenet* 20:269, 1986.
199. Quesenberry P, Temeles O, McGrath H, et al: Long term marrow cultures: Human and murine systems. *J Cell Biochem* 45:273, 1991.
200. Emerson SG, Palsson BO, Clarke MF: The construction of high efficiency human bone marrow tissue ex vivo. *J Cell Biochem* 45:268, 1991.
201. Messner HA, Fauser AA: Culture studies of human pluripotent hematopoietic progenitors. *Blut* 41:327, 1981.
202. Estorv Z, Grunberger T, Freedman MH: Clinical utility of marrow cell tissue cultures in acute leukemia of childhood. *Am J Hematol* 23:51, 1986.
203. Schulze E: The value of long-term bone marrow culture for the establishment of purging methods in bone marrow transplantation. *Acta Histochem Suppl* 39:489, 1990.

3 ABNORMAL MORPHOLOGY: GENERAL CONSIDERATIONS

Pathologic evaluation of bone marrow requires careful examination of all bone marrow preparations. Abnormal cytologic features such as megaloblastic and dysplastic changes, cytoplasm/nucleus maturation asynchrony, maturation arrest, abnormal M:E ratios and changes in the proportions of hematopoietic subtypes are best evaluated by examination of the bone marrow smears. Structural alterations such as hypercellularity, hypocellularity, fibrosis, atrophy, necrosis, granuloma, metastasis, vascular alterations and bone changes are best demonstrated on tissue sections.

Marrow smears are the primary source for bone marrow cytology. Unlike touch preparations, they contain more cells, display a higher quality of staining and demonstrate more cellular details and less artifact.

In examination of bone marrow smears, one should avoid overcrowded areas and fields with increased numbers of smudge cells and bare nuclei. Also, less attention should be paid to the areas which are distant from marrow particles and may represent marrow dilution with peripheral blood and shrinkage artifact. Megakaryocytes, mast cells and histiocytes have a tendency to adhere to the stromal matrix and tissue particles.

ABNORMAL ERYTHROID MORPHOLOGY

Conditions associated with defective erythropoiesis (vitamin B_{12} deficiency, refractory anemia, erythroleukemia) or compensatory erythroid hyperplasia secondary to rapid destruction of red blood cells (hemolytic anemia) are usually associated with various degrees of abnormal morphology in erythroid series. Megaloblastic changes are characterized by an increase in cell size and cytoplasm/nucleus maturation asynchrony, with retardation of progressive condensation of nuclear chromatin (Figure 3-1). These

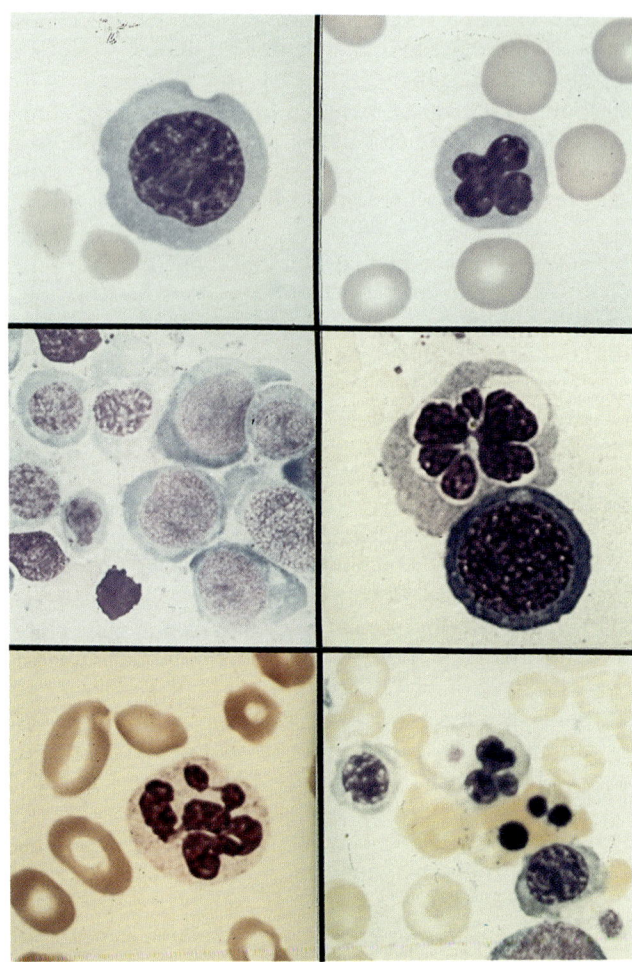

Figure 3-1. Megaloblastic changes are demonstrated by increased cell size and nuclear/cytoplasmic asynchrony of the erythroblasts, ovalomacrocytosis of the red blood cells and hypersegmentation of the neutrophils (left, top to bottom). Congenital dyserythropoietic anemias are associated with nuclear bi- and multilobulation (right, top to bottom).

changes are seen in vitamin B_{12} or folate deficiencies, myelodysplastic syndrome, erythroleukemia, congenital dyserythropoietic anemia and other conditions[1-8] (Table 3-1). The primary cause of megaloblas-

Abnormal Morphology: General Considerations

Table 3-1 Major Causes of Megaloblastic Erythropoiesis

1. Vitamin B_{12} deficiency
2. Folate deficiency
3. Orotic aciduria, Lesch-Nyhan syndrome
4. Myelodysplastic syndrome, erythroleukemia
5. Congenital dyserythropoietic anemia
6. Drugs
    A. Causing defective DNA synthesis
        i. Antipurines (e.g., mercaptopurine, thyoguanine, azathioprine)
        ii. Antipyrimidines (e.g., fluorouracil, azauridine, cytarabine)
        iii. Others: hydroxyurea, cyclophosphamide, procarbazine, acyclovir, arsenic
    B. Uncertain etiology
        a. Anticonvulsant therapy
        b. Chronic alcoholism

tic changes, in most instances, is defective DNA synthesis, which leads to ineffective erythropoiesis and production of large erythrocytes (macrocytes) (see Figure 3-1). Macrocytosis without megaloblastic changes may be seen in association with smoking, chronic pulmonary disease, pregnancy, chronic liver disease, chronic alcoholism, refractory anemia, hypothyroidism, hemolytic anemia and aplastic anemia, as well as in neonates and elderly people.[1,9-12] In iron deficiency anemia, unlike megaloblastic anemia, nuclear maturation in erythroid series is normal, but hemoglobin synthesis is defective. The polychromatophilic normoblasts may appear smalller (micronormoblasts) and show unevenly stained cytoplasm with a ragged border. Internuclear chromatin bridges and binucleation are characteristic features of congenital dyserythropoietic anemias[13,14] (see Figure 3-1). Giant mono- and multinucleated erythroblasts are frequently seen in erythroleukemia. Ringed sideroblasts (nucleated red blood cells with mitochondrial iron) are frequently seen in refractory anemias. Nuclear fragments in erythrocytes (Howell-Jolly bodies) are frequently seen in megaloblastic anemia, hemolytic anemia, leukemia and after splenectomy[15-18] (Figure 3-2). Cabot's rings are reddish-purple-stained, ring-shaped, figure-of-eight, or loop-shaped structures which are thought to represent remnants of nuclear membrane, mitotic spindle or abnormal histone biosynthesis. They are occasionally observed in erythrocytes of patients with megaloblastic anemia or lead poisoning.[19] Basophilic stippling is characterized by the presence of RNA precipitates in erythrocytes and late-stage nucleated red blood cells. These RNA aggregates appear as small, irregular basophilic cytoplasmic granules (see Figure 3-2). Basophilic stippling is observed in lead poisoning, megaloblastic anemia, myelodysplastic syndrome, leukemia and other

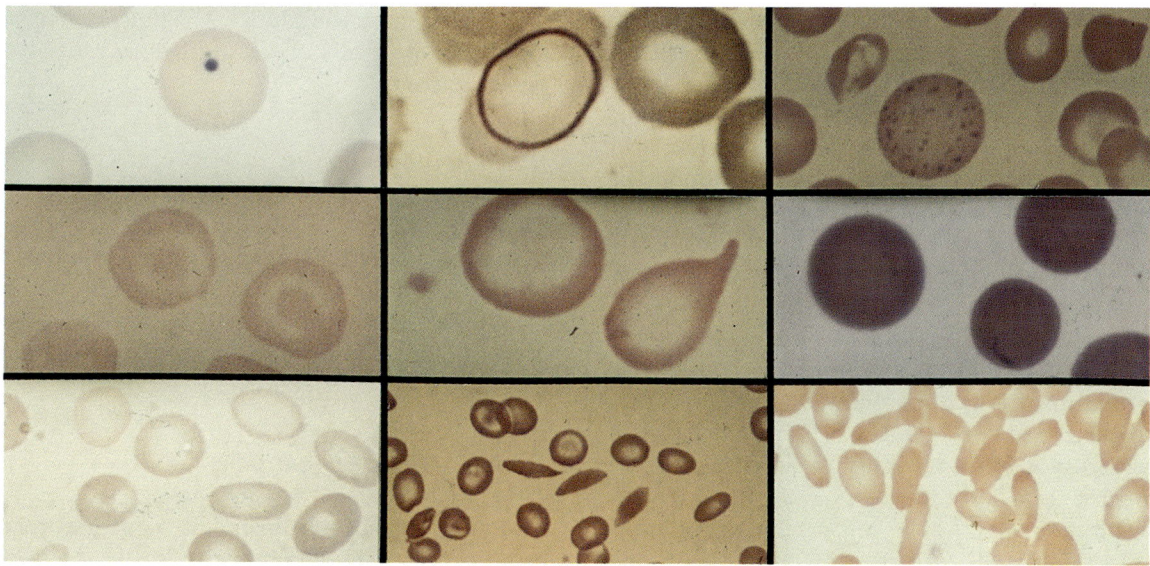

Figure 3-2. From left to right and top to bottom: Howell-Jolly body, Cabot's ring, basophilic stippling, target cells, teardrop, spherocytes, hypochromic red blood cells, sickle cells and ovalocytes.

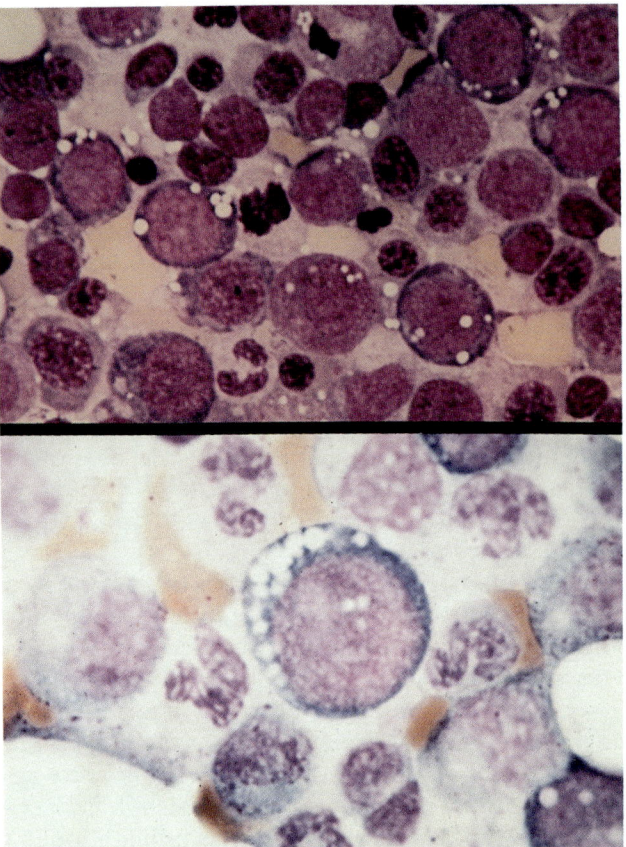

Figure 3-3. Vacuolization of the erythroblasts is frequently seen in alcoholism, riboflavin, phenylalanine and copper deficiencies, diabetic coma and chloramphenicol therapy.

forms of severe anemia.[19,20] Heinz bodies are precipitated, unstable hemoglobins which are produced in certain hemoglobinopathies, red blood cell enzyme deficiencies or drug-induced hemolytic anemias. When stained with vital stains such as crystal violet, Heinz bodies appear as cytoplasmic inclusions attached to the erythrocyte membrane. Cytoplasmic vacuolization of the erythropoietic cells has been observed in association with chloramphenicol therapy; alcoholism; riboflavin, phenylalanine and copper deficiencies; malnutrition; hyperosmolar diabetic coma; and erythroleukemia[21,22] (Figure 3-3). A spectrum of abnormal red blood cell morphology such as microcytes, macrocytes, spherocytes, ovalocytes, stomatocytes, target cells, sickle cells, teardrops, fragmented red blood cells (schistocytes) and basophilic stippling, as well as poikilocytosis (variation in shape) and anisocytosis (variation in size), which are present in a variety of anemias, are best detected in peripheral blood smear examination (Figure 3-2, Table 3-2).

ABNORMAL LEUKOCYTE MORPHOLOGY

Cytoplasmic Granules and Inclusions

"Toxic Granulation"

This term is used to describe the presence of small, dark blue cytoplasmic granules in neutrophils (Figure 3-4). These lysosomal granules are peroxidase positive and show increased alkaline phosphatase activity.[23-25] They are found in infections, burns and drug toxicity. Toxic granulation may be artifactually simulated by improper staining.

Dohle Inclusion Bodies

Dohle bodies are aggregates of rough endoplasmic reticulum which appear as oval or pear-shaped cytoplasmic inclusions in segmented neutrophils, usually associated with infectious diseases, drug toxicity, burns and aplastic anemia.[26,27] They frequently accompany toxic granulation. Dohle bodies are characteristic inclusions seen in neutrophils and giant platelets of an autosomal dominant condition called "May-Hegglin anomaly."[26,27] They stain light blue or gray with Wright's stain and bright red with methyl green pyronin.

Rider-Reilly Anomaly

This anomaly is characterized by the presence of dense azurophilic granules in neutrophils, eosinophils, basophils and, sometimes, lymphocytes and monocytes. This abnormal granulation is commonly observed in inherited mucopolysaccharidosis (Hurler's and Hunter's syndromes)[28,29] (see Figure 3-4).

Chediak-Higashi Syndrome

Chediak-Higashi syndrome is a rare, autosomal recessive disease characterized by a generalized alteration in cell membrane fluidity and fusion of cytoplasmic granules in leukocytes and platelets. This

Abnormal Morphology: General Considerations

Table 3-2 Abnormal Red Blood Cell Morphology

Abnormality	Features	Significance
Anisocytosis	Variation in RBC size	Nonspecific
Poikilocytosis	Variation in RBC shape	Nonspecific
Hypochromia and microcytosis	Small RBCs with reduced hemoglobin content	Iron deficiency, thalassemia, refractory anemia, atrensferrinemia, dialysis patients
Macrocytosis	Large RBCs	Megaloblastic anemia, alcoholism, dyserythropoiesis
Target cells	Increased surface area relative to volume	Thalassemia, hemoglobinopathies, liver disease, postsplenectomy
Sickle cells	Bipolar (sickle) or hollyleaf RBCs	Sickle cell anemia, Hb S/C disease, Hb S/thalassemia
Schistocytes	RBC fragments	Microangiopathic hemolytic anemia
Teardrops	Tennis racket RBCs	Myelofibrosis, severe anemias
Acanthocytes	Irregularly spiculated	Alcoholic liver disease, abetalipoproteinemia, postsplenectomy, malabsorption
Echinocytes	Spiculated RBCs with short, regular projections	Uremia, pyruvate kinase deficiency, low-potassium RBCs
Stomatocytes	Mouth-shaped RBCs	Hereditary stomatocytosis, alcoholism, liver diseases, RBC sodium pump defect
Spherocytes	Spherical RBCs with dense Hb content	Hereditary spherocytosis, immune hemolytic anemia, posttransfusion
Elliptocytes	Oval RBCs	Hereditary elliptocytosis, iron deficiency and megaloblastic anemias, thalassemia
Keratocytes	Half-moon or spindle RBCs	Microangiopathic hemolytic anemia

anomaly leads to defective degranulation of the coalesced cytoplasmic granules in neutrophils, NK cells and platelets[30-32] (see Chapter 8). The large cytoplasmic granules appear as reddish-purple granules in neutrophils and as bluish-purple in monocytes and lymphocytes (see Figure 3-4).

Auer Rods

Auer rods are rod-like cytoplasmic inclusions resulting from the fusion of primary granules. They are peroxidase positive and are seen in immature cells in acute myelogenous leukemia (see Figure 3-4).

Absence or Reduction of Cytoplasmic Granules

Absence or reduction of cytoplasmic granules is one of the prominent features of granulocytic cells in myelodysplastic syndrome. In the neutrophil-specific granule deficiency, there is a selective defect in myeloid cell lactoferrin gene expression.[33]

Atypical Eosinophils

Eosinophils containing eosinophilic and atypical basophilic granules have been reported in a subtype of acute myelomonocytic leukemia (M4), accompanied by the inversion of chromosome 16 (p13q22)[34], and occasionally in CML[35] (see Figure 3-4). In hypereosinophilic syndrome, eosinophils may appear hypogranular and/or may show nuclear hypersegmentation.

Abnormal Cell Morphology

Pegler-Huet Anomaly

This disorder is a congenital anomaly characterized by defective nuclear segmentation in neutrophils.[36] Most nuclei are band-shaped or bisegmented. A similar abnormality is also seen in patients with myelodysplastic syndrome, CML and lymphoma.[37]

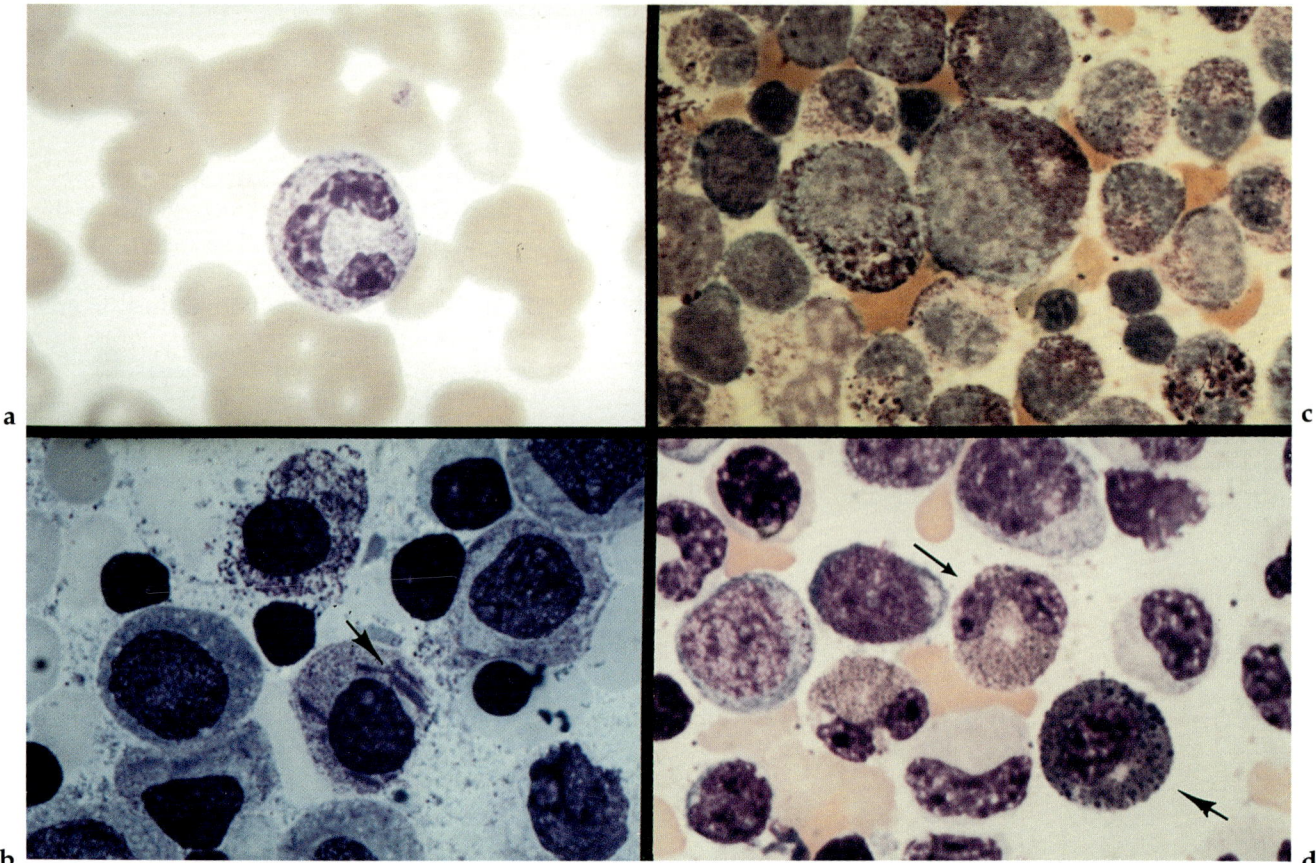

Figure 3-4. Bone marrow smears demonstrating toxic granulation in a neutrophilic stab (a), various hematopoietic cells in Alder-Reilly anomaly (b), Auer rods (c, arrow) and an atypical eosinophil with a mixture of eosinophilic and basophilic granules (d, thick arrow); a normal eosinophil is shown with a thin arrow (d).

Hypersegmented Neutrophils

Nuclear hypersegmentation (more than five lobes) in neutrophils is one of the hallmarks of megaloblastic anemia.[38,39] In normal persons, the majority of neutrophils have three-lobed nuclei, up to 20% have four lobes, and occasional neutrophils may show five lobes. Hypersegmented neutrophils are also present in chronic infection, myelodysplastic syndrome and CML (see Figure 3-1). An autosomal dominant inherited form of giant hypersegmented neutrophils has been described.[40]

Hemophagocytic macrophages

Phagocytosis of the hematopoietic cells by macrophages has been observed in a variety of neoplastic and nonneoplastic conditions[41-60] (Table 3-3). The most prominent phagocytozed cells are erythrocytes (Figure 3-5). However, erythrophagocytosis is often associated with phagocytosis of other cellular elements such as platelets and neutrophils. In a number of viral infections, such as herpes simplex virus, cytomegalovirus, Epstein-Barr virus, adenovirus, parainfluenza and measles, a significant number of reactive macrophages may display erythrophagocytosis.[47,54,57,58] The erythrophagocytic cells show abundant vacuolated cytoplasm, with one or several red blood cells or remnants of red blood cells, and contain round, oval or kidney-shaped nuclei with lacy chromatin and inconspicuous nucleoli (see Figure 3-5). In malignant histiocytosis, unlike reactive processes, phagocytic histiocytes are atypical and pleomorphic, and may show hyperchromatism, prominent nucleoli, and multinucleation.

Abnormal Morphology: General Considerations

Table 3-3 Conditions Associated with Hemophagocytosis*

1. Viral infections
   Herpes viruses (e.g., herpes zoster, herpes simplex, cytomegalovirus, Epstein-Barr virus)
   Adenovirus
   Measles (vaccine virus)
   Parainfluenza
   Rubella
   Kyasanur forest disease
2. Other infections
   Salmonellosis
   Brucellosis
   Mycobacterium tuberculosis
   Legionnaires' disease
   Rocky Mountain spotted fever
   Toxoplasmosis
   Histoplasmosis
3. Familial erythrophagocytic lymphohistiocytosis
4. Malignant histiocytosis
5. T-cell malignancies
6. Hodgkin's disease
7. Carcinoma of the stomach
8. Kawasaki's disease
9. Anticonvulsant drugs

*Adapted from Wickramasinghe SN: Blood and bone marrow, in Symmers W. st C (ed), *Systemic Pathology*. Vol 2, ed 3. London, Churchill Livingstone, 1986, p 85.

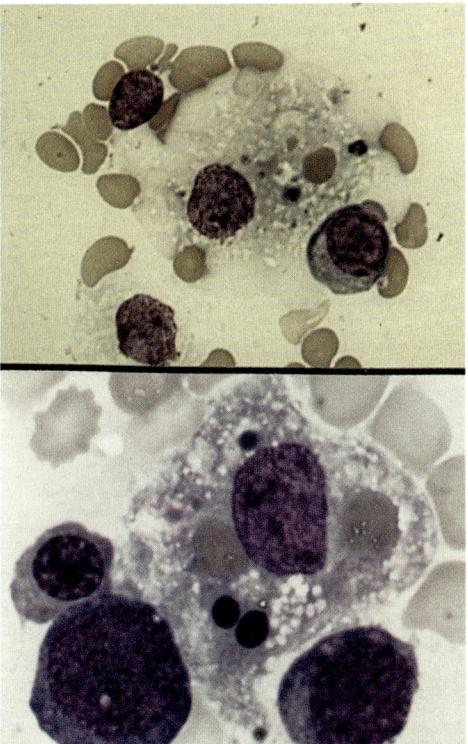

Figure 3-5. Macrophages demonstrating hemophagocytosis.

Gaucher Cells

These cells are macrophages loaded with glucocerebrosides and are characteristic of an inherited beta-glucocerebrosidase deficiency (Gaucher's disease) (see Chapter 9).[61-63] Gaucher cells are large cells with abundant pale blue, wrinkled cytoplasm (Figure 3-6). The cytoplasm is PAS and Sudan black B positive. Cells similar to Gaucher cells (pseudo-Gaucher cells) are seen in CML, acute leukemia, congenital dyserythropoietic anemia, thalassemia major and multiple myeloma, where the macrophages are loaded with lipid products derived from cell destruction[61,64] (see Figure 3-6).

Foamy Histiocytes

Foamy histiocytes are macrophages with numerous small vacuoles loaded with lipid products (Figure 3-7). These cells are seen in Niemann-Pick disease (sphingomyelin lipidosis), hypercholesterolemia, Langerhans cell histiocytosis, Wolman's disease and familial high density liproprotein deficiency[65-70] (Tangier disease).

Sea-Blue Histiocytes

Sea-blue histiocytes are histiocytes loaded with ceroid-containing granules which stain sea blue or blue-green with Romanowsky stain (see Figure 3-7). These granules vary in size and stain with Oil Red O and Sudan black B. Ultrastructurally, some of the granules may contain myelin figures (concentrically arranged membrane structures). Sea-blue histiocytes are seen in a variety of hematologic disorders such as CML, polycythemia rubra vera, erythroleukemia,

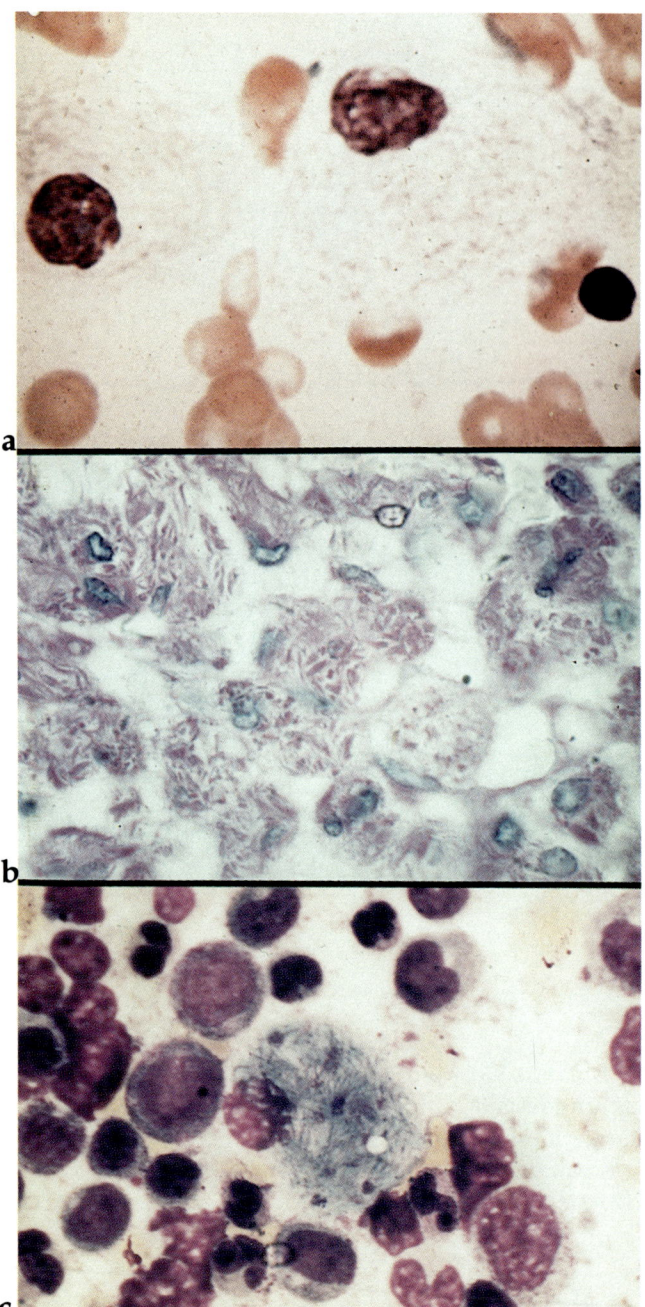

Figure 3-6. Gaucher cells with wrinkled cytoplasm (a) and PAS-positive cytoplasmic content (b). A pseudo-Gaucher cell with wrinkled blue cytoplasm and phagocytosed nuclear debris in a bone marrow smear of a patient with chronic myelogenous leukemia (c).

hemolytic anemia (thalassemia, sickle cell disease), multiple myeloma, Hodgkin's disease and other conditions such as mucopolysaccharidosis, rheumatoid arteritis and hyperlipidemia.[71-73] In some of these conditions, sea-blue histiocytes may show a wrinkled cytoplasm (pseudo-Gaucher appearance). Sea-blue histiocytosis may represent an inherited ceroid storage disease.[74]

Abnormal Lymphocytes and Plasma Cells

Atypical lymphocytes are found in the bone marrow of patients with lymphoproliferative disorders or in patients with a variety of virus infections. These lymphocytes have a diverse morphology and may appear as large cells with abundant pale blue cytoplasm, small cells with irregular nuclei and small or large cells with prominent nucleoli (Figure 3-8). In the juvenile type of neuronal ceroid-lipofuscinoses (Spielmeyer-Sjogren syndrome), approximately 20% of the circulating lymphocytes are vacuolated.

In multiple myeloma, plasma cells are often atypical and may appear large, with large nuclei, fine chromatin and prominent nucleoli, or may demonstrate erythrophagocytosis (see Figure 3-8).

Abnormal Megakaryocytes

Abnormal megakaryocytes such as small mononuclear, binuclear or bilobed megakaryocytes are frequently observed in the bone marrow of patients with myelodysplastic syndrome. These micromegakaryocytes have abundant hypogranular cytoplasm and contain one or two small round or oval nuclei (Figures 3-9 and 3-10). Abnormal megakaryocytes are frequently observed in CML, AML, primary megakaryocytosis, myelofibrosis and polycythemia rubra vera (see Figure 3-9). Megakaryocytes with disconnected nuclear lobulation appear as multinucleated giant cells. The separated nuclear lobes vary in size and shape and are unevenly distributed in a hypergranular cytoplasm. These megakaryocytes are seen more often in patients with megaloblastic anemia. Megakaryocytes with multiple cytoplasmic vacuoles are frequently seen in immune thrombocytopenic purpura and myelodysplastic syndrome. The cytoplasmic vacuoles are arranged around the periphery of the cell or within the cytoplasm around a cytoplasmic central core (Figure 3-11).

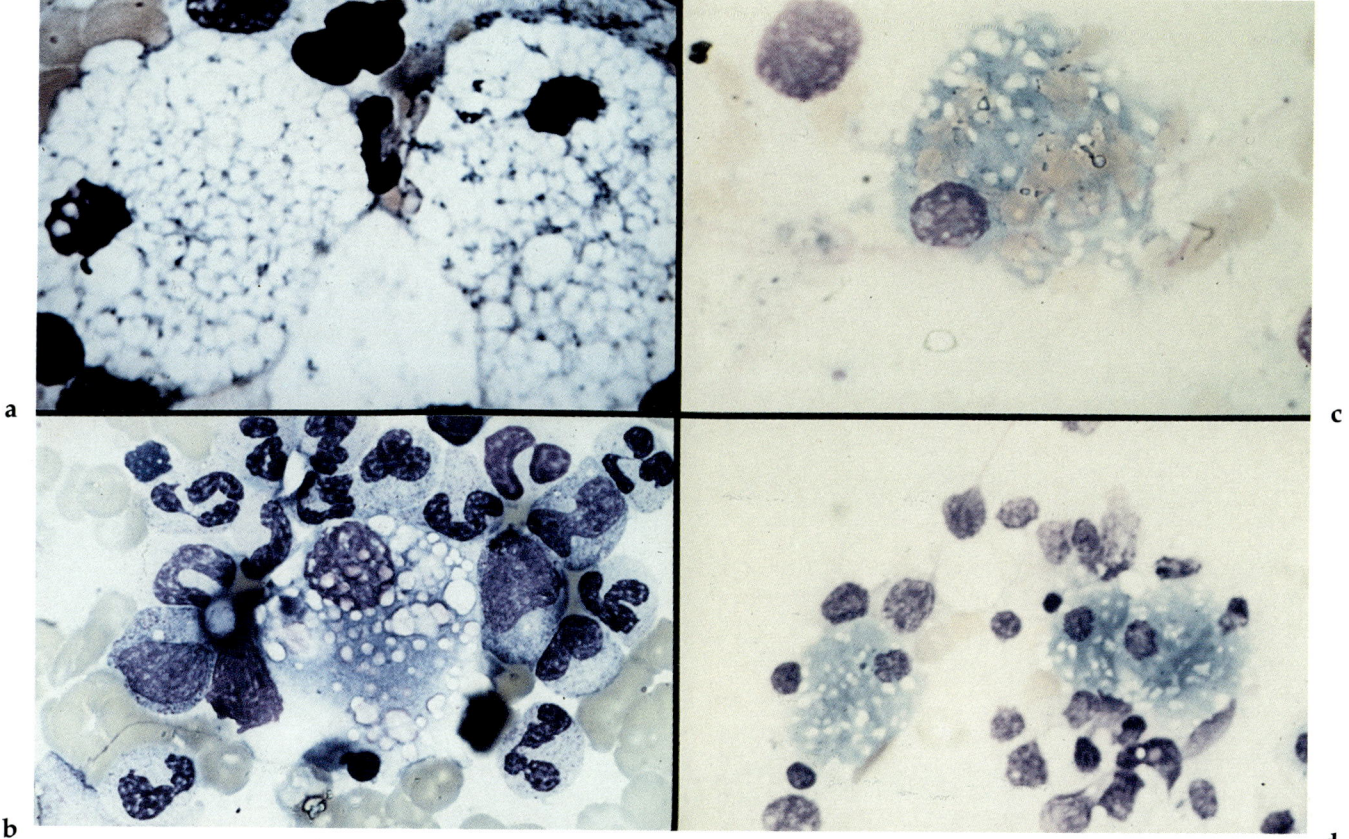

Figure 3-7. Vacuolated macrophages are seen in Niemann-Pick disease, hypercholestremia, Langerhans cell histiocytosis, Wolmans's disease and familial high-density lipoprotein deficiency (a, b). Sea-blue histiocytes are seen in a variety of hematologic disorders associated with a rapid or massive destruction of marrow cells (c, d). These cells may also show erythrophagocytic activity (c).

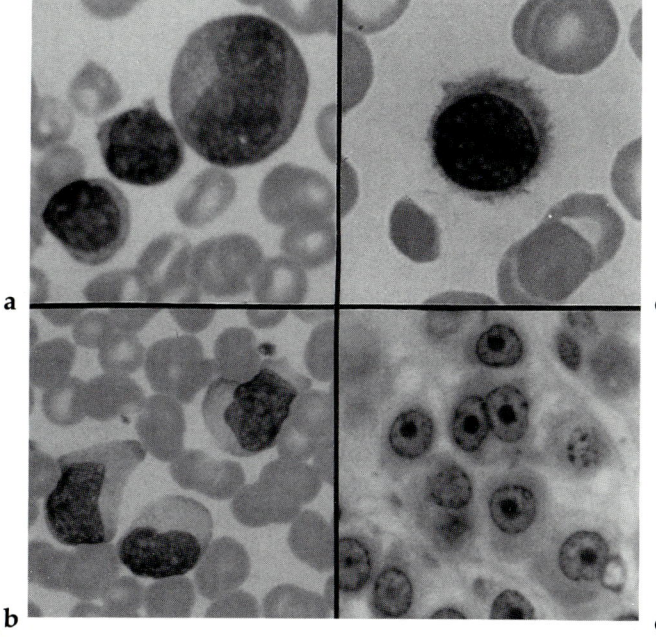

Figure 3-8. Activated lymphocytes in a patient with infectious monomucleosis, peripheral blood (a,b); a "hairy" lymphocyte from a patient with hairy cell leukemia, peripheral blood (c); immature plasma cells with prominent nucleoli in a patient with multiple myeloma, bone marrow (d).

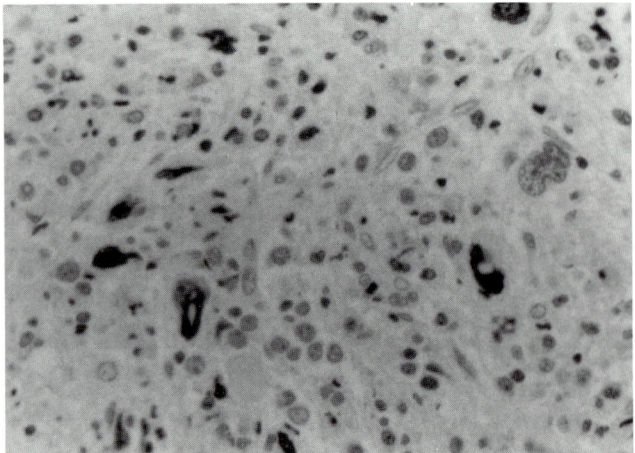

Figure 3-9. Pleomorphic megakaryocytes in the bone marrow biopsy section of a patient with primary myelofibrosis.

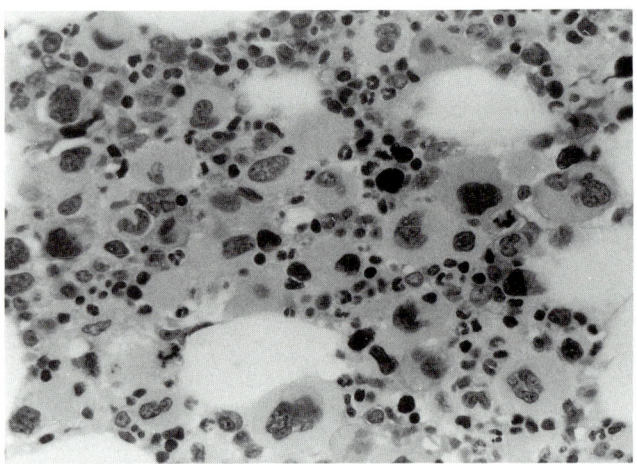

Figure 3-10. Megakaryocytes with abnormal mono- and bilobed nuclei in the bone marrow biopsy section of a patient with primary megakaryocytosis.

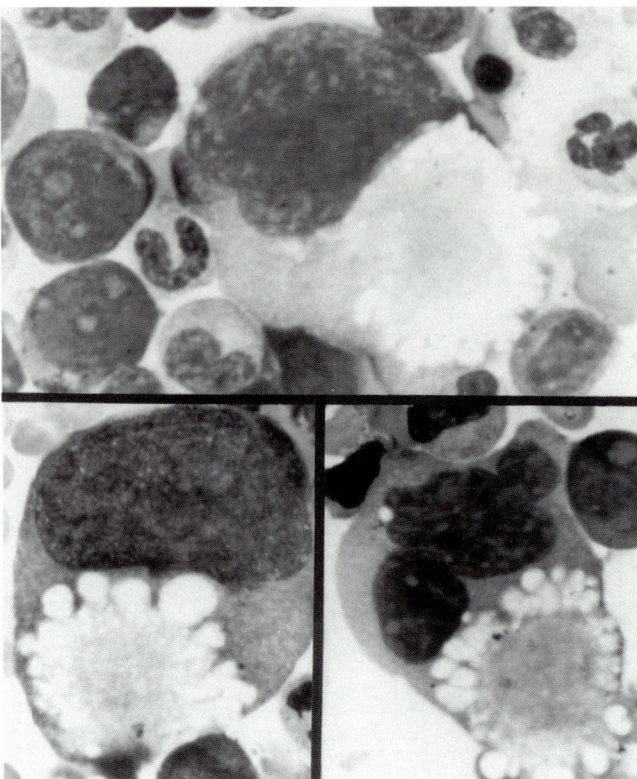

Figure 3-11. Megakaryocytes with cytoplasmic vacuolization in a patient with myelodysplastic syndrome.

ABNORMAL BONE MARROW CELLULARITY

Assessment of bone marrow cellularity is a subjective matter and is based on the estimation of the average percentage of bone marrow space occupied by hematopoietic cells. Bone marrow biopsy specimens which are composed primarily of cortical bone (superficial specimens) may appear less cellular than those from the deeper areas. In posttransplant patients, in patients who receive chemotherapy for hematologic malignancies, and in aplastic anemia patients treated with CSFs, bone marrow cellularity is usually patchy, with densely cellular foci between markedly hypocellular areas. Thus, in these conditions, small bone marrow samples may not represent the patient's overall bone marrow cellularity. Bone marrow hypocellularity is seen in aplastic or hypoplastic anemias, Fanconi's syndrome, paroxysmal nocturnal hemoglobinuria, marrow atrophy, and rare cases of leukemias (Figure 3-12).

Bone marrow hypercellularity is associated with a variety of pathologic conditions including leukemias, myelodysplastic syndromes, infections, hemolytic anemias, megaloblastic anemias, congenital dyserythropoietic anemias, hemorrhage, polycythemias and bone marrow metastasis (Figure 3-13).

Abnormal Morphology: General Considerations

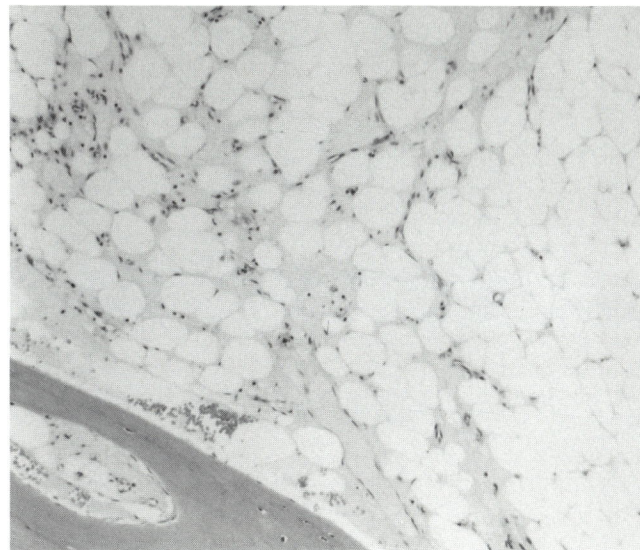

Figure 3-12. Bone marrow biopsy section of a patient with aplastic anemia demonstrating marked hypocellularity.

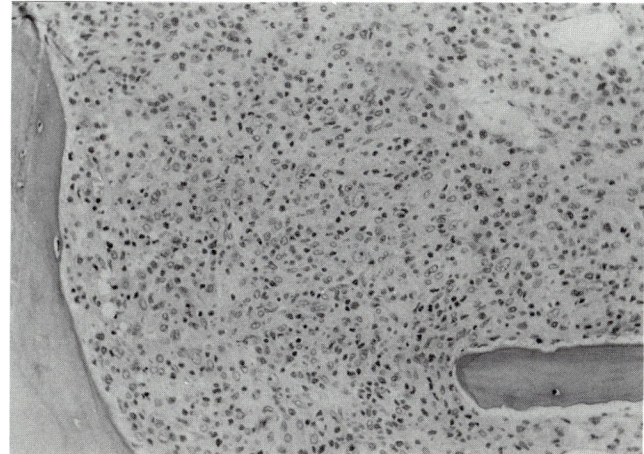

Figure 3-13. A bone marrow biopsy section demonstrating close to 100% cellularity.

BONE MARROW FIBROSIS

The fibrous matrix of the bone marrow is routinely studied by two major cytochemical stains: (1) reticulin stain, which detects a fine, fibrillar network of collagen (reticulin fibers), and (2) trichrome stain which detects a thicker fibrous matrix, which is often re-

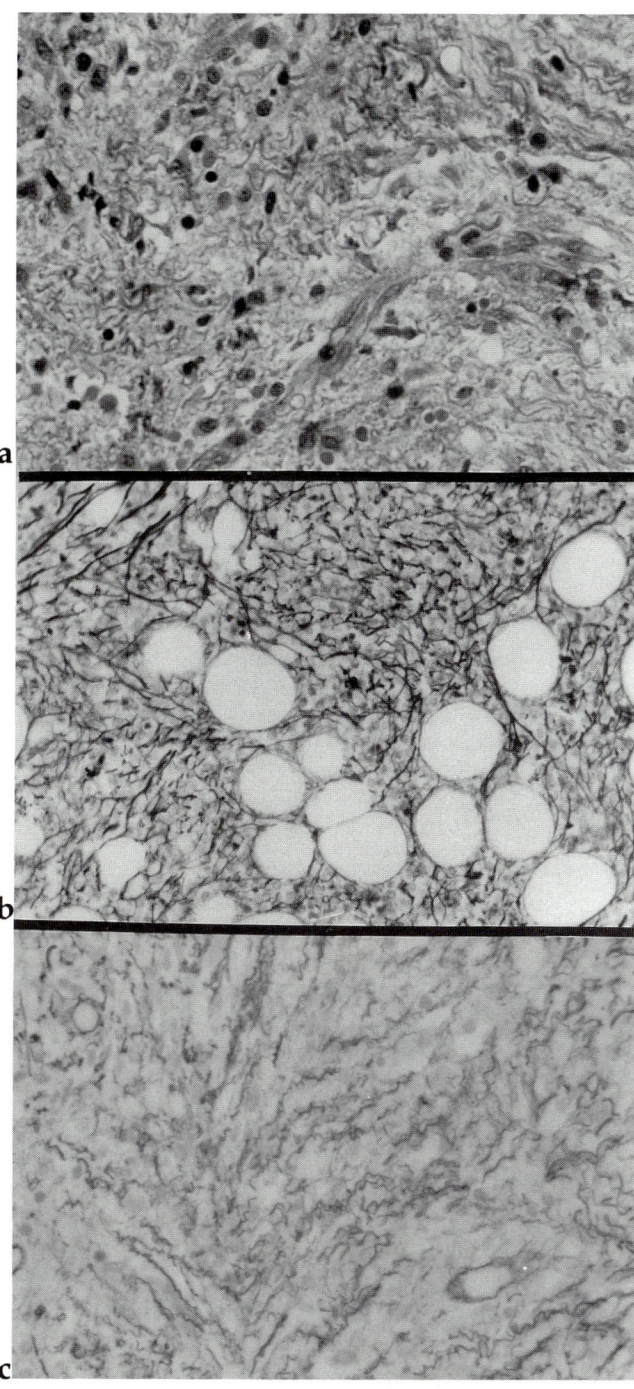

Figure 3-14. Bone marrow biopsy section of a patient with myelofibrosis. Scattered hematopoietic cells are trapped in the fibrotic marrow (a). Reticulin and Masson trichrome stains demonstrate increased amounts of reticulin fibers (b) and thick collagen bands (c).

ferred to as "mature" collagen (Figure 3-14). The mature collagen is very scanty in normal marrow, usually found in association with vascular structures.[75]

Bone marrow fibrosis is a common phenomenon seen in a variety of conditions (Table 3-4) including primary idiopathic myelofibrosis (agnogenic myeloid metaplasia), hairy cell leukemia, acute and chronic lymphoid and nonlymphoid leukemias, polycythemia rubra vera, paroxysmal nocturnal hemoglobinuria, myelodysplastic syndromes, mastocytosis, multiple myeloma and Waldenstrom's macroglobulinemia, lymphomas, Gaucher's disease, metastatic tumors, granulomas, hyperparathyroidism, osteopetrosis, osteomalacia, autoimmune connective tissue disorders, and Paget's disease, as well as in

Table 3-4 Conditions Associated with Bone Marrow Fibrosis

1. Hematopoietic disorders
    - Primary idiopathic myelofibrosis
    - Polycythemia rubra vera
    - Paroxysmal nocturnal hemoglobinuria
    - Aplastic anemia
    - Myelodysplastic syndrome
    - Chronic and acute myelogenous leukemias
    - Chronic and acute lymphoid leukemias
    - Hairy cell leukemia
    - Hodgkin's and non-Hodgkin's lymphomas
    - Multiple myeloma
    - Waldenstrom's macroglobulinemia
    - Gray platelet syndrome
    - Mastocytosis
2. Metastatic lesions
3. Storage diseases
4. Inflammatory and repair processes
    - Granulomas
    - Osteomyelitis
    - Autoimmune connective tissue disorders
    - Following bone marrow necrosis
    - Following bone marrow radiation
    - Previous bone marrow biopsy site
5. Metabolic disorders
    - Osteomalacia
    - Osteopetrosis
    - Nutritional and renal rickets
    - Primary hyperparathyroidism
6. Paget's disease

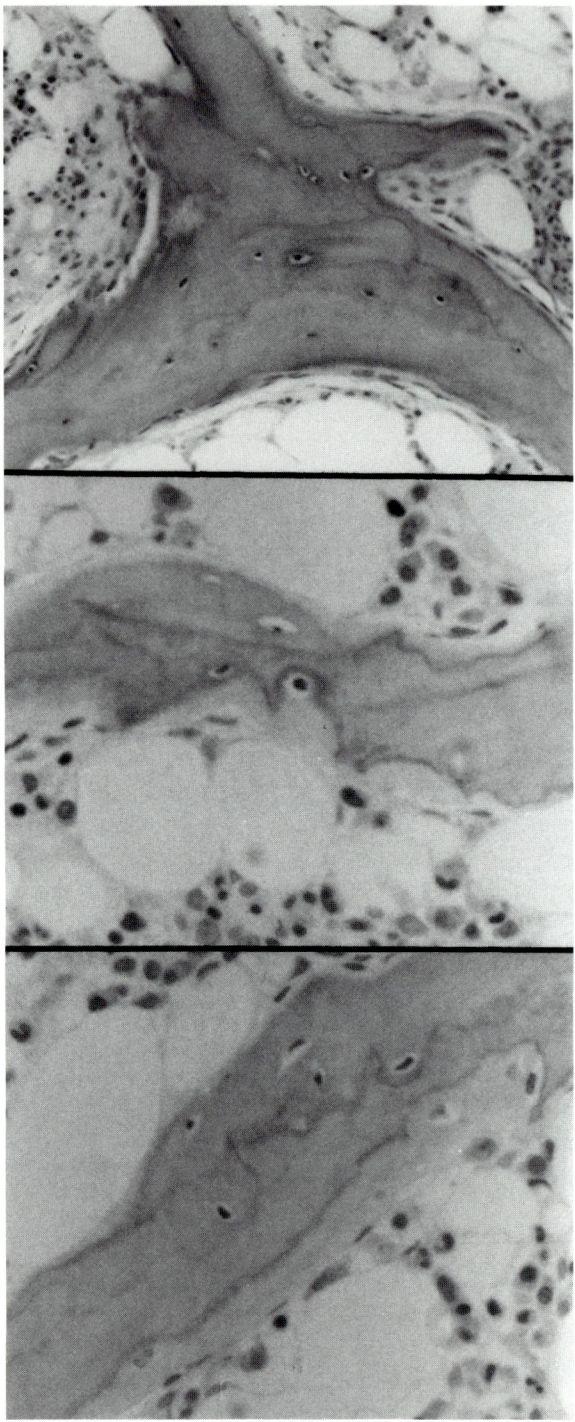

Figure 3-15. Osteoporosis and periosteal fibrosis in a patient with chronic renal disease.

repair processes following radiation therapy, necrosis and focal post-traumatic damages[76-90] (e.g., previous biopsy sites).

Bone marrow fibrosis consists of two morphologic patterns: (1) diffuse, such as in primary myelofibrosis or hairy cell leukemia, or (2) patchy or focal, such as marrow fibrosis noted in Paget's disease, hyperparathyroidism, metastatic tumors and granulomas (Figure 3-15). The fibrotic bone marrow is predominantly composed of reticulin fibers, as frequently noted in hairy cell leukemia, or may in addition demonstrate extensive deposition of mature collagen, as in primary myelofibrosis. Bone marrow fibrosis in certain conditions, such as primary myelofibrosis, metastatic carcinomas and mastocytosis, may be associated with osteosclerosis.

Deposition of fibrous matrix is increased by the proliferation and stimulation of the marrow fibroblasts. It has been suggested that the fibroblastic proliferation observed in primary myelofibrosis, essential thrombocythemia and megakaryoblastic leukemia, chronic myelogenous leukemia, polycythemia rubra vera, and gray platelet syndrome is primarily due to the release of a platelet-derived growth factor from megakaryocytes.[91,92] The monocyte/macrophage system also releases fibroblast growth factor and thus may contribute to the bone marrow fibrosis frequently noted in association with inflammatory and repair processes. There is often a fine peritrabecular fibrosis in primary hyperparathyroidism, renal failure and rickets (see Figure 3-15). Bone marrow fibrosis, if it is not extensive, can be resolved by effective treatment of the primary condition.[93]

GRANULOMAS

Bone marrow granuloma is a manifestation of a systemic chronic inflammatory reaction. Granulomas are aggregates of histiocytes which are frequently surrounded by lymphocytes, plasma cells and eosinophils. Multinucleated giant cells which result from the fusion of closely packed histiocytes may also be present. Granulomas associated with mycobacterial and fungal infections may demonstrate areas of necrosis.

Granulomas are best detected in bone marrow biopsy sections. They may also be demonstrated in bone marrow clot sections. However, it is extremely difficult to identify them in the bone marrow smears. A careful search for granulomas and microorganisms is recommended in patients with a history of fever of unknown origin, microbacterial or fungal infections, and in immunocompromised patients such as transplant patients, patients receiving chemotherapy, and patients with AIDS (Figure 3-16). Although sarcoidosis, microbacteria and fungi are the prominent causes of bone marrow granulomas,[94-98] other infectious and non-infectious conditions such as viral infections, syphilis, Q fever, typhoid fever, Legionnaires' disease, Hodgkin's disease and non-Hodgkin's lymphoma, and drug-induced inflammatory responses may lead to the formation of granulomas[99-111] (Table 3-5).

Infectious mononucleosis has been associated

Table 3-5 Conditions Associated with Bone Marrow Granulomas*

1. Infections
    Leprosy
    Tularemia
    Brucellosis
    Typhoid fever
    Legionnaires' disease
    Histoplasmosis
    Cryptococcosis
    Infectious mononucleosis
    Cytomegalovirus
    Herpes zoster virus
    Rocky Mountain spotted fever
    Q fever
    Mycoplasma
2. Sarcoidosis
3. Hematologic malignancies
    Hodgkin's disease
    Non-Hodgkin's lymphoma
    Multiple myeloma
4. Autoimmune connective tissue disorders
5. Drug-dependent inflammatory responses
    Phenytoin
    Procainamide
    Oxyphenbutazone
    Chlorpropamide

*Adapted from Wickramasinghe SN: Blood and bone marrow, in Symmers W. st C (ed), *Systemic Pathology*. Vol 2, ed 3. London, Churchill Livingstone, 1986, p 99.

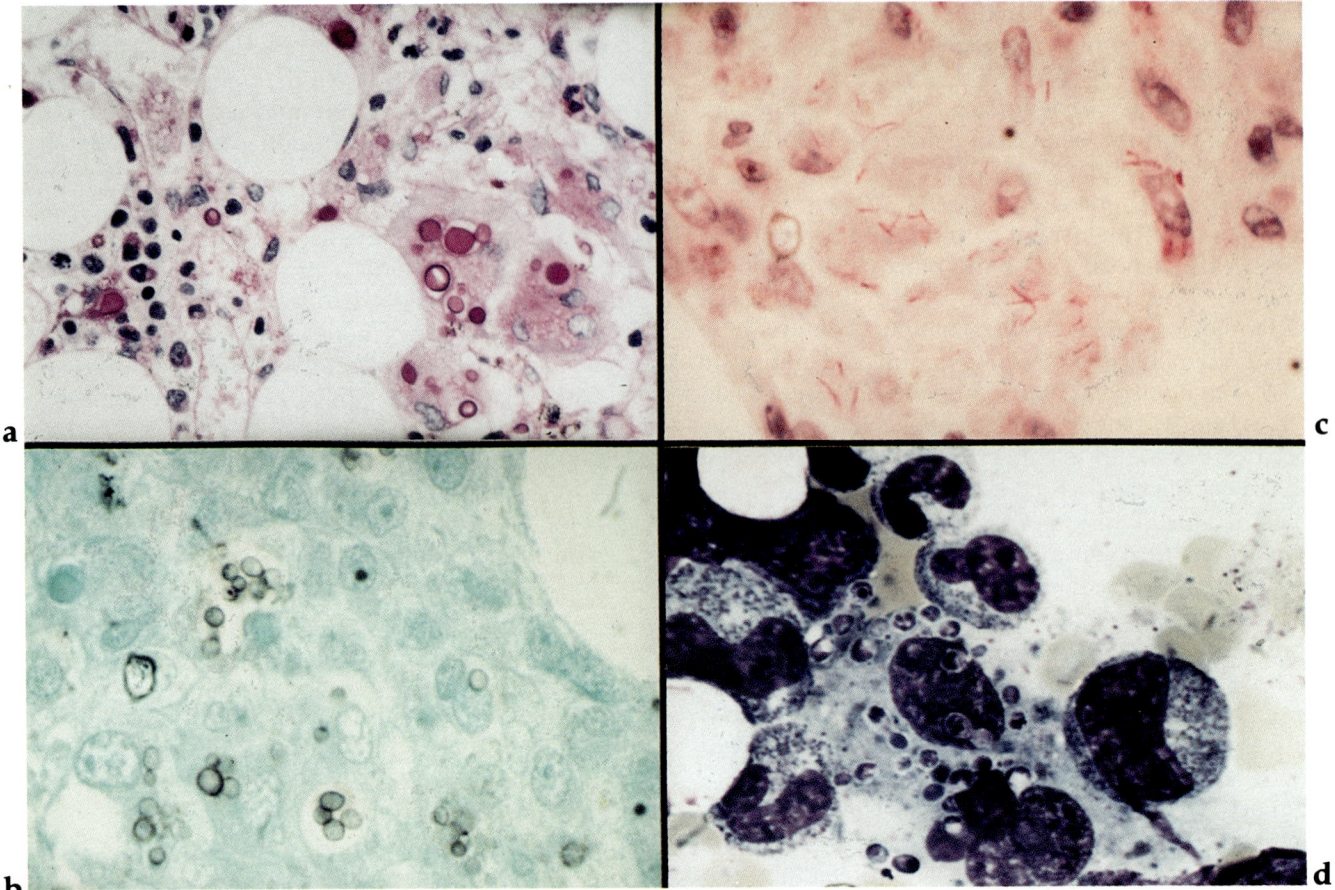

Figure 3-16. Bone marrow biopsy specimen demonstrating histiocytes containing *Cryptococcus neoformans*; PAS stain (a) and silver stain (b). *Micobacterium avium-intracellulare* demonstrated with an acid-fast stain in a bone marrow biopsy section of a patient with AIDS (c). A bone marrow smear showing a histiocyte loaded with *Histoplasma capsulatum* (d).

with granulomatous formation in bone marrow.[94,105,112,113] These granulomas are usually non-necrotizing and smaller than the granulomas of tuberculosis or sarcoidosis, and rarely demonstrate multinucleated giant cells.[94,105,112] In Q fever, especially when the disease is severe and prolonged, small granulomas may appear in bone marrow. These granulomas are composed of epithelioid histiocytes radially arranged around a fatty tissue containing fibrinoid necrosis (ring granulomas).[100,114] Similar granulomas have also been observed in patients with *Mycobacterium avium-intercellulare* (Figure 3-17). The characteristic feature of bone marrow involvement in lepromatous leprosy is the presence of clusters of foamy histiocytes containing lepra bacilli ("dirty" histiocytes)[115] (Figure 3-18). In immunocompromised conditions such as AIDS, granulomas may consist of only a small, poorly defined aggregate of epithelioid (closely packed) histiocytes with a finely granular cytoplasm[116] (Figure 3-19). Lipogranulomas which consist of aggregates of vacuolated, fat-containing histiocytes are frequently observed in bone marrow

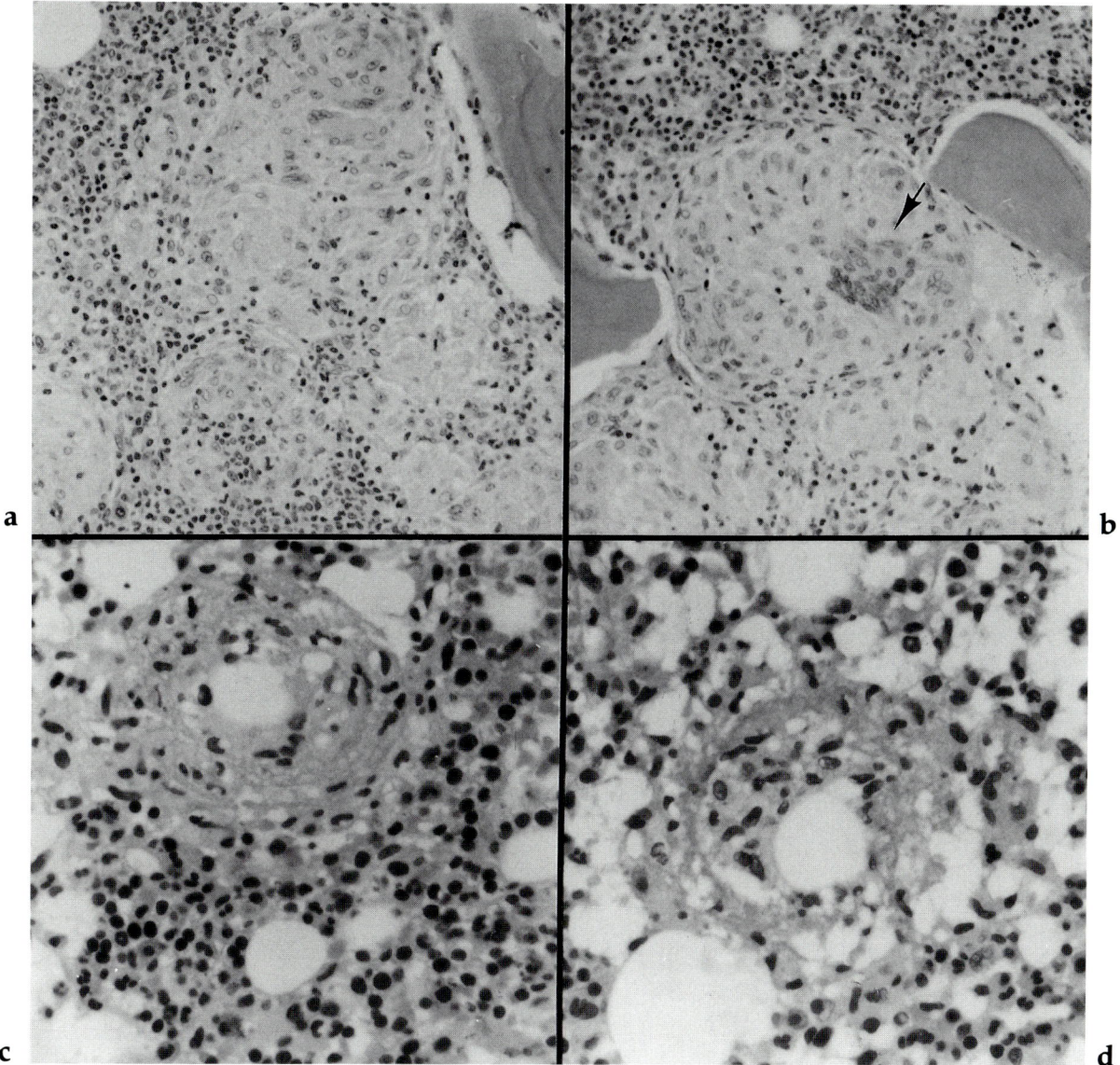

Figure 3-17. Several small granulomas composed of epithelioid histiocytes (a, b) and one multinucleated giant cell (b, arrow) are present. Granulomas with a central area of necrotic fat (ring granulomas) have been observed in Q fever and M *avium-intracellulare* (c, d).

with lymphoid aggregates or plasmacytosis.[117] Patients with Hodgkin's disease or non-Hodgkin's lymphoma may demonstrate bone marrow granulomas. However, the presence of granulomas in such patients does not necessarily indicate bone marrow involvement with the neoplastic process.[94,102,107,108]

Certain hematologic disorders (mast cell lesions, large cell lymphomas, lymphomas with histiocytic component) and metastatic carcinomas composed of cells with abundant cytoplasm (renal cell carcinoma, hepatoblastoma, pheochromocytoma) may resemble granulomas (Figure 3-20).

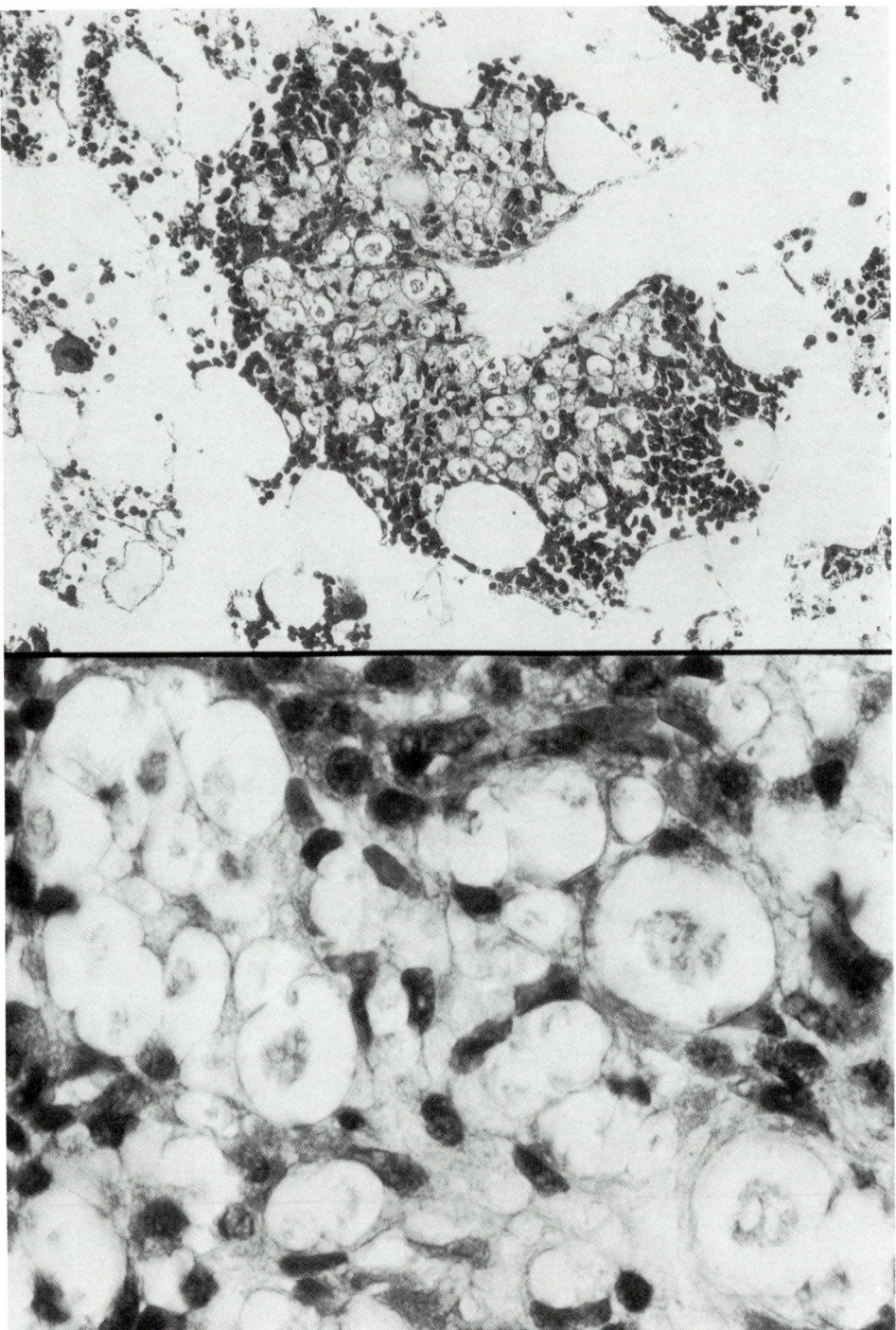

Figure 3-18. Granulomas composed of aggregates of foamy ("dirty") histiocytes are characteristic of lepromatous leprosy. From Suster S: Non-granulomatous involvement of the bone marrow in lepromatous leprosy. *Am J Clin Pathol* 92:797, 1988, with permission.

Abnormal Morphology: General Considerations

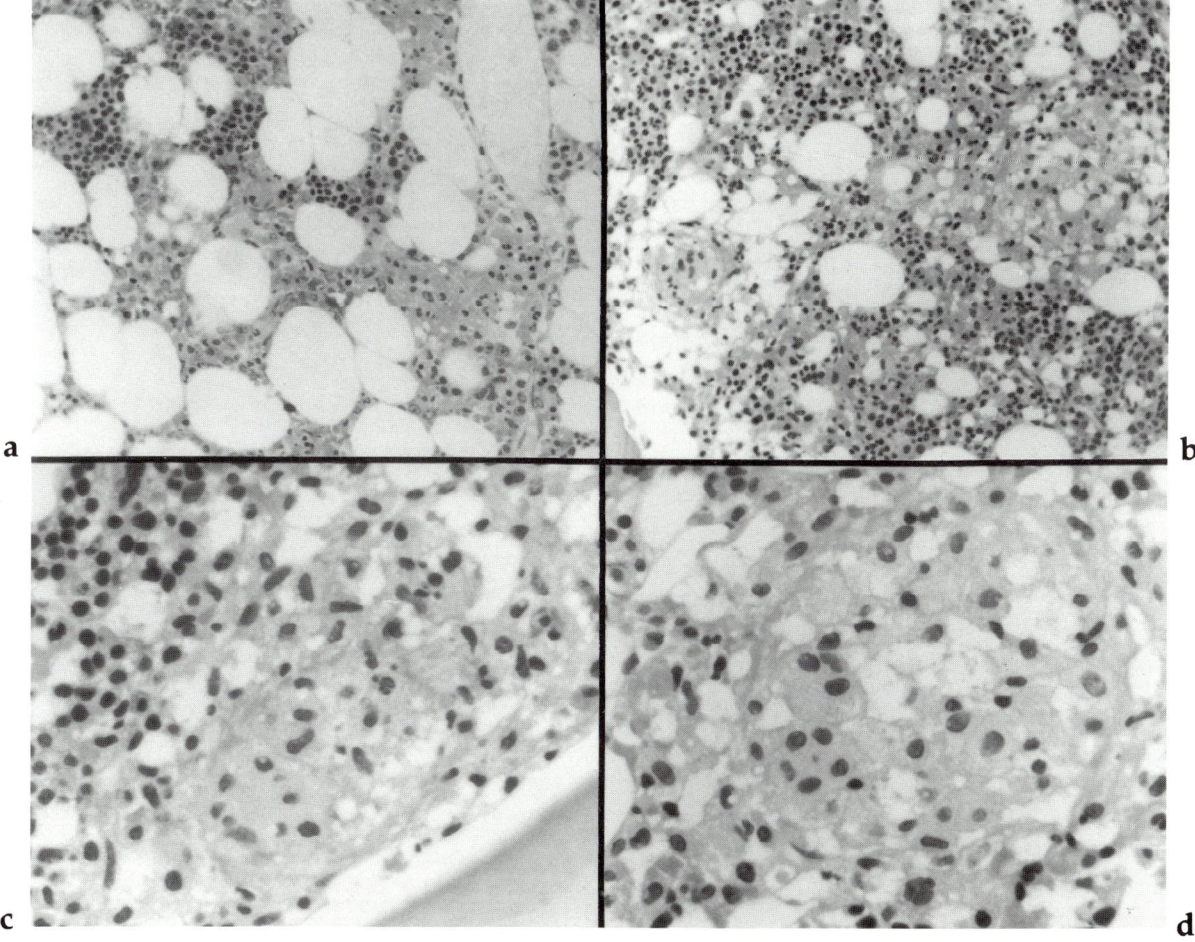

Figure 3-19. Small granulomas composed of epithelioid histiocytes in AIDS patients; low power (a, b), high power (c, d).

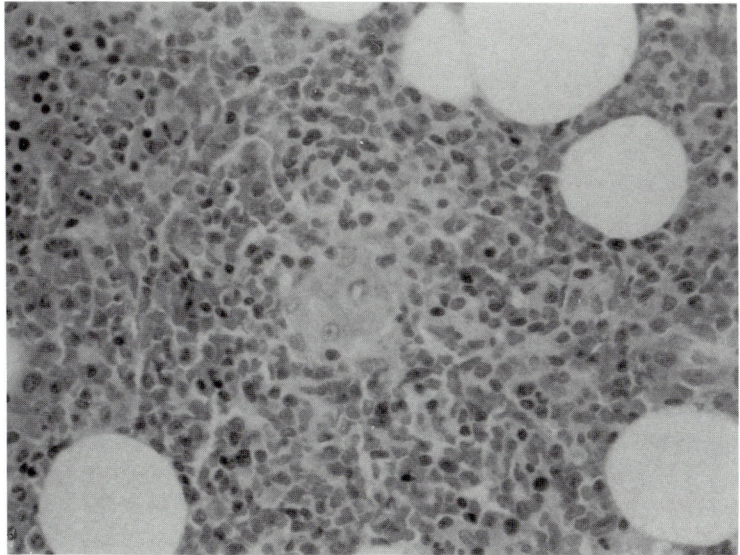

Figure 3-20. Bone marrow biopsy section from a patient with Lennert's lymphoma composed of a small cluster of epithelioid histiocytes surrounded by atypical lymphocytes, resembling a granuloma.

BONE MARROW CHANGES IN ACQUIRED IMMUNODEFICIENCY SYNDROME

Acquired immunodeficiency symdrome (AIDS) and AIDS-related complex (ARC) are disorders caused by the human immunodeficiency virus (HIV), a T-lymphotropic retrovirus.[118,119] Bone marrow examination is a common procedure and provides information regarding dysplastic hematopoiesis, lymphoproliferative disorders and disseminated opportunistic infections in patients with AIDS.

Bone marrow biopsy reveals a normo- or hypercellular marrow, often with an elevated M:E ratio, a myeloid left shift and mild to severe dysplastic changes in one or all hematopoietic lines.[120-123] The presence of scattered macrophages with erythrophagocytosis is a frequent feature. A polyclonal lymphoplasmacytosis is common, sometimes with activated lymphocytes and immature plasma cells. In rare cases, plasmacytosis is very prominent (Figure 3-21). There may be a mild to moderate eosinophilia. Reticulin fibrosis and gelatinous transformation of marrow are frequent features.[120,122] HIV DNA sequences have been detected in bone marrow precursor cells with the use of a radioactive-labeled cDNA probe and an in situ hybridization technique[116] (Figure 3-22). Patients with AIDS or ARC may demonstrate an immune-associated thrombocytopenia (ITP-like syndrome) with increased marrow megakaryocytes and peripheral thrombocytopenia.[124,125] Azidothymidine (AZT)-treated patients may show megaloblastic changes or bone marrow hypocellularity, with reduction of the erythroid, granulocytic and/or megakaryocytic lines, though megakaryocytes are least frequently affected.[126]

Approximately 30% of AIDS patients with lymphoma show bone marrow involvement.[127] AIDS-associated lymphomas are mostly high-grade B-cell lymphomas, frequently of the immunoblastic or small, noncleaved lymphocytic (Burkitt's) type. Bone marrow involvement with Kaposi's sarcoma is uncommon.[120,128]

Because of the association of opportunistic infection with AIDS, special stains and marrow cultures are routinely performed in these patients. *M. avium-intracellulare*, *Pneumocystis carinii*, and *Cryptococcus*

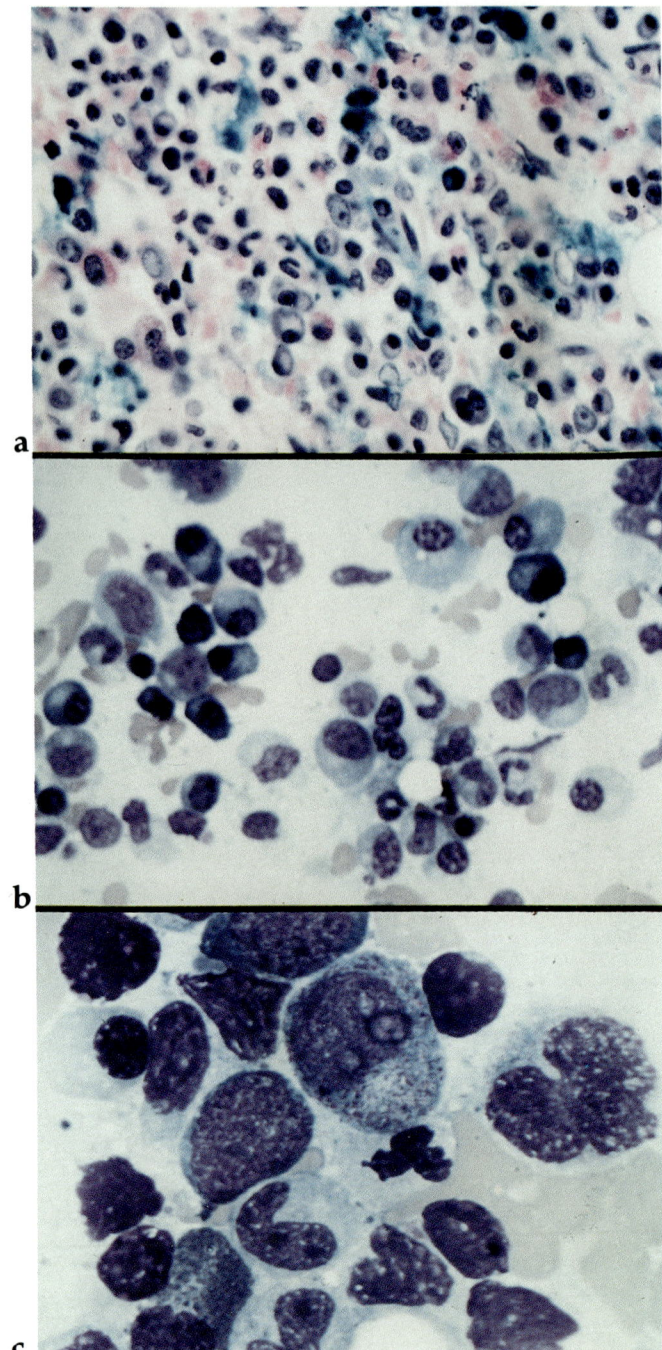

Figure 3-21. Plasmacytosis and eosinophilia are common bone marrow findings in AIDS patients (a, b), often in association with myelodysplasia (c).

Abnormal Morphology: General Considerations

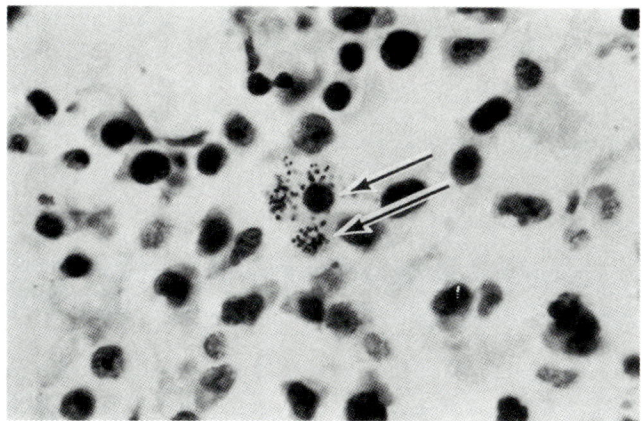

Figure 3-22. HIV DNA demonstrated in bone marrow erythroblasts and erythrocytes by an in situ hybridization technique using a 3H-labeled cDNA probe. From Sun NJC et al: Bone marrow examination in patients with AIDS and AIDS related complex (ARC). Morphologic and in situ hybridization studies. *Am J Clin Pathol* 92:589, 1989, with permission.

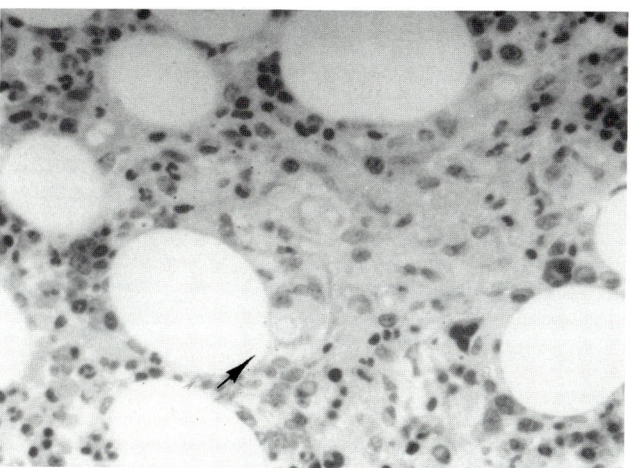

Figure 3-24. C. neoformans is one of the opportunistic infections frequently associated with AIDS. This figure shows a small granuloma with histiocytes containing cryptococci in the bone marrow biopsy section of an AIDS patient.

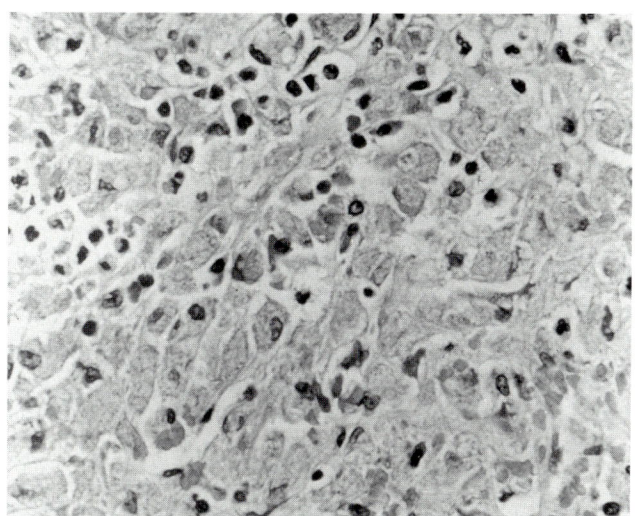

Figure 3-23. Sheets of foamy/granular histiocytes in the bone marrow of an AIDS patient with *M. avium-intracellulare*.

species are frequent pathogenic organisms. The infected bone marrow usually shows aggregates of foamy epithelioid histiocytes (granulomas) containing microorganisms (Figures 3-23 and 3-24). These granulomas vary in size and often contain no or small number of lymphocytes.

GELATINOUS TRANSFORMATION

Gelatinous transformation of the bone marrow is characterized by the accumulation of hyaluronic acid (gelatinous material), fat atrophy, and associated focal bone marrow hypoplasia.[129] This condition has frequently been mistaken for edema, necrosis or amyloidosis. The bone marrow involvement is usually patchy, and the involved areas are hypocellular and composed of an amorphous glassy or finely granular or fibrillar light pink to light blue substance (H&E stain) which reacts positively with alcian blue (particularly at high pH) and PAS stains (Figure 3-25). In Wright-stained bone marrow smears, this mucoid material is bluish-pink and is mixed with scattered adipocytes (see Figure 3-25).

Gelatinous transformation of the bone marrow has been observed in a variety of chronic debilitating disorders such as anorexia nervosa and other forms of starvation, malignancies, tuberculosis, chronic renal disease and ulcerative colitis.[130-133] However, not all cachectic patients demonstrate marrow gelatinous transformation. The mechanism of this degenerative process is not known, and factors other than malnutrition may play a role in its pathogenesis.

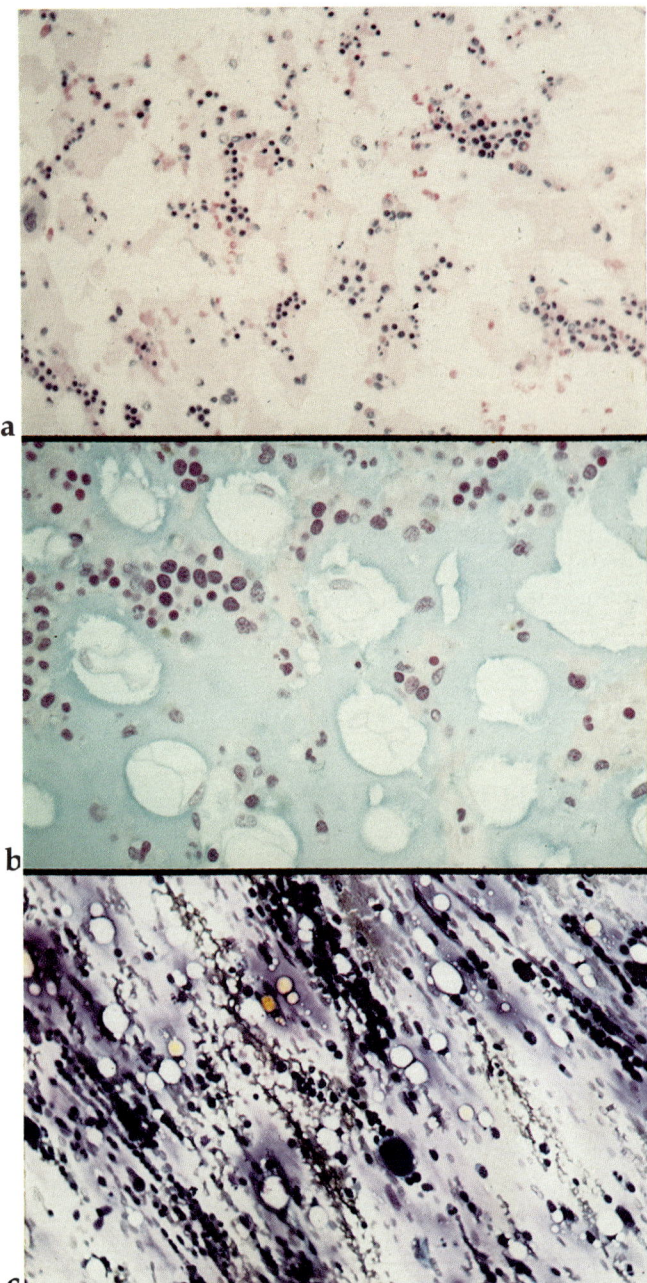

Figure 3-25. Gelatinous transformation of bone marrow fatty tissue. Biopsy sections are hypocellular (a, b) and show a homogeneous substance replacing fatty tissue. The substance stains light pink with H&E (a) and light blue with alcian blue (b) stains. The bone marrow smear (c) shows abundant bluish-pink substance mixed with scattered adipocytes and hematopoietic cells (Wright's stain).

Gelatinous transformation of the bone marrow may be reversible. This reversal has been observed in patients with anorexia nervosa when their nutritional status has been improved,[133] as well as in starved rabbits after restoration of their nutrition.[134]

BONE MARROW NECROSIS

The incidence of bone marrow necrosis in the literature varies from 0.5% to 37%.[135-143] However, extensive bone marrow necrosis is infrequent and is usually associated with life-threatening illnesses such as hematologic malignancies, bone marrow metastasis and AIDS.[140-144] The most prominent cause of bone marrow necrosis is ischemia. Ischemia results from (1) vascular occlusion by deformed red blood cells (sickle cell anemia), fibrin clot (disseminated intravascular coagulation, thrombotic throbocytopenic purpura), vascular invasion by fungi in mucormycosis or tumor emboli and tumor compression, or (2) inadequate blood supply and nutrition in rapidly growing tumors and in patients who suffer from circulatory failure, severe anemia, hyperparathyroidism or starvation.[135-146] Bone marrow necrosis is also caused by infections (gram-positive and gram-negative bacteria, Q fever, typhoid fever, diphtheria, tuberculosis, histoplasmosis) and toxic agents (chemotherapy).[135,140,141,147,148] Extensive bone marrow necrosis in patients with cancer may be associated with elevation of TNF activity in plasma.[142]

Bone marrow necrosis may cause bone pain. Extensive marrow necrosis is often associated with a leukoerythroblastic blood condition (presence of immature erythroid and myeloid cells in peripheral blood) and pancytopenia. Bone marrow tissue sections show necrotic bone and bone marrow in which often the architectural framework is still preserved and shadows of cells are recognized (coagulation necrosis) (Figure 3-26). Fibrinoid necrosis, characterized by accumulation of amorphous cell debris, is observed less frequently and is usually associated with infections. Aspirated necrotic bone marrow contains pyknotic nuclei and blurred outlines of cells in a background of amorphous granular material.

Since hematologic malignancies and metastatic tumors are the most frequent causes of bone marrow necrosis, the presence of necrosis in bone marrow samples of patients with a history of malignant dis-

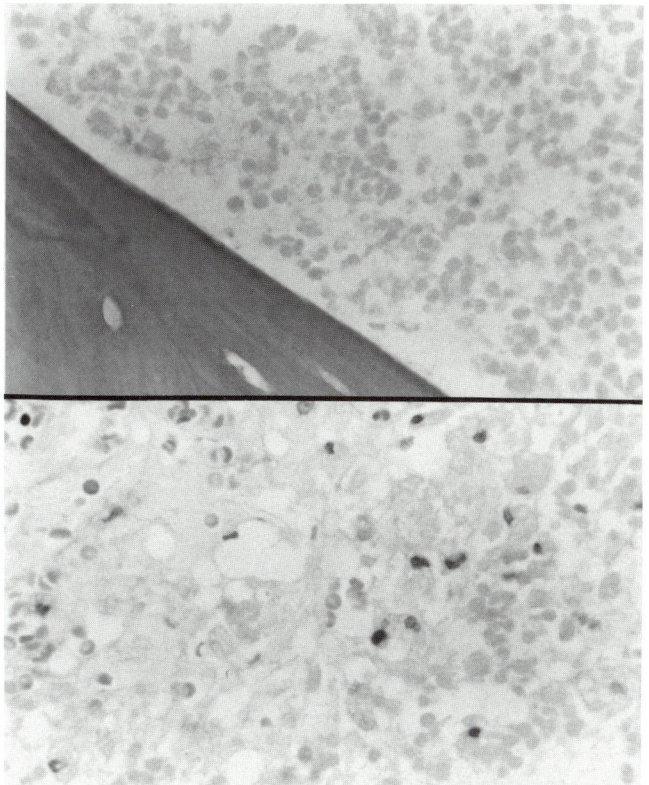

Figure 3-26. Bone marrow biopsy section demonstrating coagulation necrosis of the bone marrow.

ease is highly suggestive of bone marrow involvement. In such cases, additional sections and/or samples are recommended. The presence of bone marrow necrosis after induction chemotherapy in acute leukemia indictes a poor prognosis.[130] Extensive marrow necrosis may be associated with extramedullary hematopoiesis, probably as a compensatory process.[149]

Reversal of bone marrow necrosis is associated with removal of the cell debris by macrophages, formation of granulation tissue (a young, highly vascular connective tissue) and new bone formation.

LEUKEMIAS AND LYMPHOMAS

These disorders are discussed in detail in Chapter 6. In leukemias, the bone marrow is usually hypercellular and is diffusely infiltrated by leukemic cells. Bone

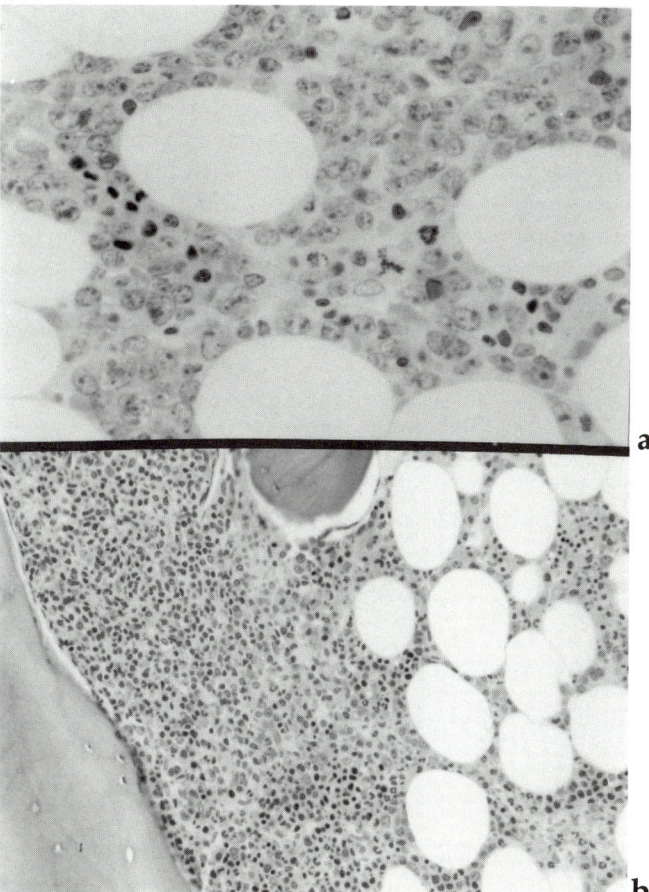

Figure 3-27. Bone marrow biopsy section demonstrating diffuse marrow involvement with a large cell lymphoma (a) and paratrabecular involvement in a small cleaved cell lymphoma (b).

marrow involvement with lymphoma may be focal or diffuse (Figure 3-27).

BONE MARROW METASTASIS

Bone marrow tissue sections are superior to bone marrow smears for the detection of metastatic tumors.[150-152] The intercellular organization of tumor cells such as glandular structures and rosettes, and tumor-associated stromal alterations such as fibrosis, are usually not detected in marrow smears. However, in some cases, such as neuroblastoma or rhabdomyosarcoma, tumor cells may be readily detected in bone marrow smears and not in clot or biopsy sections. Bone marrow biopsy sections have a higher detection rate of metastasis than aspirated bone marrow clot sections, because aggregates of tumor cells trapped in dense fibrous tissue may not be aspirable. All marrow samples prepared with various techniques, such as tissue sections, touch preparations and smears, should be thoroughly examined for the detection of metastatic tumors.[152-154]

Metastatic tumor cells tend to clump together and appear as clusters (Figure 3-28). They are usually larger than hematopoietic cells and may be associated with areas of fibrosis or necrosis. An inflammatory response evidenced by the presence of macrophages, lymphocytes and plasma cells may be seen adjacent to the metastatic site. In bone marrow smears, metastatic clusters are usually well defined and are often found at the periphery of the marrow particles. Small, round cell tumors (oat cell carcinoma, neuroblastoma, retinoblastoma, rhabdomyosarcoma and Ewing's sarcoma) may resemble hematopoietic blast cells. However, they are usually larger than the

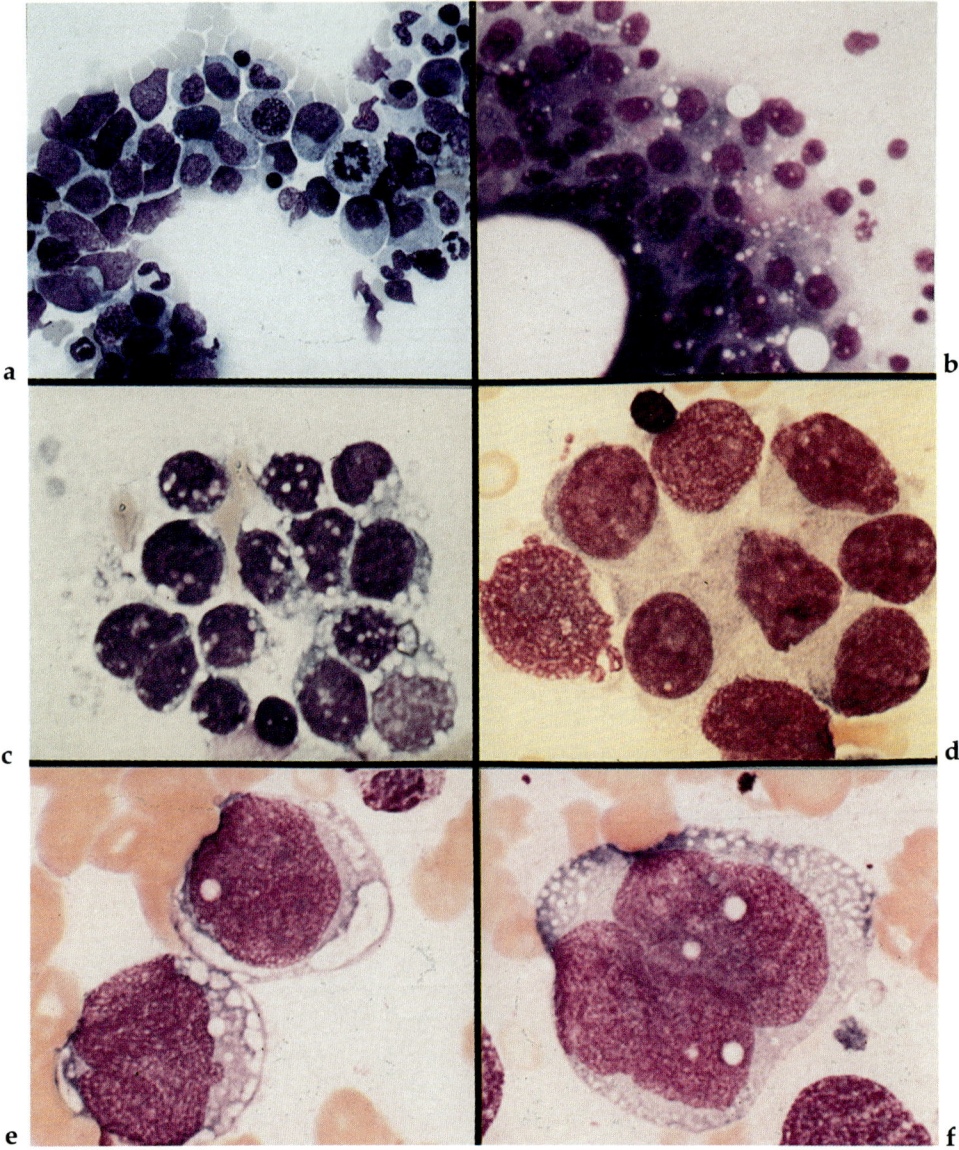

Figure 3-28. Bone marrow smears showing metastatic tumors including oat cell carcinoma (a), hepatoblastoma (b), Ewing's sarcoma (c), neuroblastoma (d), adenocarcinoma (e), and giant cell carcinoma of the lung (f).

Abnormal Morphology: General Considerations

hematopoietic blasts, often show significant nuclear pleomorphism, and may also show characteristic morphologic structures, such as an organoid pattern (oat cell carcinoma) and rosette formation (neuroblastoma) (Figures 3-28, 3-29 and 3-30). In addition, small cell tumors may demonstrate specific features when studied by electron microscopy, grown in culture or analyzed for phenotypic expressions and cytogenetic abnormalities. For example, the diagnosis of a metastatic neuroblastoma is established by demonstrating the outgrowth of neurites in tissue culture, the existence of secretory granules by electron microscopy, and the presence of cellular catecholamines and neurofilaments by immunocytochemistry.[154-156]

The presence of bone marrow fibrosis in patients with a history of malignancy is strongly indicative of metastatsis. Metastatic carcinomas, especially breast tumors, are frequently associated with bone marrow fibrosis. Fibrosis is usually patchy, is formed around the metastatic focus and extends into the tumor. Clusters and strands of tumor cells are often trapped in a dense, highly collagenized, fibrous tissue. This dense fibrosis may make the detection of small metastatic foci difficult. In such cases, examination of additional tissue sections (deeper cuts) is strongly recommended. As discussed before, metastatic carcinomas composed of cells with abundant cytoplasm and mild nuclear atypism, such as renal cell carcinoma, hepatoblastoma, pheochromocytoma, and certain hematologic disorders, such as mast cell lesions and lymphomas of the large cell or mixed cell type, may resemble granulomas (Figures 3-20, 3-31, 3-32).

Cytochemical and immunohistochemical techniques are useful in (1) distinguishing metastatic neoplasms from primary bone marrow malignancies and reactive cellular proliferations, (2) subclassification of metastatic tumors and (3) detection of small, occult

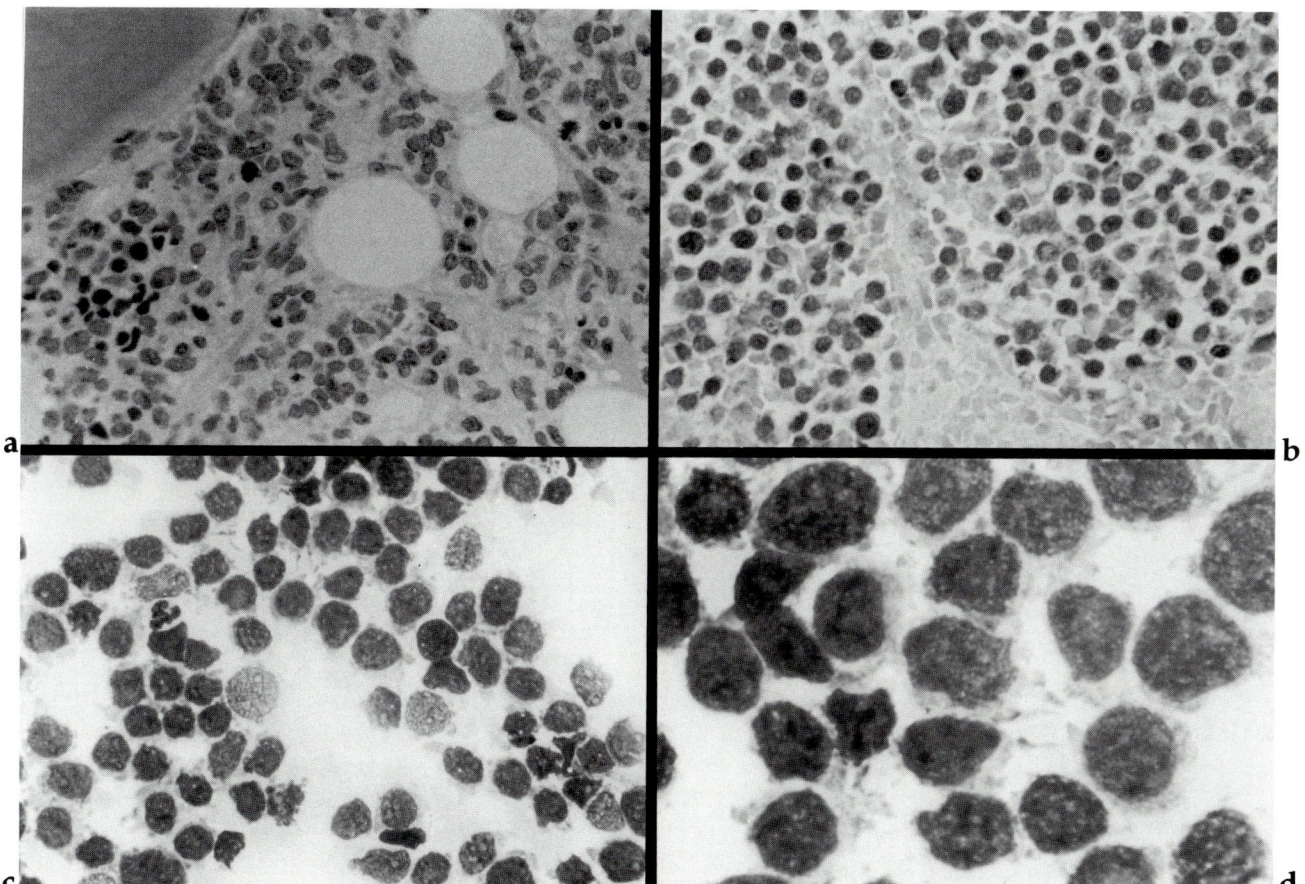

Figure 3-29. Bone marrow sample demonstrating involvement of the bone marrow with Ewing's sarcoma; biopsy section (a), clot section (b) and smear (c,d).

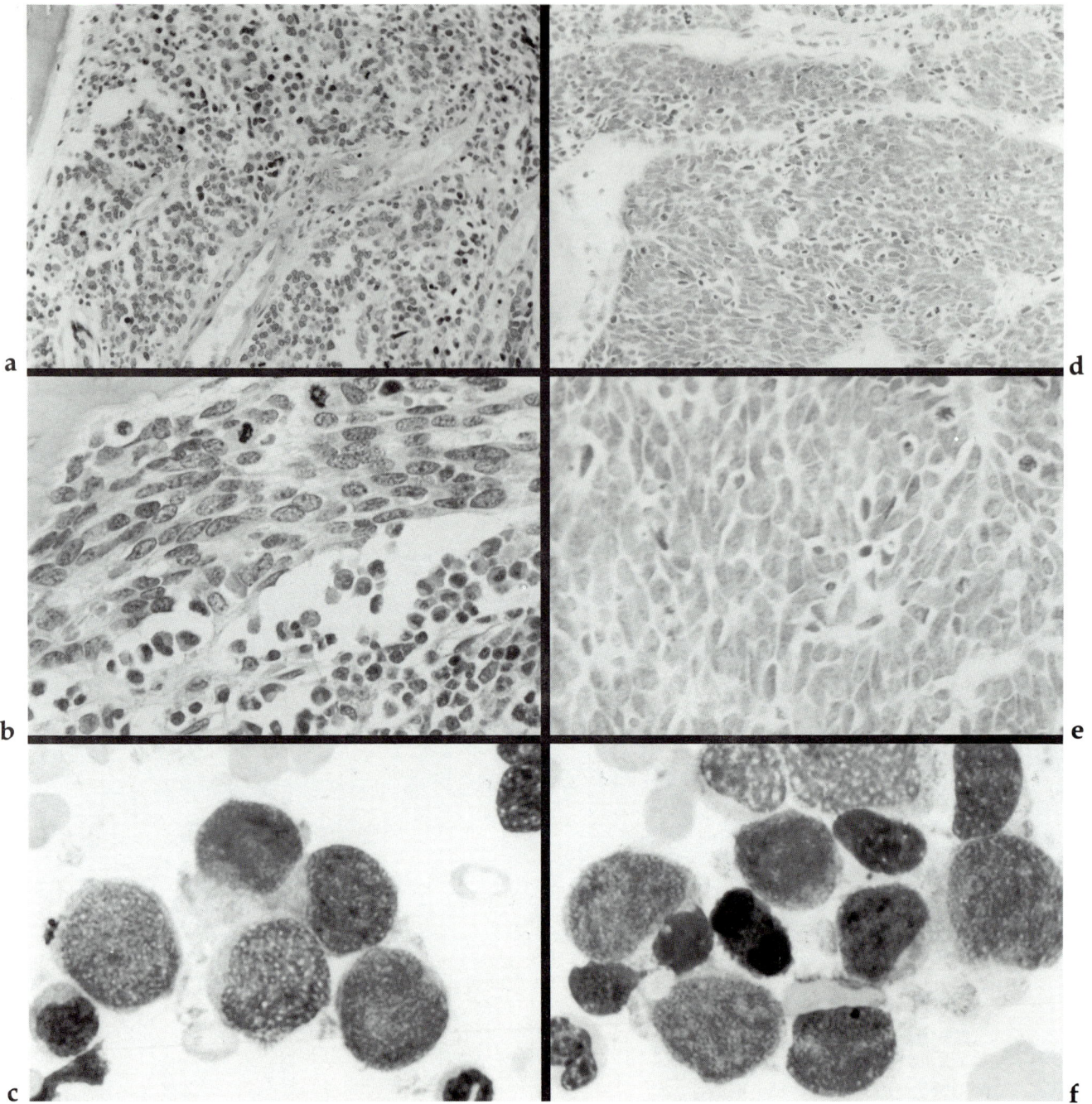

Figure 3-30. Bone marrow samples demonstrating metastatic neuroblastoma (a, b, c) and oat cell carcinoma (d, e, f); biopsy sections (a, b, d, e) and smears (c, f).

metastatic lesions (Figure 3-33). For example, histiocytic lesions are positive and metastatic carcinomas are negative for CD11c and CD68 antigens, as well as for lysozyme and alpha naphthyl butyrate esterase enzymes. Most of the ALLs are HLA-DR, TdT and CD10 positive, while these markers are not expressed in neuroblastoma, rhabdomyosarcoma and Ewing's sarcoma. Hematologic malignancies are usually positive for CD45 (common leukocyte antigen or CLA, T200, HLE), and tumors of epithelial origin

Abnormal Morphology: General Considerations

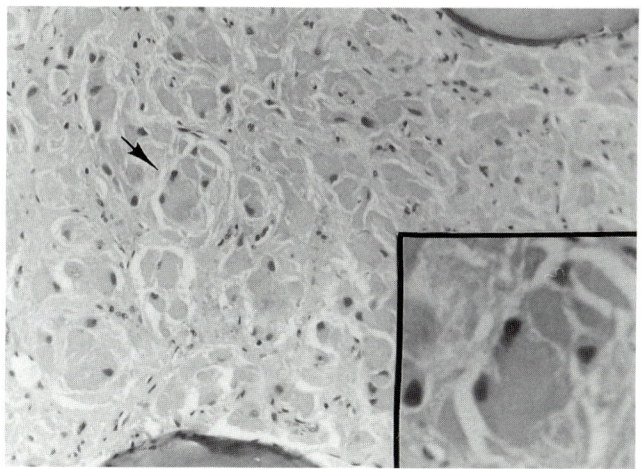

Figure 3-31. Bone marrow biopsy section demonstrating metastatic ganglioneuroblastoma. Ganglion cells are prominent (arrow and insert).

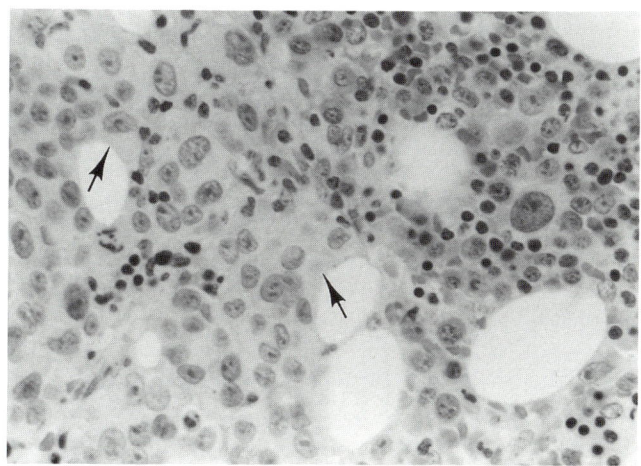

Figure 3-32. Bone marrow biopsy section demonstrating metastatic melanoma. Melanoma cells are large and pleomorphic, with abundant cytoplasm and a prominent nucleolus (arrows).

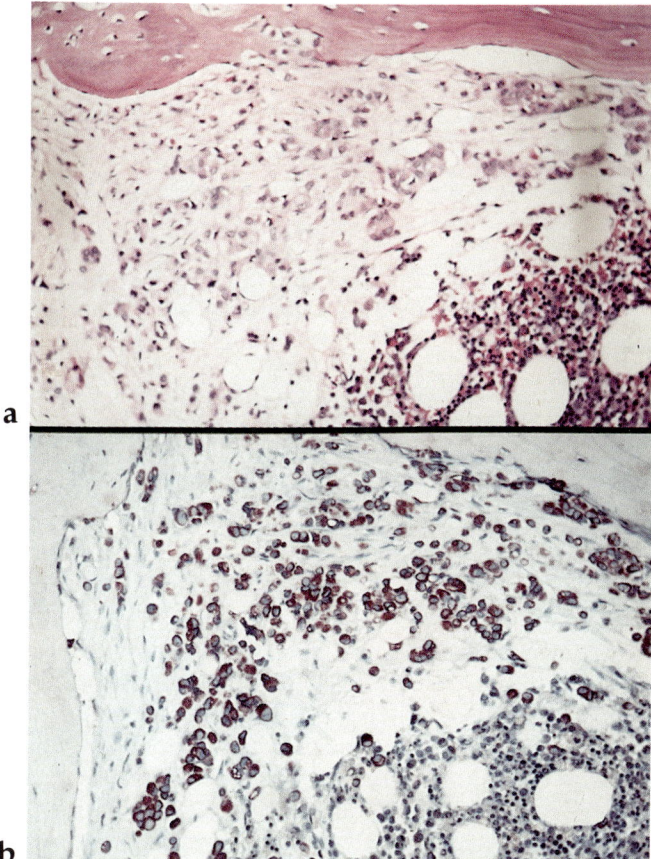

Figure 3-33. Bone marrow biopsy sample demonstrating metastatic breast adenocarcinoma. The H&E section shows several glandular structures in a fibrous stroma (a). The immunoperoxidase stain for cytokeratin shows a positive reaction in tumor cells (b).

often express cytokeratin and/or milk fat globulin. Metastatic prostatic carcinomas are positive for prostatic acid phosphatase and prostate-specific antigens. Melanoma cells are positive for S-100 protein and may show melanin pigments by Masson-Fontana stain. Metastatic rhabdomyosarcomas may demonstrate myosin, desmin or myoglobulin. Monoclonal antibodies have been used for the detection of small, occult, metastatic breast carcinomas and neuroblastomas by immunoenzyme techniques.[157-160] An automated screening method for the detection of breast metastatis in bone marrow smears by immunoenzyme staining has been recently reported.[160]

AMYLOIDOSIS

Amyloid is an extracellular deposit which appears as a hyaline, eosinophilic, amorphous material on H&E sections. The major component of amyloid is a nonbranching fibril composed of polypeptide chains, which on X-ray crystallographic analysis yield a "cross-beta" pleated sheet.[161,162] In routine histologic examination, amyloid is often recognized by

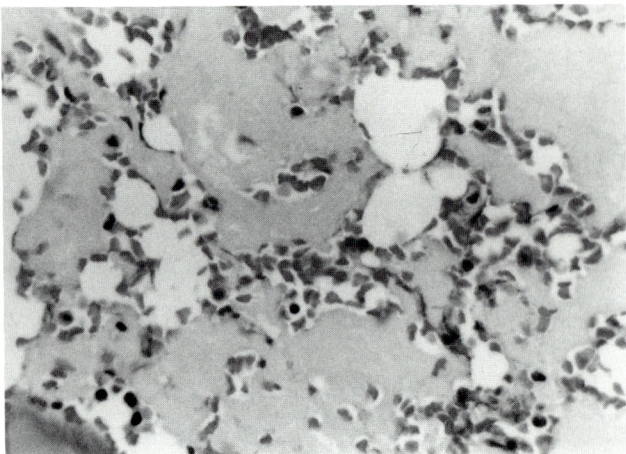

Figure 3-34. Bone marrow biopsy section demonstrating amyloid deposits.

two staining reactions: methyl violet and Congo red. Amyloid changes methyl violet from violet to rose pink and turns the red color of Congo red to orange in tissue sections. When the Congo red-stained slide is viewed under a polarizing microscope, amyloid appears as an apple green, birefringent deposit. It is also possible to detect amyloid deposits by using antibodies raised against amyloid components (anti-AA, anti-AL) by immunofluorescence or immunoperoxidase techniques.[163,164]

Bone marrow involvement with amyloidosis may be detected in the systemic forms of amyloidosis, such as primary systemic amyloidosis, amyloidosis associated with plasma cell dyscrasias (see Chapter 7) and amyloidosis secondary to chronic inflammatory diseases.[161,165-167] Amyloid deposits are usually focal and adjacent to or within the walls of small blood vessels. This vascular involvement may lead to ischemia and focal bone marrow hypoplasia. Occasionally, bone marrow involvement with amyloid is extensive (Figure 3-34).

VASCULAR CHANGES

Inflammatory vascular changes such as arteritis, arteriolitis and granulomatous vasculitis, as a systemic process, may involve bone marrow vasculature.[167,168] Similarly, atherosclerotic and thromboembolic lesions may be detected in bone marrow biopsy samples.[169] Amyloidosis may involve bone marrow vascular structures. Tumor emboli are the major sources of bone marrow metastasis and, in extensive forms, may result in microangiopathic hemolytic anemia.

BONE CHANGES

The bone–bone marrow relationship is often overlooked by pathologists and hematologists. Bone pathologists and surgical pathologists who concentrate on bone disorders may not pay adequate attention to the adjacent bone marrow tissue; on the other hand, hematopathologists and hematologists, who are searching for bone marrow disorders, may miss some clinically important bone changes. Furthermore, for evaluation of some bone disorders, undecalcified bone sections are required. This technique is not used routinely in many pathology laboratories.

In routine examination of bone marrow biopsy samples, one may detect evidence of decreased bone formation (osteopenia) or increased bone formation (osteosclerosis) in association with certain hematologic and nonhematologic conditions.

Conditions Associated with Osteopenia

Osteopenia (osteoporosis, osteolysis) may be caused by the following conditions:

1. Expansion of the bone marrow space caused by tumor infiltration, such as metastatic tumors, leukemia/lymphoma and multiple myeloma, or extensive bone marrow hypercellularity due to erythroid hyperplasia (thalassemia, vitamin B_{12}/folate deficiency).[170-174] This process is usually not accompanied by osteoclastic activity or impaired bone mineralization.

2. Imbalance of calcium metabolism, usually caused by hyperparathyroidism or renal failure. However, release of a number of mediators such as TGF-α, TNF and IL-1 is associated with bone resorption and hypercalcemia.[175] Osteolytic lesions in multiple myeloma appear to be due to the release of an osteoclastic activating factor by plasma cells.[176] Hypercalcemia associated with certain T-cell malignancies is thought to be related to the increased production of 1, 25-dihydroxyvitamin D by the tumor cells.[177]

In osteoporosis the bone marrow space is expanded at the expense of bone trabeculae. The bone trabeculae are thin and far apart. In osteomalacia the osteoid is partially decalcified. The noncalcified osteoid stains eosinophilic in plastic-embedded bone marrow biopsy sections.

Conditions Associated with Osteosclerosis

Osteosclerosis is demonstrated in bone marrow biopsy sections by increased thickness of the bone trabeculae. It is observed in primary myelofibrosis, leukemias, metastatic cancers, and mastocytosis.[21,174,178,179] Osteopetrosis, an inherited disease which occurs in both benign (autosomal dominant) and malignant (autosomal recessive) forms, is also characterized by increased bone density.[180]

References

1. Wickramasinghe SN: The deoxyuridine suppression test: A review of its clinical and research applications. *Clin Lab Hematol* 3:1, 1981.
2. Wickramasinghe SN: Annotations—kinetics and morphology of haemopoiesis in pernicious anaemia. *Br J Haematol* 22:111, 1972.
3. Reynolds EH, Laundy M: haematologic effects of anticonvulsant treatment. *Lancet* 2:682, 1978.
4. Wu A, Chanarin I, Levi AJ: Macrocytosis of chronic alcoholism. *Lancet* 1:629, 1974.
5. Girot R, Hamet M, Perignon JL, et al: Cellular immune deficiency in two siblings with hereditary orotic aciduria. *N Engl J Med* 308:700, 1983.
6. Eichner ER, Hillman RS: The evolution of anemia in the alcoholic patient. *Am J Med* 50:218, 1971.
7. Herbert V: Megaloblastic anemia. *Lab Invest* 52:3, 1985.
8. Vilpo JA: The DNA repair enzyme uracil-DNA glycosylase in the human hematopoietic system. *Mutat Res* 193:207, 1988.
9. Horton L, Coburn RJ, England JM, et al: The haematology of hypothyroidism. *Q J Med* 45:101, 1976.
10. Colman N, Herbert V: Hematologic complications of alcoholism. Overview. *Semin Hematol* 17:164, 1980.
11. Freedman BJ, Penington DG: Erythrocytosis in emphysema. *Br J Haematol* 9:425, 1963.
12. Babitz LE, Freedman ML: Anemia in the aged. *Compr Ther* 14:55, 1988.
13. Heimpel H, Wendt F: Congenital dyserythropoietic anemia with karyorrhexis and multinuclearity of erythroblasts. *Helv Med Acta* 34:103, 1968.
14. Lewis SM, Nelson DA, Pitcher DS: Clinical and ultrastructural aspects of congenital dyserythropoietic anaemia Type I. *Br J Haematol* 23:113, 1972.
15. Krause JR: The bone marrow in nutritional deficiencies. *Hematol Oncol Clin North Am* 2:557, 1988.
16. Spencer RP, Grimmond AP, Treschuk-Bahn J: Abdominal trauma with leukocytosis and Howell-Jolly bodies: Idiopathic functional asplenia. *Clin Nucl Med* 13:544, 1988.
17. Tatsumi N, Tsuda I, Matsumoto H: Maturation of Howell-Jolly bodies observed in a case of malignant histiocytosis. *Acta Cytol* 32:680, 1988.
18. Kalhs P, Panzer S, Kletter K, et al: Functional asplenia after bone marrow transplantation. A late complication related to extensive chronic graft-versus-host disease. *Ann Intern Med* 109:461, 1988.
19. Turgeon ML: *Clinical Hematology: Theory and Procedures.* Boston, Little, Brown, 1988, p 216.
20. Brown BA: *Hematology: Principles and Procedures,* ed 5. Philadelphia, Lea and Febiger, 1988, p 51.
21. Wickramasinghe SN: *Blood and Bone Marrow,* ed 3. London, Churchill Livingstone, 1986, p 77.
22. Krause JR: The bone marrow in nutritional deficiencies. *Hematol Oncol Clin North Am* 2:557, 1988.
23. Jandl JH: *Blood Textbook of Hematology.* Boston, Little, Brown 1987, p 441.
24. McCall CE, Katayama I, Cotran RS, et al: Lysosomal and ultrastructural changes in human "toxic" neutrophils during bacterial infection. *J Exp Med* 129:267, 1969.
25. McCall CE, DeChatelet LR, Cooper MR, et al: Human toxic neutrophils. III. Metabolic characteristics. *J Infect Dis* 127:26, 1973.
26. Jordan SW, Larsen WE: Ultrastructural studies of the May-Hegglin anomaly. *Blood* 25:921, 1965.
27. Cawley JC, Hayhoe FGJ: The inclusions of the May-Hegglin anomaly and Dohle bodies in infection. An ultrastructural comparison. *Br J Haematol* 22:491, 1972.
28. Pearson HA, Lorincz AE: A characteristic bone marrow finding in the Hurler syndrome. *Pediatrics* 24:280, 1964.
29. Peterson L, Parkin J, Nelson A: Mucopolysaccharidosis type VII. A morphologic, cytochemical, and ultrastructural study of the blood and bone marrow. *Am J Clin Pathol* 78:544, 1982.
30. Blume RS, Wolf SM: The Chediak-Higashi syndrome: Studies of four patients and a review of the literature. *Medicine* 51:247, 1972.
31. Targan SR, Oseas R: The "lazy" NK cells of Chediak-Higashi syndrome. *J Immunol* 130:2671, 1983.
32. Buchanan GR, Handin RI: Platelet function in Chediak-Higashi syndrome. *Blood* 47:941, 1976.
33. Lomax KJ, Gallin JI, Rotrosen D, et al: Selective defect

in myeloid cell lactoferrin gene expression in neutrophil specific granule deficiency. *J Clin Invest* 83:514, 1989.
34. Le Beau MM, Larson RA, Bitter MA, et al: Association of an inversion of chromosome 16 with abnormal marrow eosinophils in acute myelomonocytic leukemia. A unique cytogenetic clinicopathological association. *N Engl J Med* 309:630, 1983.
35. Takemori N, Saito N, Tachibana N, et al: Hybrid eosinophilic-basophilic granulocytes in chronic myeloid leukemia. *Am J Clin Pathol* 89:702, 1988.
36. Ware R, Kurtzberg J, Brazy J, et al: Congenital Pelger-Huet anomaly in triplets. *Am J Hematol* 27:226, 1988.
37. Liesveld J, Smith BD: Acquired Pelger-Huet anomaly in a case of non-Hodgkin's lymphoma. *Acta Haematol* 79:46, 1988.
38. Djulbegovi CB, Hadley T: A new algorithm for diagnosis of anemia. *Postgrad Med* 85:119, 1989.
39. Chanarin I: Megaloblastic anaemia: A perspective. *Rinsho Ketsueki* 29:1950, 1988.
40. Pittiglio DH, Sacher Ra: *Clinical Hematology and Fundamentals of Hemostasis*. Philadelphia, FA Davis, 1987, p 217.
41. Zinkham WH, Medearis DN, Obsorn JE: Blood and bone marrow findings in congenital rubella. *J Pediatr* 71:512, 1967.
42. Serck-Haussen A, Purohit GB: Histocytic medullary reticulosis: Report of 14 cases from Uganda. *Br J Cancer* 22:506, 1968.
43. Macias EG: Typhoidal cells. *Lancet* 2:927, 1975.
44. Chandra P, Chaundhery SA, Rosner F, et al: Transient histiocytosis with striking phagocytosis of platelets, leukocytes, and erythrocytes. *Arch Intern Med* 135:989, 1975.
45. Perry MC, Harrison EG, Burgert O, et al: Familial erythrophagocytic lymphohistiocytosis: Report of two cases and clinicopathology review. *Cancer* 38:209, 1976.
46. Danehbod K, Kissane JM: Idiopathic differential histiocytosis. *Am J Clin Pathol* 70:381, 1978.
47. Risdall RJ, McKenna RW, Nesbit ME, et al: Virus-associated hemophagocytic syndrome; a benign histiocytic proliferation distinct from malignant histiocytosis. *Cancer* 44:993, 1979.
48. Soffer D, Okron E, Rosen N, et al: Familial hemophagocytic lymphohistiocytosis in Israel. *Cancer* 54:2423, 1984.
49. Zuzau JP, Duran JW, Julia AF: Hemophagocytosis in acute burcellosis. *N Engl J Med* 301:1185, 1979.
50. James LS, Stass SA, Peterson V, et al: Abnormalities of bone marrow simulating histiocytic medullary reticulosis in a patient with gastric carcinoma. *Am J Clin Pathol* 71:600, 1979.
51. Kroman LY, Smith JR, Landaw SA, et al: Hodgkin's disease: Intramedullary phagocytosis with pancytopenia. *Ann Intern Med* 91:60, 1979.
52. Weisenburgher DD, Rappaport H, Ahluwalia MS, et al: Legionnaires' disease. *Arch Pathol Lab Med* 104:563, 1980.
53. Marsh WL, Bishop JW, Koening HM: Bone marrow and lymph node findings in a fatal case of Kawashaki's disease. *Arch Pathol Lab Med* 104:563, 1980.
54. Wilson ER, Malluk, A, Stagno S, et al: Fatal Epstein-Barr virus-associated hemophagocytic syndrome. *J Pediatr* 98:260, 1981.
55. Brunagelo F, Pileri S, De Solas I, et al: Peripheral T-cell lymphoma associated with hematophagocytic syndrome. *Blood* 75:434, 1990.
56. Jaffee ES, Costa J, Fauci AS: Erythrophagocytic T-Cell lymphoma. *N Engl J Med* 305:105, 1981.
57. Krause JR, Kaplan SS: Bone marrow findings in infectious mononucleosis and mononucleosis-like disease in the older adult. *Scand J Haematol* 28:15, 1982.
58. Mills MJ: Post-viral haemophagocytic syndrome. *Soc Med* 75:555, 1982.
59. Vin JAL, Kumaran TO, Marsh GW, et al: Complete recovery of histiocytic medullary reticulosis-like syndrome in a child with acute lymphoblastic leukemia. *Cancer* 51:200, 1983.
60. Reiner AP, Spivak JL: Hematophagic histiocytosis. A report of 23 new patients and a review of the literature. *Medicine* 67:369, 1988.
61. Lee RE: Histiocytic diseases of bone marrow. *Hematol Oncol Clin North Am* 2:657, 1988.
62. Goldblatt J: Type I Gaucher disease. *J Med Genet* 25:415, 1988.
63. Martin BM, Sidransky E, Ginns EI: Gaucher's disease: Advances and challenges. *Adv Pediatr* 36:277, 1989.
64. Glew RH, Basu A, LaMarco KL: Mammalian glucocerebrosidase: Implications for Gaucher's disease. *Lab Invest* 58:5, 1988.
65. Brunning RD: Morphologic alterations in nucleated blood and marrow cells in genetic disorders. *Hum Pathol* 1:99, 1970.
66. Papadimitriou JC, Chakravarthy A, Heyman MR: Pseudo-Gaucher cells preceding the appearance of immunoblastic lymphoma. *Am J Clin Pathol* 90:454, 1988.
67. Bona G, Bracco G, Gallina MR, et al: Wolman's disease: Clinical and biochemical findings of a new case. *J Inherited Metab Dis* 11:423, 1988.
68. Ordavas JM, King DC, Schaefer EJ, et al: Genetic HDL deficiency states. *Adv Exp Med Biol* 243:61, 1988.
69. Brady RO, Filling-Katz MR, Barton NW: Niemann-Pick disease types C and D. *Neurol Clin* 7:75, 1989.
70. Corbeel L: Histiocytic syndromes. *Eur J Pediatr* 148:9, 1988.
71. Vaerla-Duran J, Roholt PC, Ratliff NB: Sea blue his-

tiocyte syndrome. A secondary degenerative process of macrophages? *Arch Pathol Lab Med* 104:30, 1980.
72. Silverstein MN, Ellefson RD: The syndrome of the sea-blue histiocyte. *Semin Hematol* 9:299, 1972.
73. Sawitsky A, Rosner F, Chosky S: The sea-blue histiocyte syndrome, a review: Genetic and biochemical studies. *Semin Hematol* 9:285, 1972.
74. Zeman W: Studies in neuronal ceroid-lipofuscinosis. *J Neuropathol Exp Neurol* 33:1, 1974.
75. Prockop DJ, Kivirikko KI, Tuderman L, et al: The biosynthesis of collagen and its disorders. *N Engl J Med* 301:13, 1979.
76. McCarthy DM: Fibrosis of the bone marrow: Content and causes. *Br J Haematol* 59:1, 1985.
77. Rubins JM: The role of myelofibrosis in malignant leukoerythroblastosis. *Cancer* 51:308, 1983.
78. Bain BJ, Catovsky D, O'Brien M, et al: Megakaryocytic leukemia presenting as acute myelofibrosis—a study of four cases with the platelet peroxidase reaction. *Blood* 58:206, 1981.
79. Sawers AH, Davson J, Braganza J, et al: Systemic mastocytosis, myelofibrosis and portal hypertension. *J Clin Pathol* 35:617, 1982.
80. Smith RE, Chelmowski MK, Szabo EJ: Myelofibrosis: A review of clinical and pathologic features and treatment. *Am J Hematol* 29:174, 1988.
81. Vetgin S, Ozsoylu S: Myeloid metaplasia in vitamin D deficiency rickets. *Scand J Haematol* 28:180, 1982.
82. Boxer M, Ellman L, Geller R, et al: Anemia in primary hyperparathyroidism. *Arch Intern Med* 137:588, 1977.
83. Berton-Gorius J, Vainchenker W, Nurden A, et al: Defective alpha-granule production in megakaryocytes from gray platelet syndrome. Ultrastructural studies of bone marrow cells and megakaryocytes growing in culture from blood precursors. *Am J Pathol* 102:10, 1981.
84. Lennert K, Nagai K, Schwarze EW: Patho-anatomical features of the bone marrow. *Clin Haematol* 4:331, 1975.
85. Kundel DW, Brecher G, Bodey GP, et al: Reticulin fibrosis and bone infarction in acute leukemia—implications for prognosis. *Blood* 23:526, 1964.
86. Blayney DW, Jaffee ES, Blatter WA, et al: The human T-cell leukemia/lymphoma virus associated with American adult T-cell leukemia/lymphoma. *Blood* 62:401, 1983.
87. Failkow PJ, Jacobson RJ, Papayannopulou T: Chronic myelocytic leukemia: Clonal origin in a stem cell common to the granulocyte, erythrocyte, platelet and monocyte/macrophage. *Am J Med* 63:125, 1977.
88. Jacobson RJ, Salo A, Failkow PJ: Agenogenic myeloid metaplasia: A colonal proliferation of hematopoietic stem cells with secondary myelofibrosis. *Blood* 51:189, 1978.

89. Kuo C, Van Voolen GA, Morrison AN: Primary and secondary myelofibrosis: Its relationship to "PNH-like defect." *Blood* 40:875, 1972.
90. Bird J, Proctor S: Malignant myelosclerosis. *Am J Clin Pathol* 67:512, 1977.
91. Castro H, Malaspina H, Rabellino EM, et al: Human megakaryocyte stimulation of proliferation of bone marrow fibroblasts. *Blood* 57:781, 1981.
92. Groopman JE; The pathogenesis of myelofibrosis in myeloproliferative disorders. *Ann Intern Med* 92:857, 1980.
93. Smith RE, Chelmowski MK, Szabo EJ: Myelofibrosis: A concise review of clinical and pathologic features and treatment. *Am J Hematol* 29:174, 1988.
94. Pease GL: Granulomatous lesions in bone marrow. *Blood* 11:720, 1956.
95. Browne PM, Sharma OP, Salkin D: Bone marrow sarcoidosis. *JAMA* 240:2654, 1978.
96. Farhi DC, Mason UG, Horsburg CR Jr: The bone marrow in disseminated *Mycobacterium avium intracellulare* infection. *Am J Clin Pathol* 83:463, 1985.
97. Lawrence C, Schreiber AJ: Medical intelligence. Leprosy's footprints in bone marrow histiocytes. *N Engl J Med* 300:834, 1979.
98. White RM, Johnson CL: Granulomatous bone marrow disease in Virginia: Study of 50 cases. *Virginia Med* 112:316, 1985.
99. Geller SA, Muller R, Greenberg ML, et al: Acquired immunodeficiency syndrome. Distinctive features of bone marrow biopsies. *Arch Pathol Lab Med* 109:138, 1985.
100. Okun DB, Sun NCJ, Tanaka KR: Bone marrow granulomas in Q fever. *Am J Clin Pathol* 71:117, 1979.
101. Nosanchuk JS: Bone marrow granulomas with acute cytomegalovirus infection. *Arch Pathol Lab Med* 108:93, 1984.
102. Vu HC, Rgwlin AM: Granulomatous lesions of the bone marrow in Hodgkin's lymphoma. *Hum Pathol* 13:905, 1982.
103. Macias EG: Typhoidal cells. *Lancet* 2:927, 1975.
104. Weisenburgher DD, Rappaport H, Ahluwalia MS, et al: Legionnaires' disease. *Am J Med* 69:476, 1980.
105. Krause JR, Brubaker D, Kaplan S: Comparison of stainable iron in aspirated and needle biopsy specimens of bone marrow. *Am J Clin Pathol* 72:68, 1979.
106. Delsol G, Pellegrin M, Familiades J, et al: Bone marrow lesions in Q fever *Blood* 52:637, 1978.
107. Falini B, Tabilio A, Avlardi A, et al: Multiple myeloma with a sarcoidosis-like reaction. *Scand J Haematol* 29:211, 1982.
108. Yu HC, Rywlin AM: Granulomatous lesions of the bone marrow in non-Hodgkin's lymphoma. *Hum Pathol* 13:905, 1982.

109. Wu HV, Kosmin A: Bone-marrow granulomata and phenytoin. *Ann Intern Med* 86:663, 1977.
110. Riker J, Baker J, Swanson M: Bone marrow granulomas and neutropenia associated with procainamide. *Arch Intern Med* 138:1931, 1978.
111. Andersson DEH, Langworth S, Newman HC, et al: Reversible bone marrow granulomas—adverse effect of oxyphenbutazone therapy. *Acta Med Scand* 207:131, 1980.
112. Martin MF: Atypical infectious mononucleosis with bone marrow granulomas and pancytopenia. *Br Med J* 2(6082):300, 1977.
113. Hovede RF, Sundberg RD: Granulomatous lesions in bone marrow in infectious mononucleosis; comparison of changes in bone marrow infectious mononucleosis with those in brucellosis, tuberculosis, sarcoidosis and lymphatic leukemia. *Blood* 5:209, 1950.
114. Pellegrin M, Rizzoli R: Granulomatous hepatitis in Q fever. *Hum Pathol* 77:51, 1980.
115. Suster S, Cabello-Inchaustic B, Robinson MJ: Nongranulomatous involvement of the bone marrow in lepomatous leprosy. *Am J Clin Pathol* 92:797, 1988.
116. Sun NJC, Shapshak P, Lachant NA, et al: Bone marrow examination in patients with AIDS and AIDS related complex (ARC). Morphologic and in situ hybridization studies. *Am J Clin Pathol* 92:589, 1989.
117. Rywlin AM, Ortega RD: Lipid granulomas of the bone marrow. *Am J Clin Pathol* 57:457, 1972.
118. Gallo RC, Salahuddin SZ, Popovic M, et al: Frequent detection and isolation of cytopathic retroviruses (HTLV-111) from patients with AIDS and at risk for AIDS. *Science* 224:500, 1984.
119. Biberfeld P, Chayt KJ, Marselle LM, et al: HTLV-III expression in infected lymph nodes and relevance to pathogenesis of lymphadenopathy. *Am J Pathol* 123:436, 1986.
120. Castella A, Croxon TS, Mildvan D, et al: The bone marrow in AIDS—a histologic, hematologic, and microbiologic study. *Am J Clin Pathol* 84:425, 1985.
121. Shenoy CM, Lin JH: Bone marrow findings in acquired immunodeficiency syndrome (AIDS). *Am J Med Sci* 292:372, 1986.
122. Geller SA, Muller R, Greenberg ML, et al: Acquired immunodeficiency syndrome—distinctive features of bone marrow biopsies. *Arch Pathol Lab Med* 109:138, 1985.
123. Schnider DR, Picker LJ: Myelodysplasia in the acquired immunodeficiency syndrome. *Am J Clin Pathol* 84:144, 1985.
124. Fauci AS, Macher AM, Longo DL, et al: Acquired immunodeficiency syndrome: Epidemiologic, clinical, immunologic and therapeutic-considerations. *Ann Intern Med* 100:92, 1984.
125. Nakimi TS, Boone DC, Meyer PR: A comparison of bone marrow findings in patient with acquired immunodeficiency syndrome (AIDS) and AIDS-related conditions. *Hematol Oncol* 5:99, 1987.
126. Richmann DD, Fischl MA, Grieco MH, et al: The toxicity of azidothymidine (ATZ) in the treatment of patients with AIDS and AIDS-related complex. *N Engl J Med* 317:192, 1987.
127. Duggan MJ, Weisenburger DD, Sun NCJ, et al: Bone marrow findings in immunodeficiency syndromes. *Hematol Oncol Clin North Am* 2:637, 1988.
128. Conran RM, Granger E, Reddy VB: Kaposi's sarcoma of bone marrow. *Arch Pathol Lab Med* 110:1083, 1986.
129. Michael P: Gelatinous degeneration of the bone marrow. *J Pathol* 33:533, 1930.
130. Seaman JP, Kjeldsberg CT, Linker A: Gelatinous transformation of the bone marrow. *Hum Pathol* 9:685, 1978.
131. Tavassoli M, Eastlund TD, Vam LT, et al: Gelatinous transformation of bone marrow in prolonged self-induced starvation. *Scand J Haematol* 16:311, 1976.
132. Pearson H: Marrow hypoplasia in anorexia nervosa. *J Pediatr* 71:211, 1967.
133. Mant M, Faragher BS: The hematology of anorexia nervosa. *Br J Haematol* 23:737, 1972.
134. Tavassoli M: Differential response of bone marrow and extramedullary adipose cells to starvation. *Experientia* 30:424, 1974.
135. Brown CH: Bone marrow necrosis. A study of seven cases. *John Hopkins Med J* 131:189, 1972.
136. Norgard MJ, Carpenter JT, Conrad ME: Bone marrow necrosis and degeneration. *Arch Intern Med* 139:905, 1979.
137. Kiraly JF, Wheby MS: Bone marrow necrosis. *Am J Med* 60:361, 1976.
138. Kinney TR, Koch PA, Gottlieb RP, et al: Bone marrow necrosis in children. *Clin Pediatr* 16:565, 1977.
139. Conrad ME, Carpenter JT: Bone marrow necrosis. *Am J Hematol* 7:181, 1979.
140. Brada M, Bellingham AJ: Bone marrow necrosis and Q fever. *Br Med J* 281:1108, 1980.
141. Cassileth PA, Brooks SJ: The prognostic significance of myelonecrosis after induction chemotherapy in acute leukemia. *Cancer* 60:2363, 1987.
142. Knupp C, Pekala PH, Cornelius P: Extensive bone marrow necrosis in patients with cancer and tumor necrosis factor activity in plasma. *Am J Hematol* 29:215, 1988.
143. Maisel D, Lim JY, Pollock WJ, et al: Bone marrow necrosis: An entity often overlooked. *Ann Clin Lab Sci* 18:109, 1988.
144. Spivak JL, Bender BS, Quinn TC: Hematologic abnormalities in the acquired immune deficiency syndrome. *Am J Med* 77:224, 1984.

145. Rose MS: Apparent necrosis of bone marrow in a patient with disseminated intravascular coagulation postpartum. *Lancet* 2:730, 1973.
146. Tavassoli M: Bone marrow necrosis secondary to hyperparathyroidism. *J Miss State Med Assoc* 24:39, 1983.
147. Katzen H, Spagnolo SV: Bone marrow necrosis from miliary tuberculosis. *JAMA* 244:2438, 1980.
148. Davies SF, McKenna RW, Sarosi GA: Trephine biopsy of the bone marrow in disseminated histoplasmosis. *Am J Med* 67:617, 1979.
149. Carloss H, Winslow D, Kastan L, et al: Bone marrow necrosis: Diagnosis and assessment of extent of involvement by radioisotope studies. *Arch Intern Med* 137:863, 1977.
150. Ingle JN, Tormey DC, Tan HK: The bone marrow examination in breast cancer—diagnostic considerations and clinical usefulness. *Cancer* 41:670, 1978.
151. Singh G, Krause JR, Breitfeld V: Bone marrow examination for metastatic tumor—aspirate and biopsy. *Cancer* 40:2317, 1977.
152. Anner RM, Drewinko B: Frequency and significance of bone marrow involvement by metastatic solid tumors. *Cancer* 39:1337, 1977.
153. Ihde DC, Simms EB, Matthews MJ, et al: Bone marrow metastases in small cell carcinoma of the lung: Frequency, description, and influence on chemotherapeutic toxicity and prognosis. *Blood* 53:677, 1979.
154. Reynolds CP, Smith RG, Frenkel EP: The diagnostic dilemma of the "small round cell neoplasm." *Cancer* 48:2088, 1981.
155. Andres TL, Kadin ME: Immunologic markers in the differential diagnosis of small round cell tumors from lymphocytic lymphoma and leukemia. *Am J Clin Pathol* 79:546, 1983.
156. Kemshead JT, Goldman A, Fritschy J, et al: Use of panels of monoclonal antibodies in the differential diagnosis of neuroblastoma and lymphoblastic disorders. *Lancet* 1:12, 1983.
157. Berger U, Bettelheim R, Mansi J, et al: The relationship between micrometastasis in the bone marrow; histopathologic features of the primary tumor in the breast cancer and prognosis. *Am J Clin Pathol* 90:11, 1988.
158. Beck D, Maritaz O, Gross N, et al: Immunocytochemical detection of neuroblastoma cells infiltrating clinical bone marrow samples. *Eur J Pediatr* 147:609, 1988.
159. Thor A, Viglione MJ, Ohuchi N, et al: Comparison of monoclonal antibodies for the detection of occult breast carcinoma metastasis in bone marrow. *Breast Ca Res Treat* 11:133, 1988.
160. Mansi JL, Mesker WE, McDonnell T, et al: Automated screening for micrometastases in bone marrow smears. *J Immunol Methods* 112:105, 1988.
161. Glenner GG: Amyloid deposits and amyloidosis. The beta-fibrilloses (first of two parts). *N Engl J Med* 302:1283, 1980.
162. Glenner GG: Amyloid deposits and amyloidosis. The beta-fibrilloses (second of two parts). *N Engl J Med* 302:1333, 1980.
163. Levo Y, Livni N, Laufer A: Diagnosis and classification of amyloidosis by an immune-histological method. *Pathol Res Pract* 175:373, 1982.
164. Elghentany MT, Saleem A: Methods for staining amyloid in tissues: A review. *Stain Technol* 63:201, 1988.
165. Stone MJ: Amyloidosis: A final common pathway for protein deposition in tissues. *Blood* 75:531, 1990.
166. Kawkins PN: Amyloidosis. *Blood Rev* 2:270, 1988.
167. Enos WF, Pierre RV, Rosenblatt JE: Giant cell arteritis detected by bone marrow biopsy. *Mayo Clin Proc* 56:381, 1981.
168. Rywlin AM: *Histopathology of the Bone Marrow*. Boston, Little, Brown, 1976, p 180.
169. Pierce JR, Wren MC, Cousar J: Cholesterol embolism: Diagnosis antemortem by bone marrow biopsy. *Ann Intern Med* 89:937, 1978.
170. Thomas LB, Forkner CE Jr, Frei E, et al: The skeletal lesions of acute leukemia. *Cancer* 14:608, 1961.
171. Neiman RS, Li HC: Hypercalcemia in undifferentiated leukemia. *Cancer* 30:942, 1972.
172. Pootrakul P, Hungsprenges S, Fucharoen S, et al: Relation between erythropoiesis and bone metabolism in thalassemia. *N Engl J Med* 304:1470, 1981.
173. Raisz LG: What marrow does to bone. *N Engl J Med* 304:1485, 1981.
174. Kiely JM, Silverstein MN: Metastatic carcinoma simulating agnogenic myeloid metaplasia. *Cancer* 24:1041, 1969.
175. Mundy GR: Incidence and pathophysiology of hypercalcemia. *Calcif Tissue Int* 46(Suppl):S3, 1990.
176. Mundy GR, Raisz LG, Cooper RA, et al: Evidence for the secretion of an osteoclast-stimulating factor in myeloma. *N Engl J Med* 291:1041, 1974.
177. Fetchich DA, Bertolini DR, Sarin P, et al: Production of 1,25-dihydroxyvitamin D by human T cell lymphotropic virus-1 transformed lymphocytes. *J Clin Invest* 78:592, 1986.
178. Sawers AH, Davidson J, Baraganza J, et al: Systemic mastocytosis, myelofibrosis and portal hypertension. *J Clin Pathol* 35:617, 1982.
179. Janin A, Nelken B, Dufour S, et al: Acute monoblastic leukemia with osteosclerosis and extensive myelofibrosis. *Am J Pediatr Hematol Oncol* 10:319, 1988.
180. Marks SC: Osteopetrosis—multiple pathways for the interception of osteoclast function. *Appl Pathol* 5:172, 1987.

4 BONE MARROW HYPOPLASIA

Bone marrow hypoplasia is mostly due to a reduction and/or a defect in pluripotential stem cells or their microenvironment and is characterized by markedly hypocellular marrow and pancytopenia. In this category, the following disorders are included: (1) constitutional aplastic anemia, (2) acquired aplastic anemia, (3) paroxysmal nocturnal hemoglobinuria and (4) hypoplastic myelodysplasias and leukemias (Table 4-1). Constitutional and acquired aplastic anemias and paroxysmal nocturnal hemoglobinuria are discussed in this chapter. Marrow hypoplasias associated with myelodysplastic syndromes and leukemias, and monolinear hypoplasias such as pure red blood cell aplasia or agranulocytosis, are discussed in other chapters.

CONSTITUTIONAL APLASTIC ANEMIA

Constitutional or familial aplastic anemias are autosomal recessive disorders found with an unusually high prevalence in the Afrikaans population of South Africa.[1] Peak incidence is between the ages of 5 and 10, and males are affected twice as frequently as females.

Etiology and Pathogenesis

Familial aplastic anemia is considered one of the diseases with cellular defects in the ability to repair DNA damage, leading to spontaneous enhancement of chromosomal breakage.[2-4] This enhancement is significantly increased in homozygotes when the drugs diepoxybutane (DEB) and mitomycin C (MMC) are used.[5] Cultured bone marrow cells, lymphocytes and fibroblasts from patients with constitutional aplastic anemia often show cytogenetic abnormalities such as chromosome gaps, breaks, constrictions, exchanges and translocations.[6]

Pathology

In the early stages of the disease, bone marrow may appear hyper- or normocellular, but eventually it becomes markedly hypocellular, with small foci of hematopoietic cells, predominantly erythroid. There are increased proportions of plasma cells, lymphocytes and mast cells[7] (Figure 4-1). The morphologic findings are not pathognomonic for familial aplastic anemia and are frequently seen in acquired aplastic anemia.

Peripheral blood examination reveals pancytopenia. The anemia is usually normocytic normochromic, but there may be an increase in the number of fetal hemoglobin-containing red blood cells or in the amount of fetal hemoglobin.[7,8] Similar findings have been reported in acquired aplastic anemia.[8]

Clinical Aspects

Familial aplastic anemia has two clinical manifestations: with physical abnormalities (Fanconi anemia) and without physical abnormalities (Estern-Dameshek anemia). Associated physical abnormalities include brown skin pigmentation, hypoplastic thumb or radius, splenic and renal hypoplasia and microcephaly.

Patients with familial aplastic anemia have an increased risk of developing acute myelomonocytic and monocytic leukemias.[8,9]

ACQUIRED APLASTIC ANEMIA

The bone marrow hypoplasia in acquired aplastic anemia has been associated with exposure to a wide spectrum of chemical and physical agents and to a variety of diseases. However, because of the widespread exposure to an unlimited number of chemicals

Bone Marrow Hypoplasia

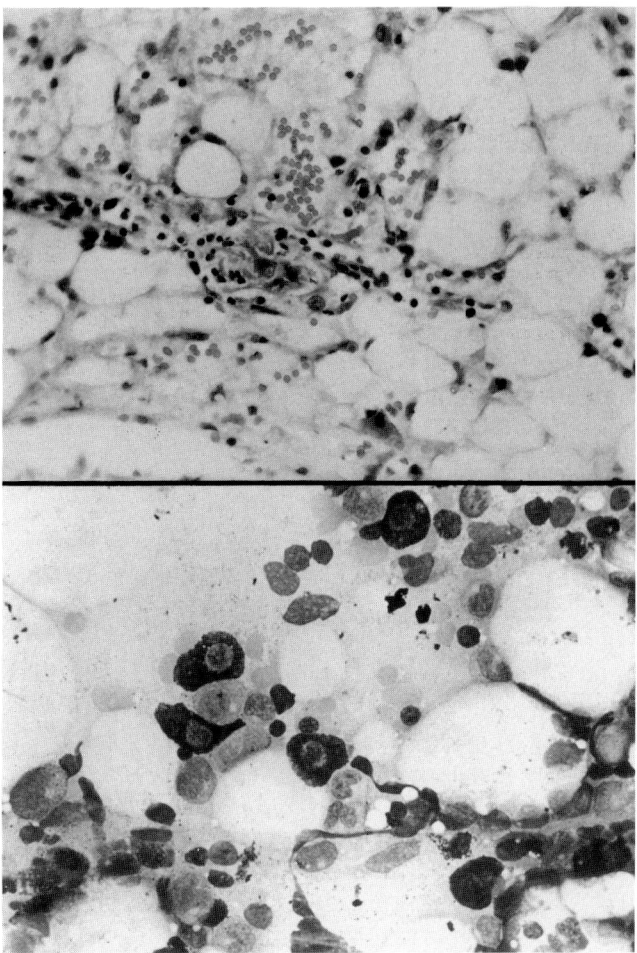

Figure 4-1. In advanced Fanconi anemia, bone marrow is markedly hypocellular and often shows increased numbers of mast cells.

Table 4-1 Classification of Aplastic Anemia

1. Constitutional (familial, congenital)
   A. Fanconi anemia
   B. Estern-Dameshek anemia
2. Acquired
   A. Idiopathic (no known etiology)
   B. Secondary
      i. Chemical and physical agents
         a. Drugs and other chemicals
         b. Radiation
      ii. Infectious
         a. Viral: hepatitis, Epstein-Barr virus, influenza
         b. Others: tuberculosis, dengue fever
      iii. Immunologic (humoral and/or cellular)
      iv. Metabolic (pancreatitis, pregnancy)
3. Paroxysmal nocturnal hemoglobinuria
4. Hypoplastic preleukemias and leukemias

such as insecticides, fertilizers and food additives, the causative factors are not detected in 50 to 75% of acquired aplastic anemia. Thus, this disease is divided into two major groups: (1) idiopathic aplastic anemia (with no known etiology) and (2) secondary aplastic anemia (see Table 4-1).

Etiology and Pathogenesis

The exact mechanism(s) of the development of acquired aplastic anemia is not known. However, damage to bone marrow stem cells and/or stromal cells by agents otherwise considered harmless could be due to the presence of several factors, such as severely depleted normal stem cells, excessive acquired vulnerability of the marrow cells, or development of an immunologic process damaging to the bone marrow cells. For example, repeated exposure to alkylating agents may lead to an irreversible reduction in the number of bone marrow stem cells.[10,11] Stem cell regeneration after repeated marrow depletion declines and eventually leads to complete bone marrow failure.[12] Successful theraputic effects of antithymocyte globulin and the frequent need for immunosuppressive drugs in identical twin transplants strongly suggest that a cell-mediated immunologic disorder plays a role in the pathogenesis of aplastic anemia in many patients.[13,14] T-cell-mediated inhibition of colony formation has been demonstrated in some patients with aplastic anemia.[15,16] Activity of these lymphocytes may be due to a primary autoimmune mechanism or may be secondary to a pathogenic stimulus.[17] Lymphocytes may act directly on the stem cells or may affect other accessory cells that are involved in cellular interactions required for the production of growth factors.[15-18] Cultures of bone marrow cells from patients with aplastic anemia demonstrate a reduction in or lack of committed progenitor cells of all lines.[59,60] This may be due to deficiency of the functional committed progenitor cells or to immune-mediated suppression of proliferation of progenitor cells.[61]

A wide variety of *drugs* such as chloramphenicol, phenylbutazone, acetylsalicilic acid and phenytoin may play a role in the development of aplastic anemia[19,20] (Table 4-2). Of these drugs, chloramphenicol is perhaps the best-documented one.[21,22] The toxic effect of chloramphenicol on bone marrow may be reversible or irreversible. The reversible toxic effects are common and are associated with increased serum iron, accumulation of iron in the mitochondria of erythroblasts (ringed sideroblasts) and vacuolization of marrow precursor cells.[23-27] These effects may be related in part to the binding of the chloramphenicol to rRNA coded for by mitochondrial DNA.[28,29] The irreversible stage appears to be associated with damage to the genetic structure of the hematopoietic stem cells, leading to sustained aplastic anemia. This stage develops weeks or months after exposure to the drug and is not dose related.[30-34]

A wide variety of *nonpharmacologic chemicals* such as alanine dyes and organic solvents have been reported in association with aplastic anemia. Benzene (benzol) and benzene metabolites suppress DNA synthesis and inhibit proliferation of hematopoietic progenitor cells.[35-39] In humans, benzene exposure has been associated with aplastic anemia, hemolytic anemia, myelodysplastic syndrome and acute myelogenous leukemia.[40-42]

Radiation may impair hematopoietic stem cells and the bone marrow microenvironment, leading to aplastic anemia. Lethal or sublethal amounts of total body irradiation, high doses of local therapeutic radiation, and long-term continuous exposure to small amounts of radiation have been reported as possible etiologic factors in aplastic anemia.[43-46]

Viral infections have been associated with aplastic anemia, probably by direct involvement of marrow stem cells. The aplastic anemia associated with viral hepatitis is usually severe and refractory.[47,48] Other viruses, such as the rubella virus, Epstein-Barr virus, HIV and parvovirus B19, may also cause bone marrow hypoplasia.[49-53b]

Pathology

Bone marrow examination of biopsy sections reveals a fatty marrow with a cellularity often less than 25% (Figure 4-2). Islands of hematopoietic cells may be randomly distributed throughout the marrow. These islands are usually predominantly erythroid and show decreased numbers of megakaryocytes (Figures 4-3 and 4-4). Bone marrow smears are hypocellular and consist predominantly of stromal tissue with scattered hematopoietic cells (see Figure 4-4). Erythroid dysplasia is a common finding, with nuclear/cytoplasmic asynchrony, nuclear lobulation, nuclear budding or fragmentation and megaloblastic changes.[54] Occasionally, the aspirated marrow sample may contain a cellular fragment, giving the wrong impression of a normocellular or even hypercellular marrow. For this reason, bone marrow biopsies are more suitable for establishment of the diagnosis of aplastic anemia. Some cases show increased proportions of macrophages, plasma cells, lymphocytes and mast cells. There may be evidence of erythrophagocytosis or hemophagocytosis, especially in early stages of the disease. Hemosiderin-containing macrophages are found in the late stages due to heavy transfusion therapy. Lymphocytes, plasma cells and macrophages either appear as well-defined aggregates or are diffusely interspersed within the marrow stroma. There are controversial reports regarding the clinical significance of the extent of marrow inflammatory cells in patients with aplastic anemia.[56, 57]

Table 4-2 Commonly Used Drugs Which May Play a Role in the Development of Aplastic Anemia*

1. Antibacterial drugs
    Chloramphenicol, sulfonamides, streptomycin, tetracycline, isoniazid, penicillin
2. Antidiabetic drugs
    Chlorpropamide, tolbutamide
3. Antiepileptic drugs
    Phenytoin, methioine, methsuximide, paramethadione, phenacemide, troxidone
4. Anti-inflammatory drugs and analgesics
    Phenylbutazone, oxyphenbutazone, indomethacin, sodium diclofenac, gold salts
5. Antimalarial drugs
    Mepacrine, chloroquine, pyramethamine
6. Others
    Allopurinol, chlorpromazine, chlorthiazide meprobamate, organic arsenicals

* Adapted from Tabulation of reports compiled by the panel on hematology of the registry on adverse reactions. Council on Drugs, American Medical Association, May 1965 and June 1967; and de Gruchy GC: *Drug Induced Blood Disorders.* Oxford, Blackwell Scientific Publications, 1975; and The International Agranulocytosis and Aplastic Anemia Study: Risks of agranulocytosis and aplastic anemia. A first report of their relation to drug use with special references to analgestics. *JAMA* 256:1749, 1986.

Bone Marrow Hypoplasia

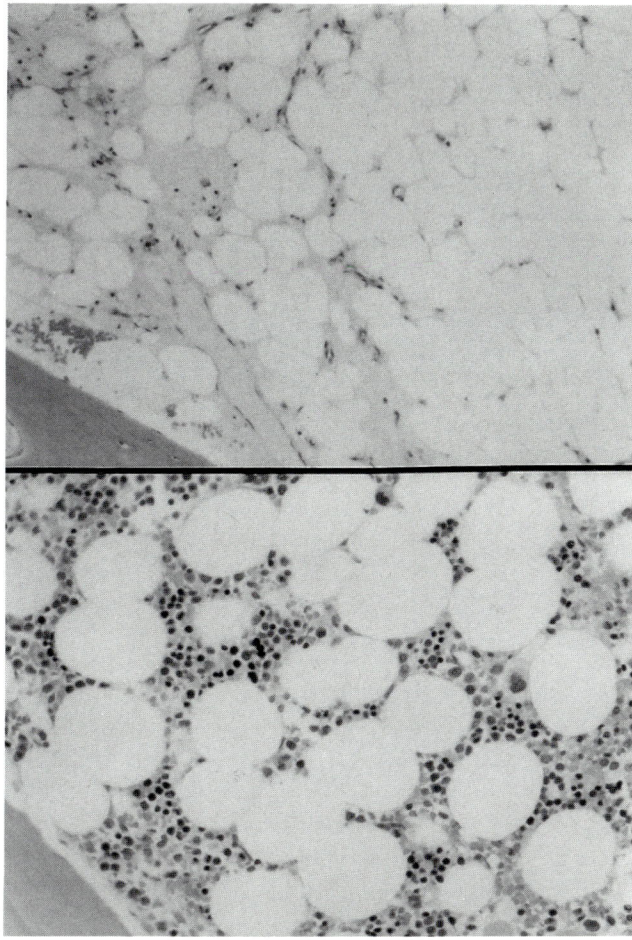

Figure 4-2. Patients with aplastic anemia may show various degrees of bone marrow hypocellularity ranging from extremely severe to moderate.

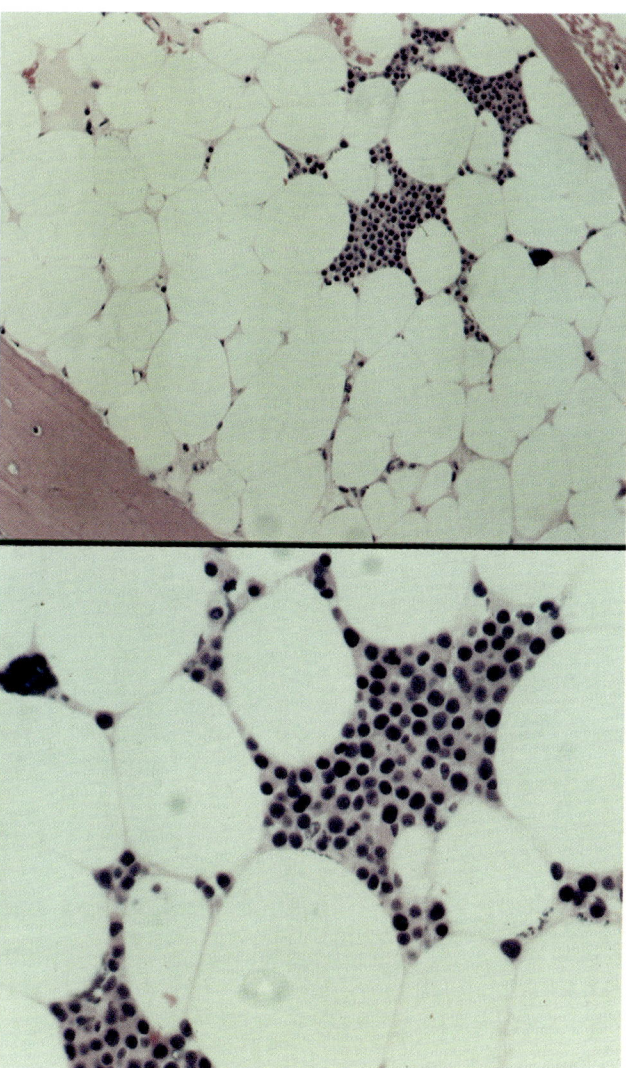

Figure 4-3. Bone marrow biopsy section from a patient with aplastic anemia demonstrating small clusters of hematopoietic, predominantly erythroid, cells.

Peripheral blood examination reveals pancytopenia. There is anemia with reticulocytopenia. Anemia is normochromic and normocytic, but macrocytosis and anisocytosis may be present, particularly when there is some residual hematopoietic activity in the marrow. Platelets, neutrophils, eosinphils and basophils are also reduced, and neutrophils may show "toxic" granulation. The LAP score is often elevated. The lymphocyte count is normal or low, and there may be an increased proportion of activated suppressor T-lymphocytes, as shown by a rise in the number of $CD8^+$ $CD25^+$ cells.[57]

Availability of the recombinant growth factors has opened a new avenue in the treatment of aplastic anemia. Patients with severe refractory anemia have shown considerable improvement during administration of growth factors such as GM-CSF. They show a continuous rise in the absolute number of peripheral blood neutrophils, eosinophils and monocytes, with a progressive increase in bone marrow cellularity. The most prominent topographic observation in the bone marrow during GM-CSF therapy is frequent clustering of myeloid cells close to the bone trabeculae. The paraosteal localization of the myeloid precursors may reflect a higher concentration of stem

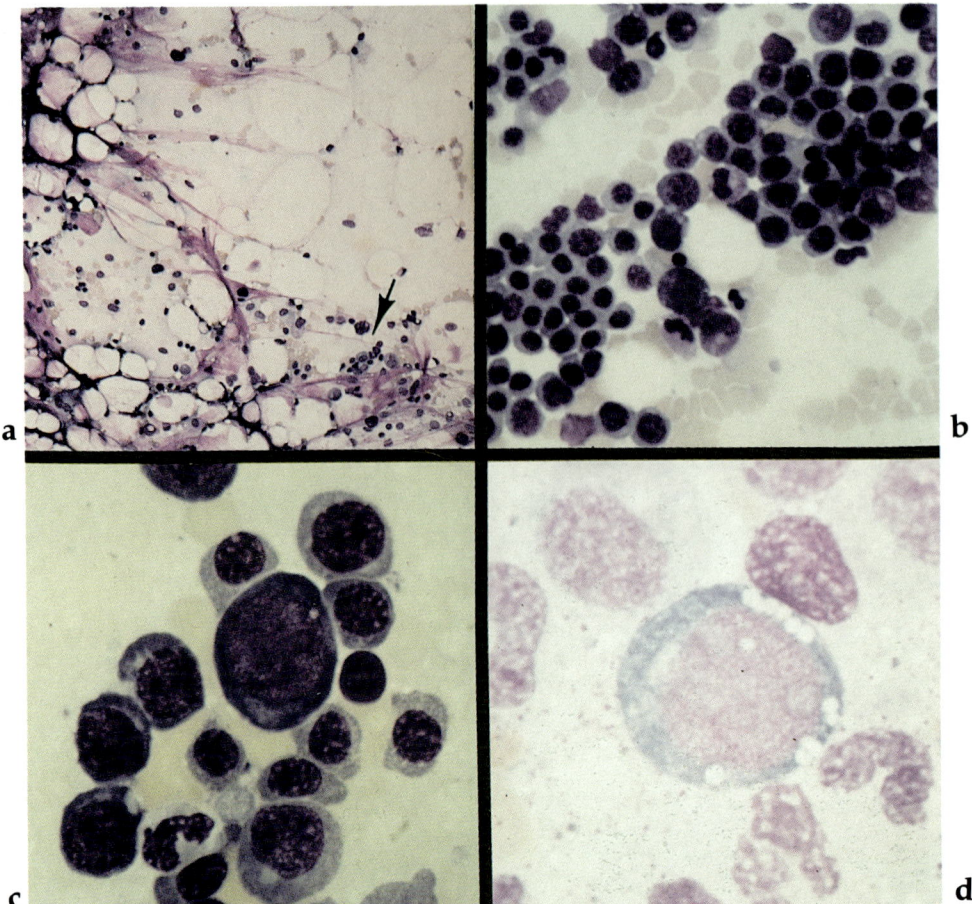

Figure 4-4. Bone marrow smears demonstrating (a) aplastic anemia. Severely hypocellular marrow with a few clusters of hematopoietic cells (arrow); (b, c) hematopoietic clusters are predominantly of an erythroid series; (d) vacuolated erythroblasts are seen in drug- or virus-induced aplastic anemias.

cells and/or stromal cells in the bone marrow adjacent to the bone trabeculae or a higher concentration of growth factors[58] (Figure 4-5).

Clinical Aspects

The clinical features of aplastic anemia are nonspecific and are usually related to pancytopenia. Pallor, fatigue, recurrent infections and purpura are common features. Lymphadenopathy and splenomegaly are unusual. Severe aplastic anemias are often idiopathic or posthepatitic,[59-61] and are charactereized by extreme pancytopenia and profound marrow hypoplasia (Figure 4-6), as outlined below[62,63]:

1. Peripheral blood
   Pancytopenia with at least two of the following:
   Neutrophils <500/µl
   Platelets <20,000/µl
   Reticulocytes <1% (corrected for hematocrit)
2. Bone marrow
   Severe hypcellularity: <25% normal
   or
   Moderate hypocellularity: 25–50% normal, with fewer than 30% of the remaining cells hematopoietic

The outcome of untreated severe aplastic anemia is very poor, with a 1-year survival of about 20%. Bone marrow transplantation and immunosup-

Bone Marrow Hypoplasia

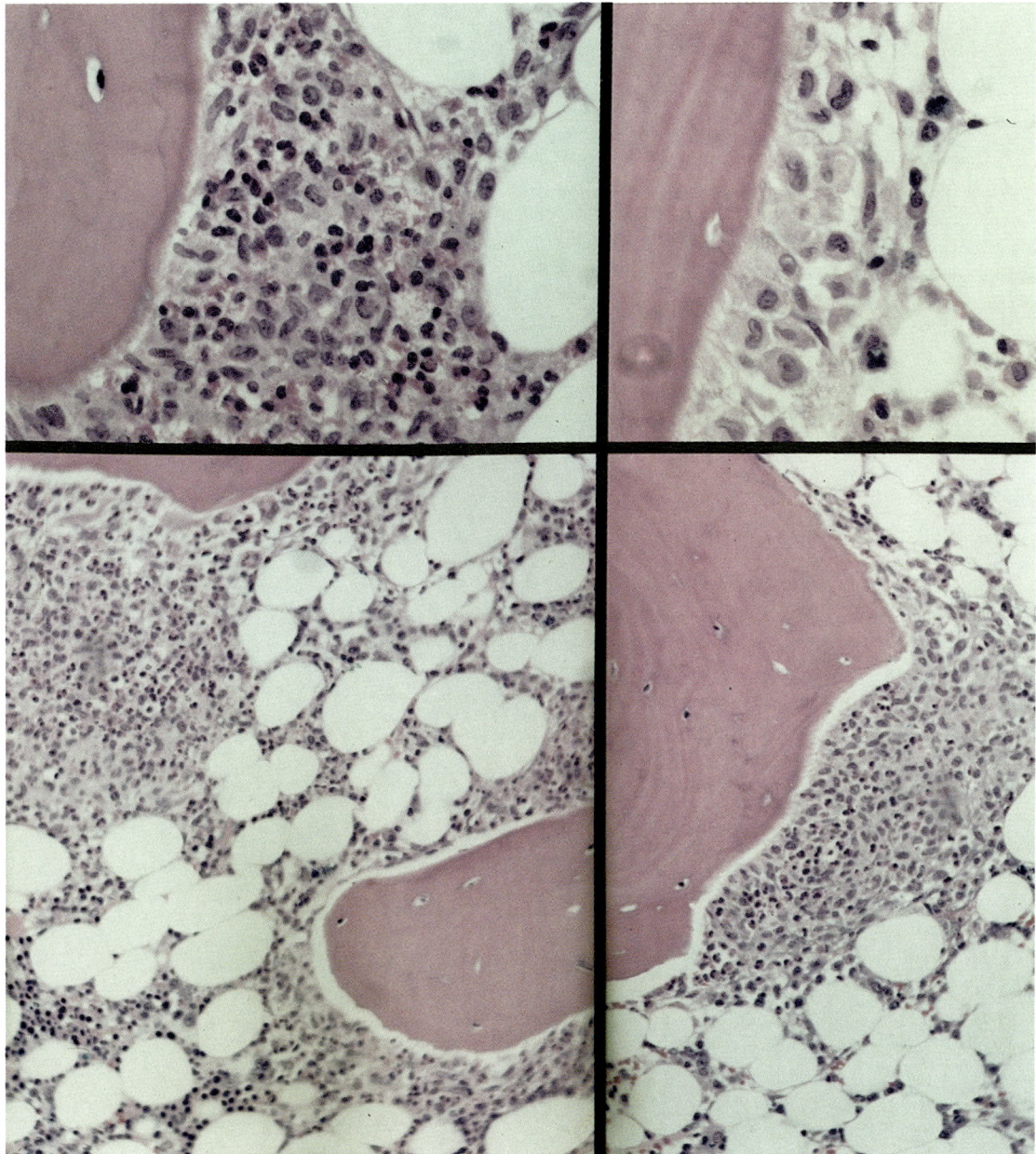

Figure 4-5. Bone marrow biopsy sections obtained 2–4 weeks after GM-CSF therapy in a patient with severe aplastic anemia. Clusters of granulocytes are often found adjacent to the bone trabeculae.

pressive therapy have significantly improved the outcome. One-year survival in patients who receive bone marrow transplants ranges from about 45 to 75%. The best results are obtained in patients younger than 20 years, in untransfused recipients and when the donor is an HLA-identical sibling.[64,65] Immunosuppressive therapy may give comparable results, especially in patients older than 20 years.[65] Hematopoietic growth factors may also play an important role in the treatment of aplastic anemia. Current clinical trials of recombinant growth factors such as GM-CSF, G-CSF and IL-3 on aplastic anemia patients demonstrate at least a temporary proliferative marrow response to these factors.[58,66-68]

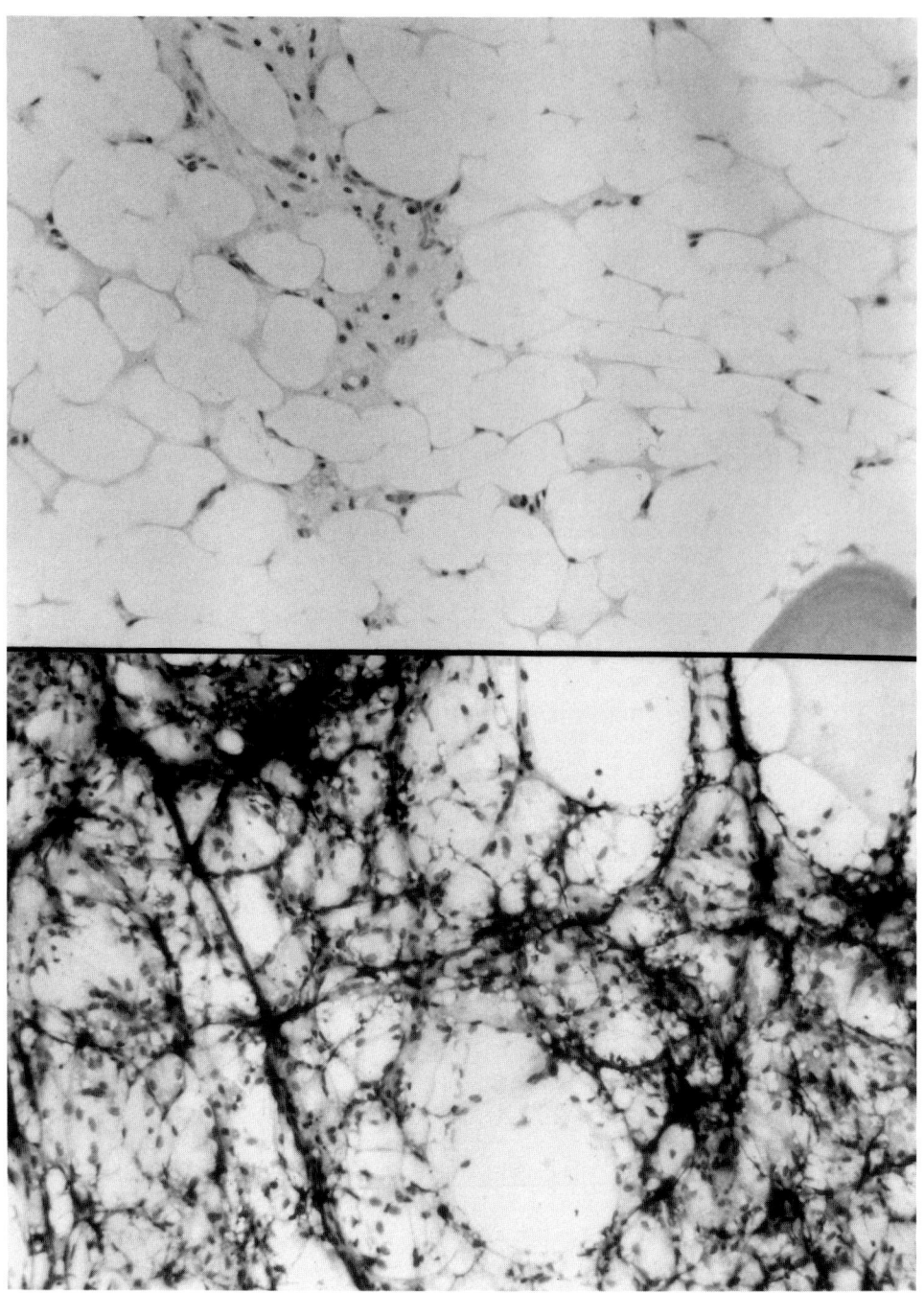

Figure 4-6. Bone marrow biopsy section and smear of a patient with severe aplastic anemia.

PAROXYSMAL NOCTURNAL HEMOGLOBINURIA

Paroxysmal nocturnal hemoglobinuria (PNH) is an acquired disorder of the hematopoietic stem cells characterized by the formation of defective erythrocytes, leukocytes and platelets due to deficiency of a number of surface membrane phosphatidylinositol-linked proteins.[69-78] The protein deficiencies are of three major categories: (1) Complement regulatory proteins including decay accelerating factor (DAF,

CD55), membrane inhibitor of reactive lysis (MIRL, CD59) and C8 binding protein; (2) membrane enzymes consisting of acetylcholinesterase, alkaline phosphatese and 5'-ectonucleotidase, and (3) other membrane-associated proteins such as lymphocyte function antigen-3 (LFA-3), CD14 and CD16.[69-79]

PNH is characterized by various degrees of hemolytic anemia (and often hemoglobinura) due to increased sensitivity of the affected RBCs to complement, venous thrombosis in unusual sites, and deficient hematopoiesis.[78]

Etiology and Pathogenesis

The etiology of PNH is not known. The lack of several membrane-associated proteins in PNH suggests a common posttranslational defect rather than genetic deletion.[79] It has been demonstrated that these proteins are attached to the membrane by glycosyl phosphatidylinositol. PNH may be in part the result of some defects in the protein attachment processes. The cause of increased red blood cell sensitivity to complement seems to be the lack of expression of DAF and MIRL. DAF accelerates the rate of destruction of erythrocyte-bound complement (C3 or C5) activators; in the presence of DAF, the enzyme complexes C3bBb and C4b2a are dissociated and therefore have short half-lives of activity.[79-82] Cells that are deficient in DFA lack the capacity to control activation of the alternative pathway of complement, and as a consequence, enhanced suseptibility to complement-mediated lysis.

MIRL regulates the activation of the membrane attack complex (C5b-9), and diminishes the rate of assembly of the polymerized C9 complex.[79] MIRL seems to play a more important role than the DFA in the protection of RBCs against complement activation.[80]

In vitro studies have demonstrated that two clones of pluripotent stem cells are present in the bone marrow of PNH patients: a defective (PNH) clone and a clone which is not defective in expressing membrane proteins.[83,84] However, in most instances, the non-PNH clone does not show a growth advantage over the defective PNH clone. In vitro studies show a marked decrease in erythroid and myeloid precursor cells in the bone marrow and peripheral cultures of PNH patients, supporting the strong clinical association between PNH and aplastic anemia.[85] Because of this close association, it has been suggested that the second non-PNH clone in the PNH bone marrow is most commonly an aplastic anemia clone.[85]

Pathology

Bone marrow in most instances is hypocellular, with features very similar to those of aplastic anemia. However, some cases may show marrow hypercellularity. There is erythroid preponderance, and stainable iron is often absent.

Peripheral blood examination commonly reveals a very severe anemia with a mild to moderate reticulocytosis. There is evidence of increased sensitivity to complement lysis, confirmed by positive sucrose hemolysis and Ham's acid hemolysis tests. Granulocytopenia and thrombocytopenia are frequent features. The LAP is low. PNH is distinguished from aplastic anemia by the following features: reticulocytosis, hemosiderinuria and hemoglobinuria, and a positive Ham's acid hemolysis test.

Clinical Aspects

The disease may affect patients at any age, and the severity of the clinical findings may vary considerably. The peak incidence is between 25 and 35 years. The most prominent feature of PNH is the complement-induced hemolysis, which is sometimes associated with hemoglobinuria. Hemoglobinuria is most commonly irregular, but in its classical form it is cyclic and occurs during sleep.

In addition to the hemolytic anemia and hemoglobinuria, PNH patients may demonstrate iron deficiency (loss of hemosiderin and hemoglobin in the urine), bleeding (thrombocytopenia), thrombosis (probably due to platelet activation by complement) and abnormal renal function.

In the majority of PNH patients, the defect is permanent and leads to aplastic anemia. Occasional cases of PNH with spontaneous recovery have been reported.[86] A positive Ham's acid hemolysis test and intravascular hemolysis have been noted in a number of patients with myeloproliferative disorders or myelodysplastic syndromes, suggesting an association between PNH and these disorders.[87] PNH has also been reported in association with acute nonlymphoid leukemia, suggesting that PNH is a preleukemic disorder.[88-90]

References

1. Rosendorf J, Berstein R, MacDugall L, et al: Fanconi anemia: Another disease of unusually high prevalence in the Afrikaans population in South Africa. *Am J Med Genet* 27:793, 1987.
2. Saunders EF, Freedman MH: Constitutional aplastic anemia: Defective hematopoietic stem cell growth in vitro. *Br J Haematol* 40:277, 1978.
3. Poon PK, O'Brien RL, Parker JW: Defective DNA repair in Fanconi's anemia. *Nature* 250:223, 1974.
4. Timme TL, Moses RE: Review: Diseases with DNA damage—processing defects. *Am J Med Sci* 295:40, 1988.
5. Rosendorf J, Bernstein R: Fanconi's anemia—chromosome breakage studies in homozygotes and heterozygotes. *Cancer Genet Cytogenet* 33:175, 1988.
6. Gordon-Smith EC, Rutherford TR: Fanconi anemia—constitutional, familial aplastic anemia. *Bailliere's Clin Haematol* 2:139, 1989.
7. Fanconi VG: Die familiare panmyelopathie. *Scheweiz Med Wochen* 94:1309, 1964.
8. Shahidi NT, Gerald PS, Diamond LK: Alkali-resistant hemoglobin in aplastic anemia of both acquired and congenital types. *N Engl J Med* 266:177, 1962.
9. Auerbach AD, Weiner MA, Warburton D, et al: Acute myeloid leukemia as the first hematologic manifestation of Fanconi anemia. *Am J Hematol* 12:289, 1982.
10. Lohrman HP: Tolerance of hemopoiesis for repeated cytotoxic drug therapy. *Blut* 39:237, 1979.
11. Morley A, Blake J: An animal model of chronic aplastic marrow failure.1. Late marrow failure after busulfan. *Blood* 44:49, 1974.
12. Hellman S, Botnick LE, Hannon EC, et al: Proliferative capacity of murine hematopoietic stem cells. *Proc Natl Acad Sci USA* 75:490, 1978.
13. Speck B, Gratwohl A, Nissen C, et al: Treatment of severe aplastic anemia. *Exp Hematol* 14:126, 1986.
14. Champlin RE, Feig SA, Sparkes RS, et al: Bone marrow transplantation from identical twins in the treatment of aplastic anemia: Implication for the pathogenesis of the disease. *Br J Haematol* 56:455, 1984.
15. Torok-Storb BJ, Seiff C, Storb R, et al: In vitro tests for distinguishing possible immune-mediated aplastic anemia from transfusion-induced sensitization. *Blood* 55:211, 1980.
16. Zoumbos NC, Ferris WO, Hsu SM: Analysis of lymphocyte subsets in patients with aplastic anemia. *Br J Haematol* 58:95, 1984.
17. Marmont AM: The autoimmune myelopathies. *Acta Haematol* 69:73, 1983.
18. Cuturi MC, Anegion I, Sherman F, et al: Production of hematopoietic colony-stimulating factors by human natural killer cells. *J Exp Med* 169:569, 1989.
19. Heimpel H, Heit W: Drug induced aplastic anemia: Clinical aspects. *Clin Haematol* 9:641, 1980.
20. International Agranulocytosis and Aplastic Anemia Study: Risks of agranulocytosis and aplastic anemia: A first report of their relation to drug use with special reference to analgesics. *JAMA* 256:1749, 1986.
21. Wallerstein RO, Condit PK, Kasper CK, et al: Statewide study of chloramphenicol therapy of fatal aplastic anemia. *JAMA* 208:2045, 1969.
22. West BC, DeVault GA Jr, Clement JC, et al: Aplastic anemia with parenteral chloramphenicol: Review of 10 cases, including the second case of possible increased risk with cimetidine. *Rev Infect Dis* 10:1048, 1988.
23. Weisenberger AS: Mechanisms of action of chloramphenicol. *JAMA* 209:97, 1969.
24. Rosenbach LM, Caviles AP, Mitus WJ: Chloramphenicol toxicity: Reversible vacuolization of erythroid cells. *N Engl J Med* 263:724, 1960.
25. McCurdy PR: Chloramphenicol bone marrow toxicity. *JAMA* 176:588, 1961.
26. Hara H, Koshaki M, Noguchi M, et al: Effect of chloramphenicol on colony formation from erythrocytic precursors. *Am J Hematol* 5:123, 1978.
27. Yunis AA, Miller AM, Salem Z, et al: Chloramphenicol toxicity: Pathogenetic mechanisms and the role of p-NO sub 2 in aplastic anemia. *Clin Toxicol* 17:354, 1980.
28. Wheeldon LW, Lehninger AL: Energy-linked synthesis and decay of membrane proteins in isolated rat liver mitochondria. *Biochemistry* 5:3533, 1966.
29. Kearsey SE, Craig IW: Altered ribosomal RNA genes in mitochondrial mammalian cells with chloramphenicol resistance. *Nature* 290:607, 1981.
30. Yunis AA, Bloomberg GR: Chloramphenicol toxicity: Clinical features and pathogenesis. *Prog Hematol* 4:138, 1964.
31. Plaut ME, Best W: Aplastic anemia after parenteral chloramphenicol: Warning renewed. *N Engl J Med* 306:1486, 1982.
32. Tabulation of reports compiled by the panel on hematology of the registry on adverse reactions. Council on Drugs, American Medical Association, May 1965 and June 1967.
33. de Gruchy GC: *Drug-Induced Blood Disorders*. Oxford, Blackwell Scientific Publications, 1975.
34. Heimpel H, Heit W: Drug-induced aplastic anemia: Clinical aspects. *Clin Hematol* 9:641, 1980.
35. Laskin S, Goldstein BD: Benzene toxicity, a critical evaluation. *J Toxicol Environ Health* 2(suppl):1, 1977.
36. Thnek A, Hogstedt B, Orofsson T: Mechanism of benzene toxicity: Effects of benzene and benzene metabolites on bone marrow cellularity, number of granulopoietic stem cells and frequency of micrinuclei in mice. *Chem Biol Interact* 39:129, 1982.

37. Cronkite EP, Inoue T, Carsten AL, et al: Effects of benzene inhalation on murine pluripotential stem cells. *Toxicol Environ Health* 9:411, 1982.
38. Kalf GF: Recent advances in the metabolism and toxicity of benzene. *CRC Crit Rev Toxicol* 18:141, 1987.
39. Aksoy M: Hematotoxicity and carcinogenicity of benzene. *Environ Health Perspect* 82: 193, 1989.
40. Vigliani ED: Leukemia associated with benzene exposure. *Ann NY Acad Sci* 271:143, 1976.
41. Aksoy M, Dincol K, Akgun T, et al: Hematologic effects of chronic benzene poisoning in 217 workers. *Br J Ind Med* 28:296, 1971.
42. Goldstein BD: Clinical hematotoxicity of benzene. *Adv Med Environ Toxicol* 4:51, 1983.
43. Ichimaru M, Ishimaru T: Aplastic anemia and atypical leukemia in the A-bomb survivors in control in the fixed cohort of Hiroshima and Nakasdaki 1950–1973. Hiroshima Radiation Effects Research Foundation, *Technical Report Draft Document*, 1977.
44. Lange RD, Wright SW, Tomonage M, et al: Refractory anemia occuring in survivors of the atomic bombing in Nagasaki, Japan. *Blood* 10:312, 1955.
45. Kirshbaum JD, Matsno T, Sato K, et al: A study of aplastic anemia in an autopsy series with special reference to atomic bomb survivors in Hiroshima and Nagasaki. *Blood* 38:17, 1971.
46. Court-Brown WM, Doll R: Leukemia and aplastic anemia in patients irradiated for ankylosing spondylitis. *Med Res Council Special Report 295.* London, H. M. Stationary Office, 1957.
47. Camitta BM, Nathan DG, Forman EN, et al: Posthepatitic aplastic anemia: An indication for early bone marrow transplantation. *Blood* 43:4
48. McSweeney PA, Carter JM, Green GJ, et al: Fatal aplastic anemia associated with hepatitis B viral infection. *Am J Med* 85:255, 1988.
49. Rasken AR, Richter P, Tallal L, et al: Hematologic defects of intrauterine rubella. *JAMA* 199:111, 1967.
50. Ahronheim GA, Auger F, Joncas JH, et al: Primary infection by Epstein-Barr virus presenting as aplastic anemia. *N Engl J Med* 309:313, 1983.
51. Barinski B, Armstrong G, Truman JT, et al: Epstein-Barr virus in the bone marrow of patients with aplastic anemia. *Ann Intern Med* 109:695, 1988.
52. Spivak JL, Bender BS, Quinn TC, et al: Hematologic abnormalities in the acquired immune deficiency syndrome. *Am J Med* 77:224, 1984.
53a. Young N, Mortimer P: Viruses and bone marrow failure. *Blood* 63:729, 1984.
53b. Rosenfeld SJ, Young NS: Viruses and bone marrow failure. *Blood Rev* 5:71, 1991.
54. Gordon-Smith EC: Aplastic anemia: Speculations on pathogenesis, in Lewis SM, Verwilghen RL (eds), *Dyserythropoiesis.* London, Academic Press, 1977, p 149.
55. Te Velde J, Haak HL: Aplastic anemia. Histological investigation of methacrylate embedded bone marrow biopsy specimens: Correlation with survival after conventional treatment in 15 adult patients. *Br J Haematol* 35:61, 1977.
56. Sale GE, Rajantie J, Doney K, et al: Does histologic grading of inflammation in bone marrow predict the response of aplastic anemia patients to anti-thymocyte globulin? *Br J Haematol* 67:261, 1987.
57. Zoumbos NC, Gascon P, Djeu JY, et al: Circulating activated suppressor T lymphocytes in aplastic anemia. *N Engl J Med* 312:257, 1985.
58. Naeim F, Champlin R, Nimer S: Bone marrow changes in patients with refractory aplastic anemia treated by recombinant GM-CSF. *Hematol Pathol* 4:19, 1990.
59. Singer JW, Doney KC, Thomas ED: Coculture studies of 16 untransfused patients with aplastic anemia. *Blood* 54:180, 1979.
60. Abdou NI, Verdirame JD, Amare M, et al: Heterogeneity of pathogenetic mechanisms in aplastic anemia: Efficacy of therapy based on in vitro results. *Ann Intern Med* 95:43, 1981.
61. Bancigalupo A, Van Lint MT, Congiu M, et al: Treatment of SAA in Europe 1970–1985: A report of the SAA Working Party. *Bone Marrow Transplant* 1(suppl 1):19, 1986.
62. Camitta BM, Storb R, Thomas ED: Aplastic anemia (first of two parts). Pathogenesis, diagnosis, treatment, and prognosis. *N Engl J Med* 306:645, 1982.
63. Gordon-Smith EC: Aplastic anemia—aetiology and clinical features. *Bailliere's Clin Haematol* 2:1, 1989.
64. Anasetti C, Doney KC, Storb MD, et al: Marrow transplantation for severe aplastic anemia. Long term outcome in fifty "untransfused" patients. *Ann Intern Med* 104:461, 1986.
65. Marmont AM, Bacigalupo A: Aplastic anemia: Pathogenesis and treatment. *Hematologica* 73:133, 1988.
66. Antin JH, Smith BR, Holmes W, et al: Phase 1/II study of recombinant human granulocyte-macrophage colony-stimulating factor in aplastic anemia and myelodysplastic syndrome. *Blood* 72:705, 1988.
67. Vadhan-Raj S, Buescher S, Broxmeyer HE, et al: Stimulation of myelopoiesis in patients with aplastic anemia by recombinant human granulocyte-macrophage colony stimulating factor. *N Engl J Med* 319:1628, 1988.
68. Chaplin RE, Nimer SD, Ireland P, et al: Treatment of refractory aplastic anemia with recombinant human granulocyte-macrophage-colony-stimulating factor. *Blood* 73:694, 1989.
69. Rosse WF: Paroxysmal nocturnal hemoglobinuria: The biochemical defects and the clinical syndrome. *Blood Rev* 3:192, 1989.
70. Nicholson-Weller A, March JP, Rosenfeld SL, et al: Affected erythrocytes of patients with paroxysmal noctur-

nal hemoglobinuria are deficient in the complement regulatory protein, decay accelerating factor. *Proc Natl Acad Sci USA* 80:5066, 1983.
71. Kinoshita T, Medof ME, Silber R, et al: Distribution of decay accelerating factor in the peripheral blood of normal individuals and patients with paroxysmal nocturnal hemoglobinuria. *J Exp Med* 162:75, 1985.
72. Hansch GM, Schonermark S, Roelcke D: Paroxysmal nocturnal hemoglobinuria type III. Lack of an erythrocyte membrane protein restricting the lysis of C5b-9. *J Clin Invest* 80:7, 1987.
73. Zalman LS, Wood LM, Frank MM, et al: Deficiency of the homologous restriction factor in paroxysmal nocturnal hemoglobinuria. *J Exp Med* 165:572, 1987.
74. Rosse WF: Paroxysmal nocturnal hemoglobinuria and decay accelerating factor. *Ann Rev Med* 41:43, 1990.
75. Selvaraj P, Dustin ML, Silber R, et al: Deficiency of lymphocyte function-associated antigen 3(LFA-3) in paroxysmal nocturnal hemoglobinuria. *J Exp Med* 166:1011, 1987.
76. Auditore JV, Hartman RC, Flexner JM, et al: The erythrocyte acetyl cholinesterase enzyme in paroxysmal nocturnal hemoglobulinemia. *Arch Pathol* 69:534, 1960.
77. Lewis SM, Daice JV: Neutrophil (leukocyte) alkaline phosphatase in paroxysmal noctural hemoglobinuria. *Br J Haematol* 11:549, 1965.
78. Rosse WF: Paroxysmal nocturnal hemoglobinuria and decay-accelerating factor. *Annu Rev Med* 41:431, 1990.
79. Rosse WF: Dr. Ham's test revisited. *Blood* 78:547, 1991.
80. Wilcox LA, Ezzell JL, Bernshaw NJ, et al: Molecular basis of the enhanced suseptibility of the erythrocytes of paroxysmal nocturnal hemoglobinuria to hemolysis in acidified serum. *Blood* 78:820, 1991.
81. Kinoshita T, Medof ME, Nussenzweig V: Endogenous association of decay accelerating factor (DAF) with C4b and C3b on cell membranes. *J Immunol* 136:3395, 1986.
82. Pangburn MK, Shreiber RD, Muller-Eberhard HJ: Deficiency of an erythrocyte membrane protein with complement regulator activity in paroxysmal nocturnal hemoglobulinuria. *Proc Natl Acad Sci USA* 80:5430, 1983.
83. Oni SB, Osunkoya BO, Luzzato L: Paroxysmal nocturnal hemoglobinuria: evidence for monoclonal origin of the abnormal red cells. *Blood* 36:145, 1970.
84. Rotoli B, Robledo R, Scarpato N, et al: Two populations of erythroid cell progenitors in paroxysmal nocturnal hemoglobinuria. *Blood* 64:847, 1984.
85. Rotoli B, Luzzatto L: Paroxysmal nocturnal hemoglobinuria. *Semin Hematol* 26:201, 1989.
86. Dacie JV, Lewis SM: Paroxysmal nocturnal haemoglobinuria: Clinical manifestation, hematology, and nature of the disease. *Series Haematol* 5:3, 1972.
87. Rotoli B, Luzzatto L: Paroxysmal nocturnal haemoglobinuria. *Bailliere's Clin Haematol* 2:113, 1989.
88. Holden D, Lichtman H: Paroxysmal nocturnal hemoglobinuria with acute leukemia. *Blood* 33:283, 1969.
89. Krause JR: Paroxysmal nocturnal hemoglobinuria and acute non-lymphoid leukemia. A report of three cases exhibiting different cytologic types. *Cancer* 51:2078, 1983.
90. Devine DV, Gluck WL, Rosse WF, et al: Acute myeloblastic leukemia in paroxysmal nocturnal hemoglobinuria. Evidence of evolution from the abnormal paroxysmal nocturnal hemoglobinuria clone. *J Clin Invest* 79:314, 1987.

5 MYELODYSPLASTIC AND MYELOPROLIFERATIVE SYNDROMES

Myelodysplastic and myeloproliferative syndromes are hematologic disorders characterized by clonal expansion of bone marrow multipotent stem cells leading to abnormal maturation and/or proliferation of the hematopoietic cells.[1-10] Dysplastic maturation is the hallmark of myelodysplastic syndromes, resulting in ineffective hematopoiesis and cytopenia, and hyperplasia of the bone marrow cells with peripheral leukocytosis, thrombocytosis and/or erythrocytosis is the characteristic feature of myeloproliferative disorders. All these conditions represent a preleukemic or chronic leukemic phase which may eventually evolve into an acute leukemia.[11-18]

MYELODYSPLASTIC SYNDROMES (MDS)

Myelodysplastic or dysmyelopoiesis syndromes are characterized by ineffective hematopoiesis and peripheral blood cytopenias. The ineffective hematopoiesis has been demonstrated by impaired GM colony formation and abnormal end products in in vitro experiments.[19,20] The defective pluripotent stem cells in MDS may eventually undergo additional nonrandom chromosomal damage, resulting in transformation of MDS to an acute leukemia.[21-23] The overall transformation rate depends on the subtype of MDS, ranging from 10% to over 60%.[10,11,24-26] Because of the natural history of MDS and the possibility of its evolution to an acute leukemia, MDS has also been labeled "preleukemia." However, this term is not accurate and should be used only retrospectively.

Etiology and Pathogenesis

In the majority of patients with MDS, no definitive etiologic factor is identified (primary MDS). However, in some patients, MDS evolves following prolonged courses of cytotoxic and/or radiation therapy.[27-32] Chemical- (benzene, alkalating agents) and/or radiation-induced MDS usually appears 4–5 years after exposure to these agents and has a high rate of transformation to acute leukemia.

The defect in multipotent stem cells may be associated with alteration in oncogene activities. There have been reports demonstrating mutation in the N-ras oncogene (codon 13) in patients with MDS and reporting that such patients may develop AML.[33,34]

Glucose-6-phosphate dehydrogenase isoenzyme studies and cytogenetic analyses support the clonal origin of MDS. The expansion of a genetically aberrant multipotent stem cell results in a morphologically diverse but clonally related progeny and leads to ineffective hematopoiesis.[1-6] The ineffective hematopoiesis may involve one or several hematopoietic lines, resulting in refractory anemia, granulocytopenia with granulocytes defective in phagocytosis, adhesive properties and microbicidal activities,[35] and thrombocytopenia with abnormal megakaryocytes. The abnormality may extend to the lymphoid line and results in a lymphoblastic transformation or evolution of a leukemia with a biphenotypic AML/ALL mixture.[36,37] It may also lead to humoral or cell-mediated suppression of normal hematopoietic stem cells.[38] It has been demonstrated that patients with MDS are deficient in helper T cells and NK activities.[39-41] Recent studies have shown the production and release of an inhibitor of normal granulopoiesis by bone marrow mononuclear cells of patients with MDS.[42,43]

Pathology

The ineffective and dysplastic hematopoiesis in MDS is demonstrated by mono- or pancytopenia and abnormal morphology in one or more hematopoietic lines. Patients with primary MDS usually have a hyper- or normocellular bone marrow, while the bone marrow of therapy-related MDS (T-MDS) patients shows a broad spectrum of cellularity, ranging from 5% to 100%.[28] Bone marrow of T-MDS patients commonly shows trilineage dysplasia involving granulocytic, megakaryocytic and erythroid series, and frequently demonstrates increased amounts of reticulin fibers. In one study, a marked increase in bone marrow reticulin fibers was observed in 50% of T-MDS patients compared to 13% of patients with primary MDS.[28]

There is also architectural disorganization of the hematopoietic cells in the bone marrow of MDS patients, demonstrated by peritrabecular localization of erythroid and megakaryocytic precursors (Figure 5-1) and by the presence of small clusters of blast cells in the central marrow regions.[44-46]

The quantitative and qualitative cytologic changes will now be discussed (Table 5-1).

Dyserythropoiesis

Common bone marrow findings in erythroid precursors include megaloblastoid changes, multinucleation, irregular nuclear shapes, nuclear fragmentation, and the presence of ringed sideroblasts (Figure 5-2). Peripheral blood examination often reveals aniso- and poikilocytosis with macrocytes and microcytes (Figure 5-3), basophilic stippling, Howell-Jolly bodies and, rarely, nucleated red blood cells.

Dysgranulocytopoiesis

Abnormal staining of the primary granules in the promyelocytes and myelocytes is common. There may be a few large granules or hypogranularity, with irregular distribution of the cytoplasmic basophilia. The cytoplasm in the perinuclear area may stain lighter than that in the periphery of the cells. The more mature granulocytic cells may show a marked size variation and decreased or absent secondary granules. Hyposegmentation (pseudo-Pelger-Huet anomaly), hypersegmentation and other forms of abnormal nuclear morphology such as ringed nuclei are seen (Figure 5-4).

Abnormal Megakaryocytes and Platelets

Mono- and binuclear micromegakarocytes, as well as megakaryocytes with multiple small separate nuclei, are common. Megakaryocytes with hypo- or hyperlobulated nuclei, vacuolated cytoplasm and giant or abnormal granules are frequently seen (Figures 5-5 to 5-7). Giant platelets and megakaryocytic fragments may be present in the peripheral blood (Figure 5-8). Platelets may show abnormal ultrastructural features such as variation in the shape and size of the granules and decrease or absence of the microtubules[9b] (Figures 5-8 and 5-9).

Classification

Myelodysplastic syndromes or refractory anemias are classified, according to the French-American-British

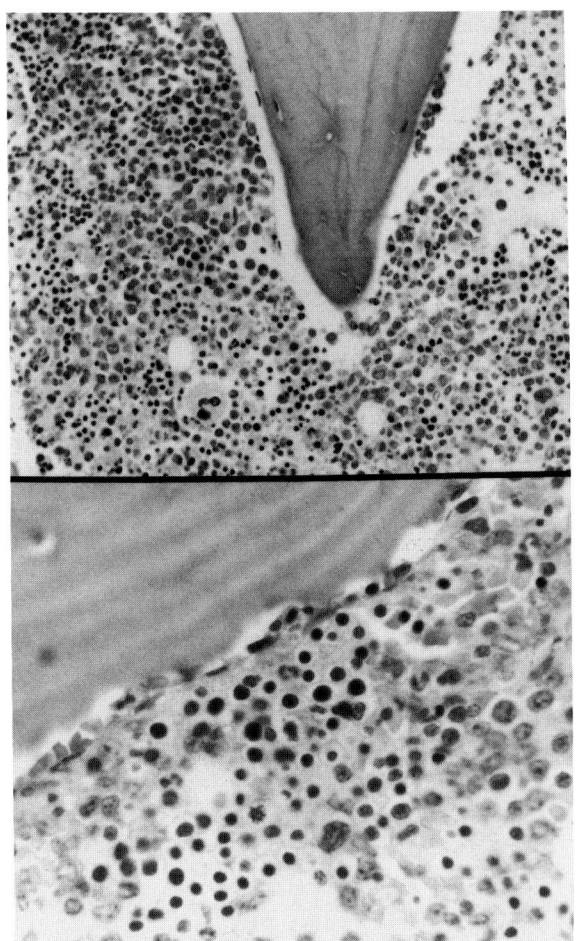

Figure 5-1. Bone marrow biopsy section from a patient with myelodysplastic syndrome (RARS) demonstrating clusters of erythroid cells adjacent to the bone trabeculae.

Table 5-1 Bone Marrow and Peripheral Blood Findings in Subtypes of MDS

Subtype	Bone Marrow	Peripheral Blood
RA	Dyserythropoiesis, blasts <5%, ringed sideroblasts <15%	Anemia, reticulocytopenia, blasts <1%
RARS	Dyserythropoiesis, blasts <5%, ringed sideroblasts >15%	Anemia, dimorphic RBCs, reticulocytopenia, blasts <1%
RAEB	Dysgranulocytopoiesis, dyserythropoiesis, dysmegakaryocytopoiesis, blasts 5–20%	Bi- or trilineage cytopenia, reticulocytopenia, blasts <5%
CMML	Increased promonocytes dysgranulocytopoiesis, dyserythropoiesis, dysmegakaryocytopoiesis, blasts 5–20%	Monocytosis >1,000/μl, reticulocytopenia, blasts <5%
RAEB-T	Dysgranulocytopoiesis, dyserythropoiesis, dysmegakaryocytopoiesis, blasts 20–30%, Auer rods	Bi- or trilineage cytopenia, reticulocytopenia, blasts >5%, Auer rods

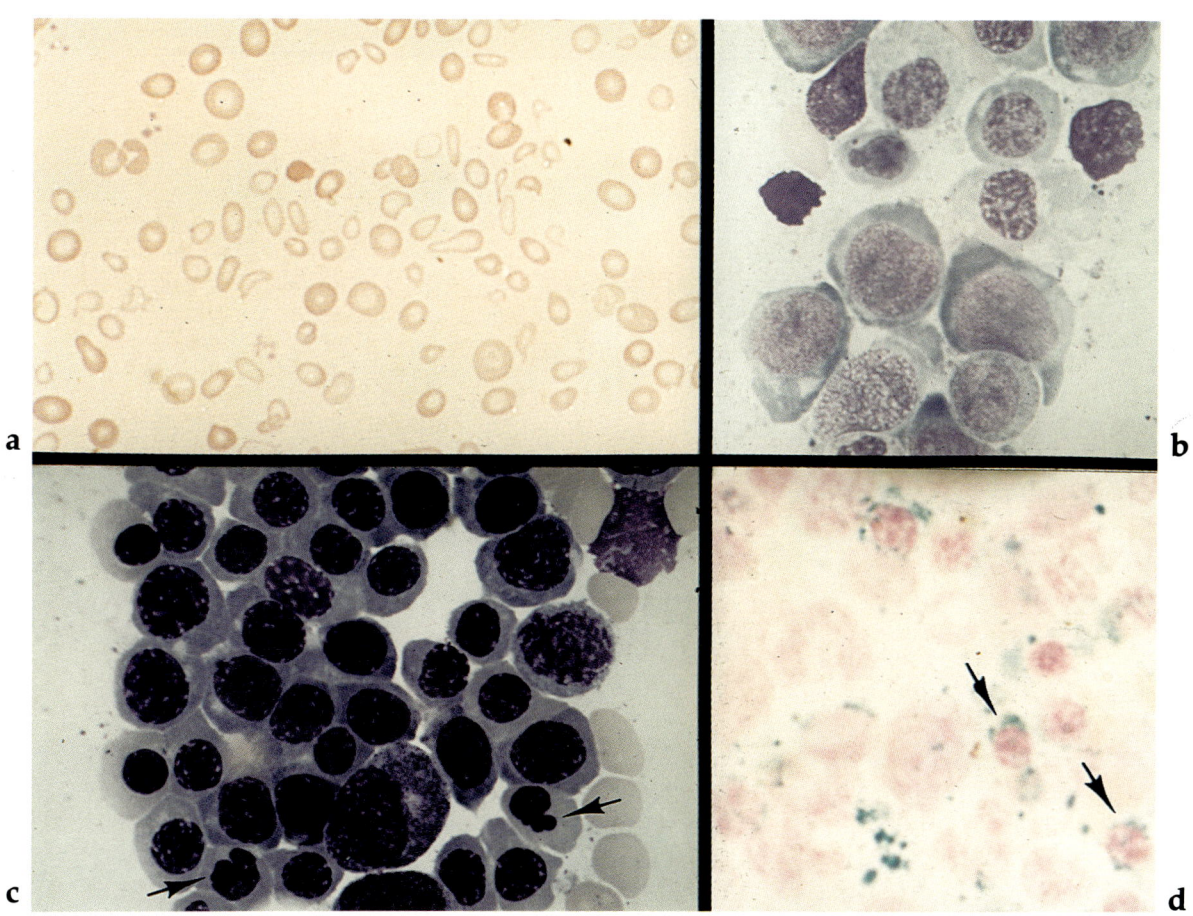

Figure 5-2. Abnormal erythroid morphology in myelodysplastic syndrome. A peripheral blood smear (a) showing marked aniso-poikilocytosis; bone marrow smears (b, c, d) demonstrating megaloblastic (b) and dysplastic (c, arrows) erythropoiesis and several ringed sideroblasts with iron stain (d, arrows).

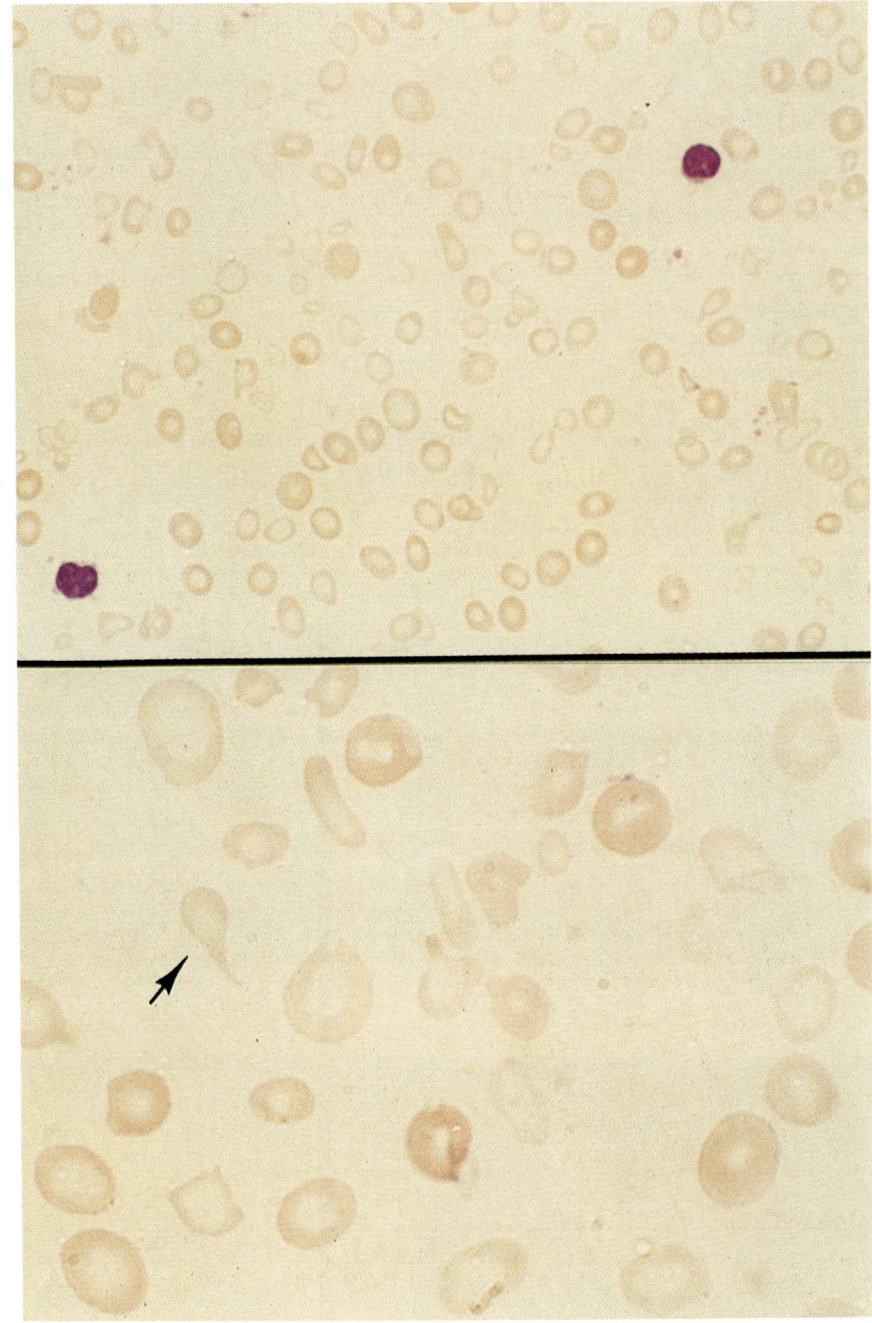

Figure 5-3. A peripheral blood smear demonstrating marked anisocytosis and poikilocytosis with the presence of macrocytes, microcytes, ovalocytes and teardrops (arrow).

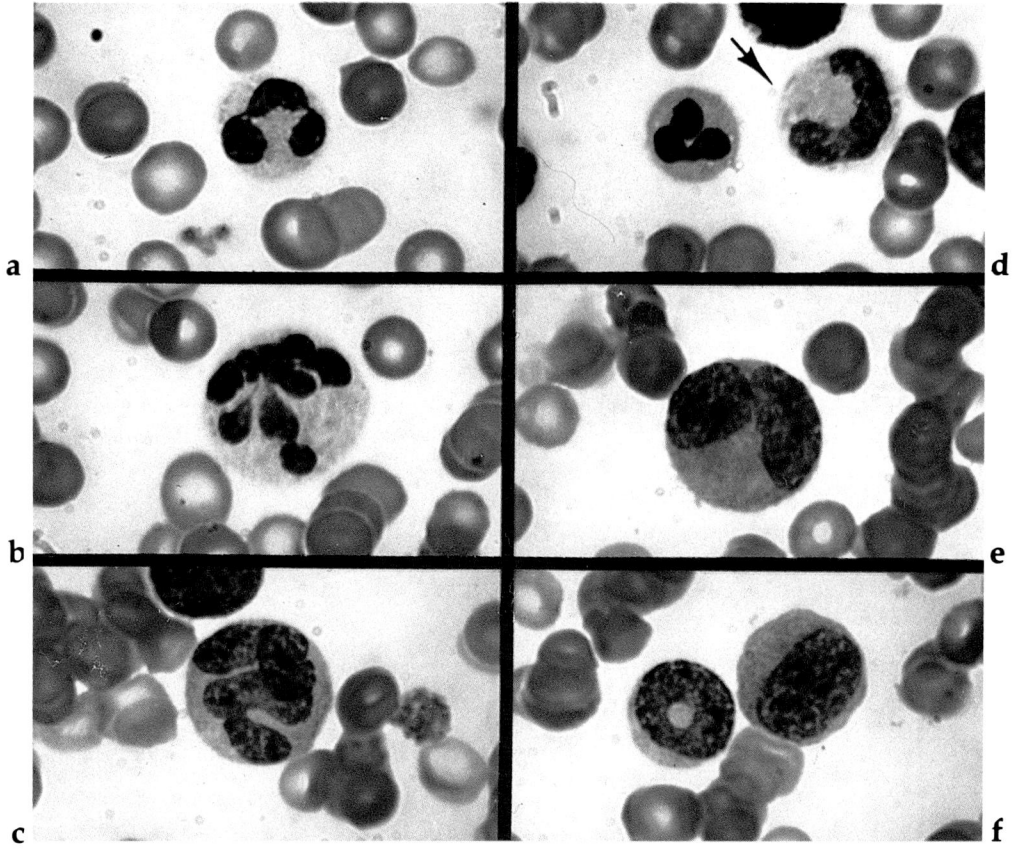

Figure 5-4. Dysplastic granulopoiesis in myelodysplastic syndromes: (a) a hypogranular segmented neutrophil; (b, c) giant hypersegmented neutrophils; (d) a hypogranular metamyelocyte (arrow); (e) a giant band, and (f) a band with a doughnut-shaped nucleus.

(FAB) Cooperative Group, into refractory anemia, refractory anemia with ringed sideroblasts, refractory anemia with excess blasts, chronic myelomonocytic leukemia and refractory anemia with excess blasts in transformation.[11,12]

Refractory Anemia (RA)

RA represents a dyserythropoietic process leading to reticulocytopenia and anemia. Patients are usually over 50 years, have normo- or hypercellular marrow with erythroid hyperplasia and stainable iron. Ringed sideroblasts are absent or rare (<15% of nucleated red blood cells), and blast cells account for less than 5% of the nucleated bone marrow cells. Erythroid dysplasia with anisopoikilocytosis is the hallmark of RA, often with absent or insignificant granulocytic and megakaryocytic dysplasia (see Figure 5-2). However, other solitary cytopenias, such as rare cases of dysgranulocytopoiesis or dysmegakaryocytopoiesis without anemia, may be included in this category. RA is the most frequent type of MDS, accounting for 25–30% of the cases, with a median survival of 50 months and a 12% rate of progression to acute leukemia.[10]

Refractory Anemia with Ringed Sideroblasts (RARS)

The characteristics of RARS are similar to those of RA, except that in patients with RARS, more than 15% of the bone marrow nucleated red blood cells are

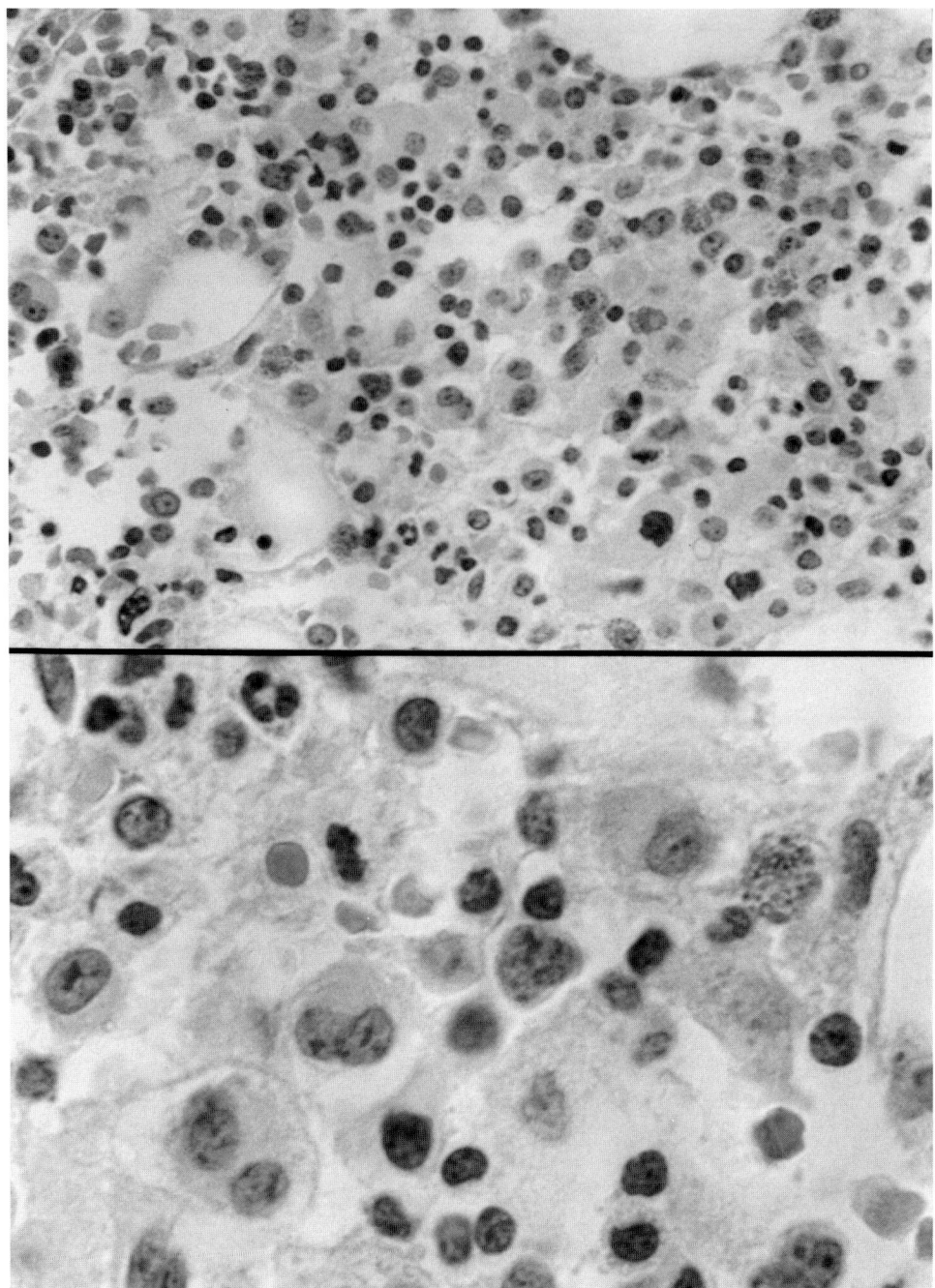

Figure 5-5. Bone marrow biopsy section from a patient with myelodysplastic syndrome (RAEB) demonstrating several mono- and binuclear micromegakaryocytes.

Figure 5-6. Bone marrow smears demonstrating the bi- and mononuclear megakaryocytes frequently seen in myelodysplastic syndrome.

Myelodysplastic and Myeloproliferative Syndromes

ringed sideroblasts (see Figure 5-3). RARS accounts for about 20–25% of MDS, with a median survival of about 50 months and <10% chance of evolving to acute leukemia. The two morphologic types of refractory anemia, RA and RARS, are associated with a much longer median survival and a lower incidence of progression to leukemia than the other subtypes of MDS.[10] (Table 5-2).

Refractory Anemia with Excess Blasts (RAEB)

This syndrome is associated with cytopenia affecting two or more of the hematopoietic lines, evidenced by disgranulocytopoiesis, dyserythropoiesis and/or dysmegakaryocytopoiesis (Figure 5-10). The bone marrow is usually hyper- or normocellular, and rarely hypocellular, with a myeloid left shift and increased myeloblasts. Myeloblasts range from >5% to <20% in the bone marrow and <5% in the peripheral blood (Figures 5-10 and 5-11). Auer rods are not seen. Ringed sideroblasts may be present but are usually <15% of the nucleated red blood cells. RAEB accounts for up to 23% of MDS, with a median survival of 11 months and a 44% chance of progression to acute leukemia.[10]

Chronic Myelomonocytic Leukemia (CMML)

The morphologic features of CMML are similar to those of RAEB, except that in CMML there is an

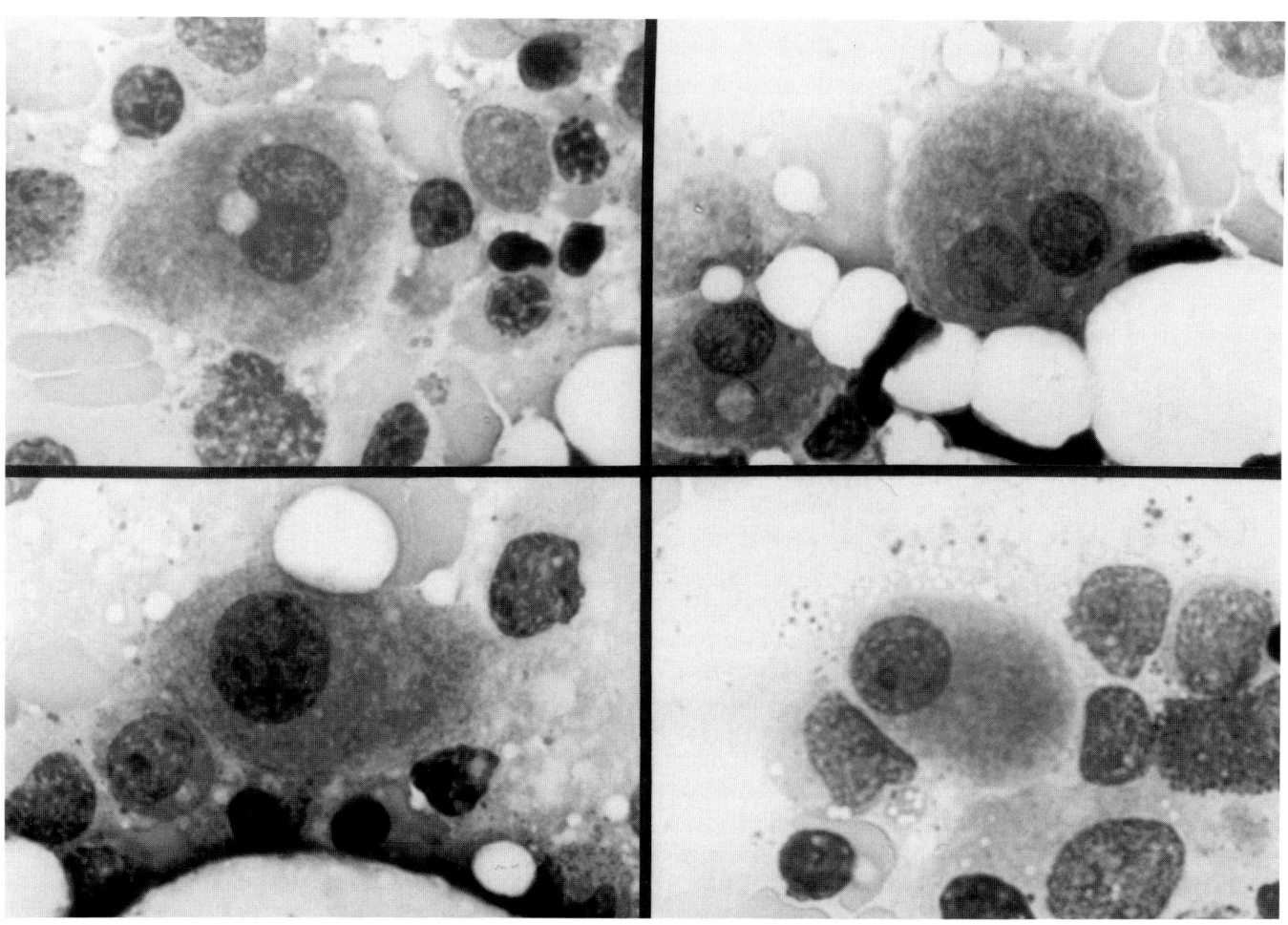

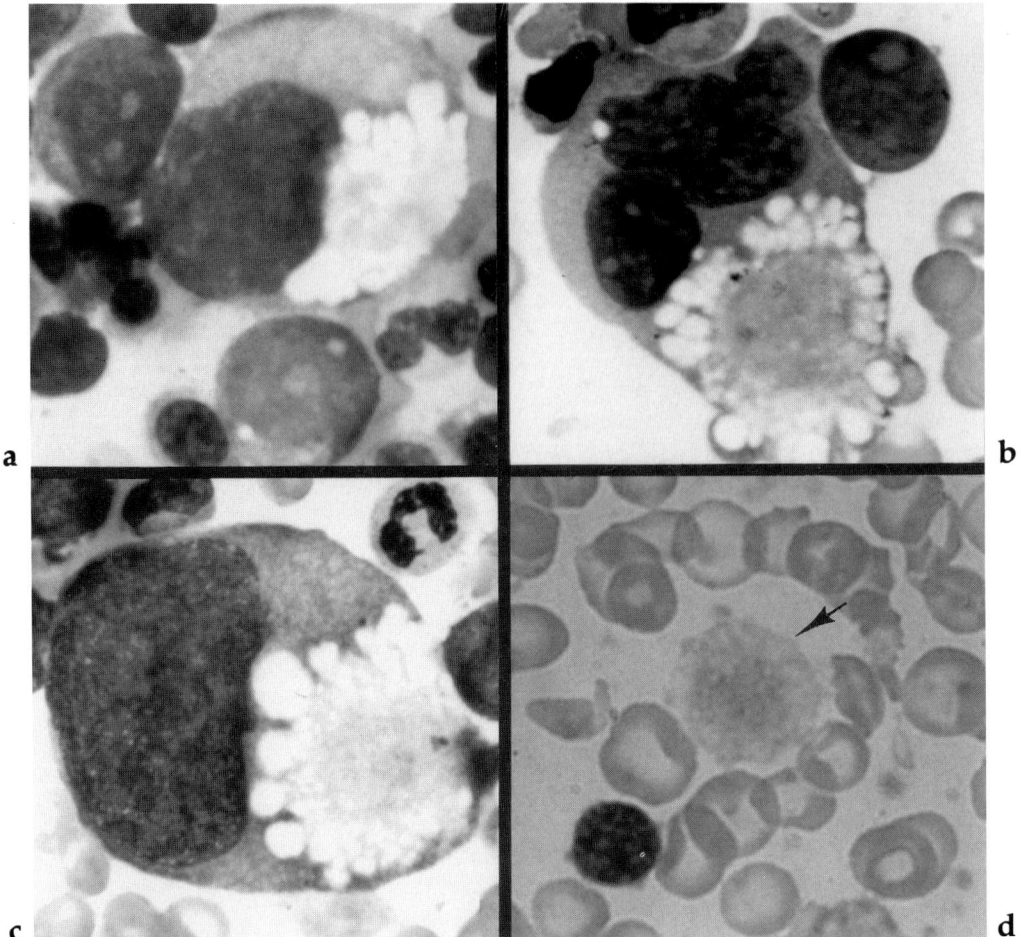

Figure 5-7. Vacuolated megakaryocytes may be present in myelodysplastic syndromes and megakaryoblastic leukemias (a, b, c); vacuoles may surround a central cytoplasmic core (b, c). This cytoplasmic core is probably the source of some of the megakaryocytic fragments found in the peripheral blood (d, arrow).

increased proportion of monocytic precursors (Figure 5-12). Identification of the monocytic precursors in the marrow may require cytochemical stains such as a nonspecific esterase stain (Figure 5-13). The defining feature of CMML is the presence of peripheral blood monocytosis of >1000/µl (Figure 5-14). Blast cells may be present in the peripheral blood but are <5% of the leukocyte differential count. CMML accounts for about 15% of MDS, with a median survival ranging from 9 to over 60 months and a 14–40% chance of progression to acute leukemia.[10,28]

Refractory Anemia with Excess Blasts in Transformation (RAEB-T)

The morphologic characteristics of RAEB-T are similar to those of RAEB, except for a higher percentage of blast cells in bone marrow and/or peripheral blood. Blasts account for >5% of the leukocytes in the peripheral blood and 20–30% of the nucleated cells in the bone marrow. Aeur rods may be present. In the recent report by the Morphologic, Immunologic, and Cytogenetic (MIC) Study Group, 9% of the MDS pa-

Myelodysplastic and Myeloproliferative Syndromes

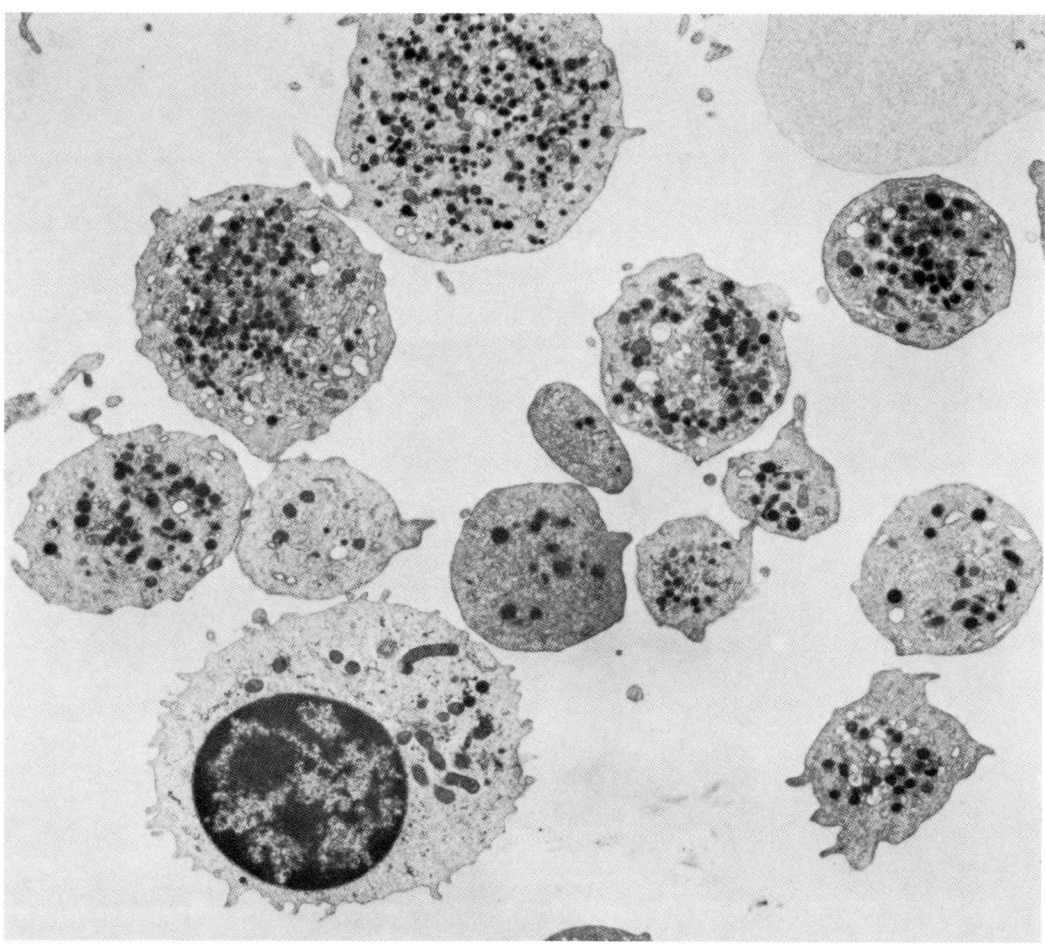

Figure 5-8. Electron micrographs of the platelets of a patient with myelodysplastic syndrome. There is marked variation in the size and granularity of the platelets. A lymphocyte is present at the lower left. From Maldonado JE: The Platelets in preleukemia and myelomonocytic leukemia. Ultrastructure, cytochemistry and cytogenetics, *Mayo Clin Proc* 50:573, 1975, with permission.

tients had RAEB-T, with a 60% rate of progression to acute leukemia and a median survival of 5 months.[10]

Cytogenetic Studies

The incidence of chromosomal aberrations in MDS ranges from 40 to 98% in various reports.[10,28] The higher figures belong to T-MDS and are usually associated with multiple chromosome abnormalities (Tables 5-3 and 5-4). The most common abnormalities in primary MDS include −5, 5q⁻, −7, 7q⁻, +8, 11q⁻ and 20q⁻. In addition, a number of translocations have been reported in primary MDS, such as t(1;3), t(2;11), t(6;9) and t(11;21) (see Table 5-4). In primary MDS, the karyotype may reveal a single abnormality at the time of diagnosis, but additional changes may occur later, especially associated with leukemic transformation of the disease.[28,47,48a,48b] By contrast, patients with T-MDS usually show multiple chromosome changes at diagnosis (see Table 5-4). The most common single chromosome abnormalities associated with T-MDS are 5q⁻, −5, 7q⁻, −7 and 12p⁻. Abnormalities of chromosomes 5 and/or 7, alone or in combination with other chromosomal aberrations,

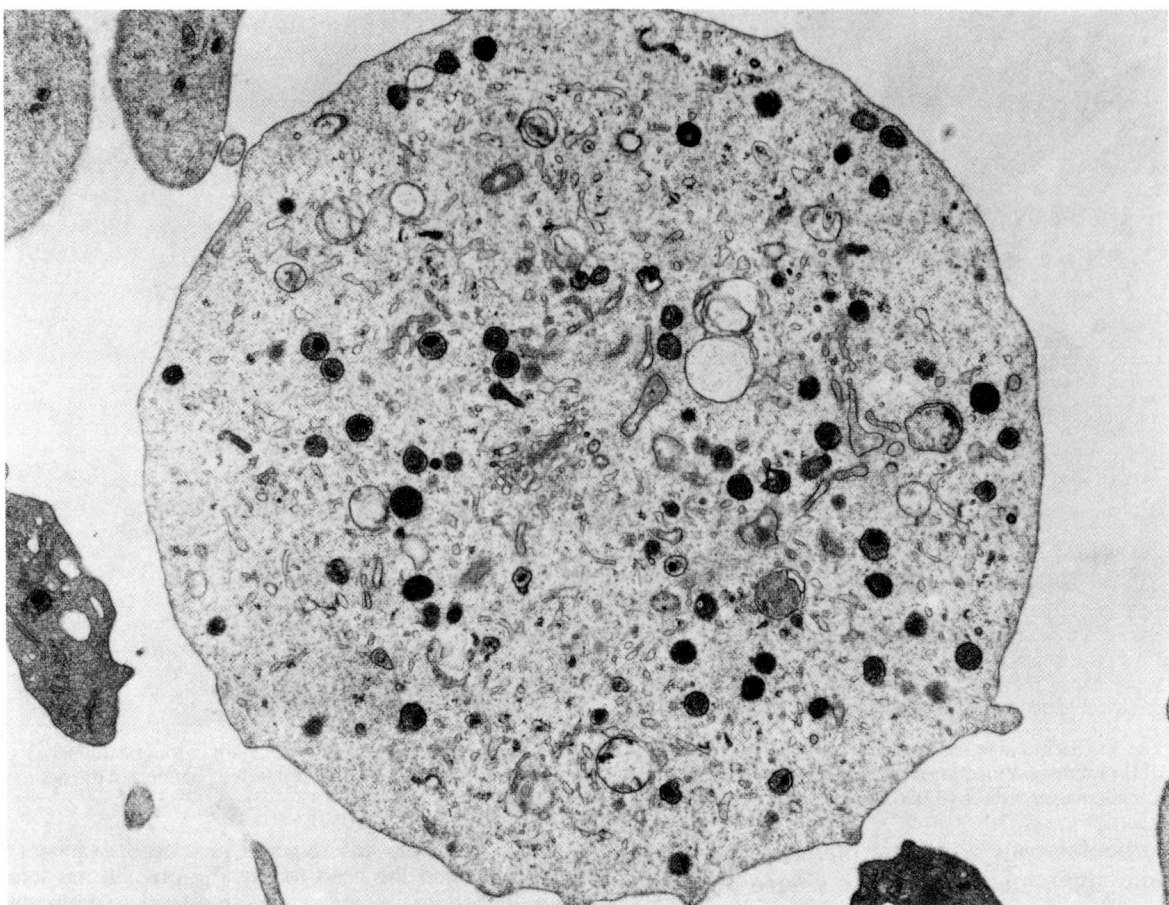

Figure 5-9. A giant platelet devoid of the peripheral band of microtubules. From Maldonado JE: The Plateletes in preleukemia and myelomonocytic leukemia. Ultrastructure, cytochemistry and cytogenetics. *Mayo Clin Proc* 50:573, 1975, with permission.

Table 5-2 Rate of Progression of Leukemia and Survival in Patients With Primary MDS*

Subtypes	Frequency (%)	Percent of Leukemic Progression	Median Survival (Months)
RA	28	12	50
RARS	24	8	51
RAEB	23	44	11
CMML	16	14	11
RAEB-T	9	60	5

* Adapted from the report of the Third MIC Cooperative Study Group: Recommendations for a morphologic, immunologic, and cytogenetic (MIC) working classification of the primary and therapy-related myelodysplastic disorders. *Cancer Genet Cytogenet* 32:1, 1988.

Myelodysplastic and Myeloproliferative Syndromes

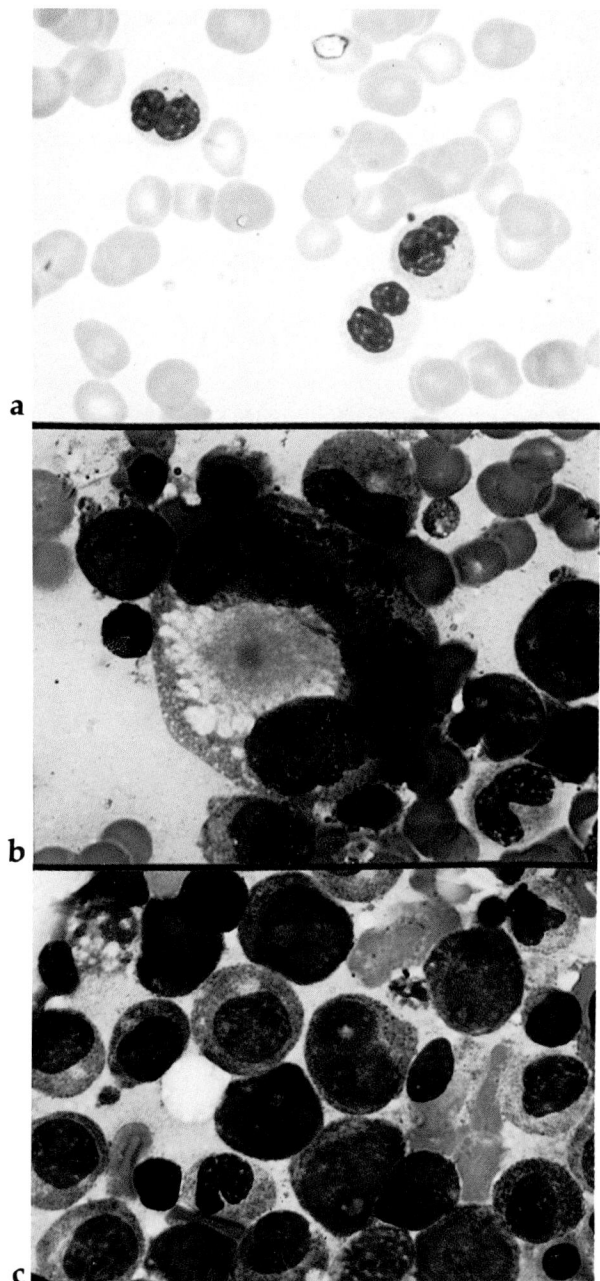

Figure 5-10. Peripheral blood and bone marrow smears from a patient with RAEB: hyposegmented neutrophils (a), a vacuolated megakaryocyte (b) and increased numbers of blast cells (c).

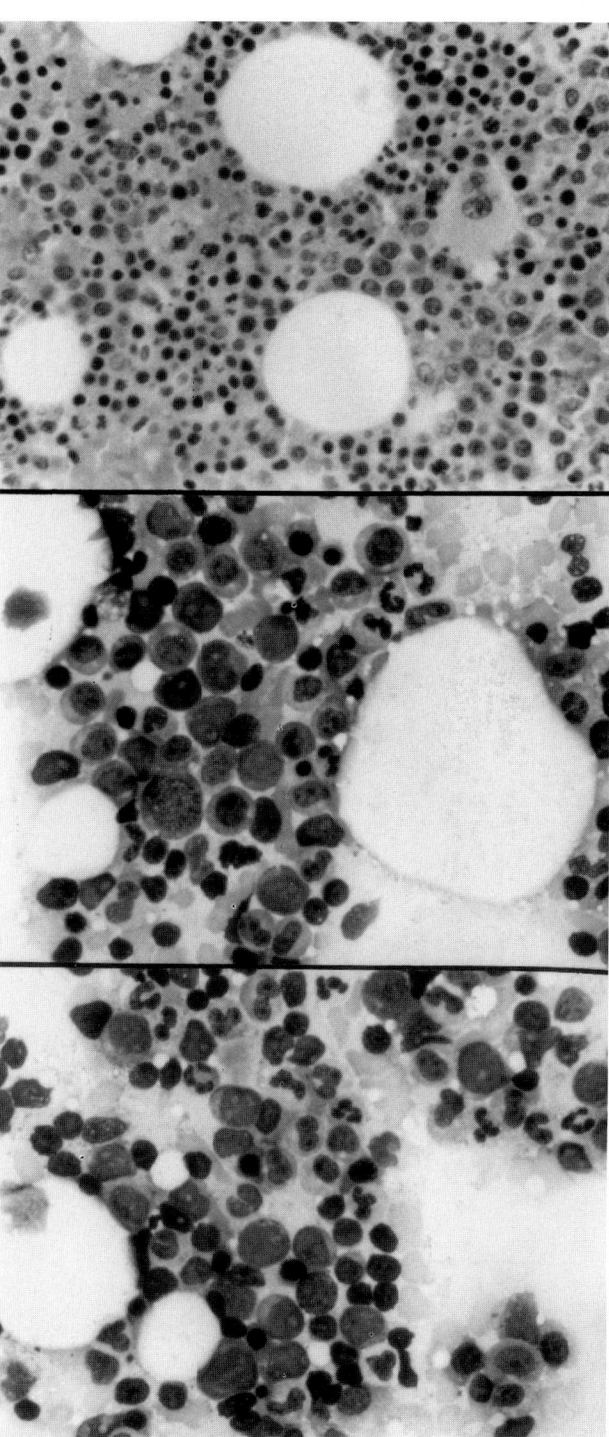

Figure 5-11. In RAEB, bone marrow demonstrates myeloid left shift and increased numbers of blast cells.

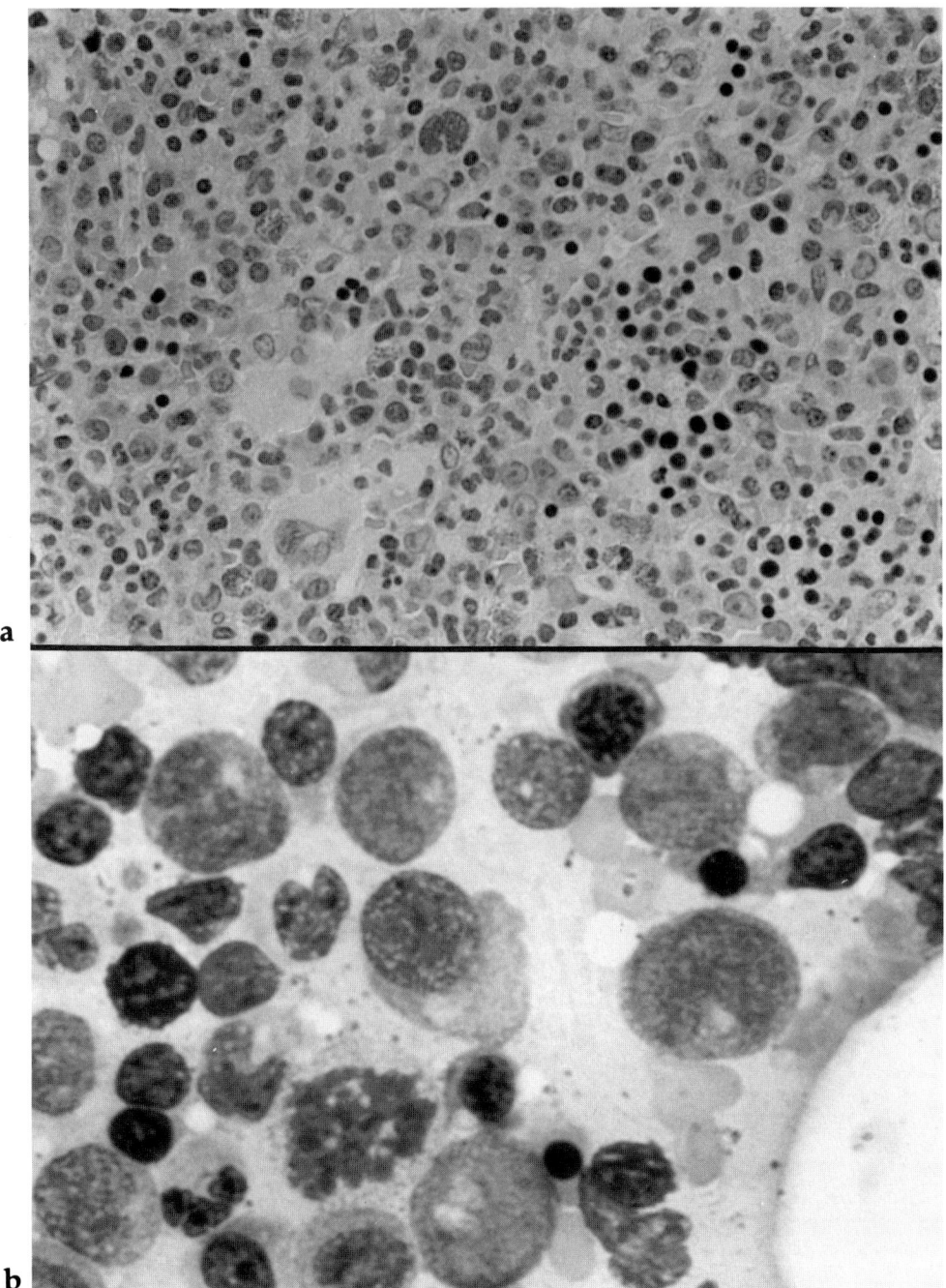

Figure 5-12. In CMML, bone marrow is hypercellular (a, biopsy) and shows increased numbers of immature myelomonocytic cells (b, smear).

Figure 5-13. Bone marrow smears from a patient with CMML demonstrating atypical monocytes (a, arrows). Several cells are nonspecific esterase positive (b, arrows).

Myelodysplastic and Myeloproliferative Syndromes

are the most common karyotypic abnormalities associated with T-MDS (see Table 5-3). In addition, various mutations in N-ras, Ki-ras and H-ras oncogenes have been reported in patients with MDS.[49c]

Two subtypes of MDS with specific chromosome abnormalities will now be briefly discussed.

The 5q⁻ Syndrome

The 5q⁻ syndrome is a disorder primarily observed in elderly women, with a female:male ratio of 2 and a median age of 65 years.[10] The main clinicopathologic features are refractory macrocytic anemia with myelodysplastic bone marrow and the presence of monolobulated micromegakaryocytes.[49b,50] The majority of patients do not show increased bone marrow blasts. 5q is the site of many genes of importance in hematopoiesis, such as GM-CSF, IL-3, IL-4 and IL-5.[48b] The major deletions in this syndrome include del(5)(q12–13q31–33), del(5)(q12q23) and del(5)(q23q32). Patients with 5q⁻ syndrome usually have a long survival.

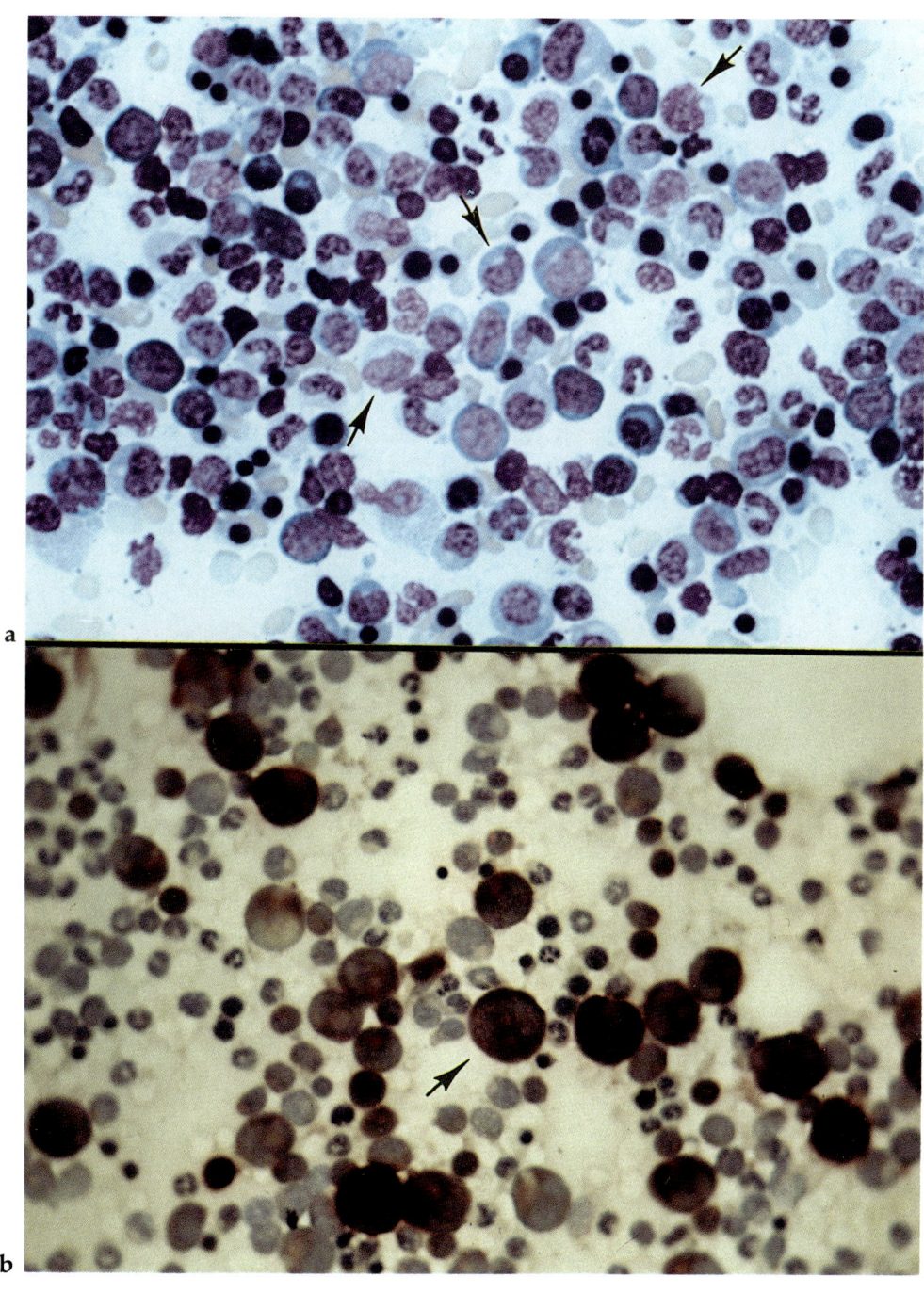

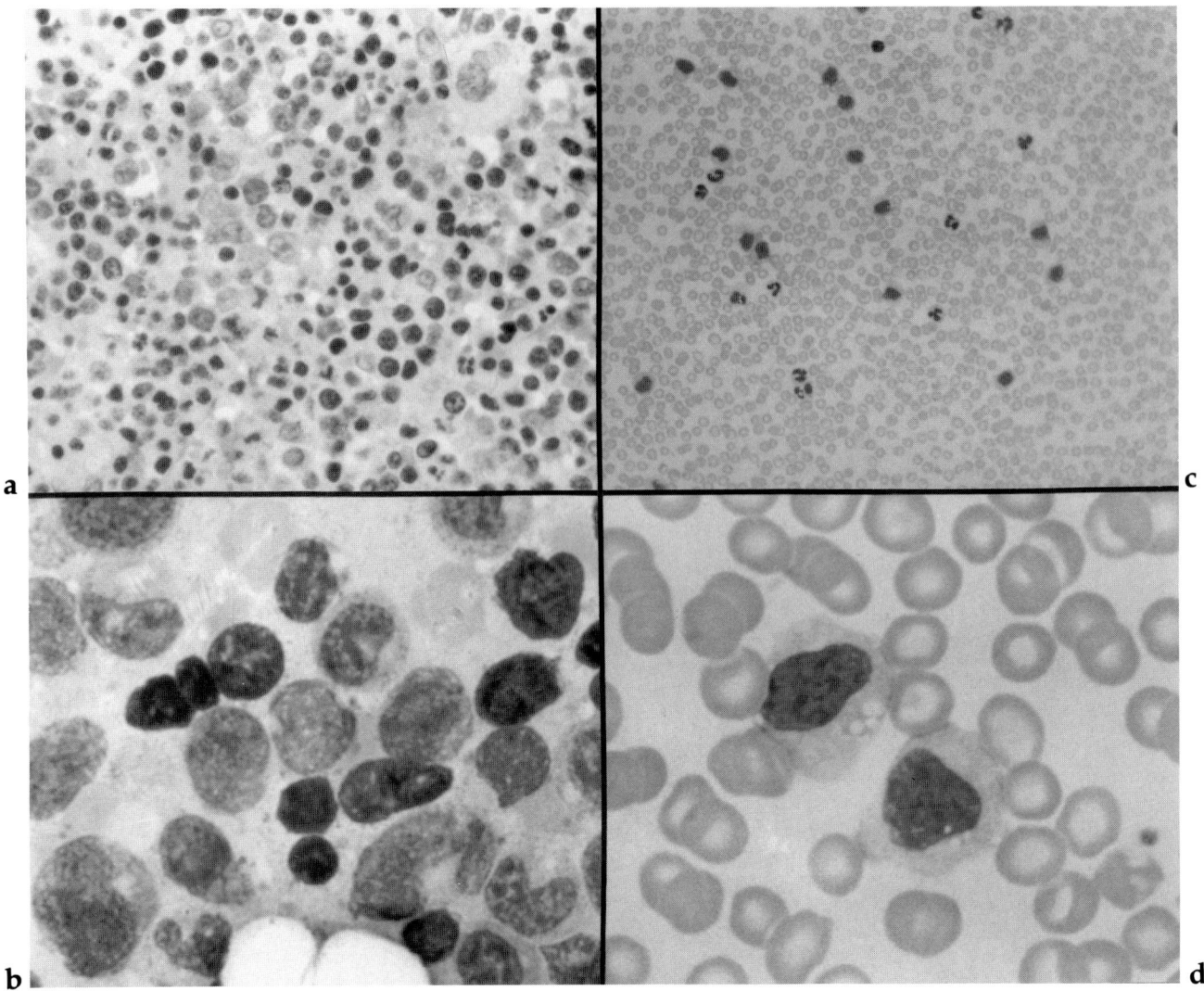

Figure 5-14. In CMML, bone marrow is hypercellular, with a myeloid left shift and increased numbers of immature myelomonocytic cells (a, b); peripheral blood shows monocytosis (c, d).

Table 5-3 Comparison of the Pathologic and Cytogenetic Features of Primary and Therapy-Related MDS*

Features	Primary MDS ($n = 48$)	Therapy-Related MDS ($n = 49$)
Median BM cellularity	80%	60%
Severe trilineage dysplasia	20%	61%
Marked increase in BM reticulin fibers	13%	50%
Transformation to AML	22%	60%
Clonal chromosome Ab	41%	98%
$-5/5q^-$ or $-7/7q^-$	12%	94%

* Adapted from Vardiman JW, et al: Myelodysplasia: A comparison of therapy-related and primary forms. *Ann Biol Clin* 43:372, 1985.

Table 5-4 Chromosome Abnormalities in Patients with MDS*

Primary	Therapy-Related
−7	del(5q)
+8	del(7q)
del(5)(q12–q34)	−5
del(7q)	−7
del(11q)	
del(12)(p11p13)	del(12p)
del(13q)	Any of the above plus:
del(20)(q11q13)	+8
	+21
	3P (del or t)
t(1;3)(p36;q21)	17q (del or t)
t(2;11)(p21;q23)	6p (del or t)
t(6;9)(p23;q34)	19p or q (t)
t(11;21)(q24;q11.2)	Xq13 (t or dup)
t(17q)	Xp11 (t)

* Adapted from the report of the Third MIC Cooperative Study Group: Recommendations for a morphologic, immunologic, and cytogenetic (MIC) working classification of the primary and therapy-related myelodysplastic disorders. Cancer Genet Cytogenet 32:1, 1988.

Monosomy 7 and 7q⁻

Unlike 5q⁻ syndrome, patients with primary MDS or T-MDS associated with 7q⁻ usually have a short survival.[51] Monosomy 7 has been observed in Fanconi's anemia, progressing to acute leukemia.[52]

Other Studies

Special Stains and Immunophenotyping

Cytochemical stains such as peroxidase, Sudan black B, nonspecific esterase and PAS are helpful in identification of the lineage of immature dysplastic cells (see Chapter 2). Peroxidase and Sudan black stains, in addition to identifying myeloblasts, provide information regarding the quantitative changes in the cytoplasmic granules of myeloid cells. Nonspecific esterase is positive in monocytic series, and PAS stain shows coarse positive cytoplasmic granules in dysplastic and leukemic erythroid precursors.

Immunophenotypic studies also provide useful information in defining the lineage association of the blast cells. For example, CD13 and CD33 are present in myeloblasts; CD11c and CD14 are strongly expressed in monocytic cells; glycophorin A is detected in erythroid precursors; and CD41a (glycoprotein IIb/IIIa), CD42a (glycoprotein I bA) and factor VIII are expressed in megakaryocytic series. Antibodies raised against CD10 (CALLA), CD19, CD20, CD5, CD7 and TdT are used for the identification of blast cells of lymphoid origin.

In Vitro Culture

Hematopoietic stem cells derived from patients with MDS demonstrate an abnormal growth pattern in culture.[53-57] Most RA and RARS patients show defective erythroid colony formation. Patients with RAEB, CMML and RAEB-T, in addition to having defective erythropoiesis, show abnormal growth of other colonies.

Clinical Aspects and Prognostic Factors

Primary or de novo MDS is usually a disease of the elderly and is uncommon under the age of 50 years, while T-MDS may arise in patients of any age. T-MDS usually appears 4–5 years following treatment of the primary disease and also has a high rate of transformation to acute nonlymphoid leukemia (see Table 5-3). An increased frequency of MDS among family members has been reported.[56]

Patients may be asymptomatic or may demonstrate mild to severe symptoms related to anemia, granulocytopenia and/or thrombocytopenia. Clinical conditions in some patients may last for years without causing any significant changes and may result in rapid deterioration in others.

Conditions reported in association with a poor prognosis include chromosome aberrations, dysplasia of all hematopoietic lines, a high percentage of micromegakaryocytes, an increased percentage of blasts in bone marrow, atypical in vitro growth of hematopoietic stem cells, DNA hypodiploidy, a decrease in bone marrow mast cells and helper T cells, and an increase in suppressor T cells and dendritic (S-100-positive) histiocytes.[57-62]

A number of modified classifications have been proposed based on a scoring system.[63,64] Low-score conditions include lack of increased blasts in bone marrow, absence of dysplastic changes in granulocytic and megakaryocytic series, and minimal pancytopenia.

Diagnosis of MDS is a clinicopathologic process, and is accomplished by obtaining proper and adequate clinical, family and environmental histories, careful peripheral blood and bone marrow examinations, and cytogenetic studies. Following are some of the recommendations of the Third MIC Cooperative Study Group regarding MDS patients[10]:

1. Clinicians are urged to take very careful clinical histories, particularly with regard to exposure to environmental cytotoxic agents.
2. Bone marrow biopsy is essential in all cases of MDS.
3. The possibility of a genetic predisposition or familial occurrence should be considered in children and young adults, particularly with RARS in children and adults and with monosomy 7 in children.

MYELOPROLIFERATIVE DISORDERS

The term "myeloproliferative syndrome" was suggested by Dameshek to describe several closely related clinicopathologic entities demonstrating bone marrow hypercellularity as the result of multilineage cell proliferation in bone marrow.[65] These entities include polycythemia rubra vera, essential thrombocythemia, agnogenic myeloid metaplasia/myelofibrosis and chronic myelogenous leukemia (CML).[13-18] The principal mechanism of a myeloproliferative process appears to be the clonal proliferation of an abnormal pluripotent bone marrow stem cell.[1-6] Polycythemia rubra vera, essential thrombocythemia and agnogenic myeloid metaplasia/myelofibrosis are discussed here; CML is discussed in Chapter 6. In addition, a transient myeloproliferative disorder associated with Down's syndrome is briefly discussed.

Polycythemia Rubra Vera (PRV)

Polycythemia rubra vera or polycythemia vera is characterized by erythrocytosis with varying degrees of thrombocytosis, leukocytosis and splenomegaly. The erythrocytosis occurs in the absence of hypoxic stimulation. The incidence of PRV ranges from 0.6 to 1.8 per 100,000,[66,67] and the median age of patients is 60 years, with only 0.1% younger than 20.[68]

Etiology and Pathogenesis

The abnormal proliferation and function of the hematopoietic cells in PRV is a clonal process demonstrated by chromosomal abnormalities and by glucose-6-phosphate dehydrogenase isoenzyme studies in patients heterozygous for the enzyme.[69-71] Clonal chromosomal abnormalities such as aberrations of chromosomes 1, 5 or 20 and trisomies 8 and 9 are reported in 10–25% of patients at diagnosis. The incidence of chromosomal abnormalities increases significantly by leukemic transformation.[69,70a] Reports of PRV in identical twins may suggest a genetic predisposition.[72-74]

The in vitro culture assays of bone marrow cells have shown some growth characteristics in PRV patients. Erythropoietin has a greater proliferative effect on the pluripotent stem cells and erythroid progenitor burst-forming units (BFU-E) of PRV patients than those of normal controls.[75,76] This increased proliferative response may lead to a gradual domination of the abnormal clone at the expense of normal progenitor cells.[77]

Clinicopathologic Features

The most common symptoms and signs in PRV patients are headache, weakness, pruritus, dizziness, splenomegaly, engorged retinal veins, and palpable liver.[68] Laboratory findings, according to the criteria proposed by the Polycythemia Vera Study Group, are divided into two major categories: category A and category B.

Category A includes (1) increased erythrocyte volume of >36 ml/kg in males and >32 ml/kg in females, (2) arterial oxygen saturation >92% and (3) splenomegaly.

Category B consists of (1) thrombocytosis with a platelet count >400,000/μl, (2) leukocytosis with a white blood cell count >12,000/μl (in the absence of fever or infection), (3) an elevated LAP score in the absence of fever or infection and (4) an serum vitamin B_{12} level >900 pg/ml or an unbound vitamin B_{12}-binding capacity >2200 pg/ml.[68]

The diagnosis of PRV is made if all three laboratory parameters from category A or if parameters (1) and (2) from category A with any two parameters from category B are present.

The bone marrow in the active erythrocytotic phase is usually hypercellular and displays hyperplasia of erythroid cells, often in association with hyperplasia of the megakaryocytic and granulocytic lines[78,79] (Figure 5-15). However, the bone marrow morphology in PRV is widely variable and offers no pathognomonic features for the diagnosis of PRV. In the majority of cases the bone marrow is packed, with over 90% cellularity and marked erythroid hyperplasia (M:E ratio <1). Megakaryocytosis is a frequent finding, and megakaryocytes often appear in clusters and show a moderate degree of pleomorphism, with a mixture of micro forms and giant forms.[80] In about 5–10% of the cases, however, the bone marrow may appear normocellular.[79] There is no correlation between the clinical course and the degree of marrow cellularity in PRV patients. Stainable iron is reduced or absent, either because of erythroid hyperplasia and iron consumption or due to iron deficiency secondary to bleeding.[81] Occasionally, PRV patients may demonstrate normal hemoglobin and hematocrit values, or even evidence of anemia as a result of hemorrhagic complications.

PRV in about 15% of the patients evolves into a condition, which clinicopathologically, is very similar to agnogenic myeloid metaplasia. This phase is referred to as "postpolycythemic myeloid metaplasia" or "spent phase."[15,82,83] Characteristic features of this phase are normalization of the red blood cell mass, presence of teardrops and leukoerythroblastosis in the peripheral blood, bone marrow fibrosis and increased splenomegaly.

Morphologic changes in bone marrow similar to those in PRV are seen in patients with erythrocytosis secondary to hypoxemia, hypovolemia or erythropoietin production by nonhematopoietic tumors such as cerebellar hemangiomas, renal cell carcinomas and hepatocellular carcinomas. In these conditions, the enhanced stimulation of erythropoiesis is caused by increased release of erythropoietin. Absolute erythrocytosis associated with increased level of erythropoietin is called *"secondary polycythemia."*

Essential Thrombocythemia (ET)

ET is a chronic, persistent thrombocytosis with no known etiology.[84-86] The age distribution is quite broad, ranging from 20 to 84 years, with rare incidents in children.[84,87] However, most patients are older than 50 years. Studies by Bellucci et al. suggest a bimodal distribution: a small peak in younger women (around 30 years) and a major peak in older adults.[88]

Etiology and Pathogenesis

ET is a clonal disorder of pluripotent hematopoietic stem cells, with primary involvement of the megakaryocytic lineage.[89] In vitro culture studies demonstrate increased numbers of megakaryocytic colony-forming units (CFU-Meg) and their ability to grow

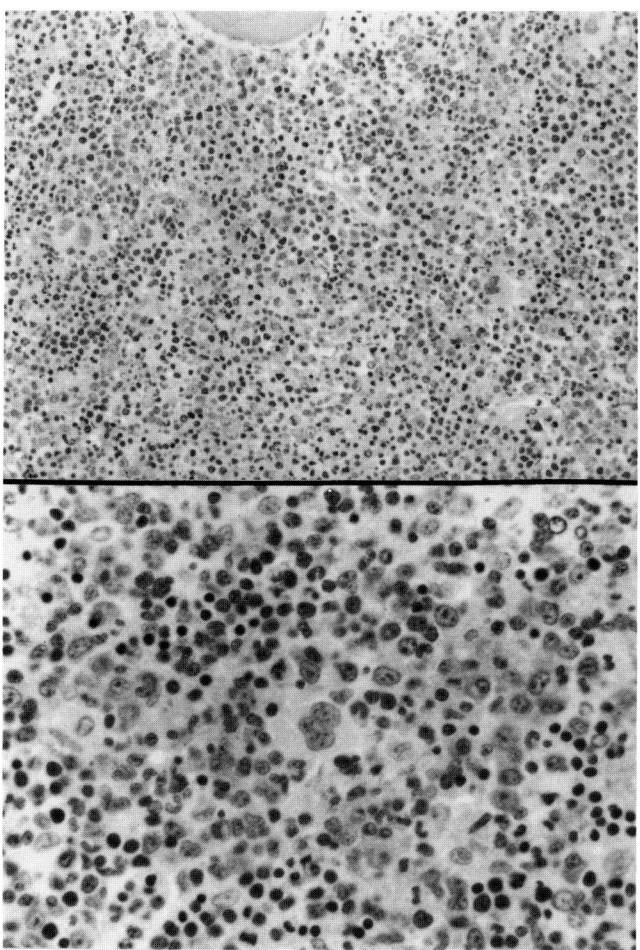

Figure 5-15. Bone marrow biopsy section from a patient with PRV demonstrating bone marrow hypercellularity with erythroid preponderance.

autonomously without added growth factors.[90-92] No etiologic factor has been identified. Only a few familial forms have been reported.[93,94]

Clinicopathologic Features

ET is a diagnosis of exclusion characterized by persistent thrombocytosis in excess of 600,000/μl (often >1,000,000/μl), lack of evidence for iron deficiency anemia or PRV as the primary cause of thrombocytosis, absent Ph or rearranged bcr, and absent or focal marrow fibrosis without splenomegaly and leukoerythroblastic reaction.[84,88,95-97] In the majority of ET patients, abnormal platelet function has been reported, leading to thrombotic or hemorrhagic complications.[98-102] However, up to one-fifth of ET patients are asymptomatic, and the only abnormal finding is an unexplained thrombocytosis.[88] Laboratory findings, such as elevated white blood cell count, LAP scores, and serum vitamin B_{12}, urate and cholesterol levels, overlap with those of PRV.[84,88]

The bone marrow is hypercellular, though some patients may show normocellular marrow.[84] Bone marrow morphology is highly variable and, according to most investigators, noncharacteristic. There is evidence of either a trilineage hyperplasia similar to that of PRV[84,103] or a monolinear megakaryocytosis, with or without significant cytologic abnormalities[104,105] (Figure 5-16). Recent studies by Thiele et al., however, demonstrated some morphologic features useful in the differential diagnosis of ET.[106]

According to these investigators, bone marrow of patients with ET, unlike that of other myeloproliferative disorders, had a normal amount of erythroid and granulocytic component, with no evidence of increased reticulin fibers. In addition, the megakaryoctes in ET were larger and showed a higher frequency of emperipolesis (internalization of hematopoietic cells) than other subtypes of myeloproliferative disorders.

Bone marrow morphology in ET, however, may resemble conditions which are associated with compensatory or reactive megakaryocytosis such as immune thrombocytopenic purpura and iron deficiency anemia. Some cases of PRV which show marked megakaryocytosis with insignificant erythroid hyperplasia (PRV in spent phase) may also imitate ET.[107]

Peripheral blood studies may reveal platelet aggregates with giant platelets and/or atypical forms, megakaryocytic fragments and a mild neutrophilia.[96,98] Occasionally, a few immature granulocytic cells are identified. Some ET patients demonstrate an increased erythrocyte mass which may be masked by hemorrhage or iron deficiency at diagnosis.[84]

Approximately 5% of ET patients may show chromosomal aberrations in hematopoietic precursor cells, and some may develop chromosomal abnormalities later, at the time of blast transformation.[84,108] A 21q⁻ abnormality has been described in ET,[109,110] and an autosomal dominant familial form of ET has been reported.[111]

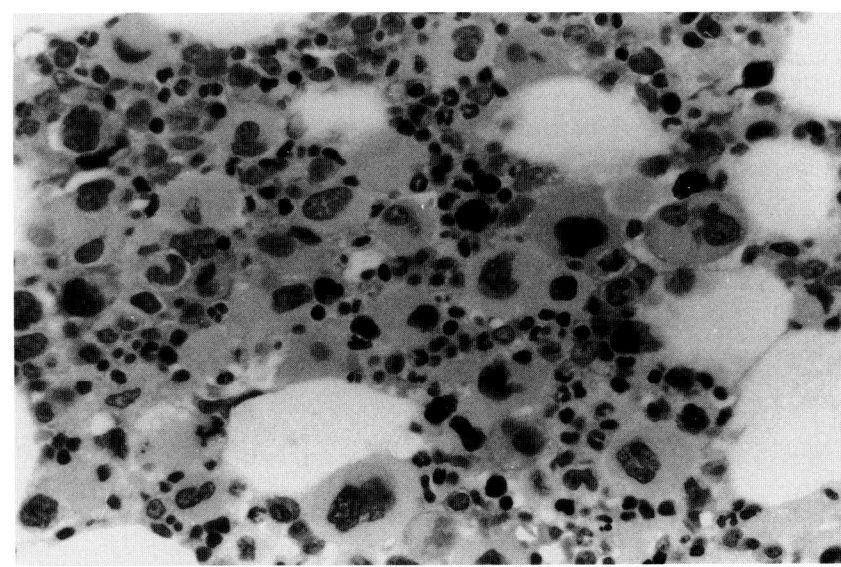

Figure 5-16. Bone marrow clot section from a patient with primary thrombocytosis demonstrating a large number of megakaryocytes.

Myelofibrosis with Extramedullary Hematopoiesis

Myelofibrosis with extramedullary hematopoiesis (agnogenic myeloid metaplasia, idiopathic myelofibrosis, myelofibrosis with myeloid metaplasia) is a chronic myeloproliferative disorder characterized by bone marrow fibrosis, extramedullary hematopoiesis, leukoerythroblastic peripheral blood (presence of nucleated red blood cells and immature myeloid cells in peripheral blood, often in association with an elevated white blood cell count), poikilo- and anisocytosis, and splenomegaly[5,112,113] (Figures 5-17 and 5-18).

Etiology and Pathogenesis

Idiopathic myelofibrosis (IMF) is a clonal disorder with unknown etiology involving multipotent hematopoietic stem cells.[14] The bone marrow fibroblasts

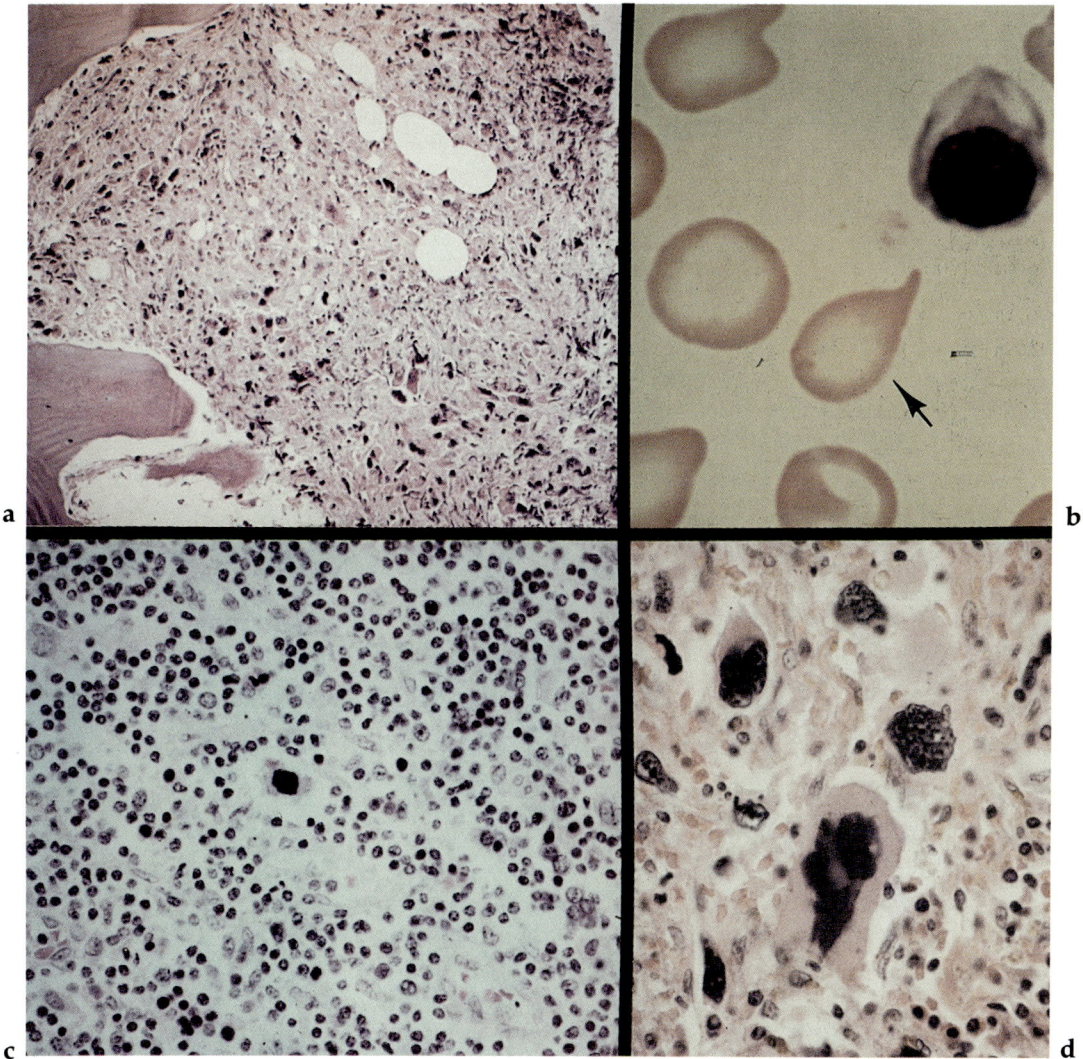

Figure 5-17. Myelofibrosis with extramedullary hematopoiesis. (a) Bone marrow biopsy section demonstrating marrow fibrosis and numerous megakaryocytes; (b) peripheral blood smear showing a teardrop (arrow) and a nucleated red blood cell; sections of a lymph node (c) and the spleen (d) demonstrate extramedullary hematopoiesis.

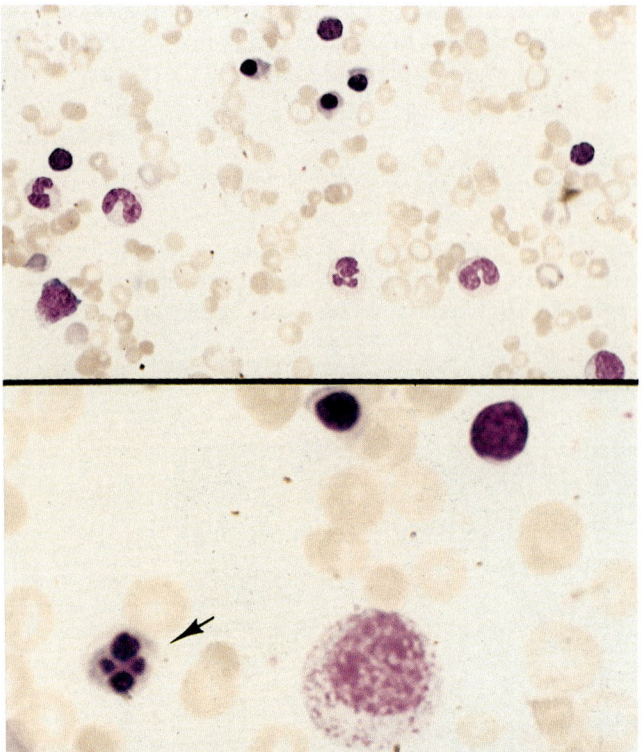

Figure 5-18. Peripheral blood smear with a leukoerythroblastic pattern demonstrated by the presence of nucleated red blood cells and immature myeloid cells. A dysplastic nucleated red blood cell with a quadrilobed nucleus is present (arrow).

are not part of the neoplastic clone, and fibroblastic proliferation appears to be a secondary phenomenon. It has been suggested that fibroblastic proliferation in IMF is due to the release of platelet-derived growth factor (PDGF) from alpha granules of the abnormal megakaryocytes and platelets.[114,115] A report of elevated plasma and decreased platelet content of platelet factor 4 and beta-thromboglobulin in IMF patients by Sacchi et al. suggests excessive release of alpha granular proteins in this disorder.[116] Advanced myelofibrosis is often associated with osteosclerosis.

Extramedullary hematopoiesis is characterized by the presence of nucleated red blood cells, myeloid precursors, and megakaryocytes outside bone marrow and peripheral blood. This phenomenon is commonly found in the spleen and liver but is also observed in lymph nodes, ascitic fluid, skin, synovium, small bowel wall, pericardium and the central nervous system[117-123] (see Figure 5-17). One of the suggested mechanisms for the extramedullary hematopoiesis in IMF is the increased access of the hematopoietic precursors to the circulation due to the alteration in the structure of the marrow stroma.[124-126] CFU-Meg, BFU-E, CFU-E, and megakaryoblasts have been identified in peripheral blood of patients with myelofibrosis.[124,125]

Several etiologic or predisposing factors have been suggested, including environmental, toxin and radiation exposure, immunologic disorders and genomic instability. An increased incidence of IMF has been reported in persons exposed to solvents and thorium dioxide, and in survivors of the Hiroshima atomic bomb explosion.[127-129] Several cases of chemotherapy-induced IMF have been described in patients receiving therapy for Hodgkin's disease and CML.[130,131] However, it is not clear whether myelofibrosis in these patients is secondary to therapy or is a rare manifestation of the original disease. IMF has also been reported in association with Immunologic disorders. The presence of antinuclear antibodies, rheumatoid factors, lupus anticoagulant, positive direct Coombs test, circulating immune complexes, and platelet-associated immunoglobulins has been demonstrated by several investigators.[132-137] The significance of abnormal immunologic markers in the pathogenesis of IMF is not clear.

Pathology

Bone marrow biopsy sections demonstrate varying degrees of cellularity and fibrosis (Figures 5-17 and 5-19). Marrow cellularity ranges from close to 100% in association with mild marrow fibrosis to markedly depleted marrow with massive fibrosis[18,126,138-140]; the bone marrow stromal matrix in IMF has excessive amounts of type I, III, IV and V collagen, fibronectin and laminin, with a predominance of type III collagen and procollagen III.[141-144] Under light microscopic examination, bone marrow fibrosis is shown by an increase in fine reticulin fibers (demonstrated by reticulin stain) and, in addition, by the presence of thick, dense, fibrous bands (demonstrated by trichrome stain) (Figures 5-19 and 5-20). The latter is usually associated with more advanced fibrosis. Bone marrow aspiration is commonly unsuccessful (dry tap), but, when successful, demonstrates a mixture of hematopoietic cells with a predominance of megakaryocytes.

The process of myelofibrosis in IMF has traditionally been divided into three stages: (1) a cellular phase with panmyelosis, megakaryocytic and

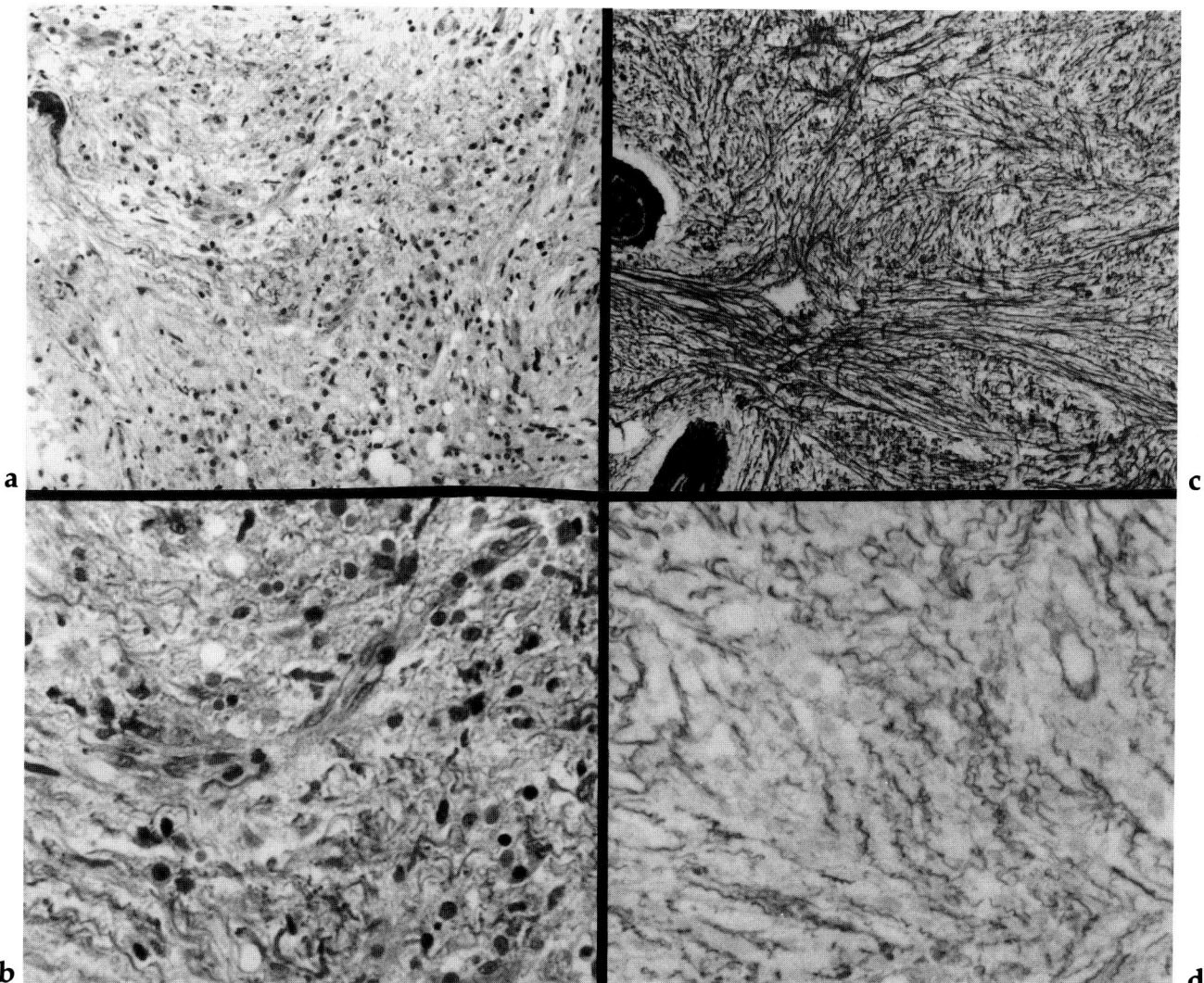

Figure 5-19. Bone marrow biopsy sections demonstrating myelofibrosis. (a, b) Advanced myelofibrosis with abundent collagen fibers and scattered hematopoietic cells; (c) reticulin stain demonstrating a marked increase in reticulin fibers; (d) trichrome stain showing coarse, wavy collagen bands.

erythroid predominance, and a slight increase in reticulin fibers, (2) myelofibrosis, with only 30% of the marrow space showing hematopoietic tissue, and (3) myelofibrosis with osteosclerosis and a minimal amount of hematopoietic tissue (marrow failure).[145]

The peripheral blood findings in IMF include anisocytosis and poikilocytosis, with the presence of teardrops and nucleated red blood cells, normochromic anemia with a low or normal reticulocyte count, and an elevated white blood cell count usually exceeding 20,000/μl, with the presence of immature myeloid cells (see Figures 5-17 and 5-18). The platelet count is normal or elevated, and giant platelets are present.

Cytogenetic abnormalities are relatively common, averaging about 50%.[146,147] A variety of chromosomal abnormalities have been reported in IMF, such as trisomy 1, 8, 9, and 21; monosomy 1; loss of Y, 7q$^-$, and 13q$^-$; and interstitial deletion of 11q.[55,147-149] The cytogenetic abnormalities appear to be acquired; however, familial occurrences of IMF have been reported.[150]

IMF is a clinicopathologic entity and should not be diagnosed on the basis of bone marrow morphology

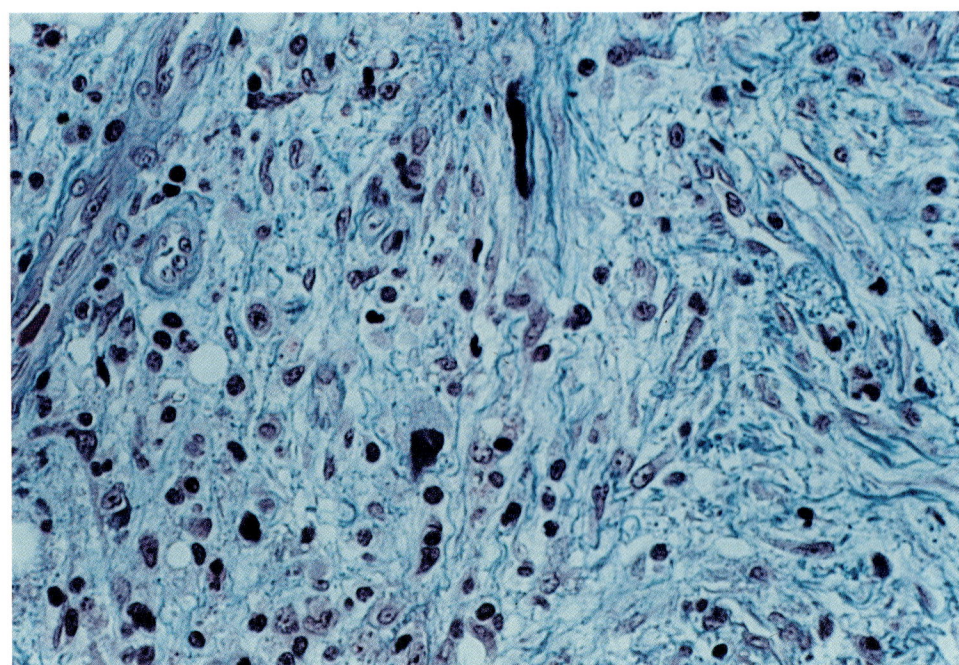

Figure 5-20. Bone marrow biopsy section stained with a trichrome stain demonstrating marked increased in collagen and scattered hematopoietic cells.

alone. There is a wide variety of conditions which may be associated with bone marrow fibrosis, such as hematologic malignancies, metastatic tumors, inflammatory and repair processes, metabolic disorders, and Paget's disease (see Table 3-1 in Chapter 3). Some of these conditions, such as metastatic carcinomas, may display extramedullary hematopoiesis and leukoerythroblastic peripheral blood. Distinguishing IMF from CML is difficult when CML is associated with marrow fibrosis.[151,152] In such cases, additional information such as lack of Ph[1] and an elevated LAP score are in favor of IMF.

IMF should be distinguished from acute myelofibrosis (malignant myelofibrosis). Acute myelofibrosis is a variant of acute leukemia (usually the megakaryoblastic type) characterized by circulating blasts, pancytopenia, minimal abnormal red blood cell morphology, minimal or absent splenomegaly, marrow fibrosis and a rapid, aggressive clinical couse (see Chapter 6).

Clinical Aspects

The average age of the patients is about 60 years, with an extremely low incidence in children. Symptoms are nonspecific and include fatigue, shortness of breath, palpitations, weight loss and discomfort or pain in the left upper abdomen due to splenomegaly.

About 25% of the patients are asymptomatic. Splenomegaly is a common feature, and hepatomegaly is present in about 70% of the patients. Bones, especially in the lower extremities, may become tender.

Several attempts have been made to correlate the clinicopathologic features with the prognosis.[153-157] The extent of erythropoietic activity may serve as an important prognostic indicator.[156,157] In a recent report by Barosi et al.,[158] where 137 patients with IMF were studied, two extreme risk groups were identified: low risk and high risk. The low-risk group (20% of the cases) comprised patients who had the diagnosis of IMF before age 45 and fewer than 24% immature myeloid cells in peripheral blood. The actuarial proportion of patients surviving at 15 years was 100% in this group. The high-risk group (30% of the cases) consisted of patients with an age at diagnosis above 45 and a hemoglobin level of <13 g/dl (associated with bone marrow erythroid hypoplasia) or more than 24% immature myeloid cells in peripheral blood.

Transient Myeloproliferative Disorder in Down's Syndrome (TMD-DS)

TMB-DS is a condition observed in neonates usually within the first month of birth and morphologically resembles acute leukemia.[159-163] It is characterized by the transient presence of blast cells in peripheral blood and increased blasts in marrow, which usually disappear spontaneously after 4–6 weeks. The percentage of blasts in the peripheral blood may exceed that in the bone marrow.[159] Major differences between TMD-DS and true leukemias in DS patients are a younger age, higher hemoglobin concentration, higher platelet and white blood cell counts, and lack of additional chromosomal abnormalities in TMD-DS patients.[159] In both conditions, blast cells are predominantly of the megakaryoctic and/or erythroid lineage.[159,163] A small proportion of patients with TMD-DS may eventually develop a true myelogenous leukemia.[164-166]

References

1. Adamson JW, Fialkow PJ, Murphy S, et al: Polycythemia vera: Stem cell and probable clonal origin of the disease. *N Engl J Med* 295:913, 1976.
2. Failkow PJ, Faguet GB, Jacobson RJ, et al: Evidence that essential thrombocythemia is a clonal disorder with origin in a multipotential stem cell. *Blood* 58:916, 1981.
3. Kay HEM, Lawler SD, Millard RE: The chromosome in polycythemia vera. *Br J Haematol* 12:507, 1966.
4. Nowell PC, Finan JB: Cytogenetics of acute and chronic myelofibrosis. *Virchows Arch (Cell Pathol)* 29:45, 1978.
5. Singal U, Prasad AS, Halton DM, et al: Essential thrombocythemia: A clonal disorder of hematopoietic stem cell. *Am J Hematol* 14:193, 1983.
6. Third International Workshop on Chromosomes in Leukemia: Report on essential thrombocythemia. *Cancer Genet Cytogenet* 4:138, 1979.
7. Degnan T, Weiselberg L, Schulman P, et al: Dysmyelopoietic syndrome. Current concepts. *Am J Med* 76:122, 1984.
8. Galton DAG: The myelodysplastic syndromes. *Clin Lab Haematol* 6:99, 1984.
9a. Galton DAG: The myelodysplastic syndromes. Part I. What are they? Part II. Classification. *Scand J Haematol* 36:11, 1986.
9b. Maldonado JE, Pierre RV: The platelets in preleukemia and myelomonocytic leukemia. Ultrastructure, cytochemistry and cytogenetics. *Mayo Clin Proc* 50:573, 1975.
10. Report of the Third MCI Cooperative Study Group: Recommendations for a morphologic, immunologic, and cytogenetic (MIC) working classification of the primary and therapy-related myelodysplastic disorders. *Cancer Genet Cytogenet* 32:1, 1988.
11. Bennett JM, Catovsky D, Daniel MT, et al: Proposals for the classification of the myelodysplastic syndromes. *Br J Haematol* 51:189, 1982.
12. Bennett JM, Catovsky D, Daniel MT, et al: Classification of the myelodysplastic syndromes. *Clin Haematol* 15:909, 1986.
13. Adamson JW, Fialkow PJ: The pathogenesis of myeloproliferative syndromes. *Br J Haematol* 38:299, 1978.
14. Jacobson RS, Salo A, Fialkow PJ: Agnogenic myeloid metaplasia: A clonal proliferation of hematopoietic stem cells with secondary myelofibrosis. *Blood* 51:189, 1978.
15. Glew RH, Haese WH, McIntyre PA: Myeloid metaplasia with fibrosis. The clinical spectrum of extramedullary hematopoiesis and tumor formation. *Johns Hopkins Med J* 132:253, 1973.
16. Bird T, Proctor SJ: Malignant myelosclerosis: Myeloproliferative disorder or leukemia? *Am J Clin Pathol* 67:512, 1977.
17. Bellucci S, Janvier M, Tobelem G, et al: Essential thrombocythemias. Clinical, evolutionary, and biological data. *Cancer* 58:2240, 1986.
18. Laszlo J: Myeloproliferative disorders (MPD): Myelofibrosis, myelosclerosis, extramedullary hematopoiesis, undifferentiated MPD, and hemorrhagic thrombocythemia. *Semin Hematol* 12:409, 1975.
19. Koeffler HP, Golde DW: Cellular maturation in human preleukemia. *Blood* 52:355, 1978.
20. Biemer JJ: The preleukemia syndrome. *Ann Clin Lab Sci* 13:156, 1983.
21. Anderson RL, Bagby GC Jr: The prognostic value of chromosome studies in patients with the preleukemic syndrome (hemopoietic dysplasia). *Leuk Res* 6:175, 1982.
22. Yunis JJ, Rydell RE, Oken MM, et al: Refined chromosome analysis as an independent prognostic indicator in de novo myelodysplastic syndrome. *Blood* 67:172, 1986.
23. Nowell PC: Cytogenetics of preleukemia. *Cancer Genet Cytogenet* 5:265, 1982.
24. Coiffier B, Adeleine P, Viala JJ, et al: Dysmyelopoietic syndromes. A search for prognostic factors in 193 patients. *Cancer* 52:83, 1983.
25. Rosenthal DS, Moloney WC: Refractory anemia and acute leukemia. *Blood* 63:314, 1984.
26. Beris P, Graf BJ, Miescher PA: Primary acquired sideroblastic and primary acquired refractory anemia. *Semin Hematol* 20:101, 1983.
27. Solal-Celigny P, Desaint B, Herrara A, et al: Chronic myelomonocytic leukemia according to the FAB classification: Analysis of 35 cases. *Blood* 63:634, 1984.
28. Vardiman JW, Le Beau MM, Albain K, et al: Myelodysplasia: A comparison of therapy-related and primary forms. *Ann Biol Clin* 43:372, 1985.

29. Cronkite E: Chemical leukemogenesis. Benzene as a model. *Semin Hematol* 24:2, 1978.
30. Kitahara M, Cosgriff TM, Eyre HJ: Sideroblastic anemia as a preleukemic event in patients treated for Hodgkin's disease. *Ann Intern Med* 92:625, 1980.
31. Pedersen-Bijergaard J, Ersboll J, Sorensen HM, et al: Risk of acute nonlymphocytic leukemia and preleukemia in patients treated with cyclophosphamide for non-Hodgkin's lymphomas. *Ann Intern Med* 103:195, 1985.
32. Kamada N, Uchins H: Preleukemic states in atomic bomb survivors. *Blood Cells* 2:57, 1976.
33. Hirai H, Kobayashi Y, Mano H, et al: A point mutation at codon 13 of the *N-ras* oncogene in myelodysplastic syndrome. *Nature* 327:430, 1987.
34. Janssen JWG, Steenvorden ACM, Lyons J, et al: ras gene mutations in acute and chronic myelocytic leukemias, chronic myeloproliferative disorders and myelodysplastic syndromes. *Proc Natl Acad Sci USA* 84:9228, 1987.
35. Boogaerts MA, Nelissen V, Roelant C, et al: Blood neutrophil function in primary myelodysplastic syndrome. *Br J Haematol* 55:217, 1983.
36. Barton JC, Conrad ME, Parmley RT: Acute lymphoblastic leukemia in idiopathic refractory sideroblastic anemia: Evidence for a common lymphoid and myeloid progenitor cell. *Am J Hematol* 9:109, 1980.
37. Eridani S, Chan LC, Halil O, et al: Acute biphenotypic leukemia (myeloid and null-ALL type) supervening in a myelodysplastic syndrome. *Br J Haematol* 61:525, 1985.
38. Jandl JH: *Blood. Textbook of Hematology*. Boston, Little, Brown, 1987, p 612.
39. Bynoe AG, Scott CS, Ford P, et al: Decreased T helper cells in the myelodysplastic syndrome. *Br J Haematol* 54:97, 1983.
40. Takagi S, Kitagawa S, Takeda A, et al: Natural killer-interferon system in patients with preleukemic states. *Br J Haematol* 58:71, 1984.
41. Anderson RW, Volsky DJ, Greenberg B, et al: Lymphocytic abnormalities in preleukemia. 1. Decreased NK activity, anomalous immunoregulatory cell subsets and deficient EBV receptors. *Leuk Res* 7:389, 1983.
42. Cukrova V, Neuwirtova R, Cermak J, et al: Leukocyte-derived inhibitory activity in patients with myelodysplastic syndrome. *Blut* 55:165, 1987.
43. Curkova V, Neuwirtova R, Cermak J, et al: Inhibitors of normal granulopoiesis produced by cells of MDS patients. *Neoplasma* 36:83, 1989.
44. Frisch B, Bartl R: Bone marrow histology in myelodysplastic syndromes. *Scand J Haematol* 36 (suppl 43):21, 1986.
45. Reddy BW: Value of altered bone marrow topography in diagnosis of myelodysplastic syndromes. *Lab Invest* 60:77A, 1989.
46. Tricot G, de Wolf-Peeters C, Vlietinck P, et al: Bone marrow histology in myelodysplastic syndromes. II Prognostic value of abnormal localization of immature precursors in MDS. *Br J Haematol* 58:217, 1984.
47. Benitez J, Carbonell F, Fayos JS, et al: Karyotypic evolution in patients with myelodysplastic syndromes. *Cancer Genet Cytogenet* 16:157, 1985.
48a. Morgan R, Hecht F: Deletion of chromosome band 13q14: A primary event in preleukemia and leukemia. *Cancer Genet Cytogenet* 18:243, 1985.
48b. Jacobs A: Genetic lesions in preleukemia. *Leukemia* 5:277, 1991.
49a. Mittelman MM, Lessin LS: Oncogenes and growth factor genes in myelodysplasia. *Hematologic Pathol* 5:37, 1991.
49b. Van den Berghe H, Vermaelen K, Mecucci C, et al: The $5q^-$ anomaly. *Cancer Genet Cytogenet* 17:189, 1985.
50. Nimer SD, Golde DW: The $5q^-$ abnormality. *Blood* 70:1705, 1987.
51. Kere J, Ruutu T, de la Chapelle A: Monosomy 7 in granulocytes and monocytes in myelodysplastic syndrome. *N Engl J Med* 316:449, 1987.
52. Carroll WL, Morgan R, Glader BE: Childhood bone marrow monosomy 7 syndrome: A familial disorder? *J Pediatr* 107:578, 1985.
53. Berthier R, Douady F, Metral J, et al: In vitro granulopoiesis in oligoblastic leukemia: Prognostic value, characterization and serial cloning of bone marrow colony and cluster forming cells in agar culture. *Biomedicine* 30:305, 1979.
54. Verma DS, Spitzer G, Dicke KA, et al: In vitro agar culture patterns in preleukemia and their clinical significance. *Leuk Res* 3:41, 1979.
55. Ruutu T, Partanen S, Lintula R, et al: Erythroid and granulocyte-macrophage colony formation in myelodysplastic syndrome. *Scand J Haematol* 32:395, 1984.
56. Li FP, Marchetto DJ, Vawter GF: Acute leukemia and preleukemia in eight males in a family: An X-linked disorder? *Am J Hematol* 6:61, 1979.
57. Milner GR, Testa NG, Geary CG, et al: Bone marrow culture studies in refractory cytopenia and "smouldering leukemia." *Br J Haematol* 35:251, 1977.
58. Greenberg PL, Mara B: The preleukemic syndrome. Correlation of in vitro parameters of granulopoiesis with clinical features. *Am J Med* 66:951, 1979.
59. Clark R, Peters S, Hoy T, et al: Prognostic significance of hypodiploid hemopoietic precursors in myelodysplastic syndromes. *N Engl J Med* 314:1472, 1986.
60. Hoelzer D: Cytobiology and clinical findings of myelodysplastic syndromes. *Recent Results Cancer Res* 106:172, 1988.

61. Jacobs RH, Cornbleet MA, Vardiman JW, et al: Prognostic implications of morphology and karyotype in primary myelodysplastic syndrome. *Blood* 67:1765, 1986.
62. Kitagawa M, Kamiyama R, Takemura T, et al: Bone marrow analysis of the myelodysplastic syndromes: Histological and immunohistochemical features related to the evolution of overt leukemia. *Virchows Arch (Cell Pathol)* 57:47, 1989.
63. Varela BL, Chuang C, Woll JE, et al: Modification in the classification of primary myelodysplastic syndromes: The addition of a scoring system. *Hematol Oncol* 3:55, 1985.
64. Mufti GJ, Stevens JR, Oscier DG, et al: Myelodysplastic syndrome: A scoring system with prognostic significance. *Br J Haematol* 59:425, 1985.
65. Dameshek W: Editorial: Some speculations on the myeloproliferative syndromes. *Blood* 6:372, 1951.
66. Modan B: An epidemiological study of polycythemia vera. *Blood* 26:657, 1965.
67. Silverstein MN, Lanier AP: Polycythemia vera 1935–1969. *Mayo Clin Proc* 46:751, 1971.
68. Berlin NI: Diagnosis and classification of the polycythemias. *Semin Hematol* 12:339, 1975.
69. Testa JR, Kanofsky JR, Rowley JD, et al: Karyotypic patterns and their clinical significance in polycythemia vera. *Am J Hematol* 11:29, 1981.
70a. Berger R, Bernheim A, Le Coniat M, et al: Chromosome studies in polycythemia vera patients. *Cancer Genet Cytogenet* 12:217, 1984.
70b. Diez-Martin JL, Graham LG, Petitt RM, et al: Chromosome studies in 104 patients with polycythemia vera. *Mayo Clin Proc* 66:287, 1991.
71. Adamson JW, Fialkow PJ, Murphy S, et al: Polycythemia vera: Stem cell and probable clonal origin of the disease. *N Engl J Med* 295:913, 1976.
72. Friedland ML, Wittels EG, Robinson RJ: Polycythemia vera in identical twins. *Am J Hematol* 10:101, 1981.
73. Burnside P, Salmon DC, Humphrey CA, et al: Polycythemia rubra vera in monozygotic twins. *Br J Med* 283:56, 1981.
74. Fairrie G, Black AJ, McKenize AW: Polycythemia rubra vera and congenital deafness in monozygotic twins. *Br J Med* 283:194, 1981.
75. Golde DW, Cline MJ: Erythropoietin responsiveness in polycythemia vera. *Br J Haematol* 29:567, 1975.
76. Zanjani ED, Lutton JD, Hoffman R, et al: Erythroid colony formation by polycythemia vera bone marrow in vitro. *J Clin Invest* 59:841, 1977.
77. Adamson JW, Singer JW, Catalano P, et al: Polycythemia vera: Further in vitro studies of hematopoietic regulation. *J Clin Invest* 66:1363, 1980.
78. Ellis JT, Peterson P: The bone marrow in polycythemia vera. *Pathol Ann* 14:383, 1979.
79. Ellis JT, Peterson P, Geller SA, et al: Studies of bone marrow in polycythemia vera and the evolution of myelofibrosis and second hematologic malignancies. *Semin Hematol* 23:144, 1986.
80. Thiele J, Moedder B, Kremer B, et al: Chronic myeloproliferative disease with elevated platelet count (in excess of 1,00,00/µl): A clinicopathological study on 46 patients with special emphasis on primary (essential) thrombocythemia. *Hematol Pathol* 1:277, 1987.
81. Ellis JT, Jensen WN, Westerman MP: Marrow iron: An evaluation of depleted stores in a series of 1332 needle biopsies. *Arch Intern Med* 61:44, 1964.
82. Silverstein MN: Postpolycythemic myeloid metaplasia. *Arch Intern Med* 134:113, 1974.
83. Silverstein MN: The evolution into and the treatment of late stage polycythemia vera. *Semin Hematol* 13:79, 1976.
84. Murphy S, Iland H, Rosenthal D, et al: Essential thrombocythemia: An interim report from the Polycythemia Vera Study Group. *Semin Hematol* 23:177, 1986.
85. Fialkow PJ, Faguet GB, Jacobsen RJ, et al: Evidence that essential thrombocythemia is a clonal disorder with origin in a multipotent stem cell. *Blood* 58:916, 1981.
86. Singal U, Prasad AS, Halton DM, et al: Essential thrombocythemia: A clonal disorder of hematopoietic stem cell. *Am J Hematol* 14:193, 1983.
87. Sceats DJ, Bailton D: Primary thrombocythemia in a child. *Clin Pediatr* 19:298, 1980.
88. Bellucci S, Janvier M, Tobelem G, et al: Essential thrombocythemias. *Cancer* 58:2440, 1986.
89. Fialkow PJ, Fauget GB, Jacobson RJ, et al: Evidence that essential thrombocythemia is a clonal disorder with origin in a multipotent stem cell. *Blood* 58:916, 1981.
90. Gewirtz AM, Bruno E, Elwell J, et al: In vitro studies of megakaryopoiesis in thrombocytotic disorders of man. *Blood* 61:384, 1983.
91. Juvonen E, Partanen S, Ruutu T: Colony formation by megakaryocytic progenitors in essential thrombocythemia. *Br J Haematol* 66:161, 1987.
92. Mazur EM, Cohen JL, Bogart L: Growth characteristics of circulating hematopoietic progenitor cells from patients with essential thrombocythemia. *Blood* 71:6, 1988.
93. Fickers J, Speck B: Thrombocythemia: Familial occurrence and transition into blast crisis. *Acta Haematol* 51:257, 1974.
94. Eyster ME, Saletan SL, Rabellino EM, et al: Familial essential thrombocythemia. *Am J Med* 80:497, 1986.

95. Lewis SM, Szur L, Hoffbran AL: Thrombocythemia. *Clin Hematol* 1:339, 1972.
96. Silverstein MN: Primary thrombocythemia, in *Hematology*, Williams WM, Beutler E, Erslev AJ, et al (eds), ed 3. New York, McGraw-Hill, 1983, p 218.
97. Wolf BC, Neiman RS: The bone marrow in myeloproliferative and dysmyelopoietic syndromes. *Hematol Oncol Clin North Am* 2:669, 1988.
98. Silverstein MN: Primary or hemorrhagic thrombocythemia. *Arch Intern Med* 122:18, 1968.
99. Singh AK, Wetherley-Mein G: Microvascular occlusive lesions in primary thrombocythaemia. *Br J Haematol* 36:553, 1977.
100. Wu KK: Platelet hyperaggregability and thrombosis in patients with thrombocythemia. *Ann Intern Med* 88:7, 1978.
101. Kawwin P, McDonough M, Insel PA, et al: Platelet function in essential thrombocythemia. *N Engl J Med* 299:505, 1978.
102. Cortellazzo S, Barbui T, Bassan R, et al: Abnormal aggregation and increased size of platelets in myeloproliferative disorders. *Thromb Haemost* 43:127, 1980.
103. Iland HJ, Laszlo J, Case DC, et al: Differentiation between essential thrombocythemia and polycythemia vera with marked thrombocytosis. *Am J Hematol* 25:191, 1987.
104. Burkhardt R, Bartl R, Jager K, et al: Working classification of chronic myeloproliferative disorders based on histological, haematological, and clinical findings. *J Clin Pathol* 39:237, 1986.
105. Thiele J, Moedder B, Kremer B, et al: Chronic myeloproliferative diseases with an elevated platelet count in excess of 1,000,000/μl: A clinicopathological study on 46 patients with special emphasis on primary (essential) thrombocythemia. *Hematol Pathol* 1:227, 1987.
106. Thiele J, Schneider G, Hoeppner B, et al: Histomorphometry of bone marrow biopsies in chronic myeloproliferative disorders with associated thrombosis—features of significance for the diagnosis of primary (essential) thrombocythemia. *Virchow Arch A (Pathol Anat)* 413:407, 1988.
107. Murphy S: Thrombocytosis and thrombocythemia. *Clin Haematol* 12:89, 1983.
108. Third International Workshop on Chromosomes in Leukemia: Report on essential thrombocythemia. *Cancer Genet Cytogenet* 4:138, 1979.
109. Zaccari A, Tura S: A chromosomal abnormality in primary thrombocythemia. *N Engl J Med* 298:1422, 1978.
110. Fuscaldo KE, Erlick BJ, Fuscaldo AA, et al: Correlation of a specific chromosomal marker, 21q-, and retroviral indicators in patients with thrombocythemia. *Cancer Lett* 6:51, 1979.
111. Eyster ME, Saletan SI, Rabellino EM, et al: Familial essential thrombocythemia. *Ann Intern Med* 88:7, 1986.
112. Gilbert HS: The spectrum of myeloproliferative disorders. *Med Clin North Am* 57:355, 1973.
113. Smith RE, Chelmowski MK, Szabo EJ: Myelofibrosis: A review of clinical and pathologic features and treatment. *Am J Hematol* 29:174, 1988.
114. Castro-Malaspina H, Rabellino EM, Yen A, et al: Human megakaryocyte stimulation of bone marrow fibroblasts. *Blood* 57:781, 1981.
115. Groopman JE: The pathogenesis of myelofibrosis in myeloproliferative disorders. *Ann Intern Med* 92:857, 1980.
116. Sacchi S, Curci G, Piccinini L, et al: Platelet alpha-granule release in chronic myeloproliferative disorders with thrombocytosis. *Scand J Clin Lab Invest* 46:163, 1986.
117. Stoderstrom N, Bardman U, Lunh B: Patho-anatomical features of the spleen and liver. *Clin Haematol* 4:309, 1975.
118. Silverman JF: Extramedullary hematopoietic asctic fluid cytology in myelofibrosis. *Am J Clin Pathol* 84:125, 1985.
119. Levine LE, Pearson MG, Baron JM, et al: Extramedullary hematopoiesis. *Arch Dermatol* 120:1282, 1984.
120. Heinicke MH, Zarrabi MH, Gorevic PD: Arthritis due to synovial involvement by extramedullary haematopoiesis in myelofibrosis with myeloid metaplasia. *Ann Rheum Dis* 42:196, 1983.
121. Sharma BK, Pounder RE, Cruse JP, et al: Extramedullary hematopoiesis in the small bowel. *Gut* 27:873, 1986.
122. Vilaseca J, Arnau JM, Tallada N, et al: Agnogenic myeloid metaplasia presenting as massive pericardial effusion due to extramedullary hematopoiesis. *Acta Haematol* 73:239, 1985.
123. Lundh B, Brandt L, Cronqvist S, et al: Intracranial myeloid metaplasia in myelofibrosis. *Scand J Haematol* 28:91, 1982.
124. Partanen S, Ruutu T, Vuopio P: Circulating haematopoietic progenitors in myelofibrosis. *Scand J Haematol* 29:325, 1982.
125. Hibbin JA, Njoku OS, Matutes E, et al: Myeloid progenitor cells in the circulation of patients with myelofibrosis and other myeloproliferative disorders. *Br J Haematol* 57:495, 1984.
126. Wolf BC, Neiman RS: Myelofibrosis with myeloid metaplasia: Pathophysiologic implications of the correlation between bone marrow changes and progression of splenomegaly. *Blood* 65:803, 1985.
127. Wyatt JP, Sommers SC: Chronic marrow failure, myelosclerosis and extramedullary hematopoiesis. *Blood* 4:329, 1950.

128. Johnson SAN, Bateman CJT, Beard MEJ, et al: Long-term haematological complications of thorotrast. *Q J Med* new series XLVI, 182:259, 1977.
129. Anderson RE, Oshino T, Yamamoto T: Myelofibrosis with myeloid metaplasia in survivers of the atomic bomb in Hiroshima. *Ann Intern Med* 60:1, 1964.
130. Carrol WL, Berbeich FR, Glader BE: Pancytopenia with myelofibrosis: An unusual presentation of childhood Hodgkin's disease. *Clin Pediatr* 25:106, 1986.
131. Dameshek W: Some speculations on the myeloproliferative syndromes. *Blood* 6:372, 1951.
132. Rondeau E, Solal-Celigny P, Dhermy D, et al: Immune disorders in agnogenic myeloid metaplasia: Relations to myelofibrosis. *Br J Haematol* 53:467, 1983.
133. Lang JM, Oberling F, Giron C, et al: Autoimmunité et deficit de immunité cellulaire au course des fibroses primitives de la moelle osseuse. *Ann Immunol (Inst Pasteur)* 128:291, 1977.
134. Caligari CF, Vigliani R, Novarino A, et al: Idiopathic myelofibrosis: A possible role for immune complexes in the pathogenesis of bone marrow fibrosis. *Br J Haematol* 49:17, 1981.
135. Khumbanonda M, Horowitz HI, Eysker ME: Coomb's positive hemolytic anemia in myelofibrosis with myeloid metaplasia. *Am J Med Sci* 258:89, 1969.
136. Bernhardt B, Valletta M: Lupus anticoagulant in myelofibrosis. *Am J Med* 272:229, 1976.
137. Hasselbalch H, Paaske-Hansen O: Platelet associated IgG and IgM in myelofibrosis. *Scand J Haematol* 32:488, 1984.
138. Jackson H Jr, Parker F Jr: Agnogenic myeloid metaplasia of the spleen. A syndrome simulating other more definite hematologic disorders. *N Engl J Med* 222:985, 1940.
139. Lennert K, Nagai K, Schwarze EW: Patho-anatomical features of bone marrow. *Clin Haematol* 4:331, 1975.
140. Linman JW, Bethell FH: Agnogenic myeloid metaplasia: Its natural history and present day management. *Am J Med* 22:107, 1957.
141. Reilly JT, Nash JRG, Macki MJ, et al: Immunoenzymatic detection of fibronectin in normal and pathological haematopoietic tissue. *Br J Haematol* 59:497, 1985.
142. Apaja-Sarkkinen M, Autio-Harmainen H, Alavaikko M, et al: Immunohistochemical study of basement membrane proteins and type III procollagen in myelofibrosis. *Br J Haematol* 63:571, 1986.
143. Zuckermann KS, Wicha MS: Extracellular matrix production by the adherent cells of long-term murine bone marrow cultures. *Blood* 61:540, 1983.
144. Reilly JT, Nash JRG, Macki MJ, et al: Endothelial cell proliferation in myelofibrosis. *Br J Haematol* 60:625, 1985.
145. Ward HP, Block MH: The natural history of agnogenic myeloid metaplasia (AMM) and critical evaluation of its relationship with the myeloproliferative syndrome. *Medicine* 50:357, 1971.
146. Sandburg A: The Chromosome in Human Cancer and Leukemia. New York, Elsevier, 1980, p 358.
147. Nowell P, Jensen J, Gardner F, et al: Chromosome studies in "preleukemia"—III. Myelofibrosis. *Cancer* 38:1873, 1976.
148. Ganser S, Carbonell F: Cytogenetic studies using HPCM-stimulated short-term liquid cultures of circulating hematopoietic precursor cells in patients with myelofibrosis. *Blut* 44:111, 1982.
149. Sessarago AF, Ravazzolo R, Bianchi-Scarra Gl, et al: Coincidence between fragile site expression and interstitial deletion of chromosome 11 in a case of myelofibrosis. *Hum Genet* 63:299, 1983.
150. Patakfalvi A, Csete B, Horvath T: Familial myelofibrosis. *Hematologica* 3:217, 1969.
151. Clough V, Geary CG, Hashmi K, et al: Myelofibrosis in chronic granulocytic leukemia. *Br J Haematol* 42:515, 1979.
152. Lazzarino M, Morra E, Castello A, et al: Myelofibrosis in chronic myelogenous leukemia: Clinicopathologic correlations and prognostic significance. *Br J Haematol* 64:227, 1986.
153. Meytes D, Katz D, Ramot B: Prognostic parameters in myeloid metaplasia: Agnogenic vs. polycythemic. *Isr J Med Sci* 12:534, 1976.
154. Manoharan A, Smart RC, Pitney WR: Prognostic factors in myelofibrosis. *Pathology* 14:455, 1982.
155. Varki A, Lottenberg R, Griffith R, et al: The syndrome of idiopathic myelofibrosis. A clinicopathological review with emphasis on the prognostic variables predicting survival. *Medicine* 62:353, 1983.
156. Najean Y, Cacchione R, Castro-Malaspina H, et al: Erythrokinetic studies in myelofibrosis: Their significance for prognosis. *Br J Haematol* 40:205, 1978.
157. Nijoku OS, Lewis SM, Catovsky D, et al: Anemia in myelofibrosis: Its value in prognosis. *Br J Haematol* 54:79, 1983.
158. Barosi G, Berzuini C, Liberato LN, et al: A prognostic classification of myelofibrosis with myeloid metaplasia. *Br J Haematol* 70:397, 1988.
159. Hayashi Y, Eguchi M, Sugita K, et al: Cytogenetic findings and clinical features in acute leukemia and transient myeloproliferative disorder in Down's syndrome. *Blood* 72:15, 1988.
160. Engel PR, Hammond D, Eitzman DV: Transient congenital leukemia in 7 infants with mongolism. *J Pediatr* 65:303, 1964.
161. Okada H, Liu PI, Hoshino T, et al: Down's syndrome associated with a myeloproliferative disorder. *Am J Dis Child* 124:107, 1972.

162. Coulombel L, Derycle M, Villeval JL, et al: Characterization of the blast population in two neonates with Down's syndrome and transient myeloproliferative disorder. *Br J Haematol* 66:69, 1987.
163. Hayashi T, Hanada R, Yamaoto K, et al: Transient megakaryoblastic proliferation in a newborn infant with Down's syndrome. *Cancer Genet Cytogenet* 28:373, 1987.
164. Yokoyama S, Nito T, Irimada K, et al: Acute megakaryoblastic leukemia preceded by refractory anemia with an excess of blast cells: Leukemic transformation in an infant with Down syndrome recovering from transient abnormal myelopoiesis. *Acta Hematol Jpn* 47:62, 1984.
165. Lin HP, Menaka H, Lim KH, et al: Congenital leukemoid reaction followed by fatal leukemia; a case with Down's syndrome. *Am J Dis Child* 134:939, 1980.
166. Morgan R, Hecht F, Cleary ML, et al: Leukemia with Down's syndrome: Translocation between chromosomes 1 and 19 in acute myelomonocytic leukemia following transient congenital myeloproliferative syndrome. *Blood* 66:1466, 1985.

6 LEUKEMIAS AND LYMPHOMAS

Hematologic malignancies are the most common cancers in children and account for over 5% of all malignancies in adults. These tumors are divided into three major groups: leukemias, lymphomas and plasma cell myelomas. Leukemias arise from hematopoietic stem cells in the bone marrow and eventually extend to the peripheral blood and other tissues. Lymphomas arise in the lymph nodes, spleen or lymphoid structures of the gastrointestinal tract, skin, central nervous system (CNS), bone and other organs. The origin of neoplastic cells in the vast majority of lymphomas are cells of the lymphoid lineage, though there are rare lymphomas of histiocytic origin. The predominant site of involvement in plasma cell tumors is the bone marrow. All three categories of hematologic malignancies, particularly leukemias and lymphomas, show significant overlap. In this chapter, leukemias and lymphomas are discussed.

ETIOLOGY AND PATHOGENESIS

Three major environmental factors have been implicated in hematopoietic malignancies: (1) ionizing radiation, (2) chemicals and (3) viruses.

Ionizing radiation includes electromagnetic rays (X-rays, gamma rays) and energetic particles, protons, alpha particles, beta particles). The extent of cellular damage by ionizing radiation depends on the type of radiation, the amount and rate of absorption and distribution of the energy in the tissue, and the intervals between radiation exposures. An increased risk of leukemia has been demonstrated in atomic bomb survivors, patients exposed to radiation for diagnostic or therapeutic purposes, and persons exposed to excessive irradiation by X-rays in radiology laboratories.[1,7] The incidence of leukemias that can be attributed to diagnostic radiology is very low, accounting for about 1% of all cases of leukemias in the United States.[6,7] According to the epidemiologic studies, there is no evidence of an increased incidence of leukemia following low-dose therapeutic exposures totaling as high as 300 rads delivered to bone marrow.[8] Leukemia is one of the most frequent cancers found in atomic bomb survivors, with as much as a 24-fold increase in overall incidence.[3,4,9,10] The increased incidence of leukemia in atomic bomb survivors was first manifested in the third year after exposure, reached a peak at 6 to 8 years, and gradually returned to baseline within about 20 years.[4] The incidence of leukemia also increases following high-dose ionizing radiation therapy. The cumulative mortality studies of over 14,000 patients irradiated for the treatment of ankylosing spondylitis showed that therapy led to the development of leukemia in 52 patients, approximately 10-fold the expected figure of 5.5.[5,11]

A variety of chemicals and drugs such as benzene, toluene, alkylating agents and immunosuppressive drugs have been associated with an increased incidence of leukemia in humans. The cumulative risk of drug-induced leukemia (usually AML) is 17% within 50 months of the beginning of therapy using alkylating agents in patients with multiple myeloma,[12] 10% within 7 years of starting chemotherapy in patients with ovarian carcinoma,[13] and 10% within 9 years from the beginning of combined chemotherapy and radiation therapy in patients with Hodgkin's disease.[14] The incidence of leukemia is also reported to be higher than in the normal population in patients with a variety of other hematopoietic malignancies and solid tumors who have received alkylating agents for cancer therapy, such as non-Hodgkin's lymphoma, chronic lymphocytic leukemia, breast cancers and bronchogenic carcinomas.[14-19] Immunosuppressive therapy in transplant patients and in patients with immune-associated disorders such as multiple sclerosis, rheumatoid arthritis and nephritis may increase the risk of hematopoietic malignancies, especially AML and non-Hodgkin's lymphoma.[20-22]

The role of viruses in the induction of hematopoietic malignancies in experimental animals is well documented. In humans, Epstein-Barr virus (EBV) and a type C retrovirus known as "human T-cell lymphotrophic virus (HTLV)" are associated with certain types of lymphoid malignancies.

There is strong evidence linking EBV to the African Burkitt's lymphoma. Burkitt's lymphoma is a B-cell malignancy associated with t(8;14) translocation and amplification of *c-myc*. It has been suggested that EBV acts as a B-cell mitogen, resulting in a polyclonal B-cell proliferation. In most individuals, the EBV-induced B-cell proliferation is a self-limited process. However, in a minority, the EBV-induced B-cell proliferation continues and the risk of an acquired cytogenetic abnormality [t(8;14)] in the rapidly growing lymphoid population increases. Clonal expansion of the abnormal cell with chromosomal translocation t(8;14) results in Burkitt's lymphoma. Thus, a chronic polyclonal proliferation of lymphocytes may lead to monoclonal lymphoproliferation.[23,24]

Types I and II HTLV have been associated with subclasses of T-cell malignancies. HTLV-I has a strong tropism for CD4$^+$ cells and has been repeatedly isolated from tumor cells in patients with adult T-cell leukemia/lymphoma (ATL). One or two copies of the HTLV-I provirus are identified in the same chromosomal locations in the neoplastic cells, and antibodies against HTLV-I are detected in over 90% of patients with ATL.[25,26] HTLV-II has been recovered in rare patients with hairy cell leukemia of the T-cell type.[27]

Other etiologic factors include family background and a predisposition to certain hematologic disorders. The high frequency of concordant leukemia in identical twins; the increased incidence in high-risk families; and the association with inherited chromosomal instability syndromes such as Down syndrome, Bloom syndrome and ataxia telangiectasia raise the possibility of an inherited susceptibility to leukemias.[28-30] Bone marrow stem cell disorders such as myelodysplastic and myeloproliferative syndromes, Fanconi's anemia and PNH also have a high incidence of progression to acute leukemias.

Frequent association of recurrent chromosomal aberrations with hematopoietic malignancies strongly suggests that chromosomal abnormalities play a major role in the pathogenesis of the malignant transformation of hematopoietic stem cells. An acquired chromosomal change may result in a defect in the maturation process and/or the function of the transformed cells, as well as a lack of response to the feedback control mechanisms. In many leukemias and lymphomas, karyotypic changes are associated with relocalization of the proto-oncogenes, which may result in structural and/or functional alterations of oncogenes in different ways (see Chapter 2). For example, translocation of an oncogene next to a transcriptionally active area may lead to amplification of the oncogene (e.g., *c-myc* in Burkitt's lymphoma). Chromosomal translocation may result in fusion of an oncogene with another gene at the site of translocation, leading to the production of a fusion gene product (e.g., the *c-abl/bcr* fusion gene in CML). Chromosomal aberrations may be associated with mutation in a proto-oncogene, leading to a qualitatively different gene product (e.g., *K-ras* in leukemias).

In addition to chromosomal translocations, chromosomal deletions are frequently associated with hematopoietic malignancies, especially therapy-related leukemias. The -5, $5q^-$, -7 and $7q^-$ are examples.[31-36] Both chromosomes 5 and 7 contain sequences involved in the production of proteins which play a role in proliferation and regulation of hematopoietic stem cells.[37-40]

LEUKEMIAS

Leukemias are traditionally divided into two major groups: acute and chronic. The neoplastic cells in acute leukemias are predominantly immature and in chronic leukemias are predominantly mature. In general, patients with acute leukemia have a more aggressive clinical course than patients with chronic (mature) leukemia. However, certain chronic leukemias may also demonstrate a rapid clinical course. Leukemias are also classified into two subclasses based on their cell of origin: lymphoid leukemias and nonlymphoid or myeloid leukemias.

In general, the involved bone marrow is hypercellular and diffusely infiltrated by leukemia cells. Areas of necrosis and/or fibrosis may be present. In the majority of the cases (>60%), leukemia cells are present in the peripheral blood at diagnosis. The term "aleukemic leukemia" refers to a leukemia which shows no evidence of peripheral blood involvement.

ACUTE LEUKEMIA

Acute Lymphoblastic Leukemia

Acute lymphoblastic (lymphatic, lymphoid, lymphocytic) leukemia (ALL) represents over 75% of all leukemias in children, with a peak incidence around 4 years of age.[41,42] The incidence of ALL is higher in males than in females, though no leukemogenic role for sex hormones has been established.[43]

Morphologic Classification

The classification proposed by the French-American-British (FAB) Cooperative Group is the only universally accepted morphologic classification for acute leukemias.[44,45] According to this group, the diagnosis of ALL is made when 30% or more of the bone marrow nucleated cells are lymphoblasts. However, some hematopathologists, including the author, also diagnose acute leukemia if blasts in peripheral blood make up 30% or more of the differential count even with <30% blasts in the marrow.

The FAB classification divides lymphoblasts into three categories: L1, L2 and L3 (Figures 6-1 to 6-3).

The **L1** lymphoblasts are characterized by morphologic homogeneity, small size, scanty cytoplasm and inconspicuous nucleoli. Lymphoblasts of the **L2** type are larger, display considerable heterogeneity in morphology, have more abundant cytoplasm and show prominent nucleoli. The **L3** lymphoblasts have morphologic and immunophenotypic features identical to those of Burkitt's lymphoma cells. They are homogeneous, with deep blue, often vacuolated cytoplasm, round nuclei and one or more prominent nucleoli (Table 6-1). The most common form of ALL is L1 in children and L2 in adults. The overall incidence of L1, L2 and L3 ALLs has been reported by the FAB Cooperative Study Group as 66, 29 and 5%, respectively.[46] The original proposal by the FAB Cooperative Study Group was later modified[46] to eliminate the rate of discordance among the observers and to improve the clinical correlations.[47-50] The modified version of the FAB classification introduced a scoring system for four cytologic characteristics: (1) nuclear:cytoplasmic ratio, (2) prominence and number of nucleoli, (3) regularity of the nuclear membrane and (4) cell size.[46] (Table 6-2).

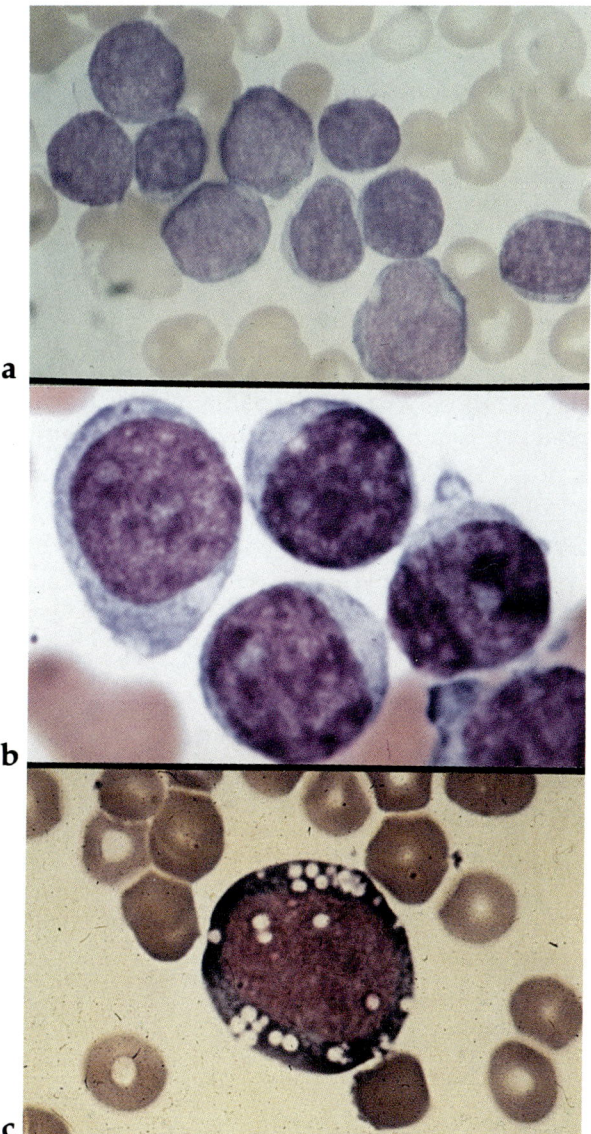

Figure 6-1. Bone marrow smears demonstrating examples of L1 (a), L2 (b) and L3 (c) ALLs.

Overall, L1 morphology is associated with a better event-free survival and induction rate than L2 morphology, and L3 morphology has the worst prognosis.[51-53]

Immunologic Classification

ALL is divided into two major categories based on immunophenotypic features: T-ALL and non-T-ALL.

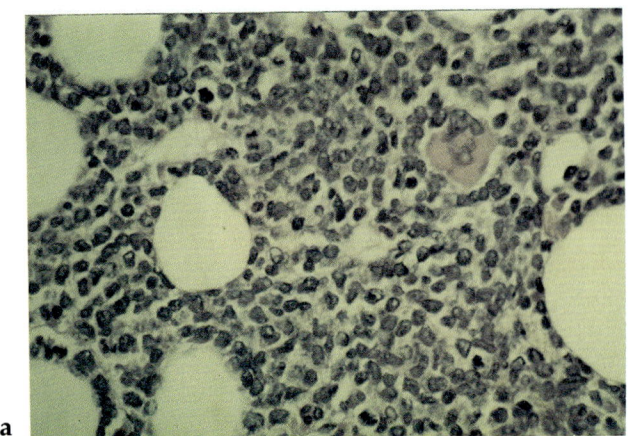
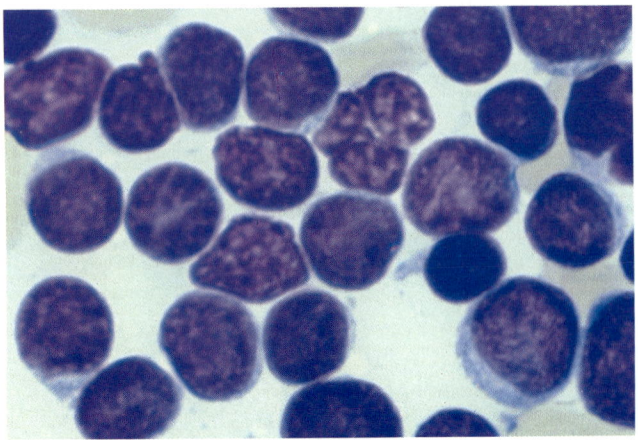

Figure 6-2. Bone marrow preparations from a patient with ALL, L1 morphology; (a) biopsy section, (b) marrow smear. (b) from Schumacher HR, Acute Leukemia. New York, Igaku-Shoin, 1990, with permission.

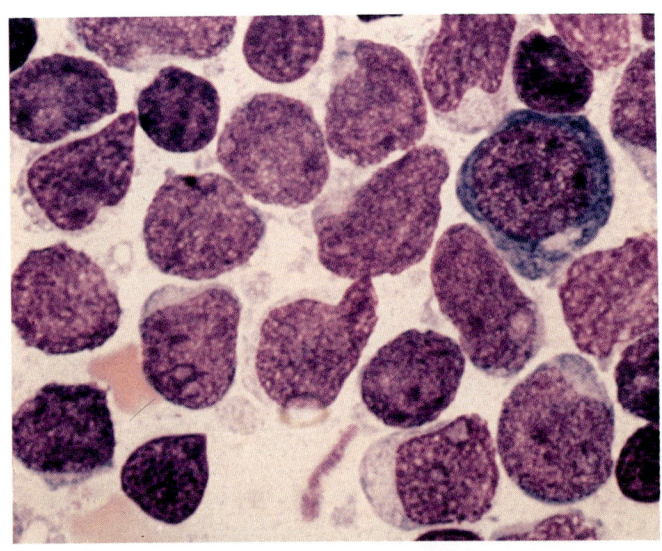

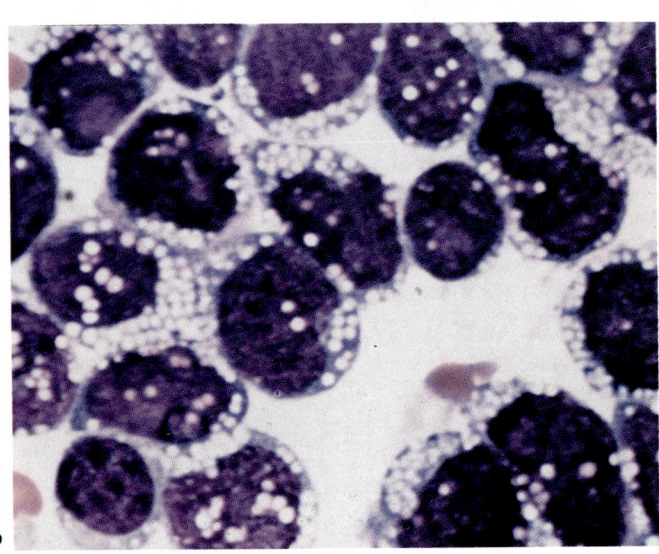
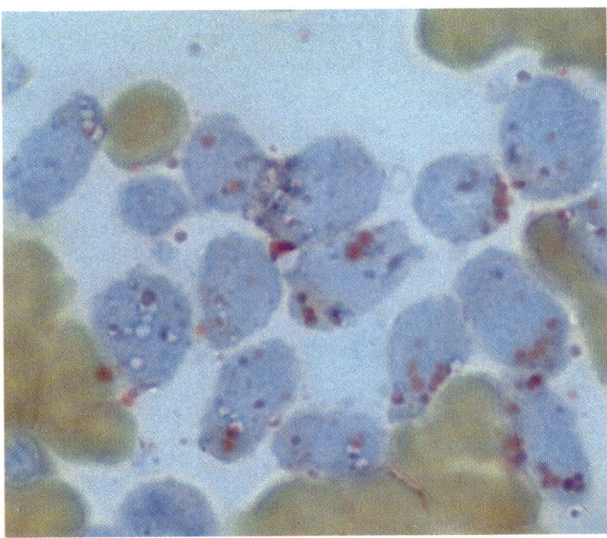

Figure 6-3. Bone marrow smears showing examples of L2 (a) and L3 (b and c) ALL. L2 lymphoblasts are large and show pleomorphic nuclei with prominent nucleoli. L3 lymphoblasts are relatively monomorphic and often show cytoplasmic vacuolization. The oil Red O stain is usually positive in L3 ALL (c). (c) from Schumacher HR; Acute Leukemia. New York, Igaku-Shoin, 1990, with permission.

Table 6-1 FAB Classification of ALL

Features	L1	L2	L3
Cell size	Predominantly small	Large, heterogeneous	Large, homogeneous
Cytoplasm	Scanty	Abundant	Moderate, deep blue, often vacuolated
Nucleus	Regular, homogeneous	Irregular, heterogeneous	Regular, homogeneous
Nucleoli	Not visible, or a few inconspicuous	One or more, prominent	One or more, prominent
Phenotype	B or T	B or T	B, SmIg+*

* Surface membrane immunoglobulin.

Table 6-2 Modified FAB Classification for L1 and L2 ALL*

Criteria	Score
High nuclear/cytoplasic ratio >75% of cells	+
Low nuclear/cytoplasmic ratio >25% of cells	−
Large cells >50% of cells	−
Irregular nuclear membrane >25% of cells	−
Nucleoli: 0–1, small >75% of cells	+
Nucleoli: 1 or more, prominent >25% of cells	−

* A total score of 0 to 2+ establishes a diagnosis of L1, and a total score of −1 to −4 establishes a diagnosis of L2.

Table 6-3 Classification of ALL Proposed by the First Morphologic, Immunologic, and Cytogenetic (MIC) Cooperative Study Group*

Type	T-ALL			
	TdT	CD7	CD2	FAB
Early T-precursor ALL t or del (9p)	+	+	−	L1,L2
T-cell ALL t(11;14) 6q−	+	+	+	L1,L2

* From First MIC Cooperative Study Group: Morphologic, Immunologic, and Cytogenetic (MIC) working classification of acute lymphoblastic leukemias. Report of the workshop held in Leuven, Belgium, April 22–23, 1985. Cancer Genet Cytogenet 23:189, 1986.

T-ALL: The T-cell phenotype accounts for about 20% of ALLs and consists of a heterogeneous group. Clinically, it is characterized by a tendency to involve older children and young adults (10–20 years old), an increased frequency of mediastinal mass, rapid progression, early relapse, marked increase in peripheral blood lymphoblasts (initial white blood cell count >100,000/μl) and a higher incidence of CNS involvement.[41,54,55] Neoplastic cells in the majority of T-ALLs express antigens which are representative of prethymocyte or early thymocyte stages in T-cell ontogeny (Table 6-3). About one-third of T-ALLs express a broad spectrum of surface antigens including antigens which represent the end stage of T-cell differentiation, such as CD3, CD4 and CD8.[56] In addition, approximately 25% of T-ALLs express phenotypic features which are unusual and cannot be mapped into the normal stages of T-cell maturation.[57,61] Some T-ALL cells (10–30%) are also CD10 and HLA-DR positive.[62-66] Since T-ALLs often express a mixture of surface antigens, it is difficult to establish their monoclonalty based on their patterns of reactivity with monoclonal antibodies, and T-cell receptor rearrangement studies are necessary (Chapter 2). However, it should be emphasized that approximately 5–15% of the non-T-cell hematopoietic malignancies may show evidence of TCR rearrangement.[67,68]

NON-T-ALL: This group of ALL accounts for over 80% of ALLs. The most frequent subtype in this category is Common ALL (pre-pre-B ALL), which expresses CD10, HLA-DR and TdT, and includes over 75% of the non-T-ALLs.[69,70] The neoplastic cells of common ALL represent an early stage of B-cell maturation. They express some of the B-specific antigens, such as CD19 and CD20 and show evidence of Ig gene rearrangement, but do not express cytoplasmic or surface membrane Ig.[71-77] A small proportion of the non-T-ALLs (5%) are less differentiated and do not express Ig or T-cell-associated antigens.[76,78] This small group, which is often referred to as "null ALL," is commonly TdT and HLA-DR positive, may express CD19 and, in most instances, represents a very early B-precursor ALL.

Another immunophenotypic category is pre-B-ALL which is defined as an acute leukemia with cytoplasmic IgM (Cμ) and forms approximately 10–15% of the non-T-ALLs. The neoplastic cells in this category, in addition to Cμ, express HLA-DR, CD19, CD10, and CD20.[76,79]

B-ALL is the most differentiated subtype, making up to 5% of the non-T-ALLs. Blast cells of this subtype express surface membrane Ig, as well as HLA-DR, CD19 and CD20.[76,79-81] B-ALL corresponds to the L3 subtype of the FAB classification. There is no correlation between the immunologic subtypes of ALL and the morphologic subtypes L1 and L2 (Table 6-4).

The most useful and widely selected markers for diagnosis and classification of ALLs are CD2, CD7, CD10, CD19 and TdT. Additional monoclonal antibodies are also used for further characterization of the leukemic cells (see Table 6-5). Some of the markers used for immunophenotyping of ALLs are not lymphoid specific, and are expressed in nonlymphoid leukemias and other cells as well. For example, CD10 has been found in kidney, fetal lung, placenta, epididymis, prostate, and neutrophils.[82] A small percentage of acute myelogenous leukemias are TdT or CD7 positive.[83-86] Also, approximately 10–30% of ALLs may express myeloid-associated antigens such as CD13 and CD33.[87-90] The ALL patients who express myeloid-associated antigens show a lower rate of complete remission.[90,91a,91b]

Cytogenetics

Approximately two-thirds of the ALL cases display characteristic chromosomal abnormalities.[92-97b] The early B-precursor ALL is often associated with t(4;11) (q21;q23) or t(9;22) (q34;q11). The ALL subtype with (4;11) translocation is CD10⁻, CD19⁺, TdT⁺, HLA-DR⁺ and may express CD24 and CD15. This subtype is frequently associated with hyperleukocytosis (white blood cell count >150,000/μl), age less than 1 year, female sex and poor prognosis.[95a]

Similarly, ALL with translocation (9;22) is often CD10⁻, TdT⁺, CD19⁺ and HLA-DR⁺, and is associ-

Table 6-4 Classification of ALL Proposed by the First Morphologic, Immunologic, and Cytogenetic (MIC) Cooperative Study Group*

Type	Non-T ALL						
	CD19	TdT	HLA-DR	CD10	Cμ	SmIg	FAB
Early B-precursor ALL t(4;11) t(9;22)	+	+	+	−	−	−	L1,L2
Common ALL 6q⁻ Near-haploid t, or del (12p) t(9;22)	+	+	+	+	−	−	L1,L2
Pre-B ALL t(1;19) t(9;22)	+	+	+	+	+	−	L1
B-cell ALL t(8;14) t(2;8) t(8;22) 6q⁻	+	−	+	±	±	+	L3

* From First MIC Cooperative Study Group: Morphologic, Immunologic, and Cytogenetic (MIC) working classification of acute lymphoblastic leukemias. Report of the workshop held in Leuven, Belgium, April 22–23, 1985. *Cancer Genet Cytogenet* 23:189, 1986.

Table 6.5 Cell Marker Studies for Acute Leukemias

	ALL	ANLL (AML)
	TdT	CD13
	CD2	CD14
	CD7	CD33
	CD10	CD41a
	CD19	Glycophorin A
Additional help:		
	T	Non-T	Myeloid
	CD1, CD3	CD20, CD22	CD11c, CD15
	CD4, CD5	CD24, CD34	CD34, CD42a
	CD8, CD16	HLA-DR	CD61, HLA-DR
	CD25, CD56	IG (K, L, ..)	

ated with a poor prognosis. The 22q chromosomal marker, known as the "Philadelphia chromosome (Ph¹)" is identified in leukemic cells of 3–5% of children and 15–25% of adults.[95b,96a,96b] As discussed in Chapter 2, in the majority of the Ph¹⁺ ALLs, the *bcr-abl* fusion gene created by (9;22) translocation encodes an mRNA of 7.0 kb, which is translated into a 190 kD protein.[95c]

Common ALL (HLA-DR⁺, TdT⁺, CD19⁺ and CD10⁺) cells may demonstrate 6q⁻, translocation or deletion of 12p, or may contain only 26–28 chromosomes (near-haploid). The hypodiploid leukemias have an unfavorable prognosis and are frequently associated with chromosomal translocations. Another frequent karyotypic feature of common ALL is hyperdiploidy. Hyperdiploidy, especially when it consists of >50 chromosomes per leukemic cell, is associated with a favorable prognosis.[95b] A small proportion of common ALL may show t(9;22).

Pre-B ALL is often associated with chromosomal translocation (1;19) or (9;22). The t(1;19) (q23;p13) is observed in approximately 25% of children with pre-B ALL and is associated with an adverse treatment outcome. This translocation results in consistent fusion of the E2A gene from chromosome 19 with the PBX1 gene on chromosome 1.[97a] The E2A/PBX1 fusion transcripts are detected in over 95% of the patients who demonstrate cytogenetic evidence of t(1;19).

The B-ALLs (L3) demonstrate three specific translocations which involve 8q24: t(8;14)(q24;q32.2) or, less commonly, either the t(2;8)(p11–p12;q24) or the t(8;22)(q24;q11). The t(8;14) translocation results in juxtaposition of the *c-myc* and *IGH* genes causing inappropriate expression of the *c-myc* gene. In some B-ALL patients there may be additional karyotypic abnormalities such as dup (1q) or t(1;19). Occasional B-ALLs may demonstrate 6q⁻.

T-ALLs expressing mature T-cell antigens often demonstrate t(11;14) or 6q⁻, and ALLs with the early T-precursor phenotype may show translocation or deletion of 9p.[97a,97b]

The Morphologic, Immunologic, and Cytogenetic (MIC) Cooperative Study Group has proposed a classification in which morphologic findings, immunophenotypic features and cytogenetic characteristics are all taken into consideration[97a, 97b] (see Tables 6-3 and 6-4).

Clinical Aspects

The greatest incidence of ALL is before age 10, especially between ages 3 and 7. Symptoms and signs are the result of bone marrow failure in the production of normal blood cells and extramedullary involvement with leukemia. Anemia, thrombocytopenia and granulocytopenia are common findings and are associated with fatigue, pallor, fever, bruisability and bleeding tendencies. Bone pain is a major complaint in about 20% of the cases. Lymphadenopathy and hepatosplenomegaly are common. The incidence of CNS and testicular involvement is rare at diagnosis but increases in relapses. Occasionally, ALL is associated with a hypereosinophilic syndrome. ALL patients with this syndrome characteristically have cytogenetic abnormalities of long arms of chromosomes 5 and 14.[98a] (see Chapter 8, page 258)

Poor prognostic factors include age younger than 1 and older than 10 years, L2 and L3 morphology, hemoglobin ≤10 g/dl, presence of a mediastinal mass, massive hepatosplenomegaly, CNS involvement and chromosome abnormalities such as t(9;22), t(4;11), t(1;19), t(8;14) and hypodiploidy.

Acute Myelogenous Leukemia

Acute myelogenous leukemia (AML) or acute nonlymphoid leukemia (ANLL) is a malignancy resulting from clonal expansion of an aberrant, committed, nonlymphoid stem cell at the CFU-S or later stages of differentiation such as BFU-E or CFU-E, CFU-GM, CFU-Meg and CFU-Eo. However, the CFU-GM is the predominant precursor cell involved in ANLL. The malignant transformation is often associated with cytogenetic abnormalities resulting in a population of abnormal cells that are not sensitive to the feedback regulators and are not capable of full differentiation. ANLL accounts for over 50% of leukemias. It represents about 80% of acute leukemias in adults and 15–20% of leukemias in children.[98b,99]

Classification

Based on the morphologic and cytochemical features of blast cells, a classification was proposed by the FAB Cooperative Group in 1976.[44] The original proposal was revised and expanded in 1985.[100,101] The FAB classification is widely accepted and has been incorporated with immunologic and cytogenetic results in numerous studies. According to the FAB classification, diagnosis of an AML is established when 30% or more of all nucleated bone marrow cells are blasts of a nonlymphoid lineage. However, some hematopathologists, including the author, also diagnose AML if the blasts in peripheral blood make up 30% or more of the differential count even with <30% blasts in the marrow.

Seven subtypes are defined by the FAB Cooperative Group and are designated as M1 through M7. M1 and M2 represent myeloblastic leukemia, M3 is promyelocytic leukemia, M4 stands for AMLs with myelomonocytic components, M5 represents monoblastic leukemias, M6 is an AML with predominance of the erythroid precursors and M7 refers to an acute leukemia of megakaryocytic lineage (Table 6-6).

MYELOBLASTIC LEUKEMIA WITHOUT MATURATION (M1): In this category, myeloblasts (sum of Type I and Type II blasts) make up 90% or more of the nonerythroid cells in the bone marrow, with at least 3% of the blast cells being MOP and/or Sudan black B positive. M1 accounts for approximately 20% of the ANLLs.[102,103]

Bone marrow is usually packed with the leukemia cells. Blast cells have a small amount of gray-blue cytoplasm, with no or a few azurophilic granules and usually no Auer rods. The nucleus shows a fine chromatin with one or more prominent nucleoli (Figure 6-4). A proportion of the blast cells usually express HLA-DR, CD13, CD33, and sometimes CD34 (see Table 6-5). In some cases, the primitive blasts display no morphologic or cytochemical features to establish a diagnosis of AML. This category is termed by some investigators "acute undifferentiated leukemia" or "AML-M0."[104,105] A proportion of the so-called acute undifferentiated leukemias demonstrate a few myeloperoxidase-containing granules by immunoelectron microscopy and thus fall into the AML-M1 category.[106a] Acute undifferentiated leukemia appears to be a heterogeneous entity and may include cases with lymphoid or mixed myeloid and lymphoid characteristics.[105,106b]

MYELOBLASTIC LEUKEMIA WITH MATURATION (M2): M2 is one of the most frequent variants, representing about 30% of ANLLs. There is evidence of partial maturation of myeloblasts to and sometimes beyond promyelocytes and myelocytes. Type I and Type II myeloblasts acount for ≥30% of bone marrow cells, but <90% of nonerythroid cells. Blast cells are commonly heterogeneous and overall larger than M1 blasts, and often show a few clusters of primary granules. The blasts express HLA-DR, CD13 and CD33, and are strongly MPO and Sudan black B positive and nonspecific esterase negative. Auer rods are usually present (Figures 6-4 and 6-5).

ACUTE PROMYELOCYTIC LEUKEMIA (M3): Approximately 5–10% of ANLLs are in the M3 category. Diagnosis of M3 is based on the presence of ≥30% promyelocytes (and myeloblasts) in bone marrow. The promyelocytes are atypical and, in the majority of cases (80%), are heavily loaded with azurophilic granules. These hypergranular promyelocytes display moderate to abundant cytoplasm and may contain one or several Auer rods (Figures 6-6 to 6-8). In occasional cases, the neoplastic cells may show morphologic features between those of promyelo-

Table 6-6 FAB Classification of Acute Nonlymphoid Leukemia

Type	Approximate Incidence	Major Features Morphology	Cytogenetic
M1	20%	Myeloblasts ≥90% of nonerythroid BM cells, infrequent Auer rods	t(9;22)(q34;q11)
M2	30%	Myeloblasts <90% of nonerythroid BM cells, frequent Auer rods	t(8;21)(q22;q22) t(6;9)(p21;q34)

M3	5–10%	≥30% promyelocytes
		Subtypes
		  Hypergranular (80%)
		  Hypo- or microgranular (20%)
			t(15;17)(q22;q11-21)

M4	30%	BM: 20–80% monocytic cells PB: >5000/μl monocytes Subtype: with >5% atypical eosinophils	t(6;9)(p21;q34) 5q⁻, 7q⁻ inv(16)(p13q22) del(16)(q22)

M5	10%	≥80% BM nonerythroid cells are monocytic Subtypes
		  M5a: monoblast predominant
		  M5b: promonocyte predominant
			t(8;16)(p11;p13)
			t(9;11)(p22;q23)
			11q⁻

M6	5%	Normoblasts ≥50% of BM cells Myeloblasts ≥30% of BM nonerythroid cells	5q⁻ 7q⁻ +8
M7	5%	≥30% megakaryoblasts Subtype: Acute myelofibrosis	t(21), +21

cytes and myelocytes. These include abundant cytoplasm with a mixture of primary and secondary granules, an eccentric round or oval nucleus and often prominent nucleoli (Figure 6-9).

Approximately 20% of M3 leukemias display promyelocytes with fine, dust-like granules and lobulated or folded nuclei (microgranular M3) (Figure 6-10). This variant may be mistaken for myelomonocytic (M4) leukemia, especially when the cells have very few microgranules.[107-109]

The M3 leukemic cells are strongly MPO and Sudan black B positive and often negative, for nonspecific esterase. They are also CD13 and CD33 positive and HLA-DR and CD14 negative. An association between the retinoic acid receptor −α (RAR −α) gene and translocation breakpoint on chromosome 17 has been suggested in M3 leukemias.[110-112]

The cytoplasmic granules in acute promyelocytic leukemia contain procoagulants which often initiate disseminated intravascular coagulation (DIC), especially during chemotherapy-induced tumor cell lysis.[113]

ACUTE MYELOMONOCYTIC LEUKEMIA (M4): Acute myelomonocytic leukemia is another common form of ANLL, representing about 30% of the total.[114,115] Diagnosis of M4 is based on both bone marrow and peripheral blood examinations. In bone marrow, nonlymphoid blast cells are ≥30% of the marrow cells. The nonerythroid population consists of a mixture of myeloid (30–80%) and monocytic (>20% to <80%) precursors (Figures 6-11 and 6-12). Peripheral blood in M4 patients often shows an absolute monocytosis (≥5000/μl), with the presence of immature and atypical forms. The leukemic blasts show considerable pleomorphism in cell size, amount of cytoplasm, cytoplasmic granularity and nuclear morphology. Auer rods are occasionally present. Cytochemical stains demonstrate MPO, Sudan black B and nonspecific esterase staining in a variable proportion of the leukemic cells. In addition, CD13, CD33 and CD14 are expressed by some tumor cells. The positivity of nonspecific esterase and CD14, together with elevated levels of serum and/or urine lysozyme, helps to identify the monocytic component

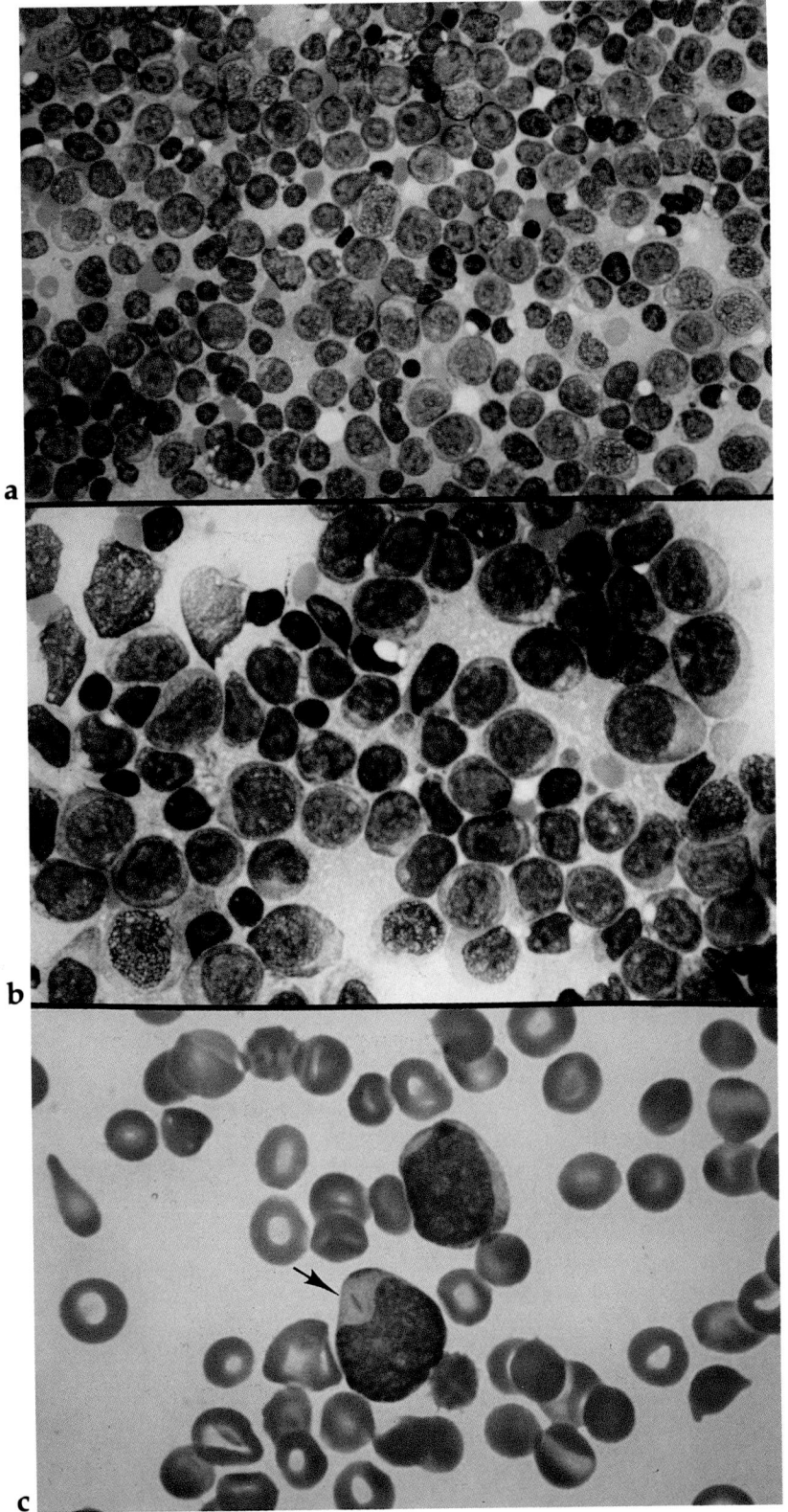

Figure 6-4. Acute myelogenous leukemia. (a and b) Bone marrow smear of a patient with AML-M1. (c) Peripheral smear from a patient with AML-M2 showing two myeloblasts, one with an Auer rod (arrow).

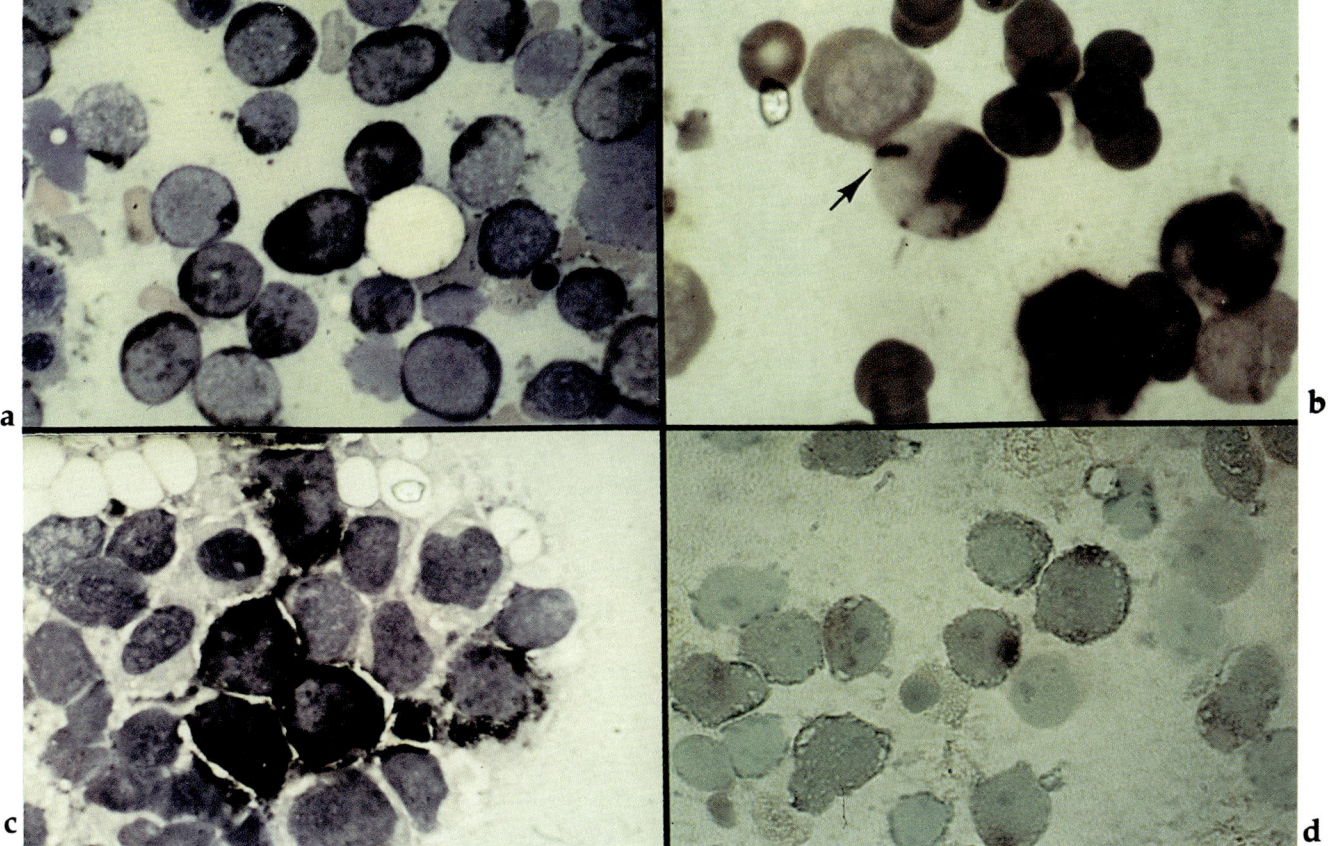

Figure 6-5. Peroxidase (a and b), Sudan black B (c), and alpha naphthyl acetate esterase (d) stains demonstrating positive blasts in a patient with AML-M2 (a–c) and a patient with AML-M7 (d). A peroxidase-positive Auer rod is noted in (b) (arrow).

in M4 leukemias and to distinguish them from the M2 category. In addition, acute leukemias with monocytic components (M4, M5), unlike other types of AML, have a tendency toward extramedullary involvement such as gingival or dermal infiltrations.

A subtype of myelomonocytic leukemia is described in association with atypical eosinophilia and abnormality of chromosome 16 (q22).[116,117] In this type of leukemia (M4Eo), 5% or more of the nonerythroid bone marrow cells are atypical eosinophils. These eosinophils are characterized by a mixture of basophilic and eosinophilic granules (see Figure 6-12), and demonstrate chloroacetate esterase and PAS (coarse granules) positivity.[103] The M4Eo subtype has a higher frequency of CNS involvement, but has a more favorable prognosis and a higher remission rate than the M4 leukemia. The most common chromosome abnormalities in this subtype are inv(16)(p13q22) and del(16)(q22).

ACUTE MONOCYTIC LEUKEMIA (M5): Acute monocytic leukemia accounts for about 10% of the ANLLs and is clonally expressed in cells committed to differentiation to the monocytic pathway.[118] The major characteristic features of M5 are a higher incidence in children and young adults, markedly elevated white blood cell counts and extramedullary involvements.[119-122] The extramedullary infiltration may involve different parts such as gums, lungs, meninges, lymph nodes, larynx, gastrointestinal tract and bladder.[120-122]

In M5 leukemia monocytic precursors comprise ≥ 30% of bone marrow cells and ≥ 80% of the nonerythroid cells. The M5 leukemia is divided into two morphologic sybtypes: M5a and M5b.

In M5a, or poorly differentiated acute monocytic leukemia, most of the leukemia cells (≥ 80%) are monoblasts. Monoblasts display abundant deep blue or gray-blue cytoplasm which is often vacuolated and

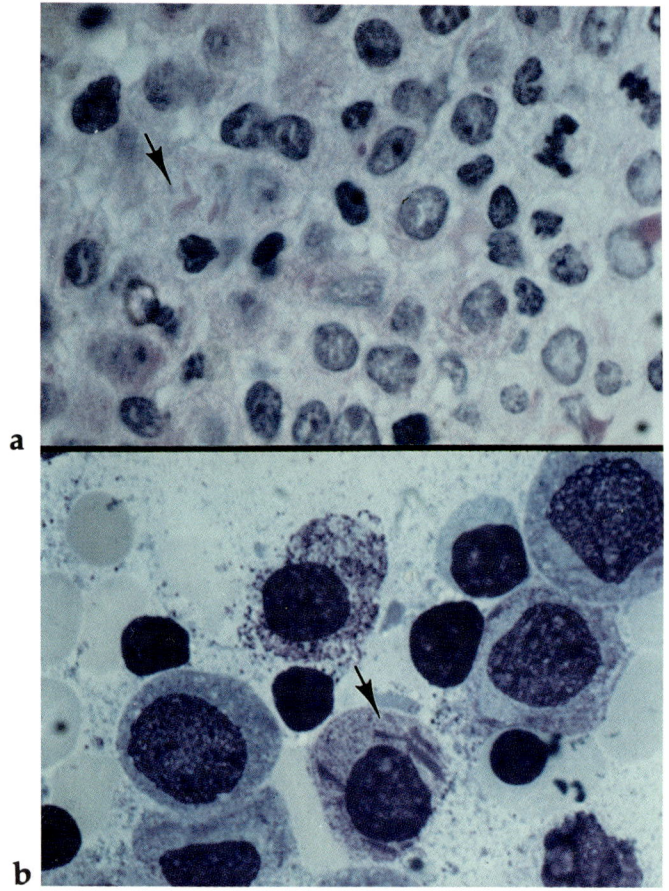

Figure 6-6. Bone marrow biopsy section (a) and smear (b) from a patient with promyelocytic leukemia (M3) showing several Auer rods (arrows).

has no or a very few azurophilic granules and no Auer rods (Figure 6-13). The nuclei are round or oblong, with one or more very prominent nucleoli.

In acute monocytic leukemia with partial differentiation (M5b), the bone marrow is replaced by a mixture of monoblasts and more mature monocytic cells. Monoblasts comprise ≥30% of bone marrow cells and <80% of the nonerythroid population. A variable proportion of leukemic cells are in further stages of maturation, and show nuclear folding and convolution (Figure 6-14). Auer rods may be detected in a small percentage of M5b leukemias.

Diagnosis of M5 leukemia is based on morphologic observations, cell marker studies (positivity for HLA-DR and CD14), positive staining for fluoride-sensitive nonspecific esterase and elevated serum and/or urine lysozyme levels.

ERYTHROLEUKEMIA (M6): Erythroleukemia (Di Guglielmo's syndrome) is a variant of leukemia which accounts for approximately 5% of de novo and 10-20% of therapy-induced (secondary) AMLs. Most M6 leukemias are preceded by a preleukemic phase (RA) characterized by anemia, megaloblastoid changes, marked bone marrow erythroid preponderance and often the presence of ringed sideroblasts. This early stage of RA evolves into an RA with excess blasts then AML-M6, and finally AML-M1 or AML-M2.[123-125] Diagnosis of M6 leukemia is defined by the FAB Cooperative Study Group based on the following two bone marrow findings: (1) ≥30% of the nonerythroid marrow cells are myeloblasts, and (2)

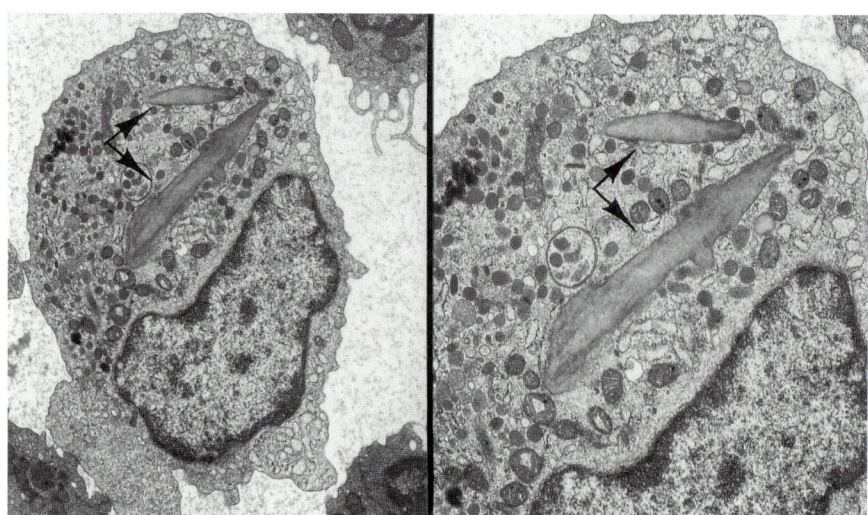

Figure 6-7. Electron microscopic photograph of a promyelocyte from a patient with AML-M3 demonstrating Auer rods (arrows).

Leukemias and Lymphomas

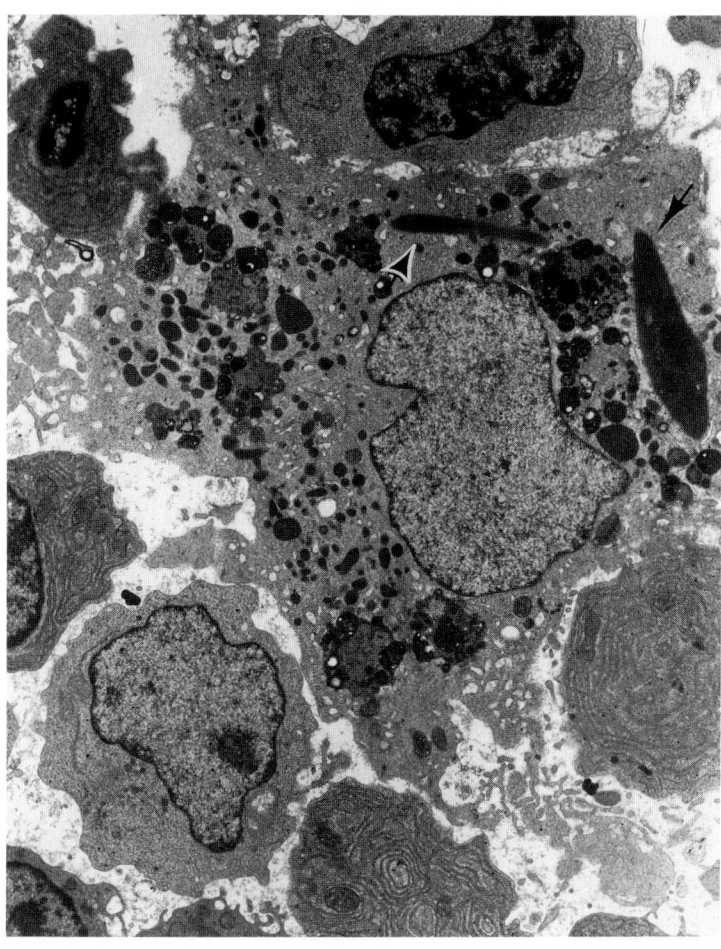

Figure 6-8. Electron microscopic photograph of a promyelocyte from a patient with AML-M3 demonstrating Auer rods (arrows).

≥50% of the bone marrow cells are nucleated red blood cells (Figure 6-15). Bone marrows with <30% blast cells fall into the category of RAEB, and bone marrows with ≥30% blasts but <50% nucleated red blood cells fit into the other subtypes of ANLL.

The erythroid precursors in M6 leukemia show marked megaloblastoid and other dysplastic changes such as bi- or multinucleated cells and giant forms. The major cytochemical and immunophenotypic characteristics of erythroid precursors in M6 are focal nonspecific esterase positivity, diffuse and/or chunk-like PAS positivity, and positive reactivity with anti-glycophorin A, anti-transferrin receptor and anti-spectrin antibodies. Patients with M6 leukemia commonly show normal to elevated serum folate and vitamin B_{12} levels, and may demonstrate a high proportion of fetal hemoglobin in electrophoresis.

MEGAKARYOBLASTIC LEUKEMIA (M7): Megakaryoblastic leukemia comprises about 5% of AMLs[101,126a-128b] and is probably the most frequent type of AML in children with Down's syndrome.[126a,126b] Megakaryoblastic leukemia has also been reported in association with mediastinal germ-cell tumors.[127a,127b] Blast cells are markedly pleomorphic, ranging from small, round cells with scanty cytoplasm, dense chromatin and inconspicuous nucleoli to large cells with abundant cytoplasm and prominent nucleoli (Figures 6-15 to 6-18). The megakaryoblasts and primitive megakaryocytes often display cytoplasmic budding, have a tendency to appear in clusters and may be closely associated with platelet aggregates (platelet shedding from the cells). The leukemia cells may express platelet-associated antigens CD41, CD42 and CD61, and are positive for platelete peroxidase (PPO). They are

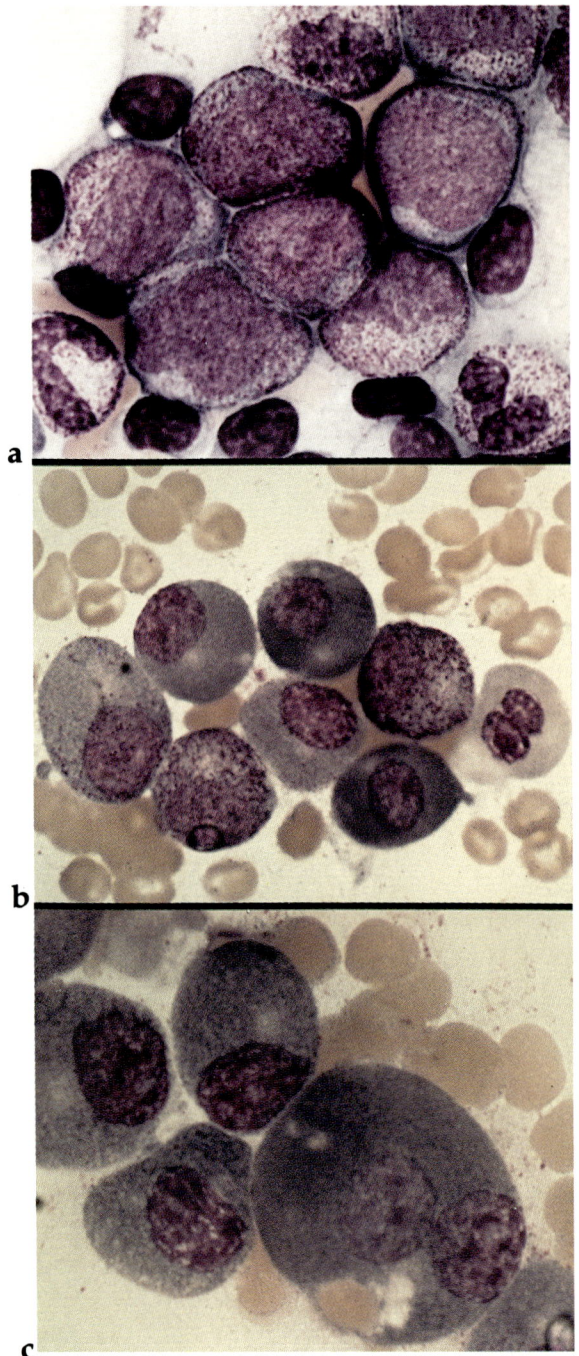

Figure 6-9. An unusual promyelocytic leukemia with clusters of early promyelocytes (a) and very late promyelocytes (b and c). A binucleated tumor cell exhibits erythrophagocytosis (c). Cytogenetic studies in this case demonstrated loss of chromosome 17.

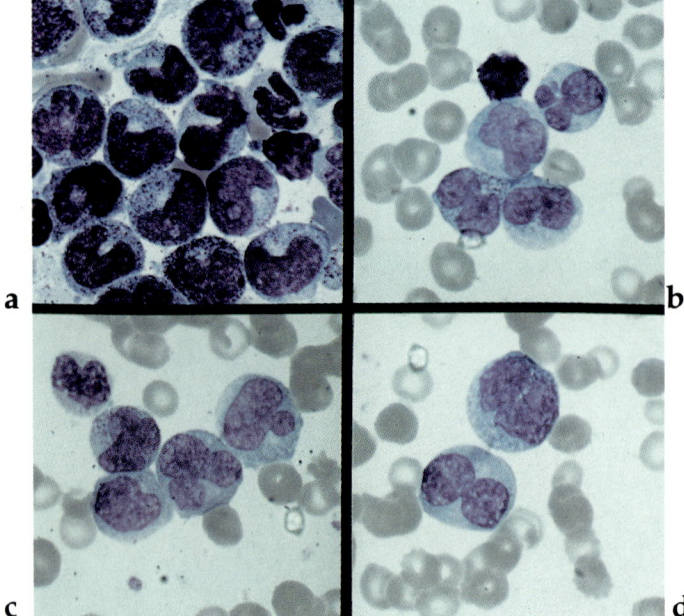

Figure 6-10. Bone marrow (a) and peripheral blood smears (b–d) from a patient with a microgranular variant of promyelocytic leukemia. Sparse granularity and nuclear folding are characteristic morphologic features.

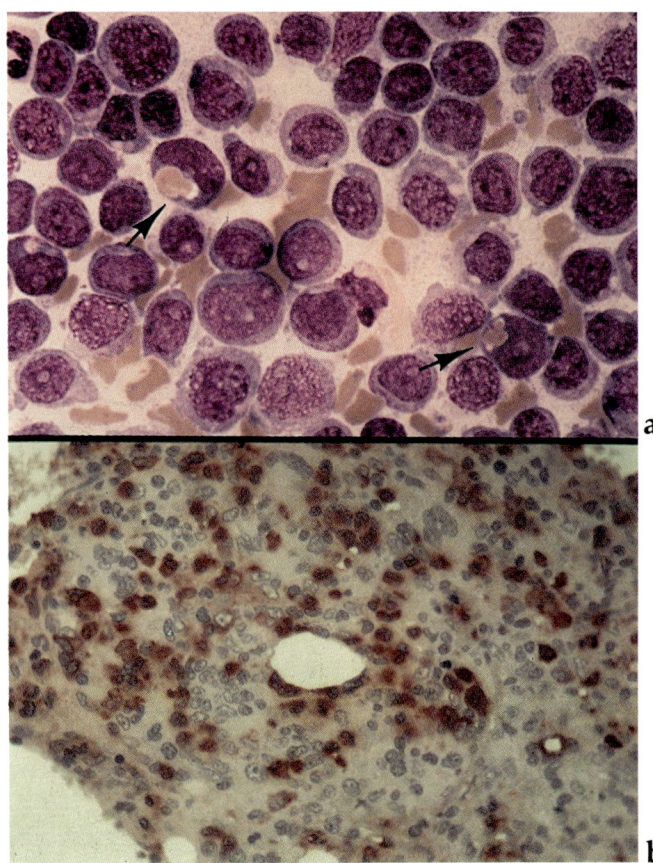

Leukemias and Lymphomas

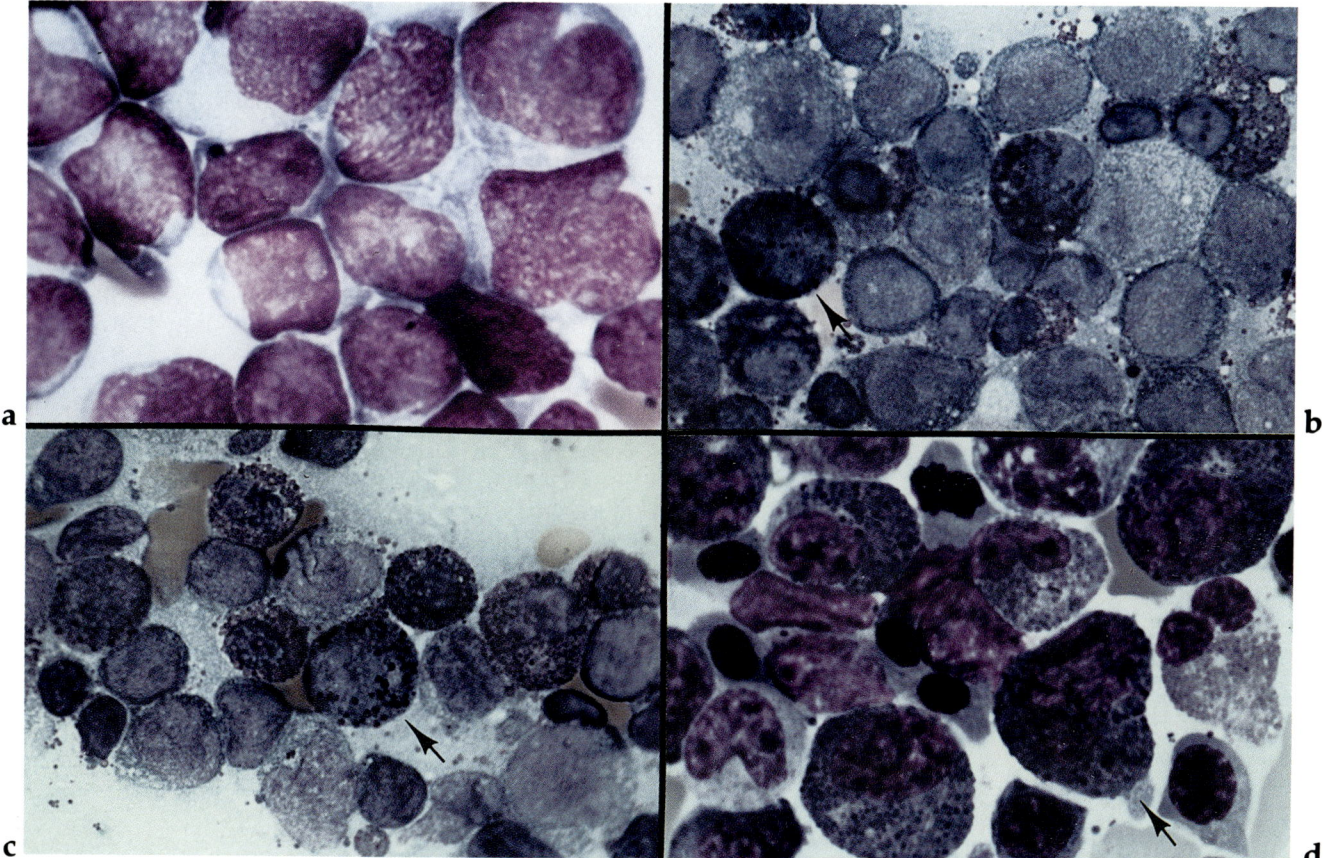

Figure 6-12. (a) A bone marrow smear displaying acute myelomonocytic leukemia (AML-M4). (b–d) Acute myelomonocytic leukemia with atypical eosinophilia (M4Eo). The atypical eosinophils contain a mixture of eosinophilic and basophilic granules (arrows).

negative for MPO, Sudan black B and alpha-naphthol butyrate esterase but may show focal positivity for alpha-naphtylacetate esterase or naphthyl AS-D acetate esterase (see Figure 6-5). This positive reactivity is inhibited by addition of fluoride. Acid phosphatase and PAS reactions are frequently positive in a localized pattern. DNA content analysis may demonstrate DNA aneuploidy.[129a]

One of the characteristic features of M7 is marrow fibrosis (Figure 6-19). The increased frequency of marrow fibrosis in megakaryoblastic leukemia and myeloproliferative disorders, as discussed before (see Chapter 5), is probably related to the release of the platelet-derived growth factor from the abnormal megakaryocytes. The marrow fibrosis in M7 may be extensive. In such cases, the bone marrow aspirates are dry and peripheral blood may contain megakaryoblasts and megakaryocytic fragments. This combination of acute leukemia and myelofibrosis represents a condition called "acute myelofibrosis (malignant myelofibrosis)."[126b-133] Acute myelofibrosis in most instances is a subtype of AML-M7; in fact, some investigators have equated acute myelofibrosis with acute megakaryoblastic leukemia.[134,135] However, other leukemias may also show extensive marrow fibrosis. Acute myelofibrosis, unlike agnogenic myelofibrosis, is characterized by an aggressive clinical course and by the presence of blast cells, pancytopenia and the lack of leukoerythroblastosis in peripheral blood. Poikiloanisocytosis and splenomegaly are minimal or lacking.[136]

Figure 6-11. Bone marrow smear (a) and lysozyme stained clot section (b) from a patient with M4 AML. A few cells show erythrophagocytosis (arrows).

156   Pathology of Bone Marrow

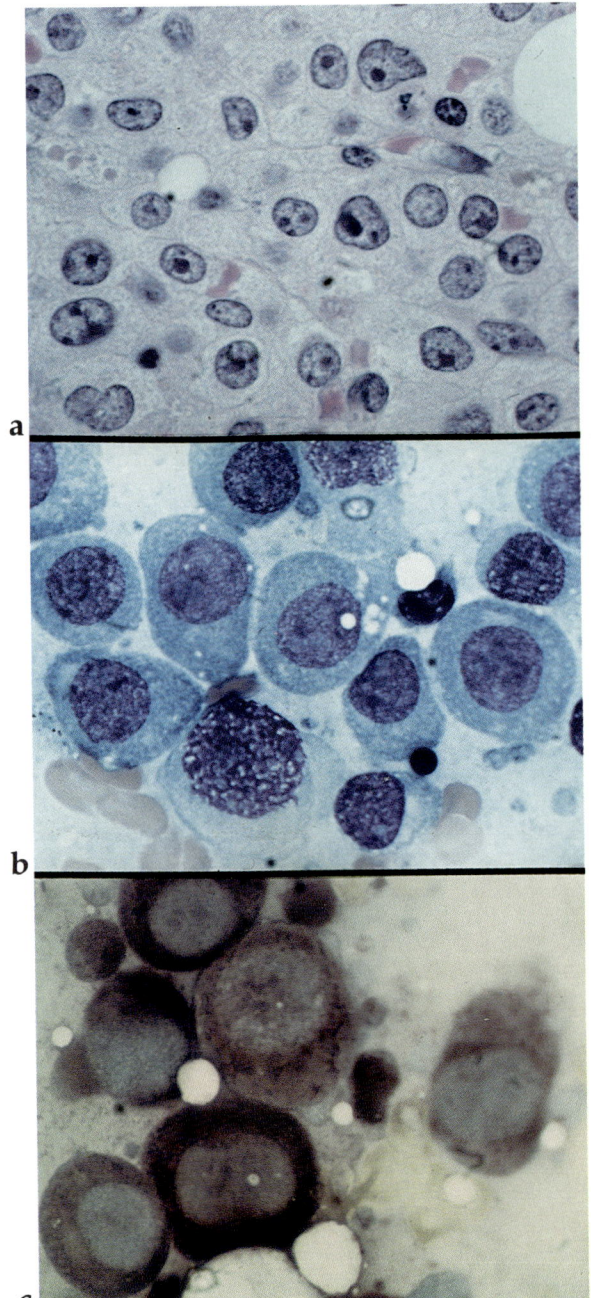

Figure 6-13. Bone marrow biopsy section (a) and smears (b and c) from a patient with monoblastic (M5a) leukemia. Blast cells are non-specific esterase positive (c).

Cyogenetics

Improved banding and culture techniques have significantly increased the detection of chromosomal abnormalities in hematologic malignancies. Many laboratories are currently able to detect chromosome abnormalities in >80% of patients with AML[137] (see Table 6-6).

The t(9;22)(q34;q11) translocation, which is the hallmark of CML (see below), is also detected in approximately 5–10% of M1 leukemias.[103] This translocation results a fusion *bcr-ab1* gene with an 8.5-kb mRNA and a 210-kD hybrid protein.

The most common cytogenetic abnormality in M2 leukemias is t(8;21)(q22;q22). The breakpoint on chromosome 8q22 is more conserved than that on chromosome 21, suggesting that the critical gene disrupted by this translocation is located on chromosome 8.[138] Translocation (8;21) often occurs in association with other chromosomal abnormalities, such as loss of the Y or X chromosome or 9q⁻. Blast cells in some AML-M2 patients may show t(6;9)(p21;q34).

The t(15;17)(q22;q11-21) has been observed in 70–100% of the patients with M3 AMLs.[137] A number of genes located within the proximity of the chromosome 17 breakpoint were considered to be involved in M3 leukemia, including C-erbB2 and C-erbA1 proto-oncogenes, myeloperoxidase gene, and the gene coding for RAR-α.[110-112,139] However, recent investigations have demonstrated that the chromosome 17 breakpoint in M3 AML is associated with RAR-α gene translocation and rearrangement.[110-112] In addition to t(15;17), M3 leukemia patients may show trisomy of chromosome 8.[103]

A variety of cytogenetic abnormalities have been reported in myelomonocytic leukemias. The most consistent ones are t(6;9)(p21;q34), 5q⁻, 7q⁻ and −7.[103] A subtype of myelomonocytic leukemia is described in association with atypical eosinophilia and abnormality of chromosome 16 (q22).[116,117] Most common chromosome abnormalities in M4Eo subtype are inv(16)p13q22) and del(16)(q22).

The most common cytogenetic abnormalities in M5 leukemias are t(8;16)(p11;p13), t(9;11)(p22;q23) and 11q⁻; in M6 leukemias, they are 5q⁻, 7q⁻ and trisomy 8; and in M7 leukemias they are translocation or trisomy of chromosome 21.[103,137]

Figure 6-14. Bone marrow biopsy section (a) and smears (b,c) from a patient with monoblastic (M5b) leukemia.

Leukemias and Lymphomas

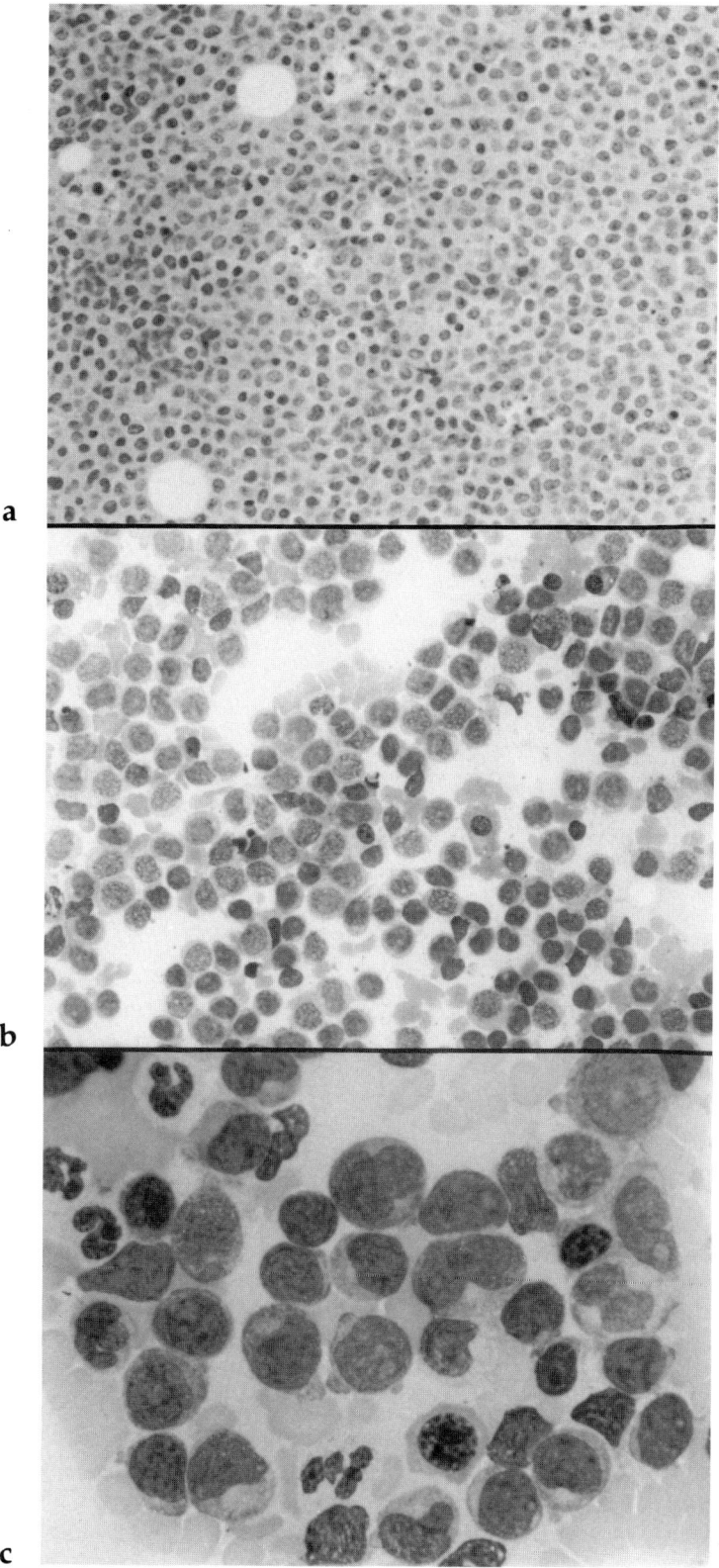

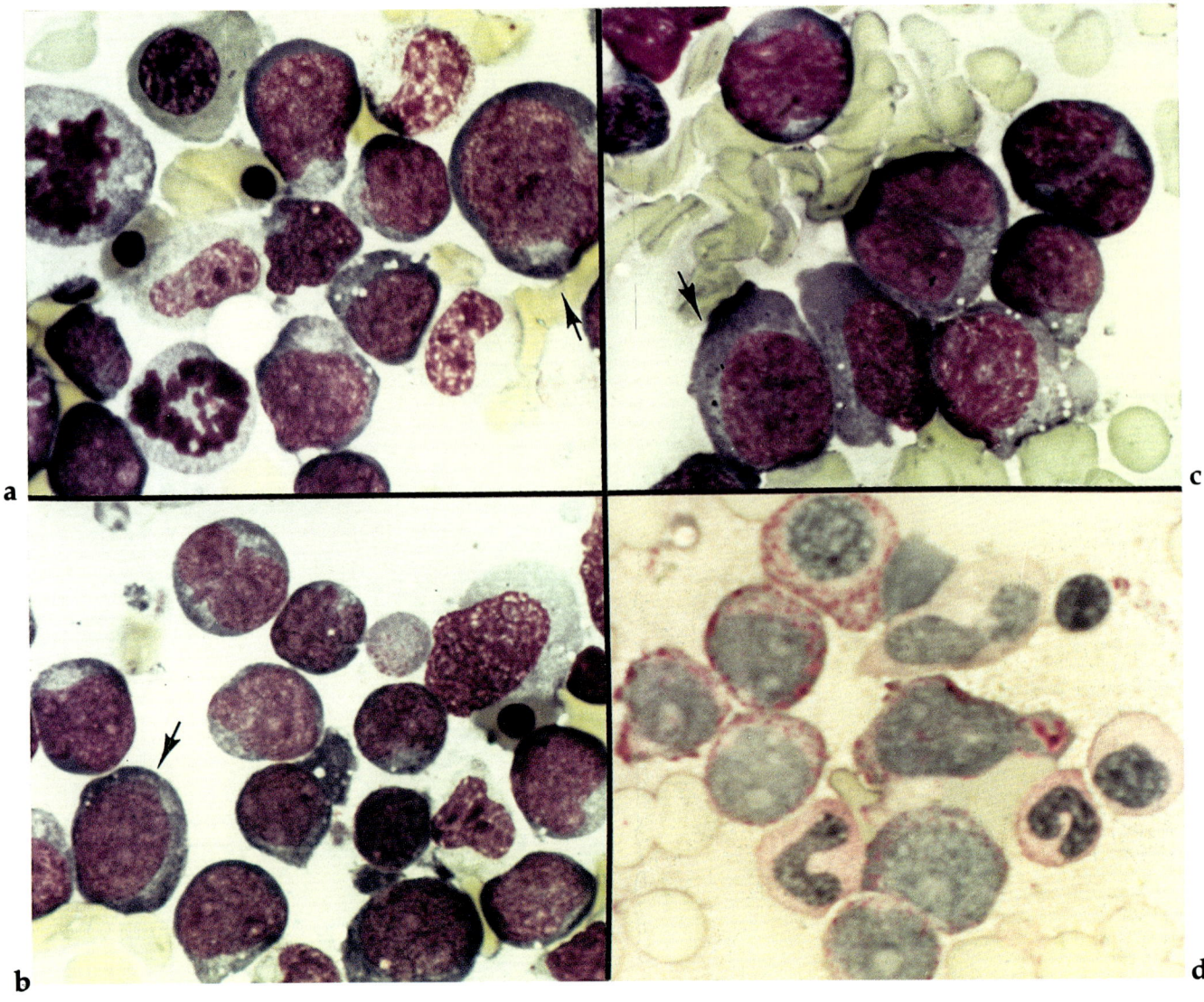

Figure 6-15. Bone marrow smears exhibiting erythroleukemia (M6). Numerous myeloblasts and erythroblasts (arrows) are present, and many show irregular and/or bilobed nuclei (a–c). Blasts display PAS-positive, coarse cytoplasmic granules (d).

Clinical Aspects

Acute nonlymphoid leukemia accounts for about 80% of acute leukemias in adults and 15–20% of acute leukemias in children, especially during the neonatal period. Clinical findings similar to those of other leukemias are related to the failure of bone marrow to produce normal blood cells and to extramedullary involvement. The most frequent symptoms and signs include pallor, fatigue, fever, easy bruising and bleeding tendencies, which are associated with anemia, granulocytopenia and thrombocytopenia. Bleeding tendencies are characteristic of AML-M3. Hepatosplenomegaly occurs in about 30% of the patients. Lymphadenopathy is rare. Extramedullary involvement is more frequent in the AML-M4 and -M5 varieties. Solid extramedullary tumors composed of AML cells are called *"granulocytic sarcomas (chloromas)."* "Chlorama" is a term that refers to the

Figure 6-17. Peripheral blood smear from a patient with AML-M7 exhibiting pleomorphic megakaryoblasts, early megakaryocytes and fragments of megakaryocytic cytoplasm (arrows).

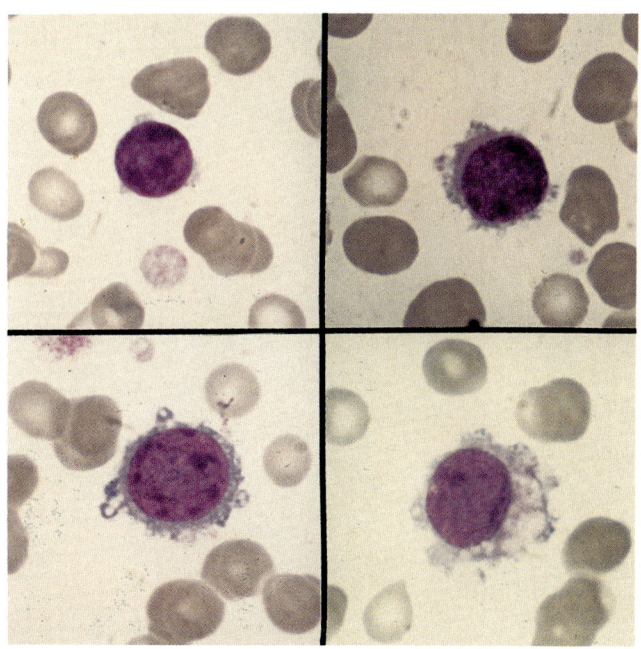

Figure 6-16. Perpheral blood smear from a patient with AML-M7 demonstrating pleomorphic megakaryoblasts with cytoplasmic budding.

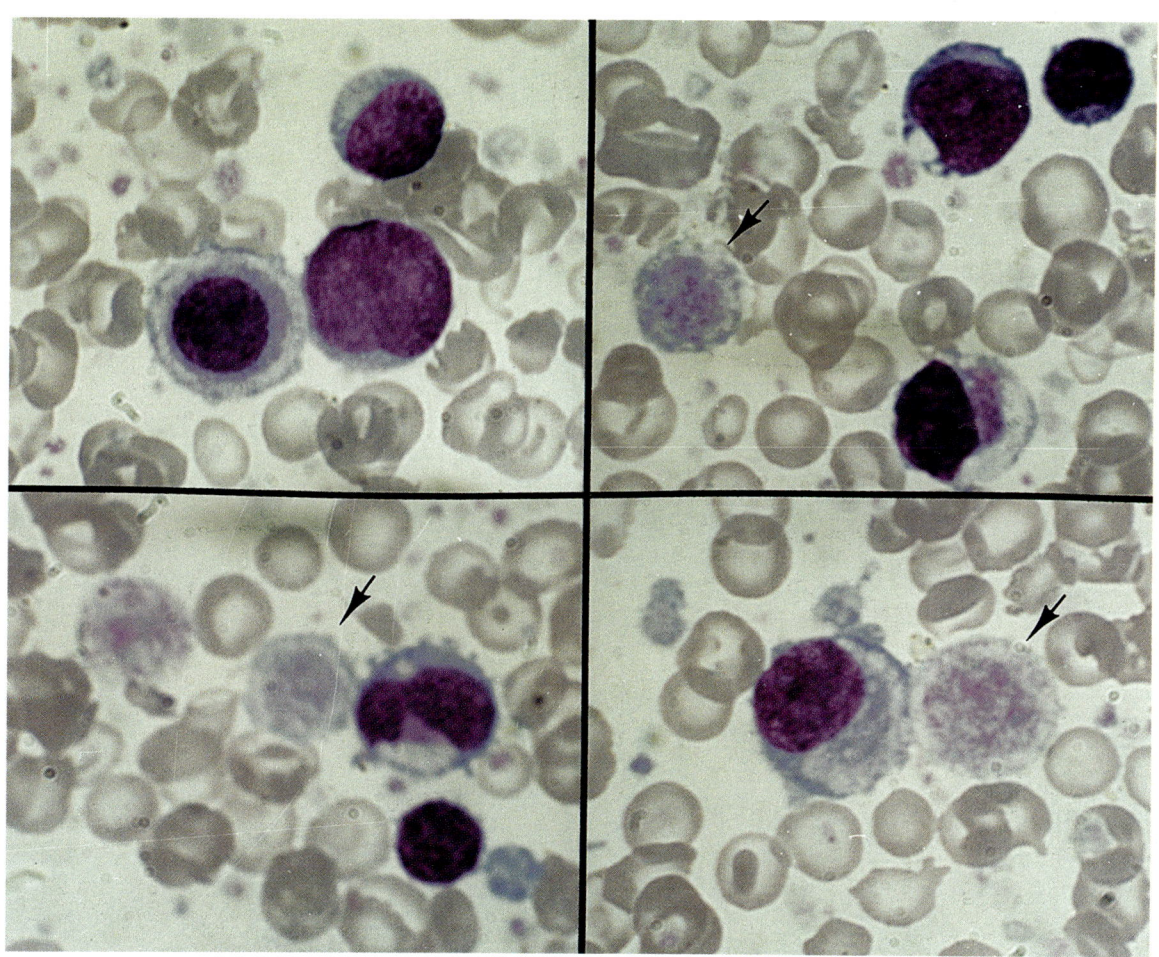

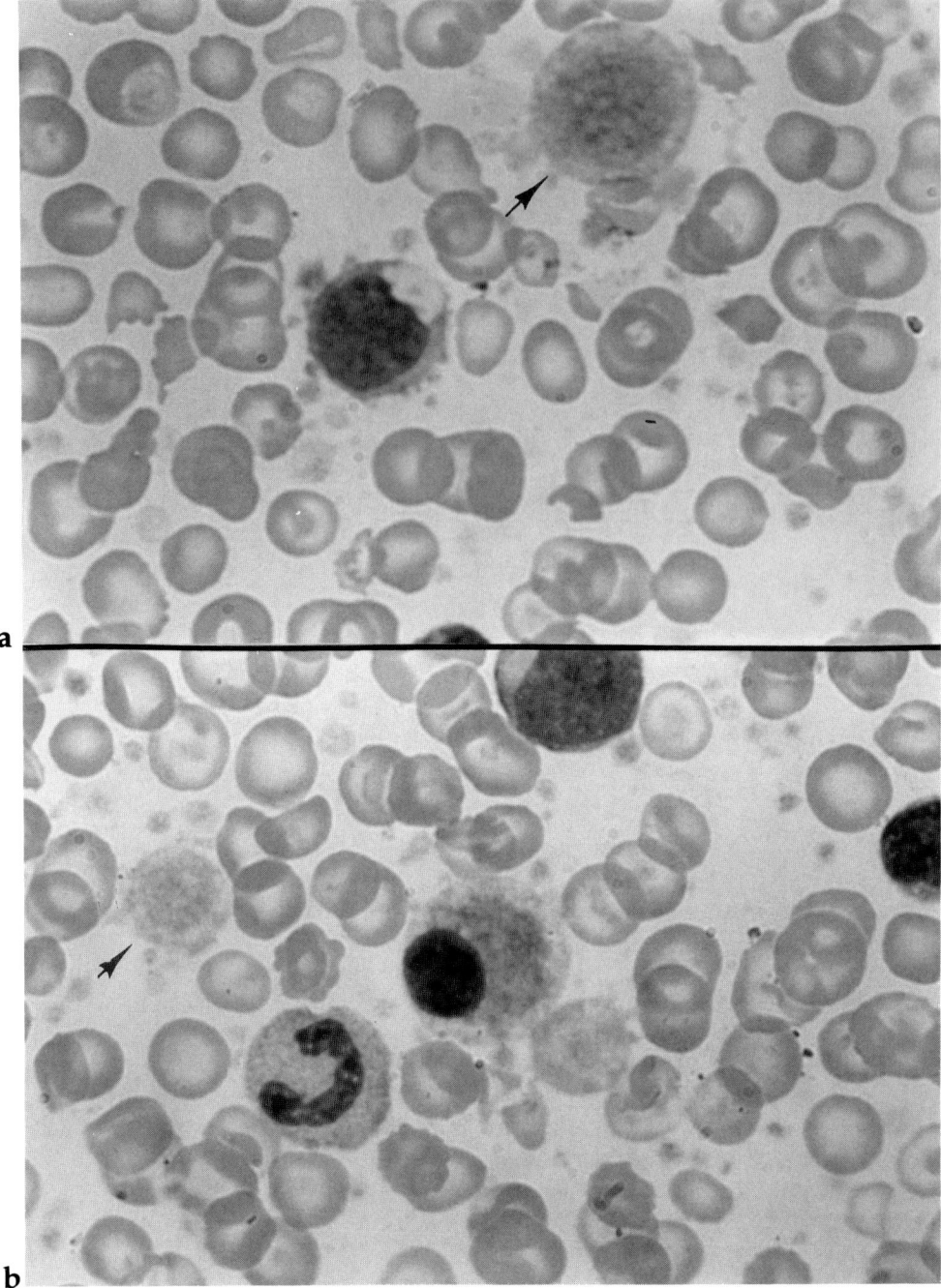

Figure 6-18. Peripheral blood smear from a patient with AML-M7 showing a vacuolated megakaryoblast (a), a micromegakaryocyte (b) and fragments of megakaryocytic cytoplasm (arrows).

green color of the tumor due to the heavy concentration of MPO in the tumor cells. Granulocytic sarcomas may be found in any location, but particularly in the paranasal sinuses, orbit, skin, CNS, and respiratory and gastrointestinal tracts.

Poor prognostic factors include old age, increased blasts in peripheral blood (>15,000/µl), thrombocytopenia (<30,000/µl), absence of Auer rods and presence of -5, -7, $5q^-$, or $7q^-$ chromosome abnormalities.

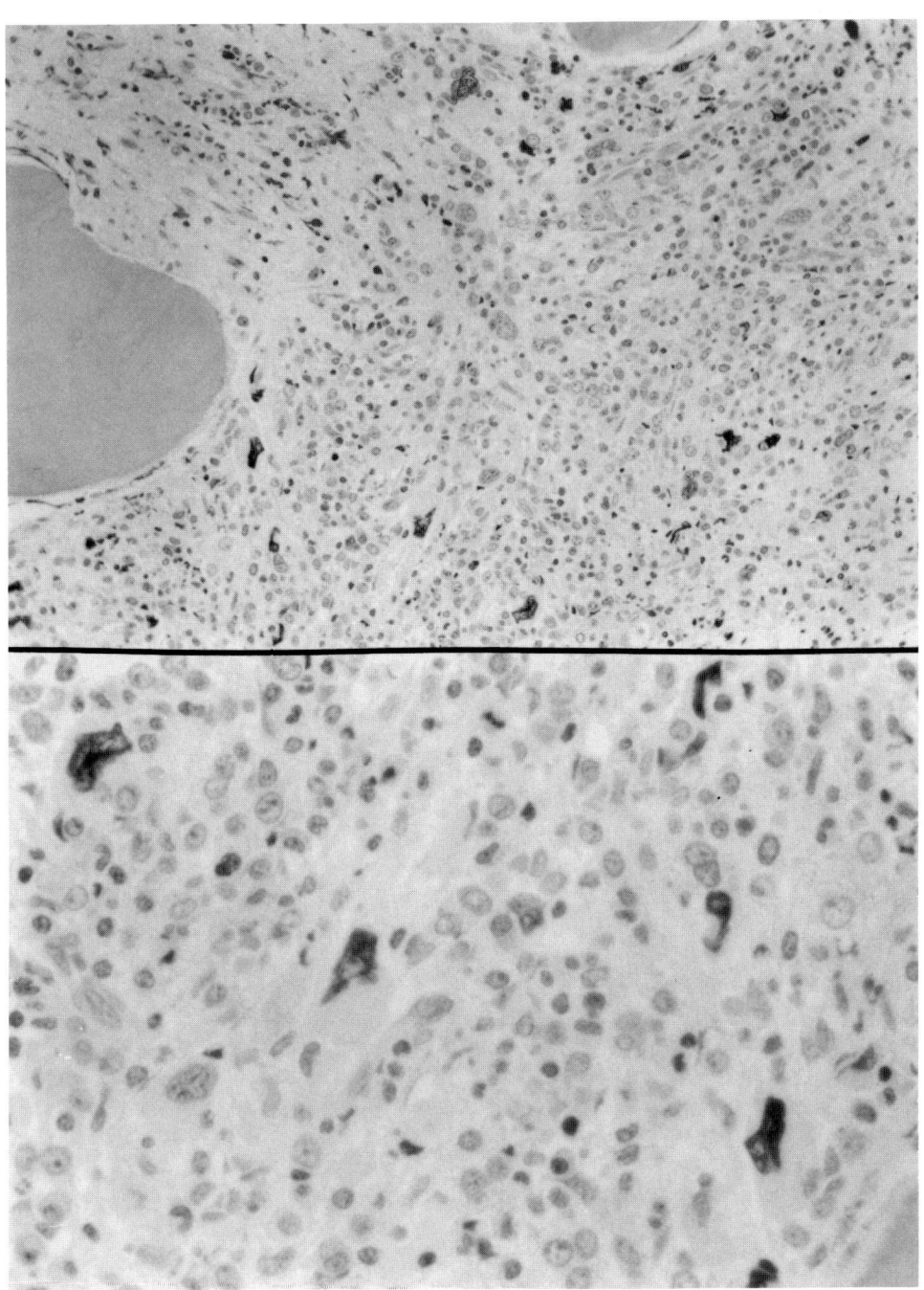

Figure 6-19. Bone marrow biopsy section from a patient with AML-M7 exhibiting marrow fibrosis with increased numbers of blast cells and abundant megakaryocytes.

Other Types of Acute Leukemia

Acute Lymphoid Leukemia of NK Phenotype

This is a rare subtype of ALL in which the blast cells express CD16, CD56 and CD57. The blasts are also CD2+ and CD8+, and may or may not express CD3.[140,141a,141b] ALL with the NK phenotype is either de novo or the result of blast transformation of large granular lymphocytic leukemia. Occasional patients may demonstrate extensive marrow fibrosis with circulating blast cells, similar to the condition referred to as "acute myelofibrosis." The blast cells have variable amounts of cytoplasm and often con-

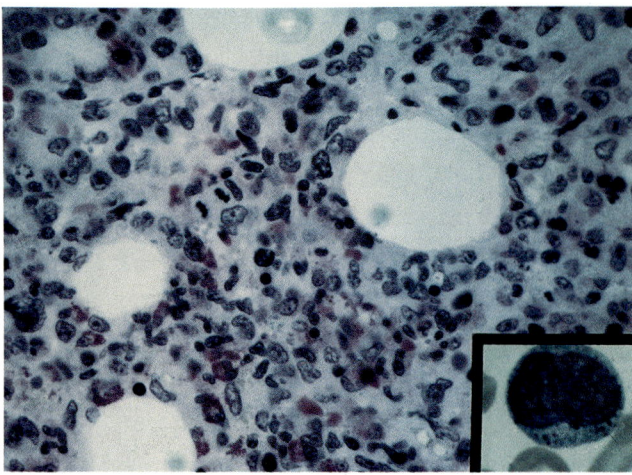

Figure 6-20. Bone marrow interstitial infiltration with blast cells in an ALL with the NK phenotype. The insert shows a blast cell with scattered azurophilic granules.

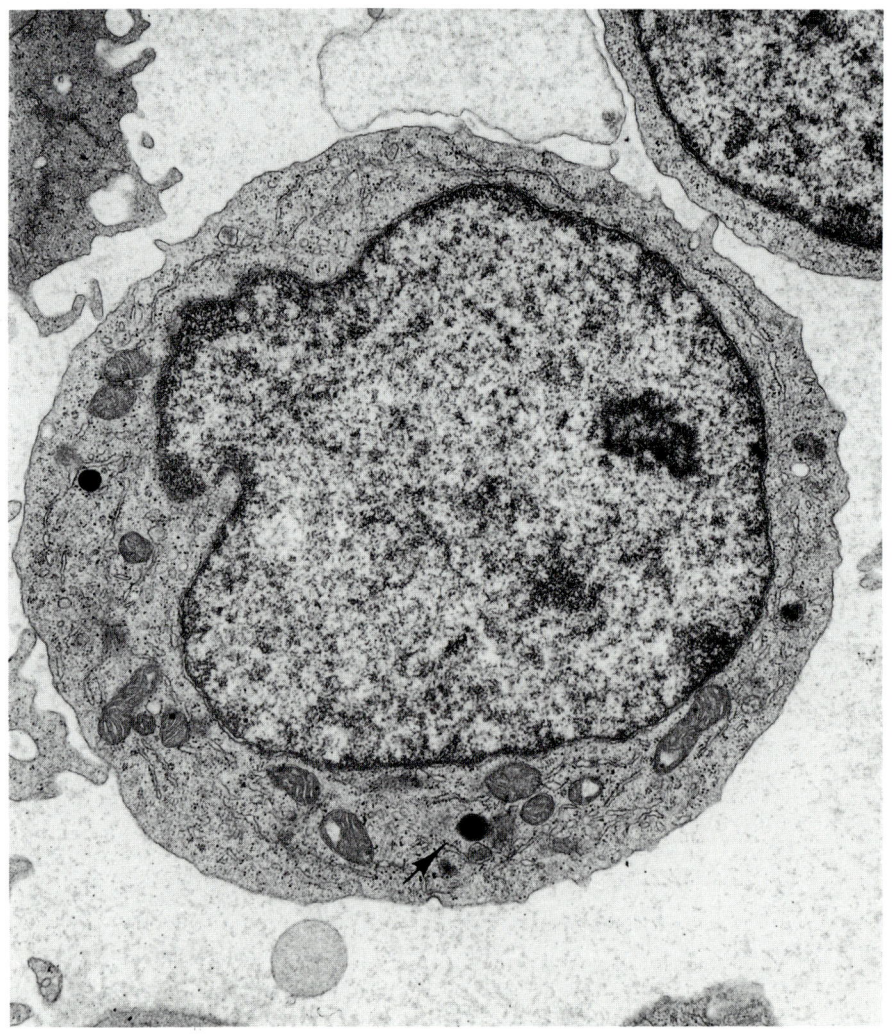

Figure 6-21. Electron microscopic photograph of a lymphoblast from a patient with NK ALL. A few small lysosomal granules are present in the cytoplasm (arrow).

Leukemias and Lymphomas

tain small numbers of azurophilic (lysosomal) granules (Figures 6-20 and 6-21).

The presence of cytoplasmic granules has also been reported in other subtypes of ALL, including common ALL and pre-B ALL[142,143a,143b] (Figure 6-22). In a recent study of over 1200 pediatric ALL cases, approximately 5% showed blasts with azurophilic cytoplasmic granules and were called *"granular acute lymphoblastic leukemia."* They were mostly of the FAB-L2 type and showed a significantly poorer outcome.[142]

Acute Basophilic Leukemia

Acute basophilic leukemia is a rare leukemia usually diagnosed on the basis of ultrastructural analysis and identification of basophilic granules in the leukemic blast cells. Recently, Peterson et al reviewed electron microscopic features of 455 acute leukemias and identified eight cases of acute basophilic leukemia.[144] Three of the cases had Ph¹ based on cytogenetic analysis. No clinical features distinguished these patients from other AML patients.

Hypoplastic Acute Leukemia

Hypoplastic acute leukemia (hypocellular acute leukemia, hypocellular bone marrow with increased blasts) is a leukemic condition characterized by marked bone marrow hypocellularity and a tendency to involve elderly persons (mainly men). Patients with hypoplastic acute leukemia are leukopenic or pancytopenic and have rare or a few blasts in their peripheral blood.[145-148] The pathogenesis of this disorder is not known, but bone marrow toxicity may play a contributing role. In a study by Gladson and Naeim,[148] a history of alcohol abuse was noted in 30% of the patients, potential exposure to toxic chemicals in 20% and a second malignancy (with a history of chemotherapy or radiation therapy) in 20%. The same study also demonstrated a history of aplastic anemia in 25% of the patients. The bone marrow is

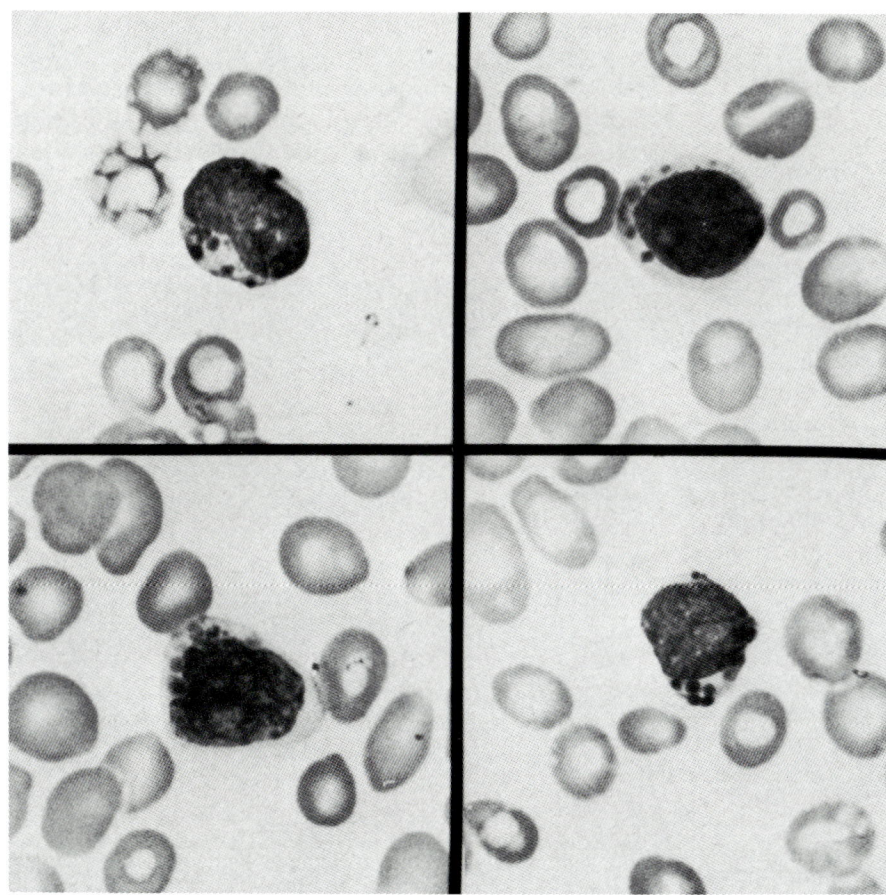

Figure 6-22. Lymphoblasts with giant cytoplasmic granules. From Yanagihara, Naeim F, Gale R, et al: Acute lymphoblastic leukemia with giant intracytoplasmic inclusions. *Am J Clin* 74:345, 1980, with permission.

hypocellular (usually > 30%), and the blast cells are the predominant cellular elements in the marrow, accounting for 30% to virtually 100% of the bone marrow cells (Figures 6-23 and 6-24). Blasts display scanty to moderate amounts of cytoplasm, round to oval nuclei with a fine chromatin, and one or more prominent nucleoli. In most morphologic studies, blast cells appear to be of myeloid origin. However, in some instances, blasts are very primitive, with negative staining for MPO and/or Sudan black B, rare or no azurophilic granules, no Auer rods, and no evidence of further differentiation toward more mature granulocytic or monocytic elements.[148] Of the 15 patients with hypocellular acute leukemia reported by Needleman et al.,[146] 14 were classified as having ANLL (10 patients M1, three patients M2 and one patient M4), and one patient was classified as having ALL-L2. All the patients reported by Beard et al.[145] and Howe and associates[147] were considered to have ANLL. In spite of the high percentage of blasts in the bone marrow, hypoplastic acute leukemia tends to remain in the smoldering phase for a long period of time before progressing to a fulminant leukemia.[145-148]

Acute Leukemia, Hand-Mirror Cell Variant

Hand-mirror cell leukemia is a morphologic varient of acute leukemia in which the leukemic cells demonstrate a cytoplasmic tail[149-152] (Figure 6-25). In most instances, this morphologic configuration is the result of ameboid movement of the neoplastic cells and is not an artifact[152,153] (Figure 6-26). The criterion proposed by some investigators for the diagnosis of hand-mirror leukemia is that ≥40% of the leukemic blast cells show hand-mirror morphology. The majority of the reported cases of hand-mirror cell leukemia are ALL.[149-152] However, the hand-mirror morphology has been observed in AMLs, as well as in lymphomas.[152,154] Most studies show no statistically significant difference in prognosis between the classic acute leukemia and the hand-mirror variant, although an increased incidence of CNS involvement and a positive correlation between the increased percentage of hand-mirror cells and a favorable prognosis have been reported.[152,155,156]

Blast Transformation of Chronic Leukemias

Progression of a chronic leukemia to an acute phase, with excessive production of blast cells, is one of the characteristic features of chronic myelogenous leukemia. A similar phenomenon also occurs occasionally in patients with chronic lymphocytic leukemia or low-grade non-Hodgkin's lymphomas. Blast transformations in chronic leukemias and lymphomas are discussed elsewhere in this chapter.

Acute Mixed Leukemias

The comprehensive multiparameter approach of studying the neoplastic cells in acute leukemias by cytochemical, immunophenotypic and molecular biology techniques has demonstrated a growing incidence of leukemias characterized by a combination of antigens and/or gene rearrangement patterns suggestive of a mixed lineage nature (Table 6-7). This group of leukemias is often referred to as "mixed lineage," or "biphenotypic" or "hybrid" leukemia.

A number of explanations for the mechanism(s) of the cell marker overlaps in mixed lineage leukemias have been proposed, including (1) *lineage infidelity*,[157] indicating that the neoplastic clone, as a consequence of its abnormal developmental program, inappropriately expresses a combination of lymphoid- and myeloid-, or myeloid- and erythroid- or B-cell and T-cell-associated antigens; (2) *lineage promiscuity*,[158] suggesting that, in normal bone marrow, differentiation and lineage commitment may be an error-prone process, and certain cells may retain features that cross over cell lineages; clonal expansion of such cells will lead to a hematopoietic malignancy with overlap features; (3) neoplasms with mixed lineage expressions are merely hematopoietic malignancies in which more than one clone of cells are affected.

A simplified approach was proposed by Gale and Ben Bassat for the classification of acute mixed (hybrid) leukemias[159] (Figure 6-27). According to their proposal, mixed leukemias are divided into two subtypes: (1) leukemias in which the individual leukemic cells express both myeloid and lymphoid features (*biphenotypic leukemias*), and (2) leukemias in which the leukemic cells are heterogeneous and display either lymphoid or myeloid features. In this group, leukemic cells are either raised from one clone with bilineage differentiation (*bilineal leukemias*) or derived from two separate clones (*biclonal leukemia*). Biphenotypic leukemias are probably the most frequent type.

Diagnosis of biphenotypic leukemia is based on the criteria established by the hematopathologist; the more restrictive are the criteria, the less frequent is the diagnosis of biphenotypic leukemia.[160-174] The

Leukemias and Lymphomas

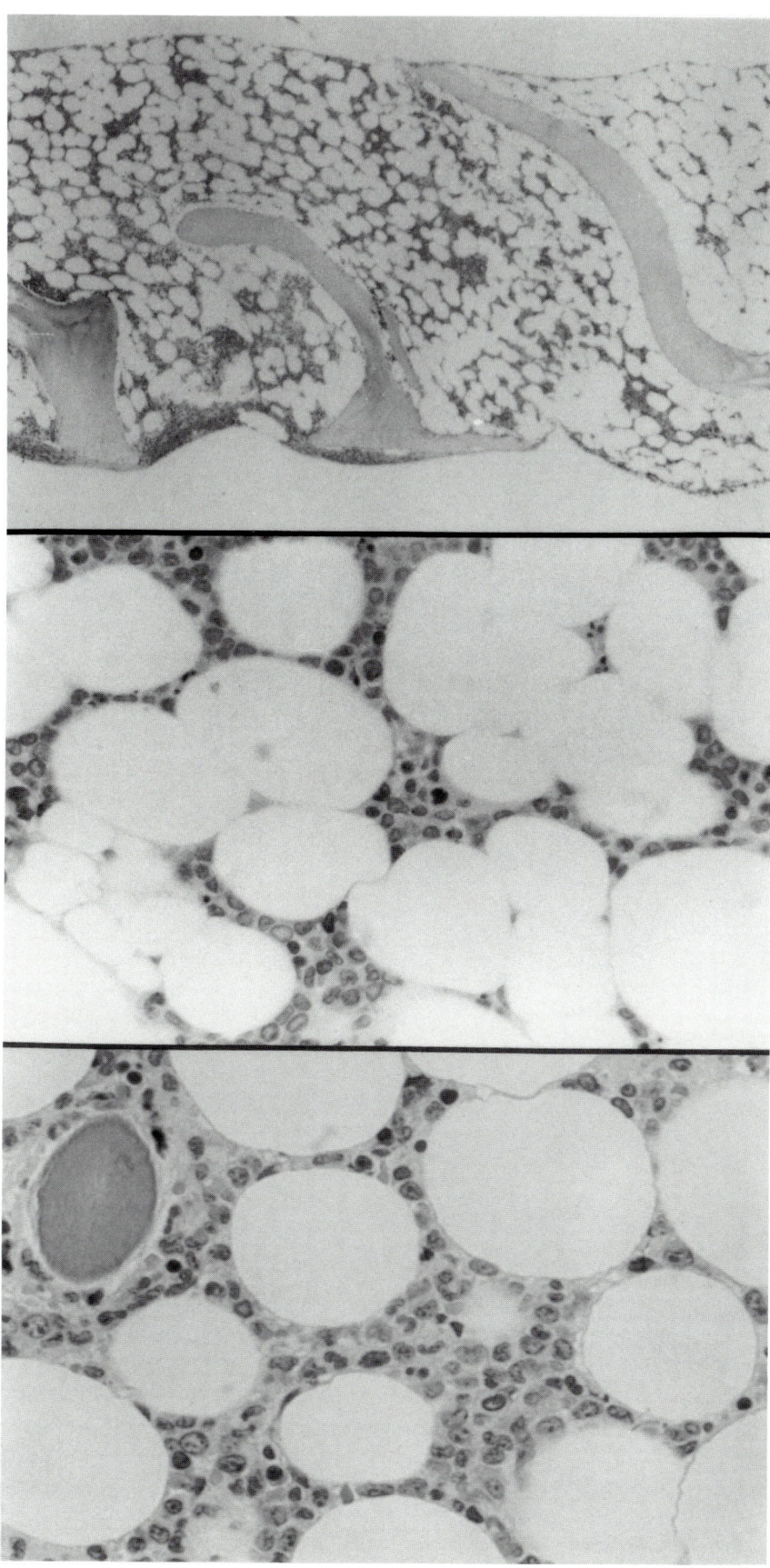

Figure 6-23. Bone marrow biopsy section demonstrating hypocellularity with increased blast cells (hypocellular leukemia).

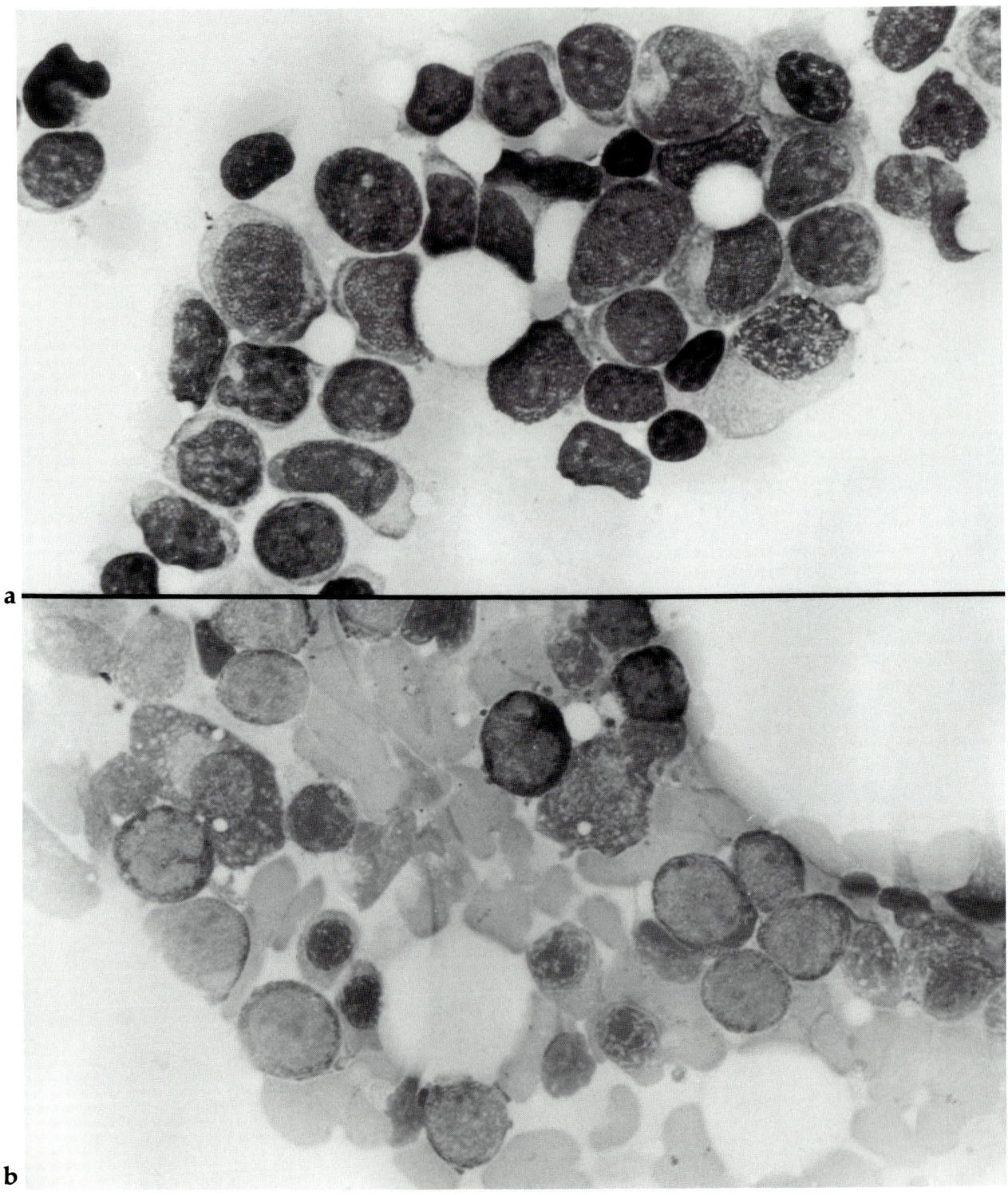

Figure 6-24. Bone marrow smears from a patient with hypocellular acute leukemia demonstrating increased myeloblasts (a) with peroxidase positivity (b).

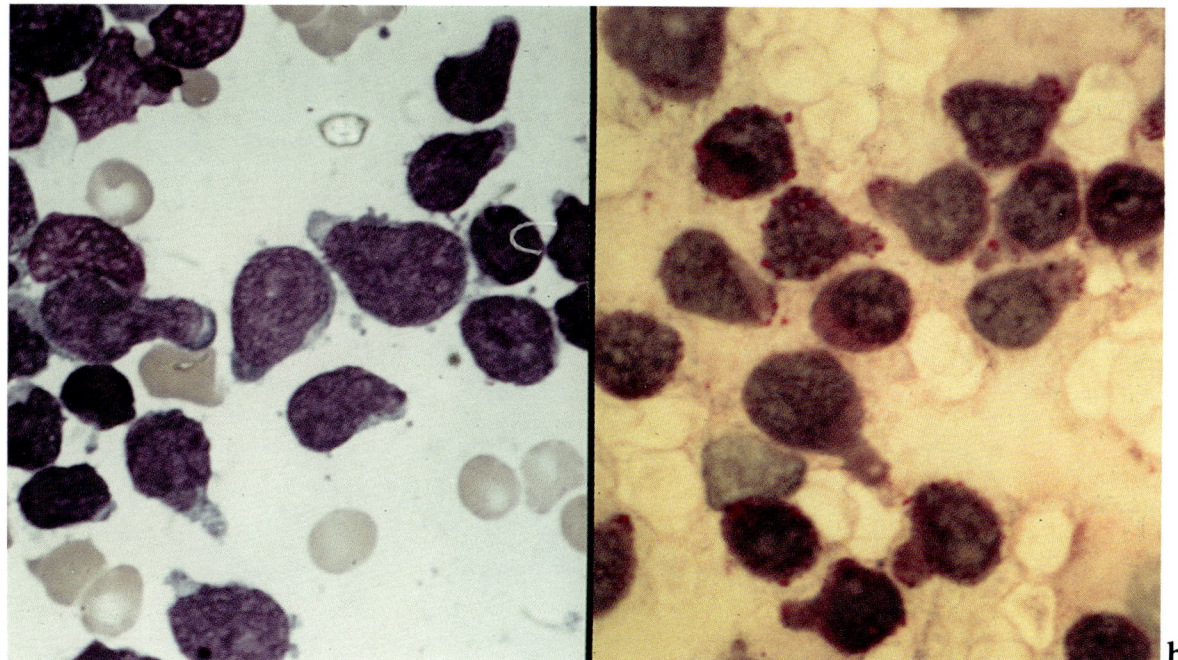

Figure 6-25. A hand mirrow variant of ALL with cytoplasmic tails (a) and coarse, PAS-positive cytoplasmic granules (b).

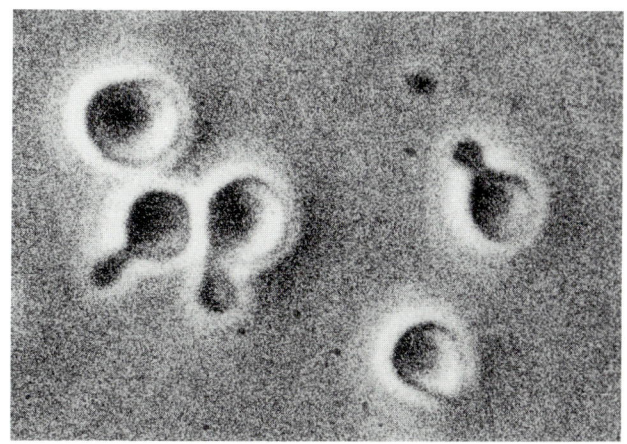

Figure 6-26. Cultured blast cells from a patient with hand mirror leukemia show prominent cytoplasmic tails due to their active mobility.

Table 6-7 Cell Markers and Gene Rearrangements Which May Overlap in Acute Myeloid and Lymphoid Leukemias*

AML
  Expression of TdT
  Expression of CD7
  Expression of CD10
  Ig or TCR gene rearrangements

ALL
  Expression of myeloid markers CD13, CD33, CD15
  Sudan black B positivity
  Ig gene rearrangement in T-ALL, and TCR gene rearrangement in B-ALL
  Leukemias with phenotypic features of both B- and T-ALL

* Adapted from Hoffbrand AV, Leber BF, Browett PJ, et al: mixed acute leukemias. *Blood Rev* 2:9, 1988.

currently available monoclonal antibodies react with antigens which are primarily differentiation associated. The majority of these antibodies are neither tumor specific nor lineage restricted, and thus may show a significant overlap in their reactivity with various lymphoid and myeloid cells. The extent of this overlapping antigenic expression should be taken into consideration when a diagnosis of acute biphenotypic or mixed leukemia is considered. For example, CD19 and CD20 appear to be B-cell-re-

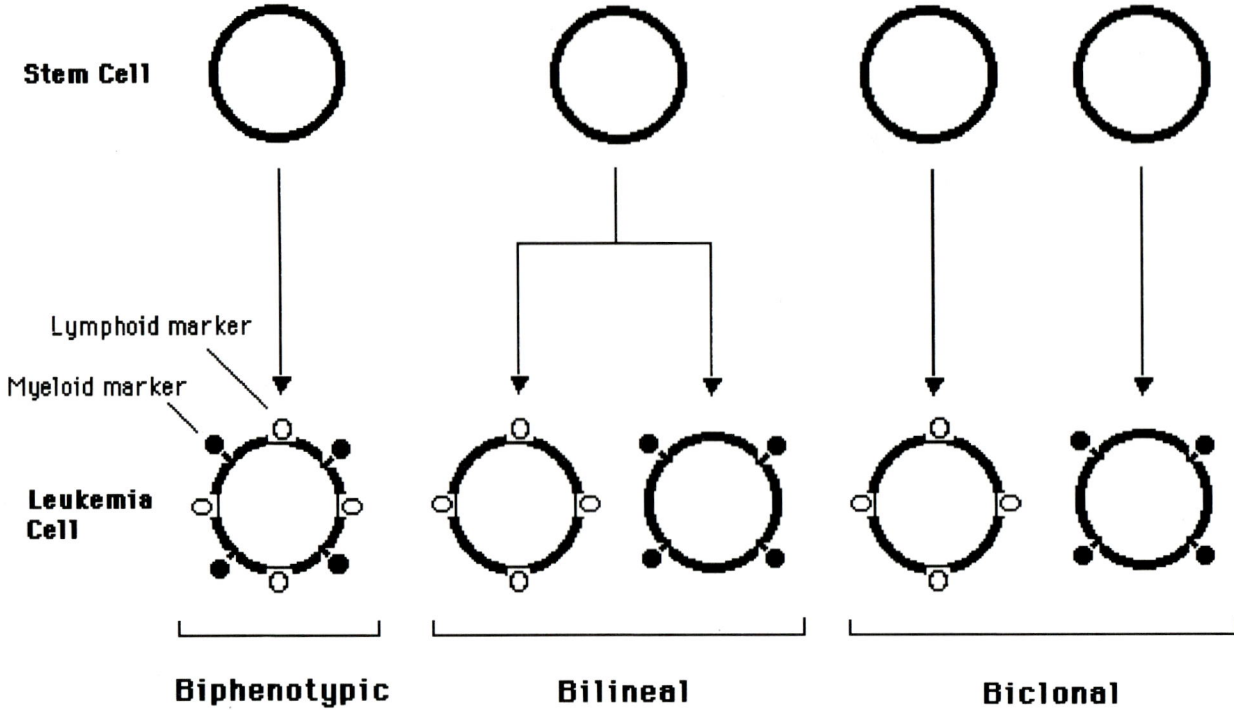

Figure 6-27. Schematic illustration of the possible mechanisms of development of acute mixed (hybrid) leukemias. Adapted from Hoffbrand et al., 1988 (Ref. 165) based on the proposal of Gale and Ben Bassat, 1987 (Ref. 159).

stricted antigens, while T-cell-associated antigens, such as CD2 and particularly CD7, have been shown to be expressed in myeloid cells. Thus, a CD19+ and/or a CD20+ AML more likely represents a true biphenotypic leukemia than a CD2+ and/or a CD7+ AML. The incidence of biphenotypic leukemia does not exceed 10% if the expression of CD2 or CD7 on AML cells is excluded as a biphenotypic feature.

Due to the lack of uniformly accepted criteria for a diagnosis of biphenotypic leukemia, it is difficult to reach a definitive conclusion regarding the clinical significance of these leukemias. However, recent studies have shown an increased incidence of CNS relapse in childhood ALL, and reduced survival with a decline in complete remissions in adult ALL, when the lymphoblasts express myeloid antigens.[90,91,162,168] A poor prognosis is also suggested for TdT-positive AMLs and for AMLs with other lymphoid features.[167,168]

A relatively large proportion of acute mixed leukemias show t(4;11) translocation.[171,172] Other possible chromosomal abnormalities in mixed leukemias include t(8;21) and 5q−.[173a,173b]

CHRONIC LEUKEMIAS

Chronic Lymphoid Leukemias

The term "chronic lymphoid leukemia" is applied to a group of leukemias in which the neoplastic cells share characteristic features of mature B or T lymphocytes by morphologic and immunophenotypic criteria. The overwhelming majority of chronic lymphoid leukemias are of the B-cell type. The T-cell variants are predominantly of the helper T-cell phenotype. Chronic lymphoid leukemia includes several well-defined clinicopathologic entities such as chronic lymphocytic leukemia, prolymphocytic leukemia, hairy cell leukemia, large granular cell leukemia, HTLV-associated leukemia and Sezary syndrome.

Chronic Lymphocytic Leukemia (CLL)

CLL is the most common form of adult leukemias in Western countries. The incidence of CLL is significantly (up to ten times) less frequent in Japanese and other Asian populations. The difference in incidence of CLL among various racial groups and the sporadic reports of high familial occurrence[175-177] suggest that genetic factors may play a role in the pathogenesis of this disorder. CLL is a disease of the elderly, with a median age of incidence of 55; about two-thirds of the patients are over 60 years of age at diagnosis.[178] The male:female ratio is 2–3:1.[179]

The defining criterion for the diagnosis of CLL is a lymphocytosis greater than 10,000/µl in peripheral blood and a bone marrow lymphocytosis of at least 30%.[180] However in some CLL patients, the peripheral blood lymphocyte count is sustained between 4000/µl to 10,000/µl. In questionable cases, particularly those with lymphocytosis <10,000/µl, cell marker studies are required for the establishment of clonal proliferation.

The neoplastic cells of B-CLL demonstrate identical bands for rearranged Ig genes on Southern blots and synthesize an identical idiotypic antibody with a single VH and VL region and a single light chain of either kappa or lambda.[181-183] Over 95% of the CLLs are of B-cell origin. T-CLLs are rare and fall into two categories: CD4+ or CD8+ subtypes. Monoclonality of T-CLLs is established by T-cell receptor gene rearrangement studies and/or cytogenetic analysis.

B-CLL

The neoplastic cells in B-CLL are typically small, with scanty basophilic, nongranular cytoplasm; regular nuclear and cytoplasmic outlines; dense nuclear chromatin with clumps of dark chromatin separated by irregular, narrow, pale spaces; and invisible or inconspicuous nucleoli,[180] (Figure 6-28). However, in about 10% of the cases, lymphocytes may show irregular, kidney-shaped or indented nuclei (Rieder cells). Overall, CLLs with irregular nuclear morphology are associated with a less favorable prognosis.[184-186]

The bone marrow is infiltrated by small lymphocytes in an interstitial or diffuse pattern. In advanced stages, the bone marrow is packed with lymphocytes, with only occasional hematopoietic clusters (Figure 6-29). A patchy or nodular pattern of bone marrow involvement is a less frequent morphologic variant (<10%) and is often associated with a more favorable prognosis.[187] Lymphadenopathy and splenomegaly are frequent findings, detected in over 85% of the patients. Other sites of involvement include the gastrointestinal tract, lungs and CNS.[188,189]

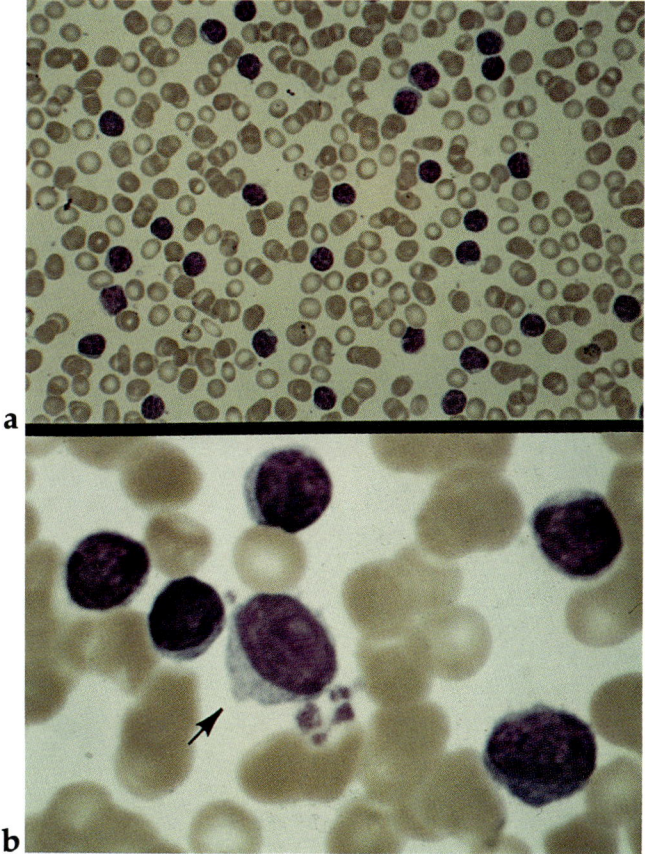

Figure 6-28. Peripheral blood smear from a patient with CLL demonstrating lymphocytosis (a) and predominance of small, round lymphocytes. A prolymphocyte is shown by the arrow (b).

The neoplastic cells of B-CLL are CD5, CD19, CD20, CD24 and HLA-DR positive and CD10, CD25, CD38 and TdT negative (Table 6-8). They may also express myelomonocytic-associated antigens, such as CD11b, CD13, and CD14.[190b] Approximately 5% of B-CLLs are CD5 negative.[191a] CLL cells express a relatively low concentration of surface membrane Ig (SmIg),[190a] but the expression is monotypic, with only one light chain, kappa or lambda, present. The low density of SmIg expressed in B-CLL cells leads to a weak fluorescence staining, a characteristic feature that could be used to distinguish B-CLL from the leukemic phase of B-cell lymphomas and from B-cell prolymphocytic leukemias. Polar redistribution of antibody-receptor complexes (cap formation) appears to be defective in the B-CLL cells.[191b] The B-CLL cells generate and release a surplus of light chain relative

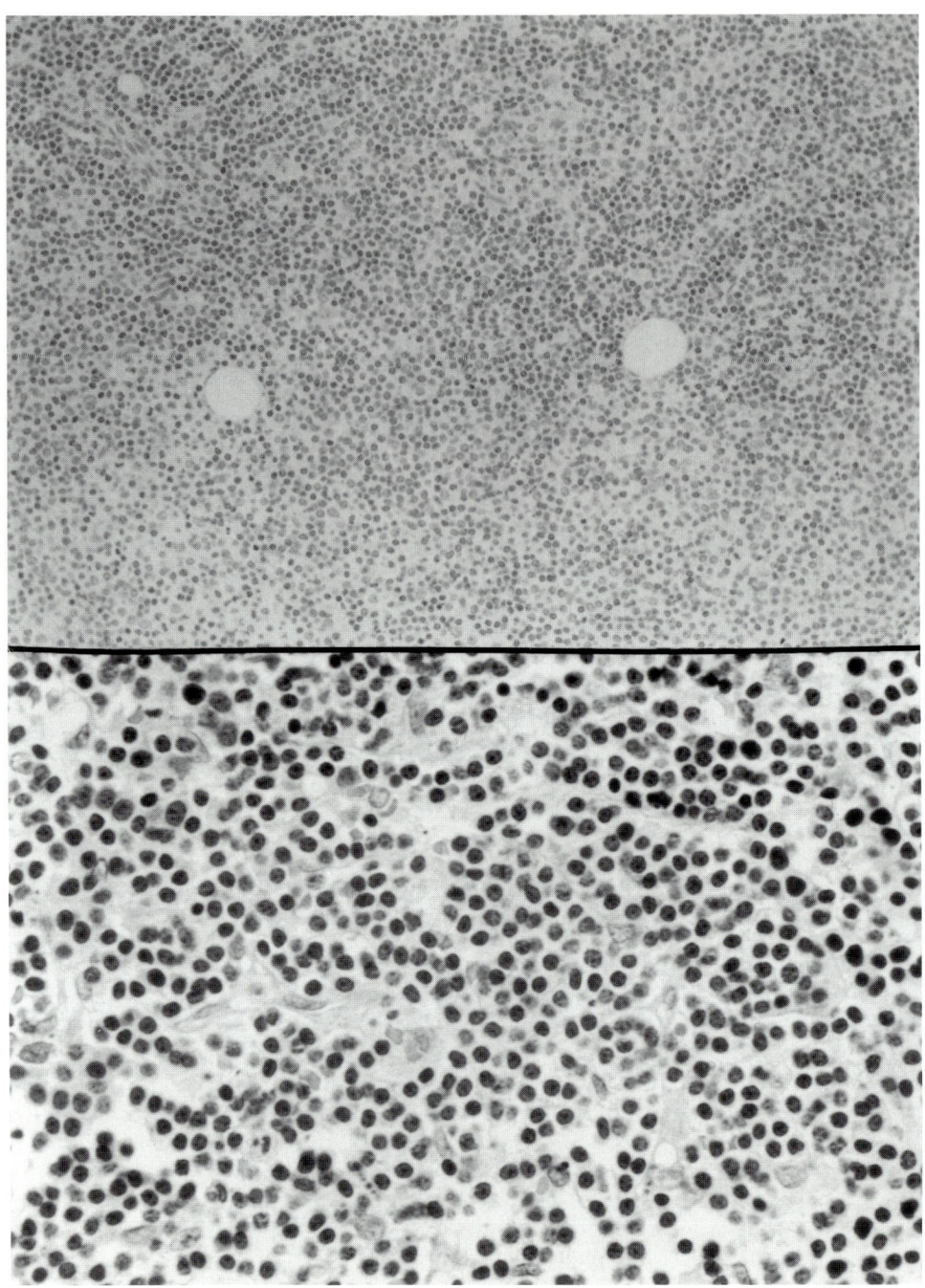

Figure 6-29. Bone marrow biopsy section from a patient with CLL demonstrating diffuse marrow involvement.

to heavy chain Ig.[192,193] The most common surface membrane phenotype in B-CLL is IgM, variably accompanied by IgD. The proliferation rate of the CLL cells is subnormal, as evidenced by a radiolabeled thymidine incorporation rate as low as 1/10th that of normal B cells. However, the exceedingly large number of CLL cells is attributed to the large pool of stem cells, the longer life span of CLL cells compared

Table 6-8 Cell Markers in Chronic (Mature) Lymphoid Leukemias*

B-cell Leukemia

Marker	CLL	PLL	HCL	Leukemic Phase of Lymphoma
SmIg	+	++	++	+
CIg	−	±	±	±
CD5	++	±	±	−
CD19/20/24	++	++	++	++
HLA-DR	++	++	++	++
FMC7/CD22	±	++	++	±
CD10	−	±	−	±
CD11c	−	−	+	−
CD25	−	−	+	−
CD35	−	−	±	−
TRAP	−	−	++	−

T-cell Leukemia

Marker	T-CLL	LGLL	T-PLL	ATLL	Sezary
Tdt	−	−	−	−	−
CD2	++	++	++	++	++
CD3	++	±	+	++	++
CD4	++	−	+	++	++
CD5	++	−	++	++	++
CD7	++	−	++	±	−
CD8	−	++	−	−	−
CD16	−	++	−	−	−
CD25	−	−	−	++	±
CD56	−	++	−	−	−

* +: weak reactions; ++: strong reactions

to normal lymphocytes, and/or an autocrine proliferating mechanism such as a self-generated growth factor.[194-198]

The disease progression in CLL leads to anemia, granulocytopenia and thrombocytopenia. Severe thrombocytopenia is usually an indicator of massive bone marrow involvement and terminal disease. Episodes of pure red blood cell aplasia have been observed in the course of B-CLL. These episodes range from 3 to 9 months and are usually associated with macrocytosis.[199,200] The mechanism of pure red blood cell aplasia in B-CLL is not well understood. However, one possibility is the reversal of the CD4:CD8 ratio and the promoting function of CD8 T cells, leading to suppression of both BFU-E and CFU-E proliferation in these patients.[201,202] Autoimmune hemolytic anemia is another hematologic complication of CLL.[203,204] The autoantibody is usually a low-affinity IgG class antibody causing a mild hemolysis in the majority of the Coombs-positive CLL patients. Approximately 50% of CLL patients develop hypogammaglobulinemia with decreased levels of all Ig classes in serum. About 5% demonstrate low serum Ig levels with a monoclonal spike, usually IgM.

A morphologic subclass of B-CLL has been introduced in the recent proposal by the FAB Cooperative Group called "CLL, mixed cell type"[180] In this category, neoplastic cells are either a mixture of small lymphocytes and prolymphocytes (>10% and <55% prolymphocyte), or a spectrum of small to large lymphocytes with rare (<10%) prolymphocytes. The former is designated as "CLL/PL" and appears to represent a more aggressive subtype of CLL.[194a,194b]

An additional subtype of B-CLL has recently been reported in which the neoplastic lymphocytes are characterized by abundant cytoplasm, strong expression of CD11c (Leu M5) antigen, and lack of tartrate-resistant acid phosphatase activity[195] (Figure 6-30). The cells are CD19 and CD20 positive, express monoclonal Ig, and are frequently CD5 positive. Splenomegaly, similar to that in patients with hairy cell leukemia, is the most frequent clinical finding in patients with CD11c+ CLL. Lymphadenopathy is rare, and the median white blood cell count is about 20,000/μl.[195]

T-CLL

Approximately 5% of the CLLs are of the T-cell phenotype. T-CLLs are divided into two major groups: CD8+ CLL and CD4+ CLL.

The CD8+ CLL has also been designated as "large granular lymphocytic (LGL) leukemia," "T lymphoproliferative disease" or "natural killer (NK) cell leukemia."[204-208] This disorder is a chronic, indolent, clonal, lymphoproliferative process characterized by a low to moderate lymphocytosis (white blood cell count ranging from 4000 to 30,000/μl) and neutropenia. Bone marrow involvement is patchy, and involvement of the other organs is unusual. Patients usually have a history of an autoimmune disorder with splenomegaly, leading to granulocytopenia as well as other cytopenias, such as thrombocytopenia or hemolytic anemia.

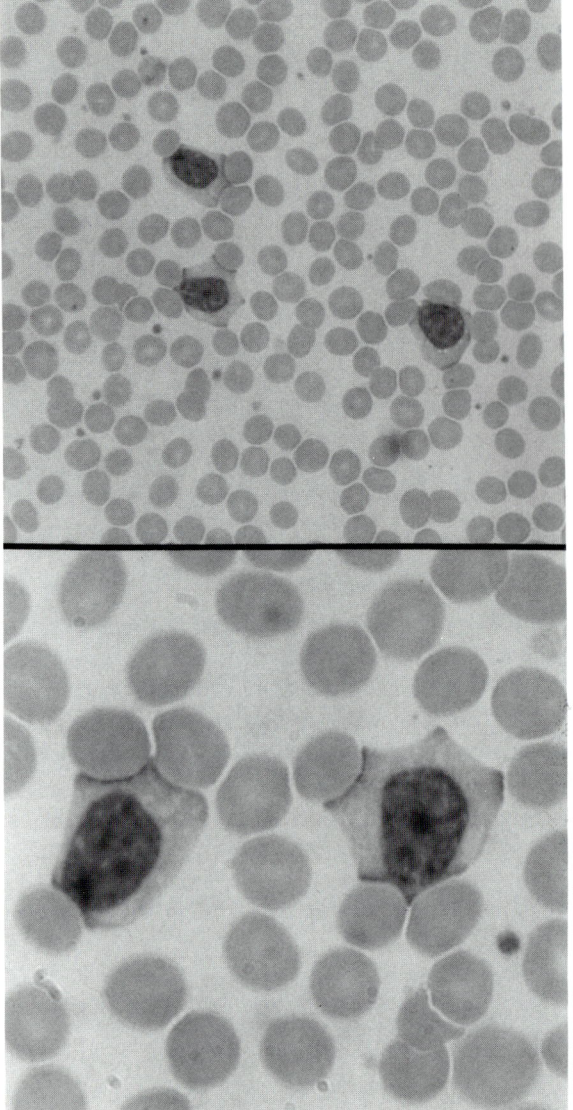

Figure 6-30. A variant of CLL characterized by large lymphocytes and abundant cytoplasm. These cells are negative for tartrate-resistant acid phosphatase and often express CD11c.

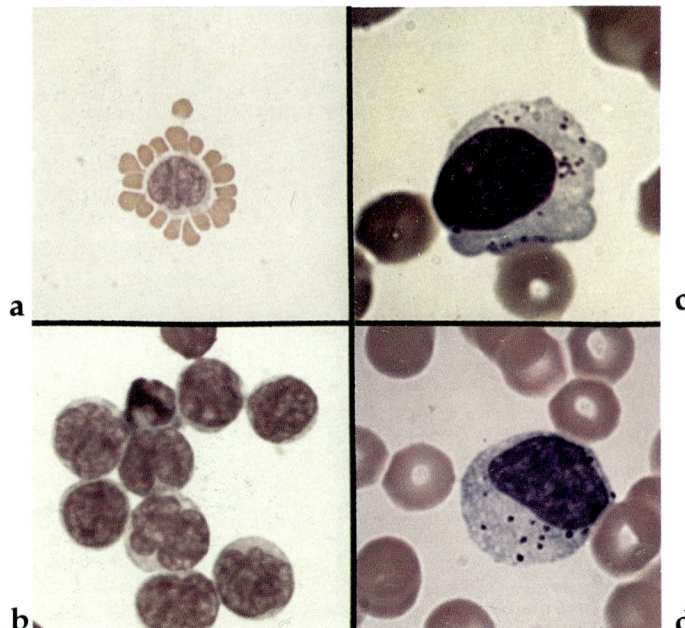

Figure 6-31. T-cell lymphoproliferative disorders. (a): An E-rosetting Sezary cell with cerebriform nucleus. (b): Convoluted lymphocytes from a patient with adult T-cell leukemia/lymphoma. (c and d): lymphocytes from a patient with large granular lymphocytic leukemia.

The CD8+ CLL cells characteristically are large lymphocytes with abundant cytoplasm and a variable number of azurophilic granules (Figure 6-31). They express receptors for the Fc portion of IgG and are involved in non-MCH-restricted cytotoxic activities.[209] The CD8+ CLL has recently been divided into two subclasses: CD3− and CD3+.[208] The CD3 negative subtype appears to represent a true NK cell leukemia. The tumor cells do not show T-cell receptor (TCR) gene rearrangement and are CD25 negative. The CD3+ leukemia represents a T-cytotoxic subtype with evidence of TCR gene rearrangement and often CD25 expression.

The CD4+ CLL represents a more bulky disease with an aggressive clinical course usually associated with marked lymphocytosis ranging from 30,000 to 700,000/μl, extensive bone marrow infiltration and frequent involvement of the lymph nodes, spleen, liver, skin and sometimes the CNS.[180,210-214] The neoplastic lymphocytes are small, with scanty, non-granular cytoplasm, round or irregular (notched, indented, convoluted or knobby) nucleus, coarse chromatin and usually no distinct nucleoli (Figure 6-32).

CD4+ CLL shares numerous clinicopathologic features with adult T-cell leukemia. However, T-CLL cells, unlike adult T-cell leukemia cells, are not infected with HTLV-1 (see below).

Cytogenetics

Chromosomal abnormalities can be detected in up to 50% of CLL patients if the CLL cells are properly

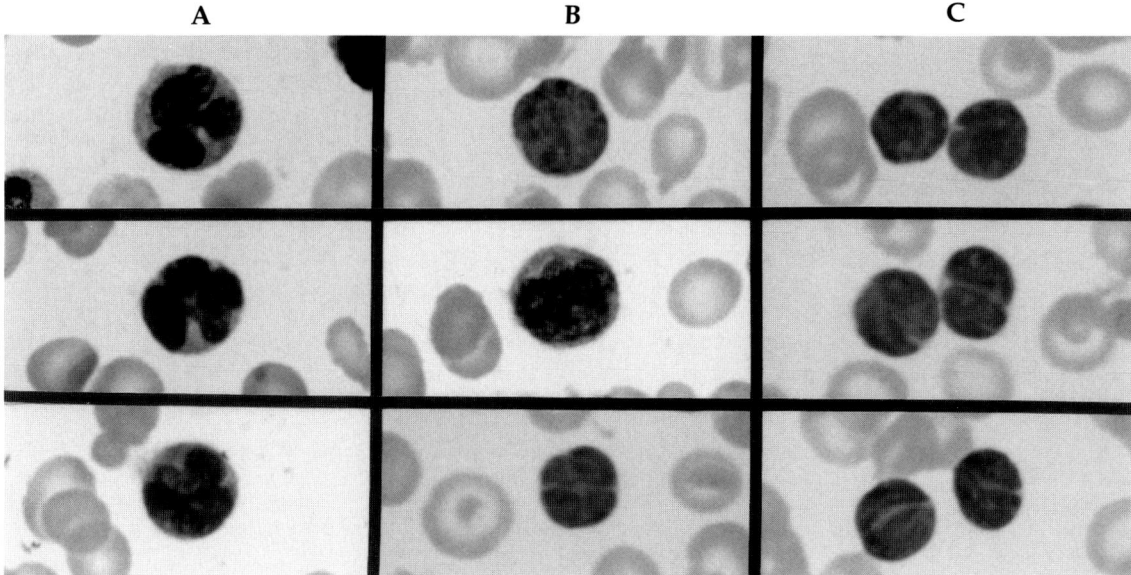

Figure 6-32. Morphologic diversity of lymphocytes observed in a variety of chronic lymphoid leukemias. Cells with cloverleaf-shaped and convoluted nuclei are more common in the T-cell variants (columns A and B), and lymphocytes with cleaved nuclei are more frequent in the B-cell types (column C).

stimulated in culture by mitogens such as pokeweed, lipopolysaccharide, TPA (12-0-tetradecanoyl-phorbol-13-acetate) and EBV.[215,216] The most common clonal chromosomal aberration in B-CLL is trisomy 12.[217,218] Other common aberrations are 14q+, structural changes on chromosomes 6, 11, and 12, and t(11;14).[215,217,219-221] The t(11;14) translocation involves rearrangement of the *bcl-1* oncogene (see Chapter 2).[221] The most frequent chromosomal aberrations in T-CLL are inv(14)(q11;q32) or t(14;14,)(q11;q32), 8q+ or structural abnormalities in chromosome 7.[221,222a] Many of the chromosomal aberrations in T cells involve 14q32.

Clinical Aspects and Prognostic Factors

CLL accounts for 30% of all leukemias in adults, and approximately 90% of the patients are over age 50. In the early stages CLL is asymptomatic (25% of the patients), but in the advanced stages it shows symptoms and signs which are the result of bone marrow and extramedullary involvement. Lymphadenopathy and splenomegaly are frequent findings occuring in 80% and 50–75% of the patients, respectively. Hepatomegaly is uncommon.

The prognostic classification, consisting of five stages originally proposed by Rai et al. for CLL[222b], has been revised and consolidated by an International Workshop on CLL into three stages: A, B, and C[223a] (Table 6-9). Stage A represents over half of the CLL patients, with a life expectancy comparable to that of the age- and sex-matched general population. Stage B accounts for about 30% of the patients, with a median survival of around 7 years. Stage C represents approximately 15% of the patients, with a median survival of about 2 years. Stage C is associated with severe anemia and thrombocytopenia. Other factors associated with an unfavorable prognosis include irregular or cleaved nuclear morphology, mixed cell type, decreased CD45RA (suppressor-inducer) T cells in B-cell CLLs,[223b] S-100[223c] and CD4 positivity in T-cell CLLs and multiple chromosomal aberrations.

Transformation of CLL to an Aggressive Lymphoid Malignancy (Richter's Syndrome)

Approximately 10% of CLL patients develop an aggressive lymphoma.[224,225] This evolution, which in essence is a form of blast transformation, appears to begin in the CLL-involved lymph nodes, where, in addition to the CLL cells, foci of large, immature lymphocytes (proliferation centers) are present. Progressive growth of the focal aggregate of transformed cells in these centers may lead to the development of

Table 6-9 Prognostic Classification of CLL*

Stage	Clinical Findings	Incidence	Median Survival
A	PB lymphocyte >4000/μl, with >40% lymphocytes in marrow, no anemia, no thrombocytopenia, fewer than three involved areas†	55%	Comparable with age- and sex-matched general population
B	Stage A plus more than three involved areas	30%	7 years
C	Stage A plus more than three involved areas, Hb <10 g/dl and platelet count of <100,000/μl	15%	2 years

* Adapted from Binet J-L, Catovsky D, Chandra P, et al: Chronic lymphocytic leukemia: Proposals for a revised prognostic staging system. Report from The International Workshop on CLL The Writing Committee, Br J Haematol 48:365, 1981.
† Areas include peripheral lymph nodes (unilateral or bilateral), spleen and liver.

an aggressive large cell lymphoma with additional chromosomal aberrations.[226-228]

Richter's syndrome is presented as a diffuse large cell (often immunoblastic) lymphoma with frequent bone marrow involvement, and sometimes peripheral blood involvement. Tumor cells in marrow smears and touch preparations appear as large blast cells with variable amounts of dark blue cytoplasm, large round or irregular nuclei, fine chromatin, and one or two prominent nucleoli. In addition to the blast cells, some cases demonstrate bizzare multi-nucleated giant cells resembling Reed-Sternberg cells. In rare cases, CLL may transform to ALL.

Prolymphocytic Leukemia (PLL)

PLL is a lymphoid leukemia characterized by a markedly elevated white blood cell count (>100,000/μl in about 80% of the cases), massive splenomegaly, and no lymphadenopathy except in the terminal stages.[229-231] PLL is less frequent than CLL and, compared to CLL, involves older people. Approximately 50% of PLL patients are over 70 years old at diagnosis.

Prolymphocyte is a large cell (larger than two red blood cells) with a variable amount of nongranular cytoplasm, a round nucleus, relatively dense nuclear chromatin and one prominent nucleolus (Figures 6-28 and 6-33). Prolymphocytes account for 55 to 70% of the white blood cells in patients with PLL.[180]

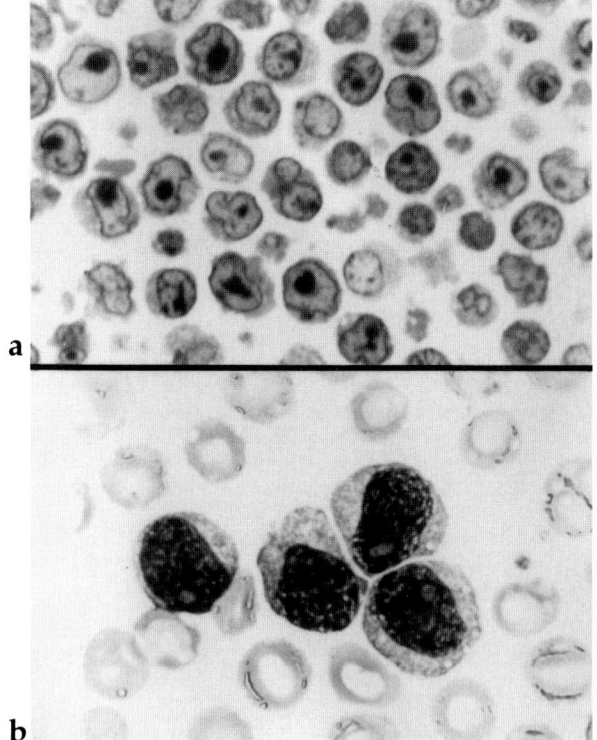

Figure 6-33. An example of prolymphocytic leukemia. The neoplastic cells are larger than normal lymphocytes and often show a prominent nucleolus. (a) A section of a methacrylate-embedded peripheral blood mononuclear pellet. (b) Peripheral blood smear.

Leukemias and Lymphomas

The pattern of bone marrow infiltration in PLL is similar to that of CLL.

The PLL cells in over 80% of the cases express immunophenotypic characteristics similar to those of B-CLL cells. However, PLL cells are CD5 negative, and show a stronger SmIg, and a higher frequency of CD22 expression than CLL cells[180] (see Table 6-8). The T-PLL usually has a helper phenotype, expressing CD2, CD3, CD4, CD5 and CD7.[180,232-236] Suppressor T-PLLs are infrequent.[235]

The most commonly reported chromosomal aberrations in B-PLL are 6q−, 14q+, t(11;14) with *bcl-1* rearrangement and t(6;12).[98,236,237] In one report, five consecutive B-PLL cases demonstrated an identical translocation between chromosomes 6 and 12 [t(6;12)(q15;p13)], suggesting a unique karyotypic subset for B-PLL.[237] Trisomy 12, the most frequent chromosomal aberration in CLL, is rare in PLL. Trisomy 8 and abnormalities of chromosome 14 are the most common chromosomal changes reported in T-PLLs.[238,239,240]

Hairy Cell Leukemia (HCL)

HCL, or leukemic reticuloendotheliosis, is a chronic neoplastic process characterized by anemia, granulocytopenia, monocytopenia, thrombocytopenia and splenomegaly.[241-246] The neoplastic lymphoid cells, with cytoplasmic "hairy" projections, are found in peripheral blood, bone marrow, spleen and other tissues (Figures 6-34 and 6-35). The disease is found more frequently in males, and the average age at onset is around 50 years (Table 6-10). No toxic, occupational or genetic predilection has been identified.[247] HCL is a chronic, indolent disease, with most patients living beyond 5 years.[248,249] Spontaneous regression of HCL has been reported in rare cases.[250]

In the majority of the patients, peripheral blood examination reveals leukopenia, with various proportions (usually 5–50%) of leukocytes being circulating hairy cells.[250] However, in some leukopenic patients, hairy cells are too few to be demonstrable.[241,250,251] In patients with elevated white blood cell counts (>10,000/μl), hairy cells usually account for the majority of the leukocytes. The proportion of HCL cells in peripheral blood fluctuates in each patient, but there is an overall tendency for these cells to increase with time.

Hairy cells are larger than mature lymphocytes and show abundant pale blue cytoplasm, often with

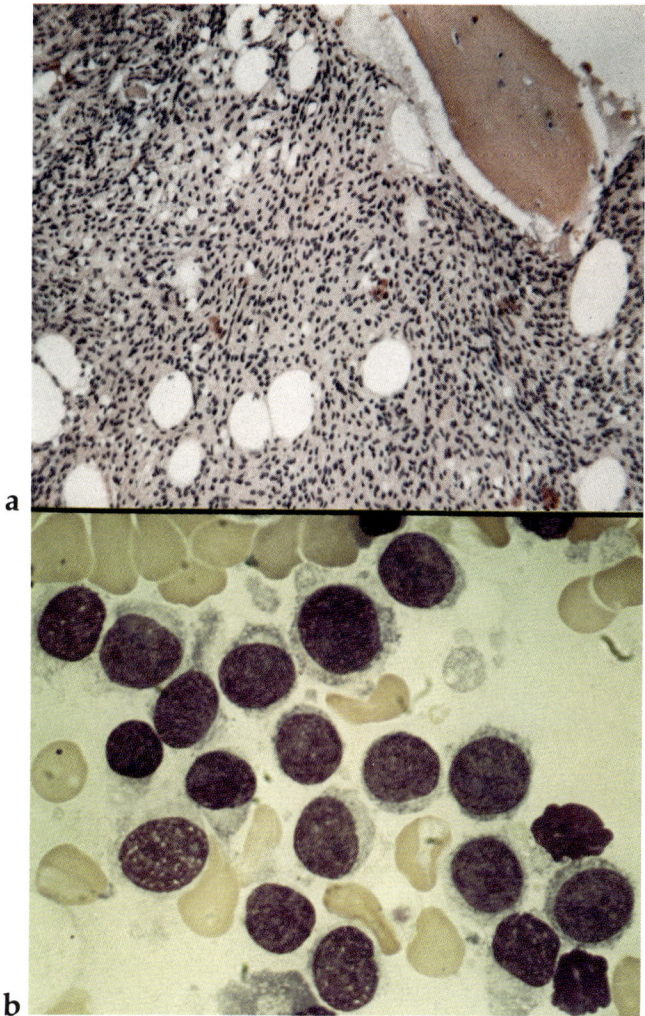

Figure 6-34. Bone marrow involvement in hairy cell leukemia is often interstitial, and tumor cells appear monomorphic, with variable amounts of cytoplasm and round or elongated nuclei; biopsy section (a) and smear (b).

an ill-defined border. Cells with the characteristic elongated (hairy) cytoplasmic projections are usually identified, though in some cases they are infrequent (Figure 6-36). The nuclei are round, oval, folded, indented or dumbbell-shaped (Figure 6-37). The nuclear chromatin is homogeneous and coarse but finer than that of the CLL cells. Rare cells may show prominent nucleoli. The hairy cytoplasmic projections are quite prominent in phase contrast microscopy or in scanning and transmission electron microscopy (Figure 6-38). In scanning electron microscopy, hairy cells

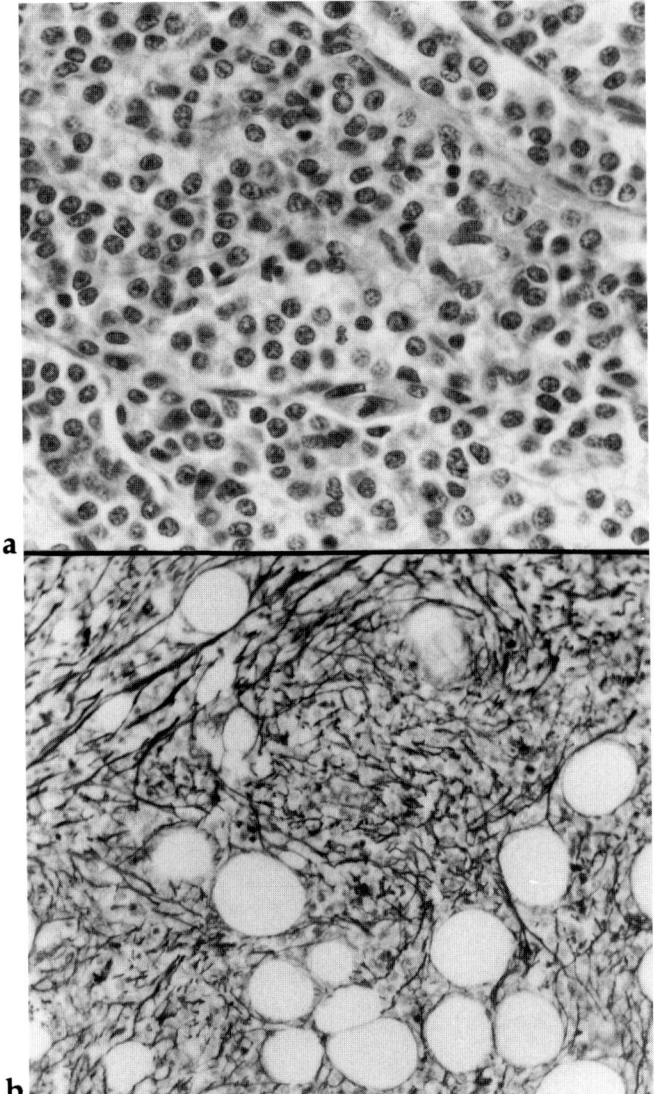

Figure 6-35. Hairy cell leukemia. (a) Section of spleen showing diffuse involvement of the red pulp. (b) Bone marrow biopsy section demonstrating a marked increased in reticulin fibers.

Table 6-10 Clinical Symptoms and Signs in Patients with HCL*

Average age	50 years
Male:female ratio	3–5:1
Most frequent complaints (%)	
Pallor	66
Fatigue	60
Upper abdominal pain	50
Fever	45
Weight loss	22
Physical findings (%)	
Splenomegaly	78
Hepatomegaly	50
Petechia and ecchymosis	33
Lymphadenopathy	16

* Adapted from Naeim F: Hairy cell leukemia: Characteristics of the neoplastic cells. *Hum Pathol* 19:375, 1988.

display microvilli and ruffles in various proportions.[252] Transmission electron microscopic studies reveal numerous mitochondria, polyribosomes, strands of rough endoplasmic reticulum, abundant cytoplasmic intermediate filaments, and rare lysosomal granules (see Figure 6-38). Cytoplasmic inclusions known as "ribosomal–lamella complexes" have been demonstrated in up to 50% of HCL cells.[253-255] However, similar structures have been demonstrated in other hematologic malignancies as well.[256]

There is some evidence that the morphology of HCL cells may correlate with the prognosis of the disease. According to Bartl and associates, patients with ovoid hairy cells have a better prognosis than those with convoluted or indented cells.[257] It has also been suggested that HCL cells with folded nuclei are more frequently associated with marrow fibrosis and severe pancytopenia than are cells with rounded or oval nuclei.[244]

The pattern of bone marrow involvement in HCL is usually interstitial or diffuse, with patchy, densely cellular areas composed primarily of tumor cells (Figures 6-34, 6-36 and 6-39). Focal or nodular marrow involvement is rare.[241,257,258] Bone marrow cellularity ranges from <25% to >90%, but in most cases the bone marrow is hypercellular. Rare cases of HCL with marked marrow hypocellularity, simulating aplastic marrow, have been reported.[259] HCL cells in tissue sections appear relatively uniform and display round, oval or irregular nuclei, often without evidence of mitotic figures or prominent nuleoli. They show abundant clear cytoplasm, creating wide nuclear spacing (see Figure 6-39). The bone marrow often reveals an increase in reticulin fibers, leading to unsuccessful bone marrow aspiration (dry tap).[246,260,261] The reticulin tends to surround the tumor cells individually or in small clusters (see Figure 6-35).

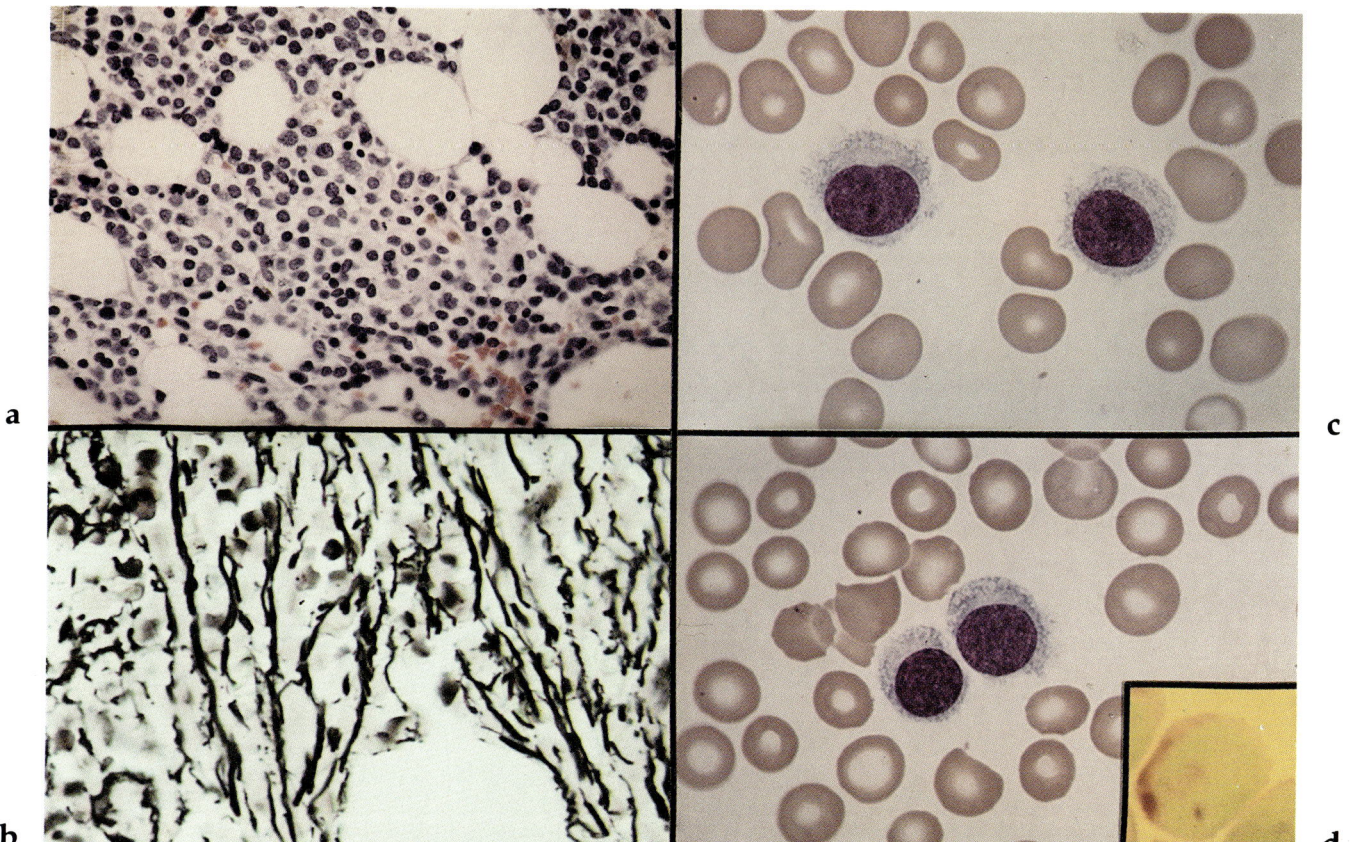

Figure 6-36. Hairy cell leukemia. Bone marrow biopsy sections demonstrating an interstitial involvement (a) and a marked increase in reticulin fibers (b); peripheral blood smears showing medium to large size lymphocytes with abundant cytoplasm and hairy cytoplasmic projections. The insert displays a hairy cell positive for tartrate resistant acid phosphatase.

In the vast majority of cases, the diagnosis of HCL is established by examination of bone marrow biopsy sections. However, in a small proportion of the cases, especially when the marrow involvement is focal, the initial bone marrow sections may not be diagnostic and additional biopsy is required.[241,257,258]

Recombinant alpha-interferon (IFN-α), which has been used successfully as a therapeutic agent for HCL, has a profound effect on the bone marrow.[262,263] IFN-α causes a decline in the size of the neoplastic mass and an increase in hematopoiesis. These changes are associated with significant improvement in hemoglobin levels and in granulocyte/monocyte and platelet counts.[263-265] Despite the remarkable therapeutic effects of IFN-α, complete remission is infrequent, and when therapy is withheld, the disease may progress gradually.[263]

Splenic involvement is one of the characteristic features of HCL, and splenomegaly is one of the most prominent clinical features. However, 20–30% of the patients may lack splenomegaly.[244,254] These patients tend to remain free from significant neutropenia, have an excellent survival rate and are usually older than the patients with splenomegaly.[254,266] HCL infiltrates the splenic red pulp in a diffuse pattern (see Figure 6-35). In the majority of the cases, this infiltration is associated with hypersplenism, contributing to the patient's pancytopenia. Occasional patients may show a platelet abnormality and dysfunction secondary to hypersplenism. Splenectomy is usually associated with immediate alleviation of the pancytopenia, but over 50% of the splenectomized patients eventually require further therapy.[267-270]

HCL involves the liver in up to 50% and the

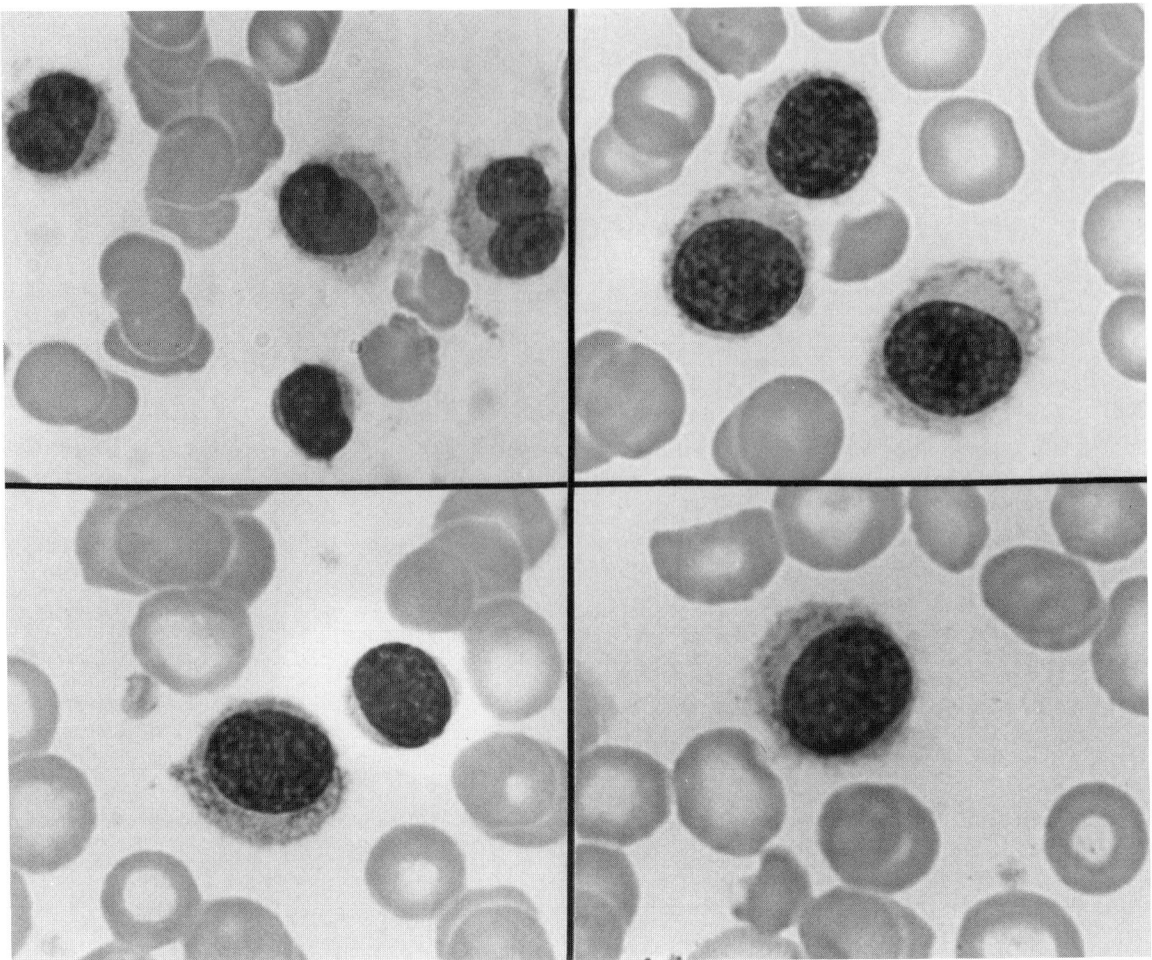

Figure 6-37. Peripheral blood smears demonstrating hairy cells with abundant cytoplasm and round, kidney-shaped, or dumbbell-shaped nuclei. "Hairy" cytoplasmic projections are noted in several cells.

lymph nodes in approximately 15–20% of the cases. Tumor invasion of other tissues, such as skin and lung, is rare.[271,272]

Cytochemical and Immunophenotypic Features

Hairy cells contain an acid phosphatase isoenzyme (type 5) that is resistant to tartaric acid[273,274] (see Figure 6-36). Although the presence of tartrate-resistant acid phosphatase (TRAP) is characteristic of HCL, cells in other conditions, such as Sezary syndrome, small and large cell lymphomas, PLL of the T-cell type, Hodgkin's disease and Gaucher's disease, may infrequently reveal TRAP positivity.[274-277]

Other reported cytochemical features include a diffuse, finely granular cytoplasmic positivity with beta-glucuronidase and acid-nonspecific esterase (alpha-naphthyl butyrate or acetate esterase).[278,279] Recent studies have demonstrated the presence of S-100 protein in hairy cells.[280,281]

In the overwhelming majority of HCL patients, the neoplastic hairy cells express the characteristics of B lymphocytes.[282-286] Immunophenotypic studies suggest that in the B-cell developmental pathway, hairy cells, similar to PLL cells, precede plasma cells.[285-287] This suggestion is supported by reported cases of HCL with osteolytic lesions or monoclonal gammopathies, by reports of patients with coexistent HCL and myeloma, and by demonstration of PCA-1 (a plasma cell-associated antigen) on the hairy cells.[286-290] Hairy cells express SmIg, HLA-DR, CD45, B cell-associated markers (CD19, CD20, CD22, CD24), CD25 and integrins (membrane adhesion

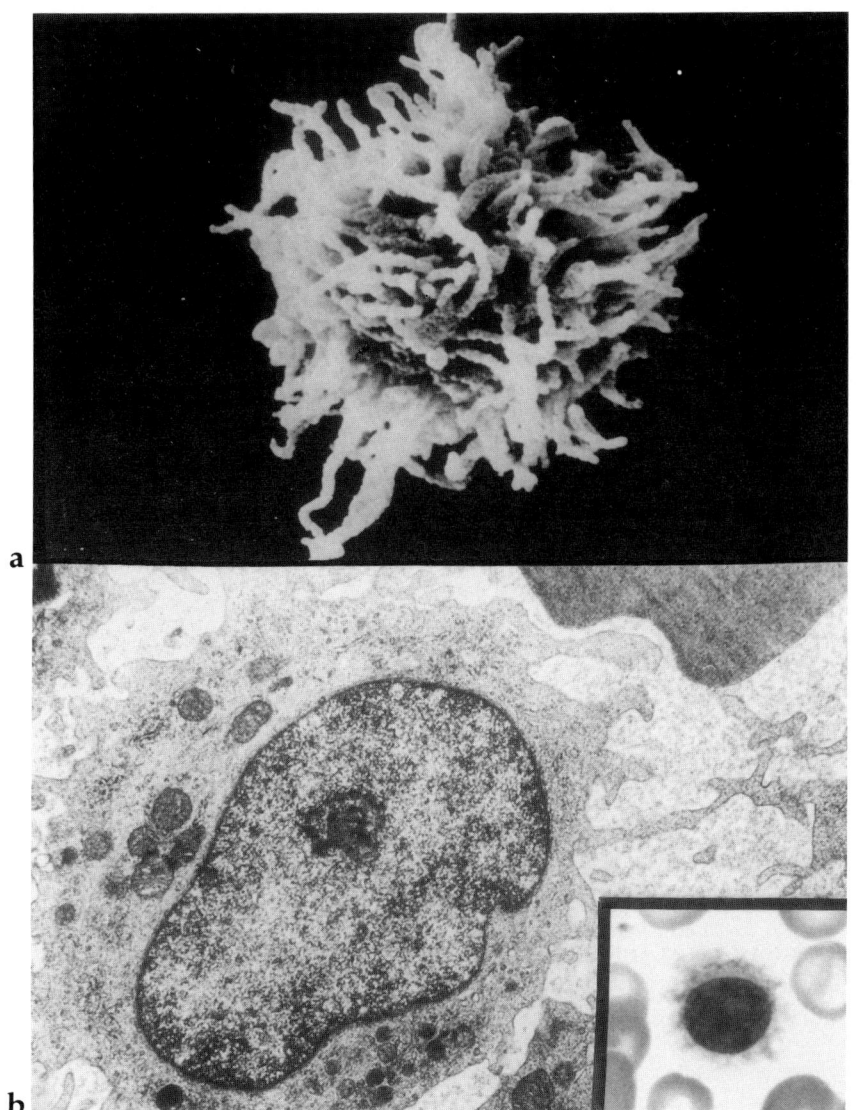

Figure 6-38. Scanning (a) and transmission (b) electron microscopic photographs of HCL cells. The insert demonstrates light microscopic features of an HCL cell with numerous cytoplasmic ("hairy") projections. (a) From Naeim F: Cytoskeletal control of redistribution of surface membrane receptors in hairy cells. *Am J Clin Pathol* 74:660, 1980, with permission. (b) From Naeim et al: Hairy cell leukemia. A heterogeneous chronic lymphoproliferative disorder. *Am J Med* 65:479, 1978, with permission.

molecules) such as CD11a, CD11c and CD18[180,251] (see Table 6-8). CD5 expression is infrequent. Monoclonality of HCL is established by monotypic expression of one Ig light chain (kappa or lambda) and Ig gene rearrangement studies.[251,291,292a] The IgG3 subclass is the most frequent surface membrane Ig (SmIg) expression reported in HCL cells.[292b] Another characteristic feature of hairy cells is that, in contrast to CLL cells, they demonstrate an enhanced ability to redistribute ligand–receptor complexes and induce cap formation.[293,294] The general consensus is that HCL represents a neoplasm of B-lymphocyte lineage. However, in addition to B-cell characteristics, HCL cells display features that are not usually shared by cells of other B-cell malignancies. These features (which are mostly observed in antigen-presenting cells) include elongated cytoplasmic projections, TRAP positivity, surface adherence and phagocytosis, expression of IL-2 receptor (CD25) and S-100 positivity.[251] Although HCL is essentially considered a B-cell malignancy, occasional cases of T-cell HCL have been reported and a few have been associated with HTLV-II.[295-299] There is a controversy over whether the scattered reported cases of "T-cell" HCL are all true HCLs or whether, in some cases, they are variants of T-cell CLL/lymphoma or represent a non-HCL lymphoid population (or cell line) in a patient with HCL.[300-303] For example, a report of an HTLV-II+ HCL turned out, in further studies, to be a case of B-cell HCL with simultaneous clonal proliferation of

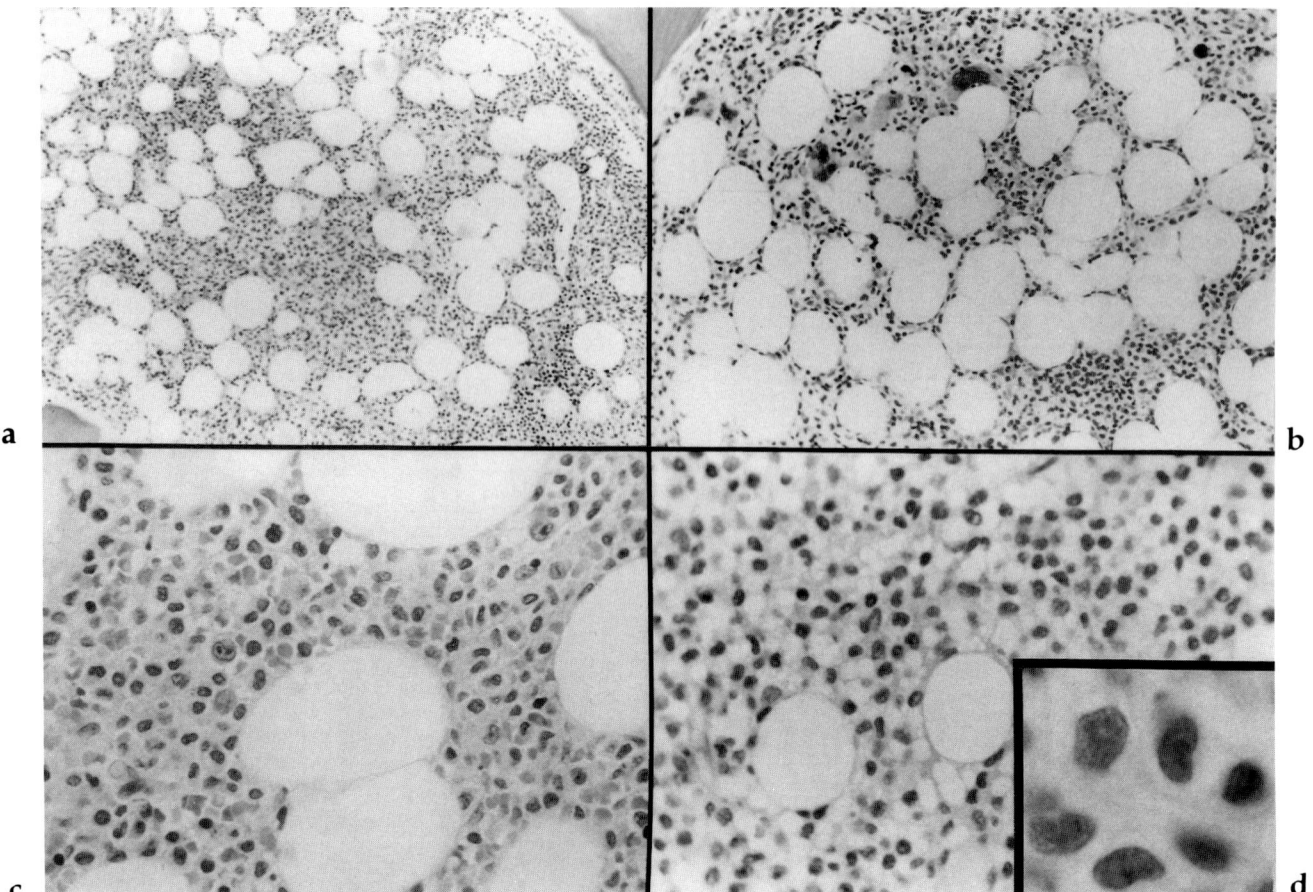

Figure 6-39. Bone marrow biopsy sections demonstrating interstitial involvement in patients with hairy cell leukemia. Under high power, the tumor cells exhibit abundant pale cytoplasm (c, d, and insert). From Naeim F: Hairy cell leukemia: Characteristics of the neoplastic cells. *Hum Pathol* 19:375, 1988, with permission.

HTLV-II-infected T cells,[301,302] and a T-cell line derived from a patient with B-cell HCL was proved to be the result of laboratory contamination.[304]

Several reports have demonstrated in vivo and in vitro phenotypic changes (from the B- to the T-cell type) in hairy cells.[305,306] There are also reports of simultaneous expression of B- and T-cell antigens ("hybrid" B/T phenotype on hairy cells).[307]

Cytogenetics

Structural and numerical chromosome abnormalities have been reported in HCL.[308-311] Common abnormalities include 6q$^-$ and trisomy of chromosomes 3, 4, 12 and 18. Patients with chromosome abnormalities appear to have a shorter survival than patients with normal karyotypes.[311]

Defective Immune Functions

Evidence of defective cell-mediated immunity in HCL has been demonstrated by several investigators based on clinical and experimental studies.[312-316] Studies on autologous and allogeneic mixed lymphocyte reactions have suggested that the responding T cells in HCL patients are defective.[312] Furthermore, absence of NK activity and a decline in the release of IL-1 have been demonstrated in these patients.[314,315] Recent studies have shown that the sera of HCL patients contain a soluble form of IL-2 receptor released by hairy cells.[317-319] The serum levels of IL-2 receptor and NK activity of peripheral blood mononuclear cells from the same patients are inversely related, suggesting that the excess IL-2 receptor in patients' serum might remove IL-2 and thus interfere with NK cell activation. Serum IL-2 receptor assays might be useful in monitoring and evaluating the response of HCL patients to IFN-α therapy.[319]

Hairy Cell Variant (HCL-V)

A variant of HCL, a relatively rare disorder, has been characterized by morphologic features intermediate between those of hairy cells and prolymphocytes.[180, 320a,320b] This variant is characterized by splenomegaly, an elevated white blood cell count usually >50,000/μl and lack of monocytopenia. The neoplastic cells have abundant basophilic cytoplasm with cytoplasmic projections, moderately condensed heterochromatin and a prominent nucleolus. In contrast to typical HCL cells, HCL-V cells are CD25 negative.

An unusual, rare morphologic variant of HCL with multilobated nuclei has been described in which the tumor cells show up to six-lobed nuclei.[321]

HTLV-1-Associated T-Cell Leukemia

This clinicopathologic entity is a T-cell malignancy transmitted by HTLV-1, a type C retrovirus with strong trophism for $CD4^+$ lymphocytes. The disorder, also known as "adult T-cell leukemia/lymphoma (ATLL)," was originally observed as an endemic disease in the adult population of southwestern Japan, in the Kyushu district and adjacent areas. It has also affected non-Japanese people, predominantly blacks living in the Caribbean and the southeastern United States.[322,323] The disease is initiated by HTLV-1 infection of the $CD4^+$ lymphocytes. The HTLV RNA is transcribed into DNA and is then randomly integrated into the host DNA. The infected T-cell population increases at first in a polyclonal fashion, and then a predominant clone emerges.[324] ATLL is extremely rare in children. The reported median age in the United States is 34 (ranging from 24 to 62).[323]

The vast majority of infected persons show no signs and symptoms, and only a small proportion (estimated at 0.01–0.1%) develop ATLL.[324,325] Thus, the clinical presentation may range from a carrier state to a subclinical form, in which patients are virtually asymptomatic and are distinguished by a mild proliferation of atypical $CD4^+$ cells, and finally to a fulminant stage.[326-331] In this stage, the disease is characterized by skin lesions, lymphadenopathy, hepatosplenomegaly, bone marrow and bone involvement, high white blood cell count with convoluted lymphocytes and hypercalcemia. Hypercalcemia and bone marrow involvement are slightly more common in American than in Japanese patients.[324,332] The disease in its fulminant form has a rapid course, with a median survival of approximately 8 months.[322,329,331]

ATLL comprises a wide spectrum of histopathologic and cytologic features. The neoplastic cells in a given patient may be predominantly small or large, or may consist of a mixture of small and large cells[323,333,334] (Figures 6-31, 6-32, 6-40 and 6-41). The morphologic hallmarks are pronounced nuclear pleomorphism and convolution (Figures 6-40 and 6-41). The nuclear chromatin is clumped or condensed, and the nuclear outline is markedly convoluted and appears "clover-leafed."[180] Nucleoli are uncommon and, if present, are not prominent. The neoplastic cells display a variable amount of basophilic, agranular cytoplasm. The morphologic features of ATLL overlap with those of Sezary syndrome, T-PLL, T-CLL and peripheral T-cell lymphomas. The diagnosis is based on a comprehensive clinicopathologic review and the demonstration of HTLV-1 infection. ATLL cells are usually positive for CD2, CD3, CD4, CD5 and CD25 and negative for TdT, CD7 and CD8 (see Table 6-8).

A variety of chromosomal aberrations have been described in ATLL, including $14q^-$ and trisomy 7.[334,335]

Sezary Syndrome

Sezary syndrome is the leukemic phase of a cutaneous T-cell lymphoma (mycoses fungoides) characterized by pruritic and pigmented erythroderma and cutaneous infiltration of neoplastic T cells in the epidermis and upper dermis.[336,337] The malignant cells are T lymphocytes, generally with a helper/inducer phenotype ($CD4^+$).[186,338,339] Cutaneous T-cell lymphoma (CTCL) is a relatively uncommon disease involving elderly people (usually over 50 years old). The incidence is higher in men than in women.

The etiology of CTCL/Sezary syndrome is not known. However, retrovirus particles and reverse transcriptase activities have been reported in cultured neoplastic cells derived from patients with this disorder.[340,341] The possibility of a new retrovirus, HTLV-V, has recently been suggested in association with CTLC.[342] A frequent history of exposure to toxic

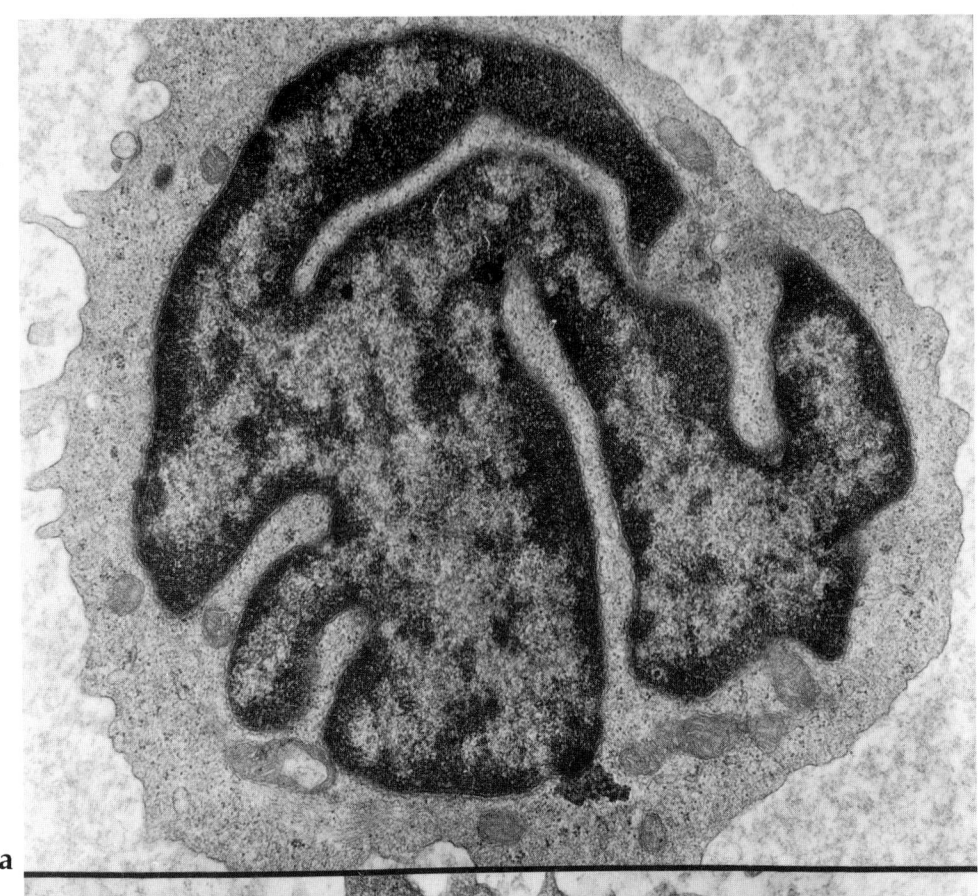

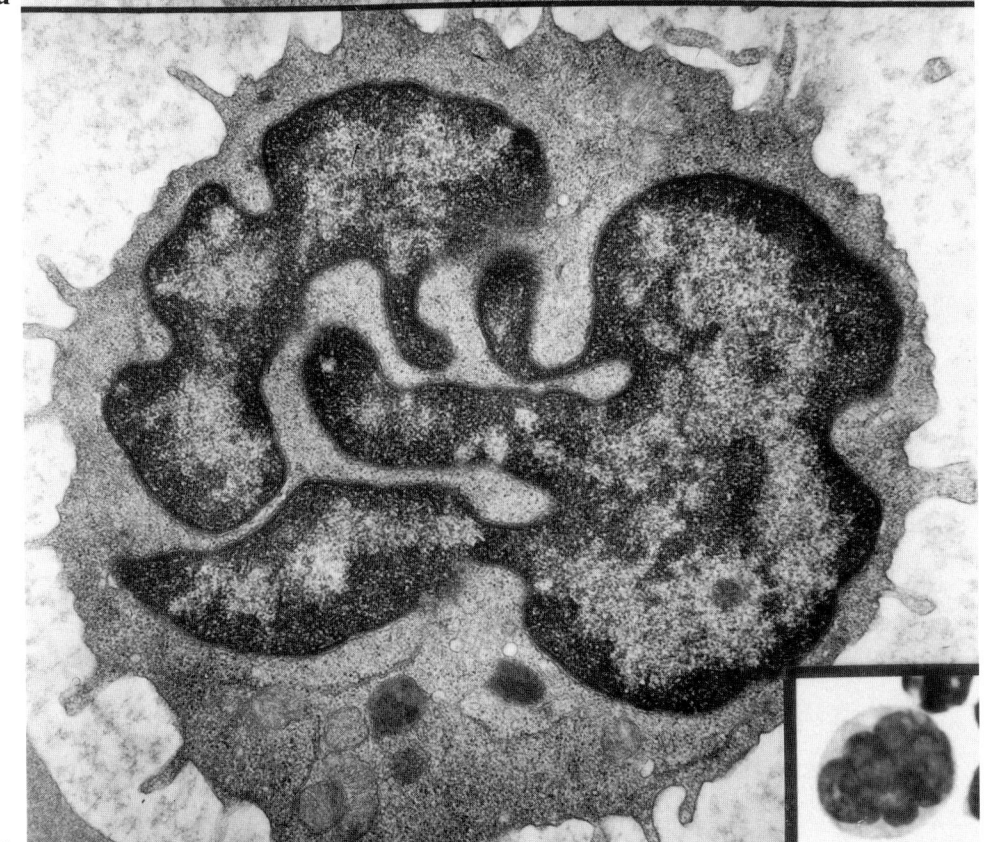

182

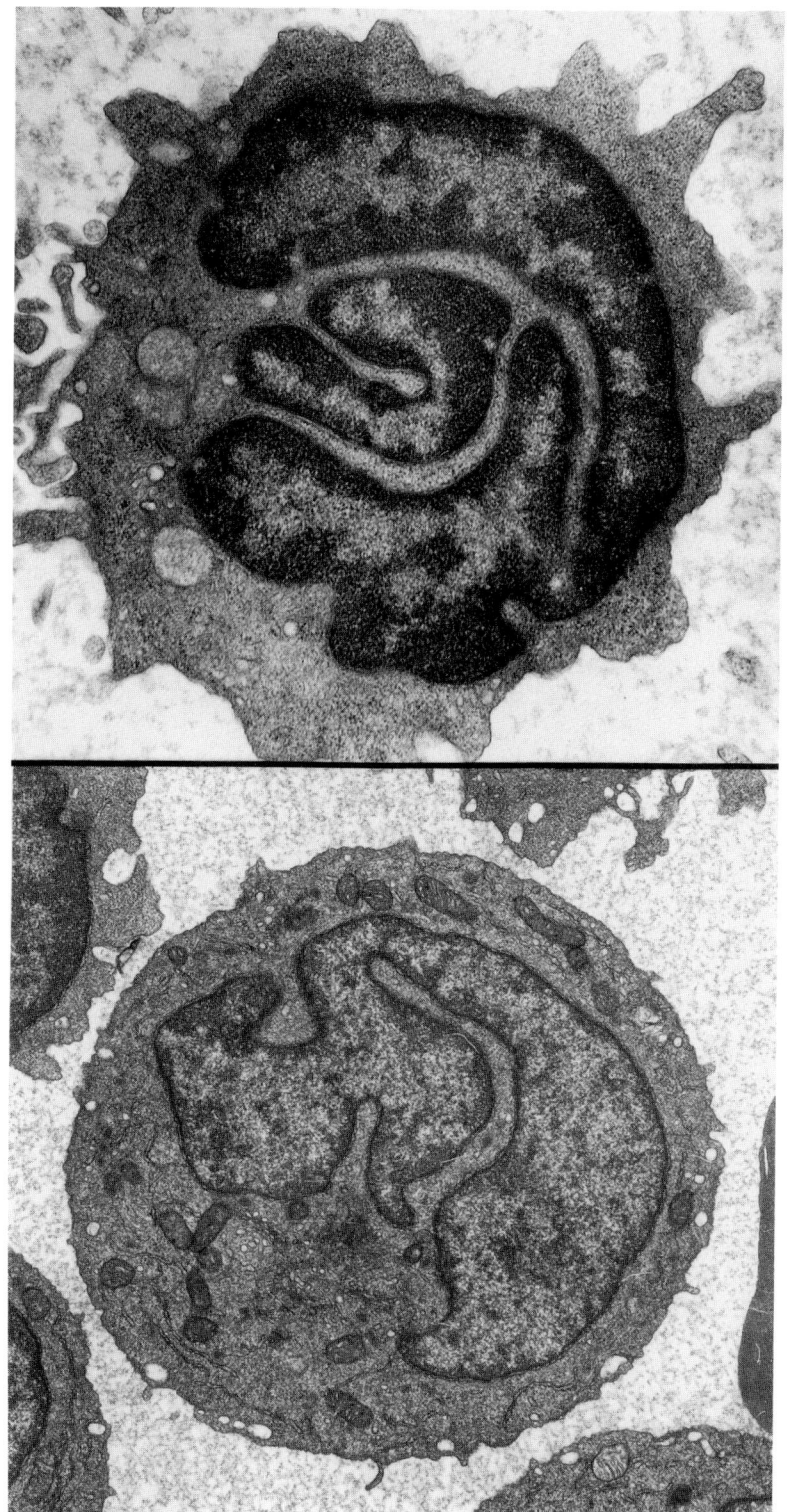

Figure 6-41. Electron microscopic features of tumor cells in a patient with adult T-cell leukemia/lymphoma demonstrating markedly convoluted nuclei.

Figure 6-40. Marked nuclear convolution of tumor cells in a patient with adult T-cell leukemia/lymphoma. (a and b) Electron microscopy, peripheral blood. Insert: light microscopy, peripheral blood.

chemicals and biologic agents has been recorded in CTCL patients, suggesting chronic immunologic stimulation leading to malignant transformation.[343,344]

The characteristic morphologic feature of neoplastic cells in CTCL, both in solid tissues and in peripheral blood, is cerebriform nuclear convolution (Figures 6-31 and 6-42). In peripheral blood smears, Sezary cells may vary in size. Overall, the small variant of the Sezary cell (also called the "Lutzner cell"), which is the size of a small lymphocyte, is more common than the large variant. The large Sezary cells are larger than neutrophils, show a narrow rim of clear basophilic cytoplasm and no azurophilic granules, and often display a near-tetraploid aneuploidy.[180] The nuclear chromatin is densely clumped, and the nucleoli are small and inconspicuous. Lymphocytes with cerebriform nuclei ("Sezary-like" cells) have been observed in the peripheral blood of healthy individuals, accounting for 1% to >6% of peripheral blood mononuclear cells.[345-348] Similar cells have also been described in a number of benign dermatoses, such as erythremic eczema, psoriasis, lichen planus and actinic reticuloid,[349-352] as well as in AIDS.[353]

Marrow involvement is detected in approximately 20% of CTCL patients, and is associated with disseminated disease and a poor prognosis.[354-357] Marrow involvement is often subtle and difficult to recognize. The neoplastic cells usually appear as small lymphoid aggregates with characteristic nuclear convolutions. Diffuse bone marrow involvement is less frequent.

Sezary cells express CD2, CD3, CD4 and CD5, and generally lack HLA-DR and CD7 (see Table 6-8). Unlike Serzary cells, the Sezary-like lymphocytes observed in benign dermatoses and AIDS are $CD8^+$.[352,353]

DNA aneuploidy is relatively frequent in CTCL and Sezary syndrome, accounting for up to 40% of the cases. Aneuploidy is often a near-tetraploid hyperdiploidy.[358,359,365] Several chromosomal aberations and breakpoints have also been reported in CTCL, including $6q^-$, $7q^-$, $9q^-$, $17p^-$ and t(10,22).[360]

Leukemic Phase of Splenic Lymphoma

Certain splenic lymphomas are associated with circulating villous lymphocytes in peripheral blood.[361] These cells are larger than CLL cells, and similar to hairy cells, have abundant cytoplasm with cytoplasmic projections. The nucleus is round or ovoid, has clumped chromatin, and may contain a small nucleolus in half of the cases.[180,361] The disease, in contrast to HCL, involves the splenic white pulp, with bone marrow infiltration in about 50% of the cases.[361,362] The splenic lymphoma cells have immunophenotypic properties similar to those of PLL cells and, unlike hairy cells, are TRAP, CD11c and CD25 negative.[180]

Leukemic Phase of Other Lymphomas

Peripheral blood involvement in non-Hodgkin's lymphomas traditionally was referred to as "lymphosarcoma cell leukemia."[363] This leukemic phase represents disseminated disease and is often characterized by an atypical lymphocytosis (usually >5000 cells/μl). The atypical lymphocytes display the cytologic features of the original neoplastic lymphoma cells. Follicular, small, cleaved-cell lymphomas are the most frequent types of lymphomas observed in the leukemic phase.[363-366] The circulating cells in these lymphomas are small, with a scanty cytoplasm and a cleaved nucleus. The nuclear chromatin is uniformly condensed, and nucleoli are either absent or barely visible.[180]

Chronic Myelogenous Leukemia (CML)

CML is a clonal disorder of the multipotent hematopoietic stem cell.[367-370] The involved clonal multipotent stem cell is capable of differentiation but is defective in response to mechanisms regulating proliferation. The result is an overproduction of end-stage hematopoietic cells, predominantly granulocytes. CML is consistently associated with Philadelphia chromosome (Ph^1), originally described as shortening of the long arm of chromosome 22.[371] Ph^1 is the result of the translocation of genetic material between chromosomes 9 and 22 [t(9;22)(q34;q11)].[372] CML appears to be a multistep evolutionary process initiated by the proliferation of Ph^1-negative clonal cells and followed by clonal expansion of Ph^1-positive cells.[373-375] This chronic stage eventually progresses to the accelerated phase and blast transformation, which are often associated with additional nonrandom chromosomal changes.[376-379] An increased incidence of CML is noted after exposure to ionizing

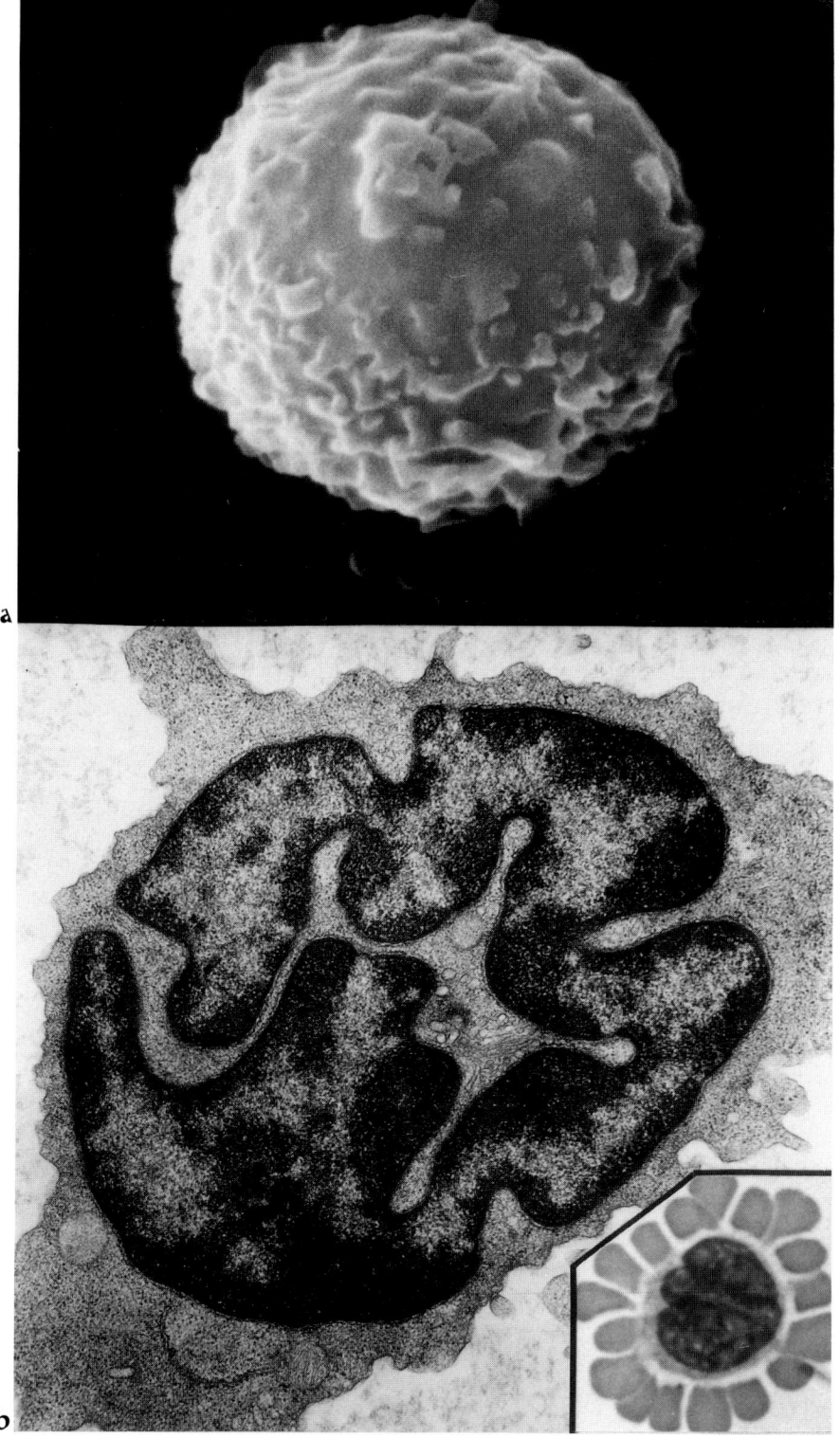

Figure 6-42. Scanning (a) and transmission (b) electron microscopic features of a Sezary cell. The insert demonstrates light microscopic features of a Sezary cell with E-rosetting and a cerebriform nucleus.

radiation, with 5- to 10-year gaps from exposure to development of CML.[380] Familial incidence is rare.[381]

Pathology

Bone marrow examination reveals a hypercellular marrow with a markedly elevated M:E ratio, usually >10:1 (Figure 6-43). Megakaryocytes are abundant and dysplastic, with a large number of micromegakaryocytes and many large, bizzare, multilobulated forms often appearing as patchy clusters. The granulocytic component in the chronic phase of the disease is mildly to moderately left-shifted. Myeloid dysplasia such as abnormal nuclear morphology, nuclear-cytoplasmic asynchrony and nuclear hypo- or hypersegmentation is a common feature. Eosinophils including precursor cells are prominent. Basophilia is also a frequent feature, but is usually less than 20%. The increased turnover of granulocytes leads to the formation of sea-blue histiocytes and pseudo-Gaucher's cells loaded with cell membrane debris, hemosiderin and/or other phagocytic particles (see Figure 6-43). Plasma cells, lymphocytes and mast cells may be increased. There may be increased formation of reticulin fibers, and the extent of fibrosis correlates with the degree of megakaryocytosis. Osteosclerosis may occur in association with marrow fibrosis.

Although the overwhelming majority of bone marrow stem cells in CML patients are neoplastic and Ph^1-positive, a normal residual stem cell pool exists which is suppressed by leukemic-inhibitory factors and the proliferative advantage of the neoplastic clone.[375,382] Long-term liquid cultures of bone marrow cells derived from CML patients provide a growth advantage of Ph^1-negative nonclonal cells over Ph^1-positive clones.[376,383] CML blast progenitor cells have a reduced capacity to adhere to the bone marrow stroma.[384] This may explain the release of premature Ph^1-positive cells into the peripheral blood of CML patients.

Peripheral blood examination reveals a marked granulocytosis with a low LAP score (see Chapter 2). The white blood cell count is commonly >50,000/μl and often greater than 100,000/ul.[375] There is a granulocytic left shift, with the presence of precursor cells in various stages of maturation similar in proportion to their relative frequency in normal bone marrow; blasts are less than 5% and promyelocytes are less than 10% of the white blood cells. The monocyte count is increased, but not proportionally to the

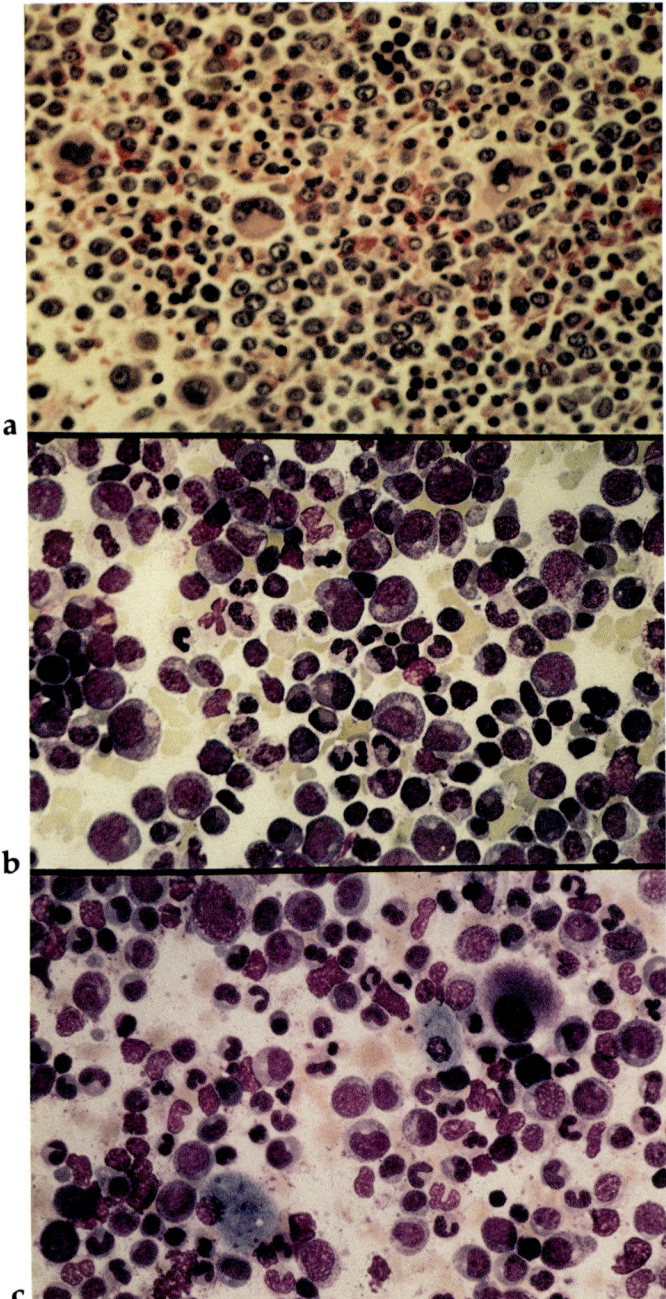

Figure 6-43. Bone marrow in chronic myelogenous leukemia; clot section (a) and smears (b and c). The M:E ratio is markedly elevated, and pseudo-Gaucher's cells are present (c).

neutrophil count. Eosinophilia and/or basophilia is common, and approximately one-third of the patients show thrombocytosis (a platelet count >700,000/μl) and one-half demonstrate anemia (Hb <12 g/dl) at diagnosis. Anemia is usually normocytic normochromic. Nucleated red blood cells and micromegakaryocytes or megakaryocytic fragments may be present in the peripheral blood. Other peripheral blood findings include elevated levels of lactic dehydrogenase (LDH), uric acid and vitamin B_{12}. Major differences between CML and leukemoid reactions are presented in Table 6-11.

CYTOGENETICS: As briefly mentioned, leukemic cells in most (95%) CML patients demonstrate a shortened chromosome 22 (Ph chromosome)[371] resulting from a reciprocal translocation between chromosomes 9 and 22 [t(9;22)(q34;q11)].[372,374,376,377,384] With this translocation, a segment of the *c-abl* proto-oncogene is translocated into the center of the BCR gene on chromosome 22. The center of the BCR gene contains six small exons and is termed *bcr*. The newly formed *bcr/abl* hybrid gene translates into an 8.5-kb mRNA and a 210-kD protein with increased tyrosine kinase activity.[385-388]

The Ph^1 chromosome is also found in about 2% of patients with AML without a history of CML, and in up to 25% of adults and 10% of children with ALL.[386] In approximately half of these cases, a *bcr/abl* hybrid protein of 190 kD rather than 210 D is found.[386,389]

ACCELERATED PHASE AND BLAST TRANSFORMATION: The evolutionary process in CML eventually leads to the expansion of a new clone which is defective in progressive differentiation. This new clonal expansion presents with increased numbers of blast cells. The accelerated phase represents the transition from the chronic phase of CML to an acute leukemia (blast crisis, blast transformation, or blastic phase).

The accelerated phase is a relatively ill-defined clinicopathologic entity often characterized by increasing degrees of anemia and thrombocytopenia, by an increased percentage of blast cells in bone marrow and/or peripheral blood (≥15% but <30%), and by 20% or more basophils.[390-392]

Blast crisis is characterized by 30% or more blasts in bone marrow and/or peripheral blood. Since CML is a disorder of pluripotent stem cells, blasts in the acute phase may represent a nonlymphoid, lymphoid or mixed lineage leukemia. Blasts in approximately 70-80% of the cases are of granulocytic origin based on morphologic, cytochemical and immunophenotypic studies. Lymphoid blast crisis accounts for 15-20% of the cases. Megakaryocytic and erythroid blast crisis are uncommon (<10%). Blast transformation is often associated with additional chromosomal abnormalities.[393,394] Recent advances in technology and availability of comprehensive multiparameter cytochemical, immunophenotypic and molecular biologic studies have increased the rate of the detection of the mixed lineage blast crisis.

Clinical Aspects

CML accounts for about 20-35% of adult leukemias.[375] The median age of occurrence is 45-50 years, and the male:female ratio is slightly greater than 1. Clinical symptoms are minimal or nonexistent in the early stages of the disease, and up to 45% of the patients may be asymptomatic at diagnosis.[375] However, clinical findings are primarily related to the

Table 6-11 Differential Diagnosis Between CML and Leukemoid Reaction

	CML	Leukemoid Reaction
Peripheral blood		
WBC	Markedly elevated Usually >100,000/μl	Elevated Usually <50,000/μl
PMNs	All stages of maturation	Almost all mature
LAP score	Reduced	Elevated
Bone marrow		
M:E ratio	>10:1	<10:1
t(9;22)	Present	Absent
Splenomegaly	Marked	Variable

increased leukemic mass and to granulocytic and platelet dysfunction. Fatigue, malaise, headache, weight loss, bleeding and right upper quadrant pain, splenomegaly and hepatomegaly are the most common symptoms and signs. Vaso-occlusive manifestations, such as CNS infarction, venous thrombosis, priapism and pulmonary insufficiency secondary to the markedly elevated white blood cell and/or platelet counts, are rare.

Approximately 60-70% of CML patients develop an accelerated phase, which lasts for 6-18 months before death or blast crisis occurs.[390,395] Overall, blast crisis develops in 70-80% of CML patients, leading to death within 3-6 months.[396] In addition to disease acceleration and blast crisis, other parameters associated with a poor outcome include coexisting of severe leukocytosis with marked thrombocytopenia, splenomegaly[391] and bone marrow fibrosis.[397]

Juvenile Chronic Myelogenous Leukemia (JCML)

JCML, or subacute myelomonocytic leukemia,[398] is a rare myeloproliferative disorder of infancy and early childhood. It is distinguished from the adult form of CML by frequent cutaneous manifestations (eczema, xanthoma, and cafe-au-lait spots), thrombocytopenia with hemorrhagic diathesis, elevated fetal hemoglobin level, marked monocytosis, lymphadenopathy, absence of Ph^1 and a relatively rapid course[399-401] (Table 6-12). JCML patients frequently show immunologic abnormalities such as strikingly high immunoglobulin levels and a high incidence of antinuclear (>50%) and anti-IgG (>40%) antibodies.[401] There are several reports indicating an association between JCML and two unrelated disorders: neurofibromatosis and persistent EBV infection.[402-404] Most of the patients with JCML are diagnosed before the age of 2 years. The median survival is about 9 months.[401]

JCML, similar to classic adult CML, appears to be a clonal disorder of multipotent stem cells and is associated with hypercellular bone marrow, splenomegaly and decreased LAP.[400,401] However, unlike adult CML, immature and abnormal monocytic and erythroid precursors are the most prominent hematopoietic components in JCML. Abnormal erythropoiesis includes the presence of high levels of fetal hemoglobin (15-50%) and low expression of the I antigen.[405,406]

The most prominent cytogenetic feature in JCML is the absence of Ph^1 chromosome. Most patients have a normal karyotype, and chromosomal aberrations, when present, are most commonly found in chromosomes 7 and 8.[405,407]

Table 6-12 Major Differences Between Juvenile and Adult Types of CML

Findings	Juvenile Type	Adult Type
Age	Usually <2 years	Usually >2 years
Skin rash	Frequent	Absent
Lymphadenopathy	Frequent	Rare
WBCs	Usually <100,000	Usually >100,000
Monocytosis	Usually present	Absent
Thrombocytopenia	Common	Uncommon at unset
RBC abnormalities		
Fetal Hb level	15-50%	Normal
Level of 1 antigen	Reduced	Normal
Normoblasts in PB	Frequent	Unusual
Immunologic abnorm.	Frequent	Unusual
Prominent clone in culture	Monocytic	Granulocytic
Ph^1 chromosome	Absent	Present
Blast transformation	Rare	Common
Median survival	<9 months	2.5-3 years

Combined immune deficiency, congenital viral infections and persistent EBV infection may present a clinicopathologic picture very similar to that of JCML. However, in none of these conditions is the fetal hemoglobin level as high as it is in JCML.

Chronic Neutrophilic Leukemia (CNL)

A rare entity termed "chronic neutrophilic leukemia (CNL)" has been reported. It is characterized by marked mature peripheral neutrophilia, hepatosplenomegaly and elevated LAP. CNL is distinguished from leukemoid reactions by the presence of hepatosplenomegaly; lack of fever, sepsis, an inflammatory process and malignancy; and a normal erythrocyte sedimentation rate.[408] Peripheral blood examinations reveal an elevated white blood cell count ranging from 50,000 to 100,000/μl, with the majority of the leukocytes being neutrophilic granulocytes and bands. Myelocytes and metamyelocytes are rare. The bone marrow is markedly hypercellular, with an elevated M:E ratio of over 4:1 and with fewer than 5% blasts and promyelocytes. The other hematopoietic components are unremarkable. Patients with CNL show a normal karyotypes. Survival, in the limited number of reported cases, ranges from 2 months to 5 years.[408-410]

Chronic Monocytic Leukemia (CMoL)

CMoL is a rare condition characterized by splenomegaly, hepatomegaly, and peripheral blood and bone marrow monocytosis.[411] Monocytosis, which often intensifies after splenectomy, consists of mature cells ranging from 1,000 to over 16,000/μl in peripheral blood and accounting for more than 50% of the bone marrow cells in most patients. Scattered leukemic cells in the bone marrow may show erythrophagocytosis. Patients are adults and more frequently male. Median survival is around 2 years.

Other Granulocytic Leukemias

Eosinophilic Leukemia (Malignant Eosinophilia, Primary Eosinophila)

This is a rare but distinct entity which represents the more aggressive end of the spectrum of disorders called "hypereosinophilic syndromes." The major problem is to differentiate the autonomous, unremitting eosinophilic leukemia from the severe, hypereosinophilic syndromes which are secondary to chronic hypersensitivity of undetermined etiology. The recommended criteria for the diagnosis of eosinophilic leukemia are marked persistent eosinophilia with the presence of immature forms, hepatosplenomegaly and lymphadenopathy, usually accompanied by anemia and thrombocytopenia.[412] However, many of these features are also present in severe hypereosinophilic syndromes. Distinguishing features in a few instances have been the presence of cytogenetic abnormalities in patients with eosinophilic leukemia. The reported cytogenetic abnormalities include Ph^1 chromosome and trisomy of chromosome 8.[413,414] However, the rare reported cases of Ph^1-positive eosinophilic leukemia may represent a variant of CML with excessive eosinophilia.

Bone marrow examination reveals a myeloid left shift, with marked eosinophilia ranging from 30 to 80%, and predominance of eosinophilic promyelocytes, myelocytes and metamyelocytes (Figure 6-44). Bone marrow fibrosis may be present.[412]

Peripheral blood examination reveals marked leukocytosis, which usually ranges from 50,000 to 200,000/μl with eosinophilia often >60%. An eosinophilic left shift is common, with the presence of eosinophilic promyelocytes, myelocytes and metamyelocytes. Anemia and thrombocytopenia are common.

Hepatosplenomegaly, lymphadenopathy, cardiomyopathy and respiratory distress are the major clinical findings. Similar to CML, eosinophilic leukemia may progress to a blastic phase and turn into AML. Eosinophilic leukemia is a rapidly fatal disease.

Mast Cell Leukemia

This is a rare leukemia with an acute clinical course. It is characterized by the presence of atypical mast cells in the peripheral blood (usually >10% of white blood cells) and diffuse, destructive infiltration of the bone marrow with atypical mast cells (Figures 6-44 and 6-45). The condition is often associated with peptic ulcer, prominent constitutional symptoms (such as fever, weight loss and weakness) and hepatomegaly.[415a] Mast cell leukemia is a leukemic manifestation of aggressive systemic mastocytosis developing in approximately 15% of the patients.[416-419] Leukemic mast cells are pleomorphic, consisting of morphologically typical mast cells mixed with less differentiated or bizzare forms. Since the cytoplasmic granules

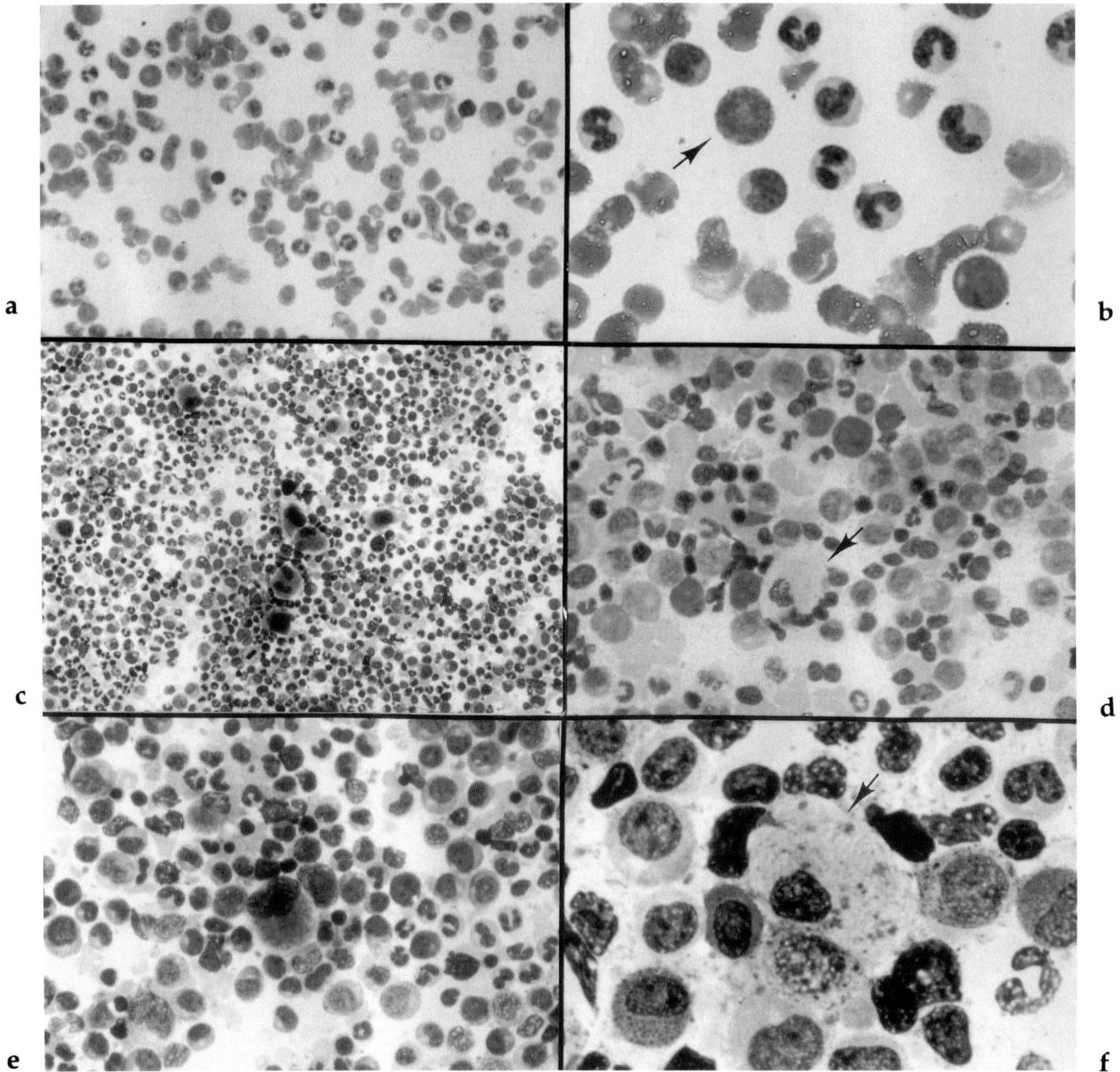

Figure 6-44. Chronic myelogenous leukemia. Peripheral blood shows a marked granulocytosis (a,b) with the presence of immature forms (b, arrow). Bone marrow is hypercellular and demonstrates an increased M:E ratio (often >10); pseudo-Gaucher cells are frequently present (d, f, arrows).

in mast cells contain histamine and heparin, the neoplastic cells may stain intensely with toluidine blue. They are MPO negative, PAS positive and usually stain positively for naphthol AS-D chloroacetate.

Mast cell leukemia is a rapidly fatal disease, with a mean survival of <6 months.[415a,415b] Mast cell leukemia, unlike other types of systemic mast cell disease, is rarely associated with urticaria pigmentosa.[415a]

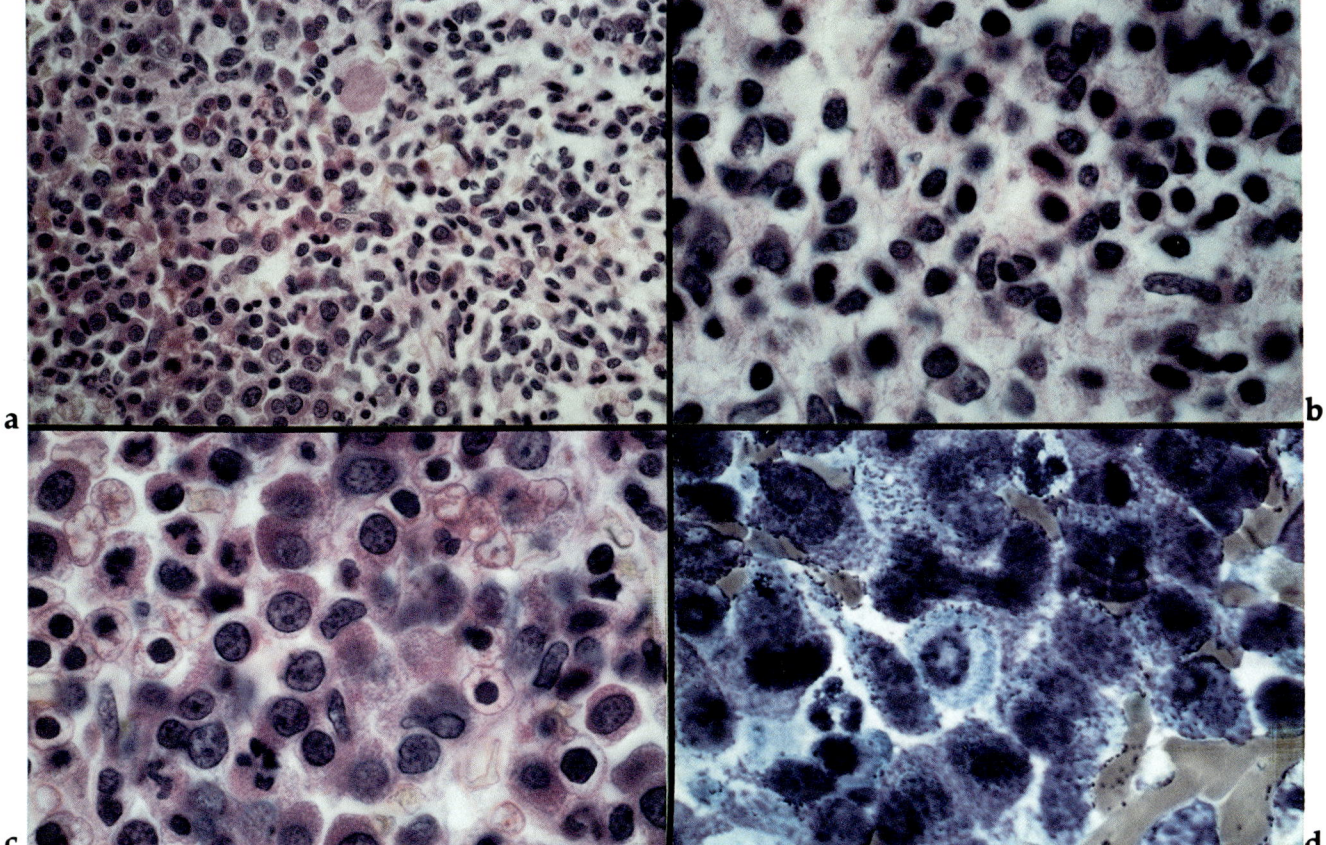

Figure 6-45. Bone marrow from a patient with malignant mastocytosis exhibiting increased marrow mast cells with atypical features; clot sections (a–c) and smear (d). Heavy cytoplasmic granules, pleomorphic nuclei, and prominent nucleoli are demonstrated in the higher-power fields (c and d).

Mast cell leukemia should be distinguished from cases of AML that arise against the background of a systemic mast cell disease. In a recent study by Travis and associates,[420] 22 of 66 patients with systemic mast cell disease were found to have hematologic disorders, including myelodysplastic syndromes in 10, myeloproliferative disorders in 5, AML in 3, lymphoma in 3, and chronic neutropenia in 1.

Basophilic Leukemia

This disease is extremely rare and is characterized by a marked basophilia with a high proportion of immature forms, an elevated leukocyte count and hypercellular bone marrow with a myeloid left shift.[421a] De novo basophilic leukemia should be differentiated from cases of CML and acute myelomonocytic leukemia associated with marked basophilia. Basophilic leukemia is Ph[1] negative. The cytoplastic granules in the basophilic precursors stain with toluidine blue. Rare AMLs may show evidence of basophilic differentiation (acute basophilic leukemia) on the basis of electron microscopic examination.[144]

MALIGNANT LYMPHOMAS

Classification

Malignant lymphomas are divided into two major subclasses: Hodgkin's disease and non-Hodgkin's lymphoma (NHL). The incidence of bone marrow involvement is significantly higher in NHL (ranging from 25 to 90%) than in Hodgkin's disease (5 to 15%).[422-427] In the majority of cases, the distribution of Hodgkin's disease and NHL in bone marrow is focal or patchy. Thus, the lesions may be missed if bone marrow samples are inadequate. The recommended size of bone marrow biopsy samples for diagnosis of lymphoma is at least 2 cm.[426] Overall, bilateral posterior iliac crest biopsy samples increase the chances of demonstrating bone marrow involvement in lymphomas.[427,428]

Hodgkin's Disease

Hodgkin's disease is distinguished from NHL by its bimodal age distribution, infrequent extranodal (bone marrow, gastrointestinal tract, CNS, skin) involvement, higher rate of localized disease at diagnosis and histopathologic features (presence of Reed-Sternberg cells in a background of inflammatory cells). The origin of the Reed-Sternberg (RS) cells and their variants is still controversial. There are reports suggesting that RS cells are of lymphoid (T-cell or B-cell) lineage, and there are also reports supporting their origin from a mononuclear macrophage system (histiocytes, dendritic cells).[429-432]

The diagnostic RS cell is described as a large, binuclear ("owl-eye" appearance) cell with abundant cytoplasm and huge, round, inclusion-like nucleoli (Figures 6-46 and 6-53). In addition to the diagnostic RS cells, several mononuclear, multinuclear and multilobular RS variants have been identified which are useful in the diagnosis and classification of Hodgkin's disease. The RS cells and their variants are intermixed with a variety of inflammatory cells including lymphocytes, plasma cells, histiocytes, eosinophils and fibroblasts. This polycellular background of inflammatory cells is an important diagnostic feature in Hodgkin's disease. In general, the lymphocytic component in Hodgkin's disease consists of small lymphocytes with round nuclei and no atypical features.

Hodgkin's disease has been classified into four groups: (1) lymphocyte predominance, (2) nodular

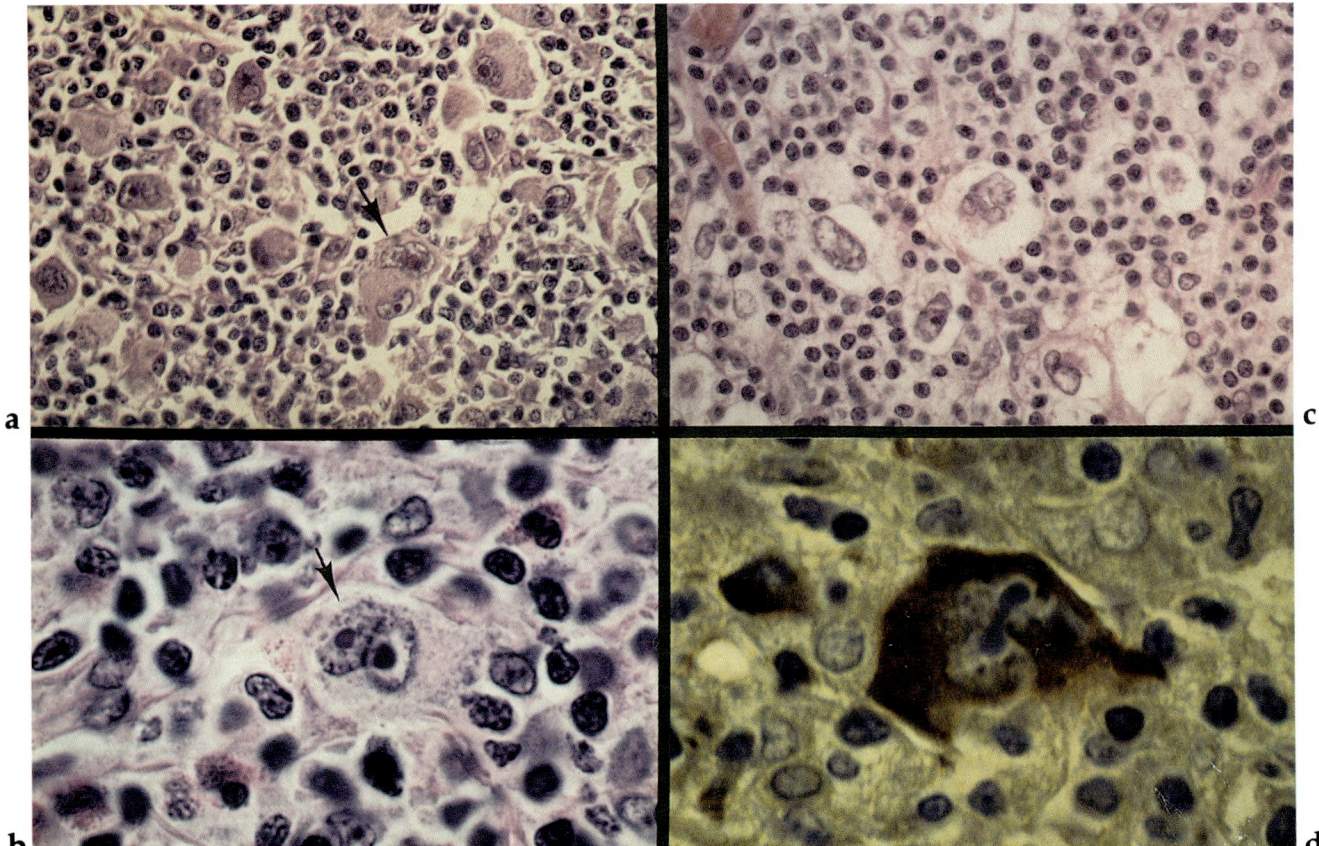

Figure 6-46. Hodgkin's disease. (a and b) Classical RS cells (arrows). (c) Lacunar cells. (d) An RS cell with strong cytoplasmic CD15 positivity; immunoperoxidase technique.

sclerosis, (3) mixed cellularity, and (4) lymphocyte depletion with the following histopathologic features:

Lymphocyte predominance accounts for about 10% of the cases and has been characterized by sparsity of neoplastic cells and predominance of lymphocytes and/or histiocytes. The neoplastic RS variants ("L and H" variants), or "popcorn" cells, are large cells with a large, delicate, multilobated nucleus, multiple small nucleoli and scant to moderate amounts of pale or basophilic cytoplasm. The pattern of lymph node involvement is nodular or diffuse. Recent investigations suggest that the nodular variant of the lymphocyte predominance Hodgkin's disease is closely related to the B-cell lymphomas and probably represents a B-cell neoplasm of low-grade malignancy.[433]

Nodular sclerosis is the most common type of Hodgkin's disease (40–70%), with a peak incidence in adolescents and young adults and a greater frequency in women. Its distinctive histopathologic features are nodular compartmentalization of the involved tissues by thick bands of collagen and the presence of *lacuner cells* (Figures 6-46 and 6-47). Lacuner cells are RS variants characterized by abundant pale cytoplasm, a large, lobulated nucleus and a small nucleolus. The cytoplasm retracts in the process of formalin fixation, creating a hole or lacuna around the cells. In some cases, the lacunar cells are expanded and appear as sheets of cohesive cells (syncytial variant). Collagen formation in the early stages is minimal (cellular phase).

Mixed cellularity is another common type of Hodgkin's disease (30–50%), characterized by the presence of numerous classic RS and RS variants (see Figure 6-46).

Lymphocyte depletion is a rare type (<5%) characterized by sparsity of lymphocytes and other reactive cells and by the presence of numerous bizzare RS variants. This type has considerable morphologic overlap with pleomorphic large cell NHLs, which are predominantly of the T-cell type.

Bone marrow involvement in Hodgkin's disease is less frequent than in NHL, accounting for about 5–15% of the cases.[434-437] Lymphocyte depletion and mixed cellularity types infiltrate bone marrow the most. Bone marrow involvement is <10% in nodular sclerosis and rare in lymphocyte predominance Hodgkin's disease.[436,437] Negative bone marrow results in patients with Hodgkin's disease often indicate lack of extranodal involvement.[436]

Diagnosis of Hodgkin's disease in bone marrow samples is made in the presence of typical RS cells and/or their variants in association with characteristic polymorphic inflammatory cells and often fibrosis (Figure 6-48). The presence of atypical large histiocytic cells with the proper background of inflammatory cells or focal fibrosis in a patient with a history of Hodgkin's disease strongly suggests bone marrow involvement, even without the presence of diagnostic RS cells.[438] Bone marrow fibrosis or necrosis in a patient with diagnosed Hodgkin's disease is suspicious for marrow involvement.

RS cells and their variants are usually $CD45^-$, $CD30^+$ (Ki-1, Ber-H2) and $CD15^+$ in mixed cellularity, nodular sclerosis, and $CD45^+$, $CD30^+$, $CD15^-$ and often $L26^+$ in lymphocyte predominance Hodgkin's disease[439,440] (see Figure 6-46).

Disorders associated with a polymorphic cellular proliferation such as granulomas, virus infections, angioimmunoblastic lymphadenopathies and pleomorphic T-cell lymphomas may mimic Hodgkin's disease.

CYTOGENETICS: There is relatively little information regarding the cytogenetic aberrations in Hodgkin's lymphoma. Several factors are responsible for this situation, including sparsity of neoplastic cells in the tissue samples and their relatively low proliferative index.[441] The frequency of detection of chromosomal abnormalities in Hodgkin's disease varies significantly among cytogenetic laboratories, ranging from 22 to 83%.[443-445] The most common chromosomal abnormalities reported in patients with Hodgkin's disease are numerical abnormalities, particularly hyperdiploidy. The major causes of hyperdiploidy in these patients, in order of frequency, are $+5$, $+2$, or $+1$, $+12$ and $+21$. Loss of chromosomes 22, 10, 13 and 21 has also been reported. The most frequent structural abnormalities involve chromosome 1 (1p or 1q).[441]

Clinical Aspects

There are four clinical stages for Hodgkin's disease (and non-Hodgkin's lymphoma) defined as follows:

Stage I   Involvement of a single lymph node region or a single extranodal tissue.

Stage II   Involvement of two or more lymph node regions on the same side of diaphragm with or without involvement of limited contiguous extranodal tissues.

Stage III Involvement of lymph node regions on both sides of the diaphragm, with or without involvement of the spleen and/or limited contiguous extranodal tissues.

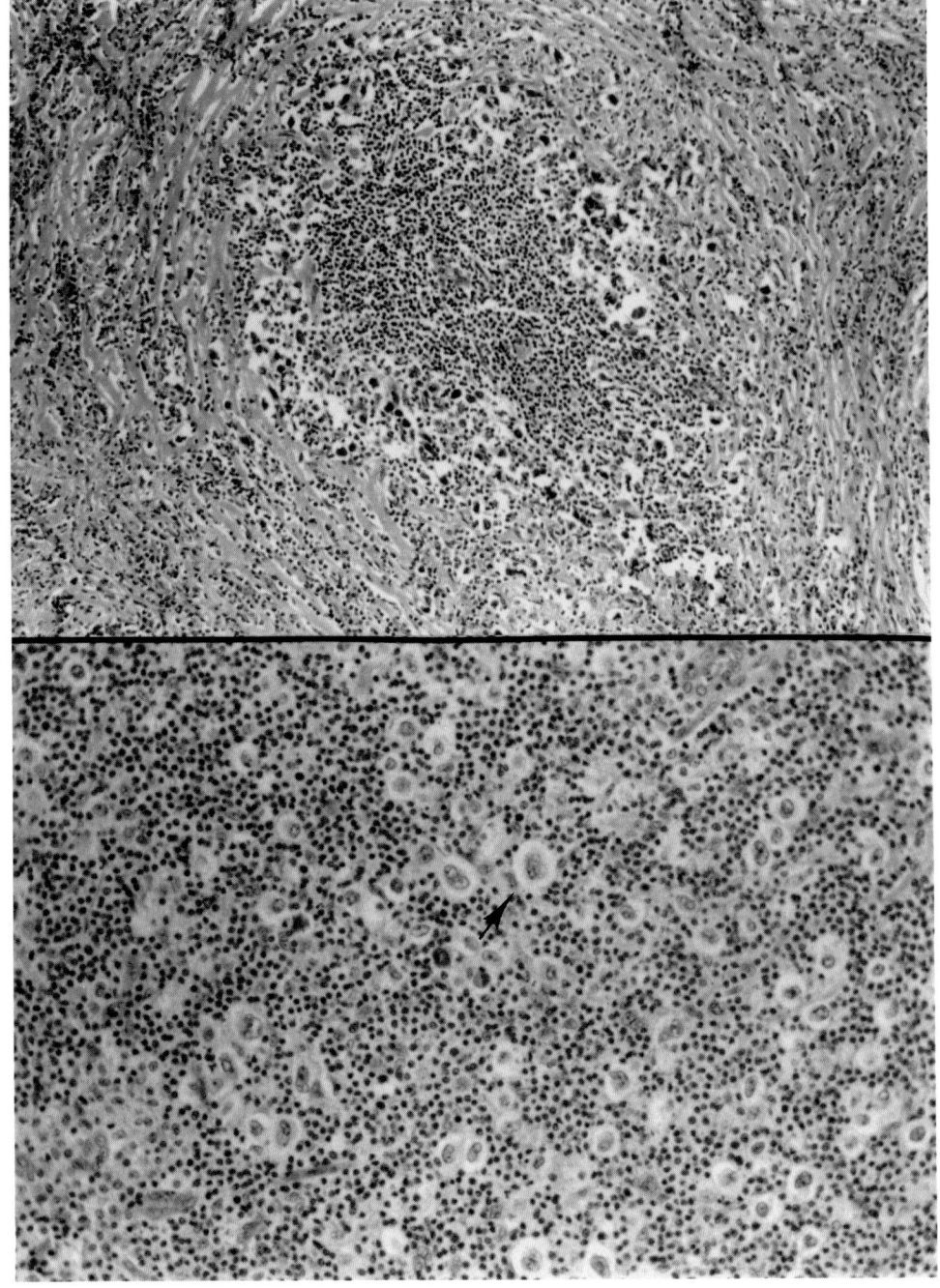

Figure 6-47. Lymph node section demonstrating nodular sclerosis Hodgkin's disease with numerous lacunar cells (arrow).

Stage IV Disseminated or multiple foci of involvement of one or more extranodal organs or tissues.

All the stages are further divided into (A) or (B) on the basis of the absence or presence of systemic symptoms, respectively. These symptoms include fever, night sweats, and/or unexplained weight loss of >10%.

The most common complaint is enlargement of the superficial lymph nodes, with involvement of the cervical, axillary and inguinal regions about 70%, 15% and 8% of the time, respectively. Mediastinal involve-

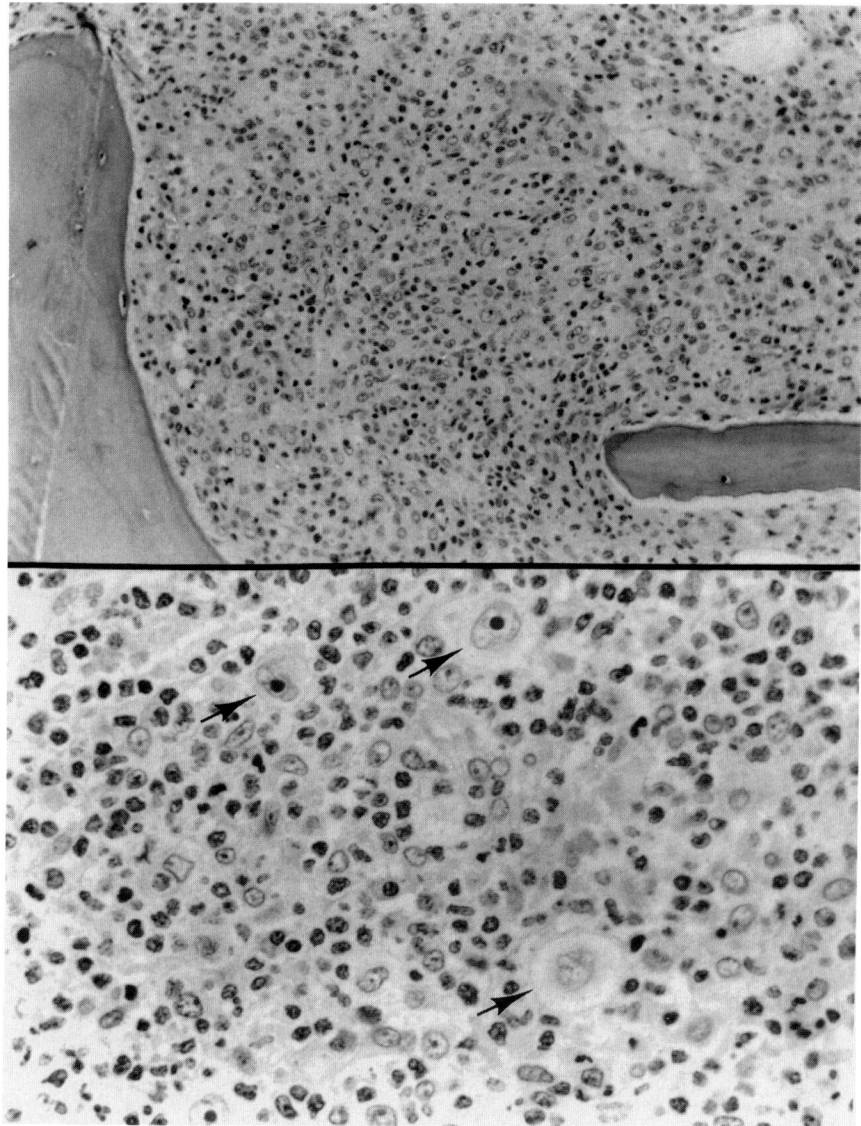

Figure 6-48. Bone marrow biopsy section exhibiting Hodgkin's disease. Several RS variants are present (arrows).

ment is reported in up to 60% and retroperitoneal involvement in about 25% of the cases. Mediastinal lymphadenopathy is one of the characteristics of nodular sclerosis. Low-grade fever and night sweats are common, particularly in the advanced stages. Modern combinations of radiotherapy and chemotherapy have resulted in very high survival rates. The cure rate for patients with early-stage disease is 90% or higher, and for patients with advanced disease is about 70%.[446] Patients with lymphocyte predominance and nodular sclerosis types usually have a localized disease and an excellent prognosis. Patients with the lymphocyte depletion type have the worst prognosis.

Non-Hodgkin's Lymphoma (NHL)

Diagnosis and classification of NHL is one of the most difficult areas in surgical pathology and has generated considerable controversy among the experts in lymph node pathology. During the last two decades, several classifications have been proposed, based on morphologic and immunophenotypic characteristics of NHL. The two most popular classifications currently used in the United States are the Rappaport classification and a classification proposed by an international panel of experts in lymph node pathology (Working Formulation)[447] (Table 6-13). the major emphasis in all proposed classifications has been correlation between the morphologic and/or immunophenotypic characteristics of the NHLs with the prognosis and response to therapy. Most of the classifications are based on two morphologic criteria: the pattern of lymph node involvement (follicular versus diffuse) and the cellular morphology (size, nuclear shape, chromatin density, nucleolus). In general, follicular lymphomas are almost always of B-cell origin and show a better prognosis than their diffuse counterparts, and those composed of small cells do better than those with large cells. By contrast, diffuse lymphomas may be either B- or T-cell types, are more aggressive than their follicular counterparts and include all highly aggressive tumors. Lymphomas composed of immature cells (prominent nucleoli and fine nuclear chromatin) are commonly aggressive. Pattern recognition is commonly made in the original lymphoid tissue (usually lymph node) and may be obscured in bone marrow biopsy samples because of patchy involvement of the bone marrow. Bone marrow involvement in NHL features a diverse morphology which includes the following patterns: focal, nodular (patchy), paratrabecular, interstitial, diffuse or a combination of these patterns (Figure 6-49). The patient's clinical history and, if possible, review of the original diagnostic tissue are of great help in the evaluation of bone marrow samples for the diagnosis of lymphomas. However, one should keep in mind that in some cases, there may be a significant difference between the involved bone marrow and lymph node morphology[448] (Figure 6-50).

Several studies have been reported regarding the incidence and morphologic characteristics of bone marrow involvement in NHLs.[427-429, 426,427] Primary involvement of bone (or bone marrow) with NHL is rare, accounting for <1% of all NHLs.[449,450] Bone marrow examination is frequently used for pathologic staging of patients with clinical stage I and stage II disease, and for posttherapy follow-up in patients with advanced disease. However, recent studies of patients with follicular small cleaved cell, diffuse large cell, and diffuse mixed lymphomas in advanced clinical stages (beyond stage II) suggest that bone marrow examination may not contribute significantly to the prognostic information or therapeutic decisions.[425]

The histopathologic features of NHLs based on the Working Formulation terminology will now be discussed.

Low-Grade Lymphomas

The most prominent members of this group of malignant lymphomas are (1) small lymphocytic, (2) follicular small cleaved cell and (3) follicular, mixed, small cleaved and large cell lymphomas. Low-grade lymphomas have a high incidence of marrow involvement.

Small lymphocytic lymphoma accounts for about 5% of NHLs and is composed of small lymphocytes with scanty blue nongranular cytoplasm, a round nucleus with dense, clumpy chromatin and an inconspicuous nucleolus (see Figure 6-29). These cells are morphologically and immunophenotypically similar to CLL cells. Small lymphocytic lymphoma and CLL are closely related diseases and in most instances appear to represent different spectrums of the same disorder, with wide overlapping features.[426,451] Bone marrow involvement is a common feature in small lymphocytic lymphoma and is observed in up to 90% of the cases.[448] Marrow involvement is most commonly interstitial or diffuse, though focal involvement with a random or paratrabecular distribution is also noted. Some cases of small lymphocytic lymphoma with massive bone marrow involvement are associated with a monoclonal gammopathy, usually of the IgM type, and may present clinical manifestations of Waldenstrom's macroglobulinemia.[451-453] The neoplastic cells in small lymphocytic lymphomas associated with IgM gammopathy often demonstrate plasmacytoid features. Most of the small lymphocytic lymphomas (>90%) are of B-cell origin. The neoplastic cells are usually IgM, CD19, CD20, CD22, CD24, HLA-DR, L26, and CD5 positive and CD10 negative.[449-451]

The two other types of low-grade lymphoma are *follicular small cleaved* and *follicular, mixed, small cleaved and large cell*, accounting for approximately 25% and 10% of all NHLs, respectively. These two categories also show a high incidence of bone marrow involvement (40–60%). The small cleaved cells are slightly larger than normal lymphocytes, and have a scanty cytoplasm and an irregular, "cleaved" nuclear contour. The nuclei have moderately condensed chromatin and small nucleoli. The large cells have two to three times the diameter of normal lymphocytes, have a rim of amphophilic cytoplasm, and show round or oval, slightly irregular vesicular nuclei with

Table 6-13 Classification of NHLs: Working Formulation Compared to the Rappaport Classification

Working Formulation	Rappaport Equivalents
Low-grade	

A. Malignant lymphoma, small lymphocytic
    Consistent with CLL
    Plasmacytoid
	Well-differentiated lymphocytic

B. Malignant lymphoma, follicular,
    predominantly small cleaved cell
    Diffuse areas
    Sclerosis
	Nodular, poorly differentiated

C. Malignant lymphoma, follicular, mixed,
    small cleaved and large cell
    Diffuse areas
    Sclerosis
	Nodular, mixed cell type

Intermediate-grade	

D. Malignant lymphoma, follicular,
    predominantly large cell
    Diffuse areas
    Sclerosis
	Nodular histiocytic

E. Malignant lymphoma, diffuse, small
    cleaved cell
    Sclerosis
	Diffuse, poorly differentiated

F. Malignant lymphoma, diffuse, mixed,
    small and large cell
    Sclerosis
    Epithelioid cell component
	Diffuse, mixed cell type

G. Malignant lymphoma, diffuse, large cell
    Cleaved cell
    Noncleaved cell
    Sclerosis
	Diffuse, histiocytic

High-grade	

H. Malignant lymphoma, large cell,
    immunoblastic
    Plasmacytoid
    Clear cell
    Polymorphous
    Epithelioid cell component
	Diffuse histiocytic

I. Malignant lymphoma, lymphoblastic
    Convoluted cell
    Nonconvoluted cell
	Lymphoblastic

J. Malignant lymphoma, small
    noncleaved cell
    Burkitt's lymphoma
    Follicular areas
	Diffuse, undifferentiated
	    Burkitt's lymphoma
	    Non-Burkitt's lymphoma

Miscellaneous	
Composite	Composite
Mycosis fungoides	Mycosis fungoides
Histiocytic	Histiocytic
Extramedullary plasmacytoma	Extramedullary plasmacytoma
Unclassifiable	Unclassifiable

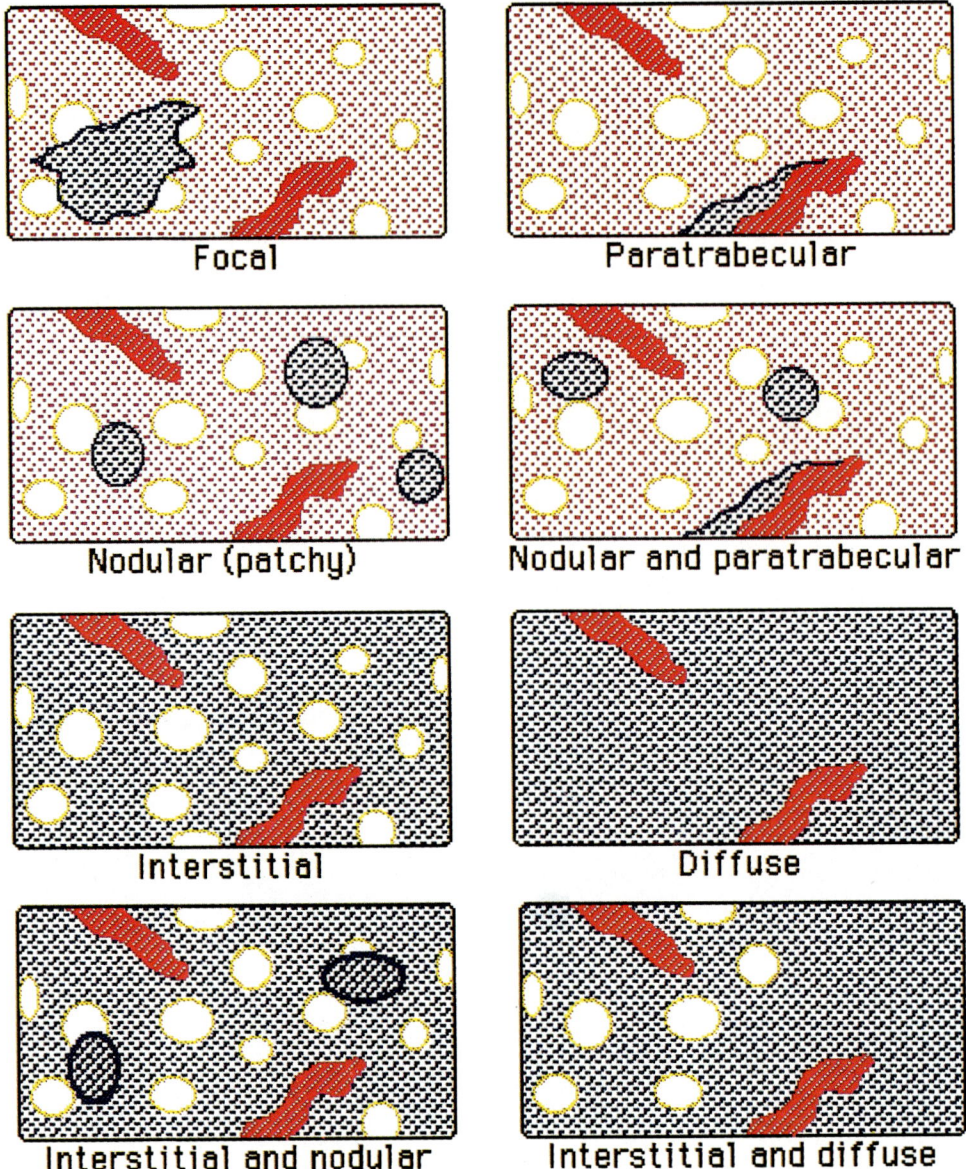

Figure 6-49. Schematic illustration of various patterns of bone marrow involvement (blue color) in lymphoproliferative disorders.

Figure 6-50. Discordant morphologic features have bee observed in lymph node and corresponding bone marrow biopsy sections of patients with lymphoma. In this figure, column A represents lymph node involvement and column B represents bone marrow involvement in patients a, b, and c. From Kluin P, Krieken JH, Kleiverda K, et al: Discordant morphologic characteristics of B-cell lymphomas in bone marrow and lymph node biopsies. *Am J Clin Pathol* 94:59, 1990, with permission.

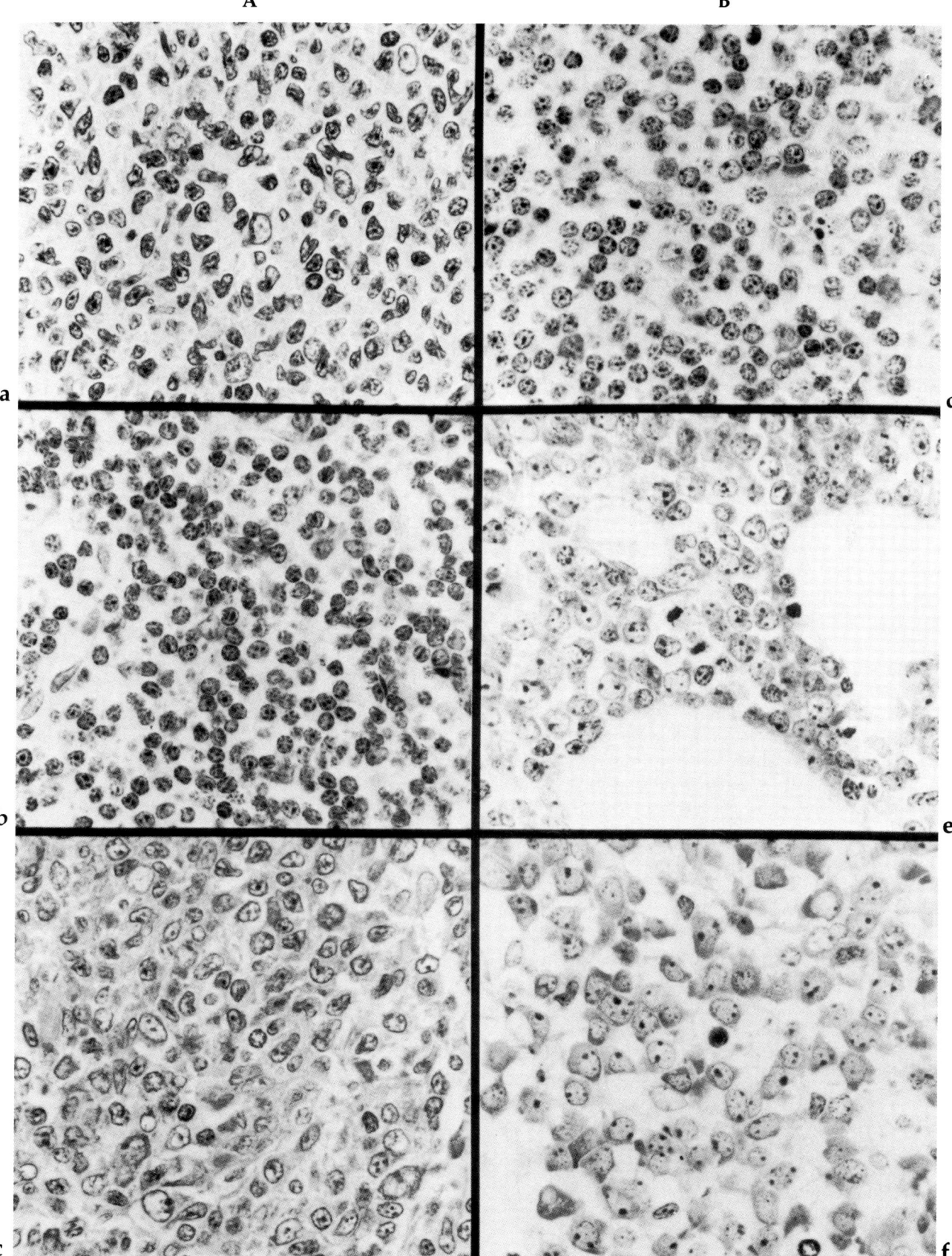

one to three basophilic nucleoli. The nucleoli are often closely apposed to the nuclear membrane.

The most frequent patterns of bone marrow involvement in these two types of lymphoma are focal, patchy and paratrebecular (Figures 6-51 and 6-52). Clusters of small or small and large, atypical lymphoid cells with irregular or cleaved nuclei and variable amounts of cytoplasm are found adjacent to the bone trabeculae, often associated with increased reticulin. In the mixed small cleaved and large cell lymphomas, the bone marrow lesions may occasionally resemble germinal centers, with centrally located larger cells surrounded by small cleaved cells. Some follicular lymphomas may show clusters of epithelioid histiocytes and thus mimic granulomas.[454,455] In such instances, careful cytologic evaluations and immunophenotypic studies may help to reach the correct diagnosis. Sometimes there may be a need for gene rearrangement studies (see Chapter 2).

Follicular lymphomas are virtually all of B-cell origin and are extremely rare in children. They express membrane IgG or IgM, are CD19, CD20, CD22, CD24, L26, LN1 (CDW75) and LN2 positive, and show Ig gene rearrangements. They are often CD5 negative and may express CD10.[451-461]

Differential diagnosis of low-grade lymphomas from benign/reactive lymphoid aggregates in bone marrow sometimes may create problems. Lymphoid aggregates are relatively common in bone marrow samples, especially in elderly people.[426] In biopsy and clot sections they appear as round or oval, well-defined, randomly distributed structures primarily composed of small, mature lymphocytes with round nuclei (Figures 6-53 and 6-54). Scattered plasma cells, macrophages and eosinophils may also be present within or around the lymphoid aggregates. Benign lymphoid aggregates are usually closely associated with small vessels.[426] In some cases, lymphoid aggregates demonstrate germinal centers, which, especially in adults, may indicate reactive lymphoid hyperplasia similar to the follicular hyperplasia in the spleen.[462]

Intermediate-Grade Lymphomas

Intermediate grade lymphomas are (1) *follicular large cell*, (2) *diffuse small cleaved cell*, (3) *diffuse mixed, small and large cell* and (4) *diffuse large cell* types, which account for approximately 5, 7, 7 and 20% of the NHLs, respectively, with an overall incidence of bone

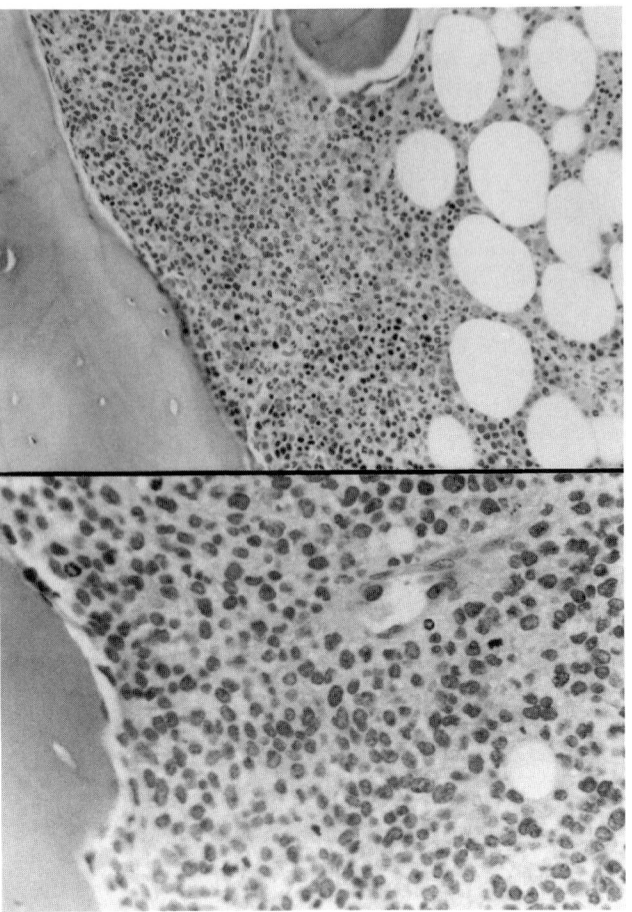

Figure 6-51. Paratrabecular bone marrow involvement in small cleaved lymphocytic lymphoma.

marrow involvement ranging from 25% to >60%[425,463] (Figures 6-52, 6-55 to 6-57). In the intermediate-grade category, T-cell lymphomas involve bone marrow more frequently than B-cell lymphomas.[426,463] The bone marrow involvement is focal, patchy or diffuse, and there is less correlation between the morphology of the lymphoma in the lymph node and the bone marrow biopsy specimens.[426] Bone marrow lesions in T-cell lymphomas are usually polymorphous, and are often mixed with reactive cells such as eosinophils, plasma cells, neutrophils and epithelioid histiocytes. The epithelioid histiocytes are particularly prominent in *Lennert's lymphomas* (T-cell lymphomas with epithelioid cell component). Increased vascularity and reticulin fibrosis are frequent findings. Because of the pleomorphic nature of the T-cell lymphomas and the frequency of interstitial marrow involvement, the neoplastic infil-

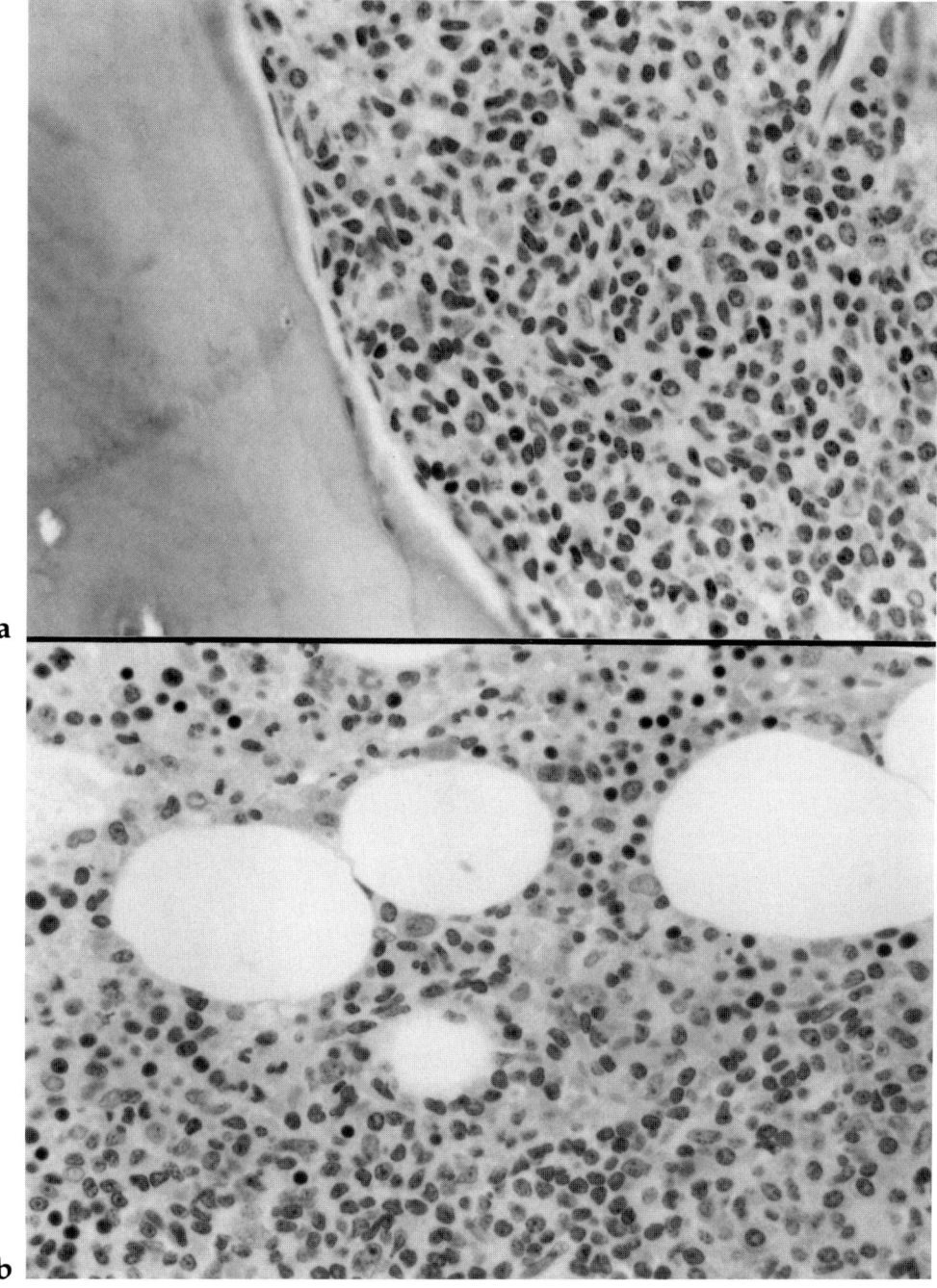

Figure 6-52. Malignant lymphoma, mixed, small and large cell type, with paratrabecular (a) and interstitial (b) bone marrow involvement.

trate blends with the normal hematopoietic cells and makes the diagnosis difficult. Also, bone marrow involvement with Lennert's lymphoma, because of the presence of epitheliod histiocytes, may mimic granuloma, particularly when the involvement is patchy and in small clusters.[463-467] The B-cell variants show monotypic surface and/or cytoplasmic Ig light chain kappa or lambda staining (predominantly of the IgM class), with evidence of Ig gene rearrangements. They express several B-cell-associated antigens such

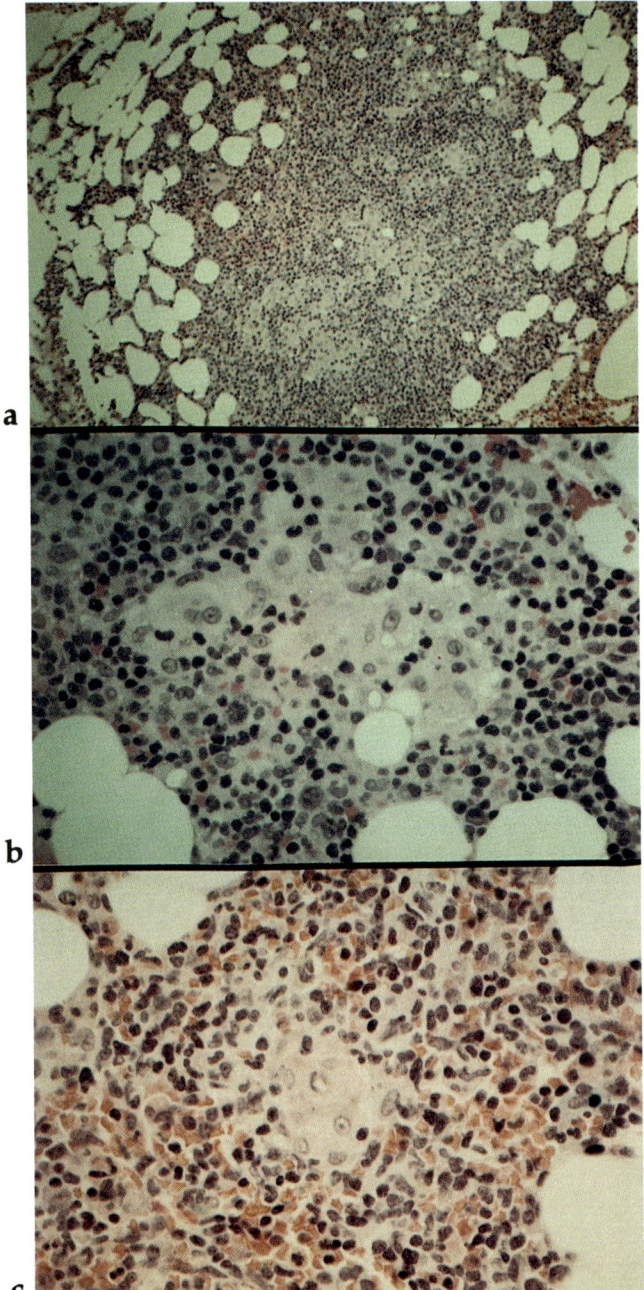

Figure 6-53. Benign lymphoid aggregates and granulomas appear as relatively well-defined nodular structures in bone marrow sections. A lymphoid aggregate composed of small clusters of histiocytes surrounded by small, round lymphocytes are demonstrated in (a) and (b). Bone marrow involvement with Lennert's lymphoma (lymphoma with epithelioid cell component) may resemble a granuloma (c).

as CD19, CD20, CD22, CD24, LN2 and L26. The T-cell variants often show a marked predominance of CD4+ cells with evidence of TCR gene rearrangements and abnormal expression of T-cell-associated antigens such as coexpression of CD4 and CD8, or lack of expression of one or several pan T-cell antigens such as CD2, CD5, CD7, UCHL1 and βF1.

High-Grade Lymphomas

These are the most aggressive NHLs. They are all diffuse and include (1) immunoblastic, (2) lymphoblastic and (3) small noncleaved cell (Burkitt's) lymphomas (Figures 6-58 to 6-60).

Immunoblastic lymphoma usually affects elderly people or immunocompromised patients such as transplant or AIDS patients.[468,469] It is characterized by large neoplastic immunoblasts with abundant cytoplasm, a large round or irregular nucleus with finely dispersed chromatin and one or two prominent nucleoli (Figure 6-58). Immunoblastic lymphomas are divided into the following categories: plasmacytoid, clear cell, polymorphous and immunoblastic lymphoma with epithelioid cell component. The plasmacytoid subtype is often of the B-cell type, and the rest are usually of T-cell origin. The polymorphous variant may contain giant RS-like cells.[463] Bone marrow involvement is usually interstitial or diffuse, and the neoplastic cells in both biopsy sections and marrow smears may be mistaken for clusters of megaloblasts. However, other changes are usually absent, and immunophenotypic analysis confirms the T- or B-cell origin of the tumor cells.

Lymphoblastic lymphomas are aggressive tumors with a high incidence of mediastinal and bone marrow involvement and rapid evolution to a leukemic phase. Morphologically, lymphoblastic lymphoma cells are indistinguishable from ALL cells.[470,471] The incidence of bone marrow involvement is about 60% at diagnosis,[448] as demonstrated by interstitial or diffuse marrow infiltration of blast cells. Nuclear convolution is a prominent feature, though it may not be present in all blasts or in all cases (see Figures 6-59 and 6-60). Nuclear chromatin is finely dispersed, and nucleoli are not prominent. Most of the lymphoblastic lymphomas are TdT positive and express one or several T-cell markers (CD1 through CD8, UCHL1, MT1, βF1). Several chromosomal translocations have been reported in lymphoblastic lym-

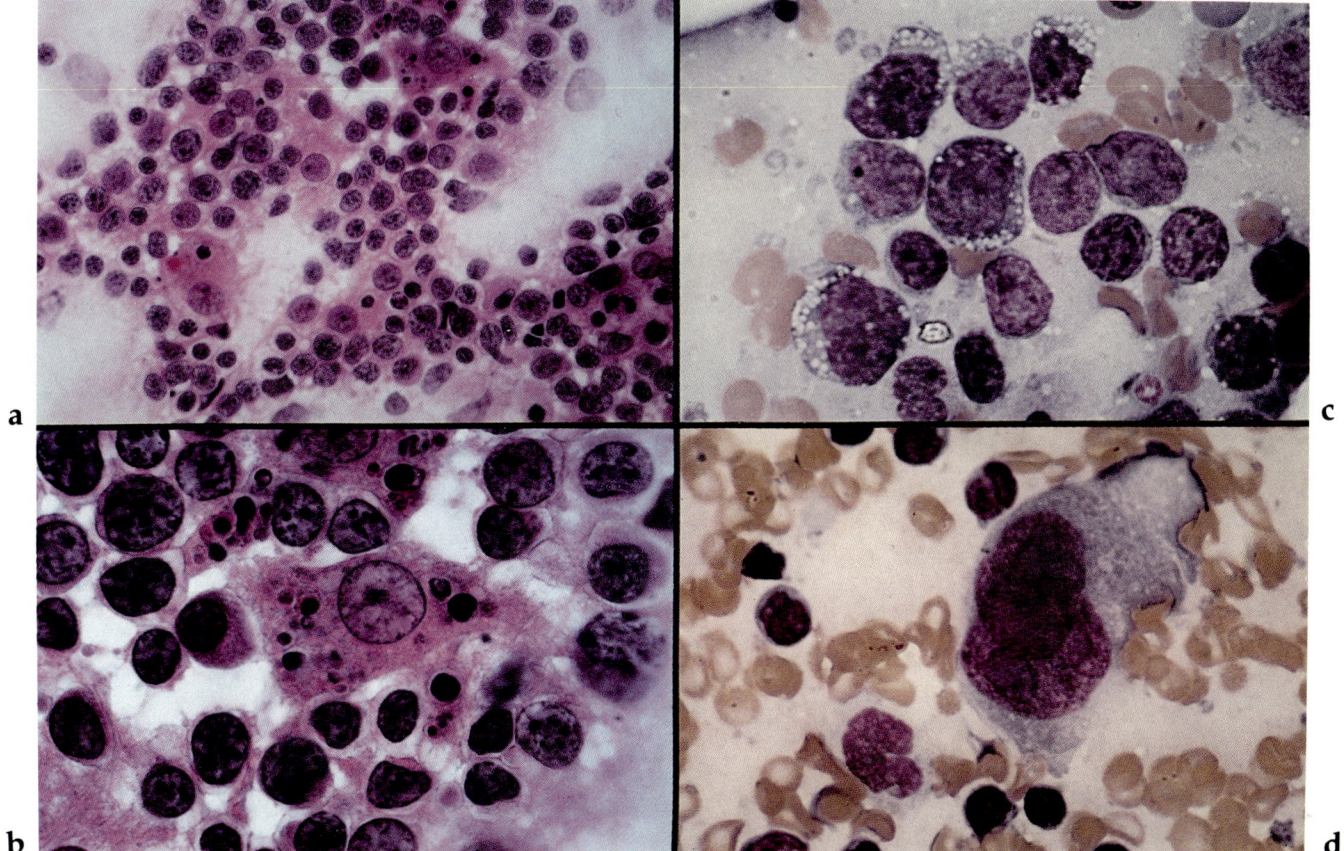

Figure 6-54. (a and b) Bone marrow biopsy touch preparation demonstrating a lymphoid aggregate with lymphocytes, a few plasma cells, and scattered macrophages containing nuclear debric (tingible body macrophages). (c) Bone marrow smear showing lymphoma, mixed, small, and large cells. (d) Bone marrow smear displaying a bilobed RS cell with prominent nucleoli.

phomas. Some involve chromosomal regions relevant to T-cell differentiation, such as T-cell receptor genes, particularly TCRA located on chromosome 14q11.[472] This is very reminiscent of the translocations of Ig genes in B-cell neoplasms.

Small noncleaved cell lymphomas (Burkitt's), in contrast to lymphoblastic lymphomas, are of the B-cell type and are composed of immature small cells with prominent nucleoli. The endemic form of small noncleaved lymphoma (African Burkitt's) predominantly involves jaw bones, while in the sporadic form (in the United States and Europe) abdominal involvement is the predominant feature. Generalized lymphadenopathy and bone marrow infiltration are common features, particularly in the sporadic form, with frequent progression to leukemia (the L3 subtype of ALL). For example, about two-thirds of Burkitt's lymphomas in the United States and Europe show bone marrow infiltration at diagnosis, while in African patients, bone marrow is involved in only about 8%.[473]

Bone marrow involvement, similar to that of lymphoblastic lymphoma, is usually interstitial or diffuse. The tumor cells show a high nuclear/cytoplasmic ratio, with scanty blue cytoplasm which is often vacuolated. Scattered macrophages throughout the tumor create the so-called starry sky pattern (see Figure 6-60). However, this pattern is not pathognomonic for Burkitt's lymphoma and may be seen in other aggressive lymphomas. The nuclei are either uniformly round or oval, with finely dispersed

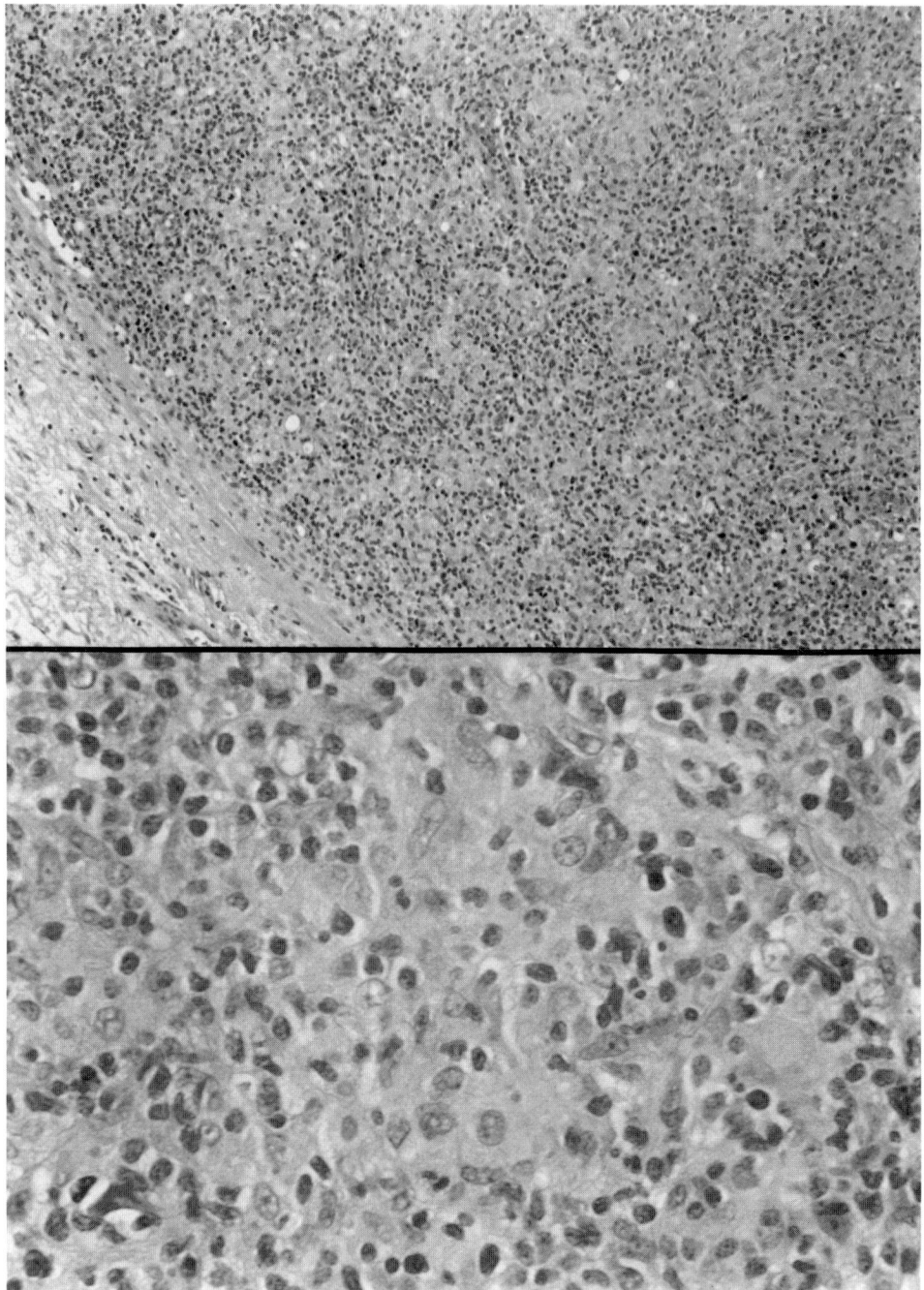

Figure 6-55. Lymph node biopsy section demonstrating a malignant lymphoma, diffuse, mixed, small and large cell, with an epithelioid cell component (Lennert's lymphoma).

chromatin and multiple discernible nucleoli, or are to some degree irregular and pleomorphic, with fine chromatin and one prominent nucleolus. Tumor cells may display cytoplasmic vacuoles which often contain neutral fat and stain with Oil Red O. Small noncleaved lymphomas are usually SmIg (kappa or lambda) CD19, CD20, L26, LN1, LN2 and CD10 positive and may express CD38 and Ki67. They also show evidence of Ig gene rearrangements.

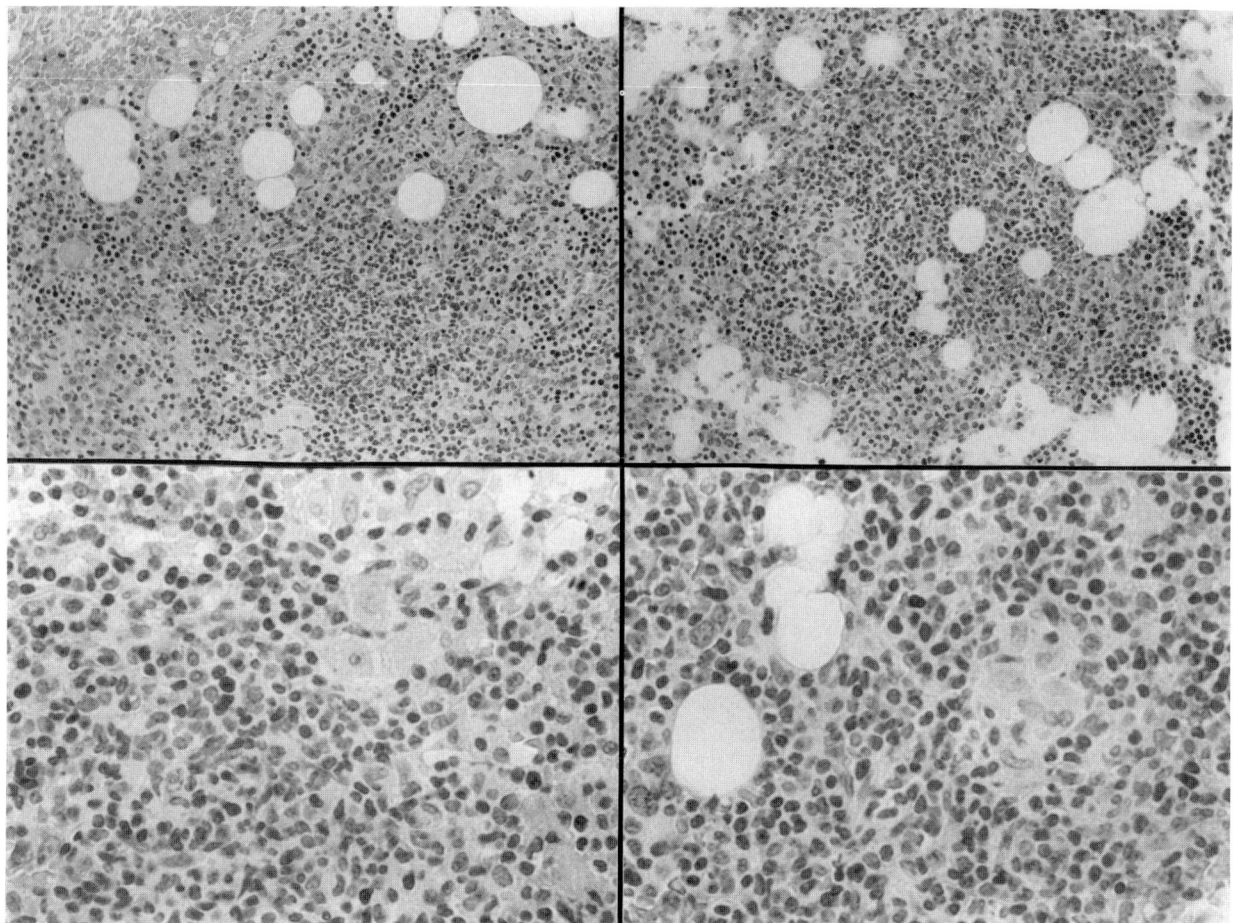

Figure 6-56. Bone marrow involvement in a diffuse lymphoma with epithelioid cell component (Lennert's lymphoma).

As discussed before (see Chapter 2), one of the characteristic features of small noncleaved cell lymphomas is the t(8;14) chromosomal translocation, in which c-myc from chromosome 8 is translocated to the Ig heavy chain locus on chromosome 14.[474,475]

CYTOGENETICS: The most significant associations of histopathology with cytogenetics involves the 8q24 and 14;18 translocations.[137,476] Over 85% of small noncleaved cell lymphomas demonstrate 8q24 translocation, which is predominantly of the t(8;14) (q24;q32) type (Figure 6-61). Another frequently associated chromosome translocation in B-cell lymphomas, particularly of the follicular type, is t(14;18) (q32;q21), which involves the bcl-2 and IGH genes (Figure 6-62) (see Chapter 2). Additional chromosome abnormalities in the karyotypes with 8q24 or 14;18 translocations are trisomy 7, 12, 21, or X, monosomy 1, 6 or 7, and 6q$^-$.[476] The most frequent T-cell-associated abnormalities are rearrangements of 14q11-13, which includes t(1;14)(q23;q11), t(11;14)(p14;q13), t(14;14)(q11;q32) and inv(14)(q11q32). These translocations involve the tcl-1, tcl-2, tcl-3 and TCRA genes (see Chapter 2).

Clinical Aspects

The low-grade and intermediate-grade lymphomas are commonly seen in the adult population. Low-grade and follicular lymphomas are rare in children. Most of the NHLs in children and adolescents are in the high-grade category, particularly lymphoblastic lymphoma and small noncleaved lymphoma. The prognosis of NHL depends on the histopathologic subtype of the tumor and the extent of dissemination.

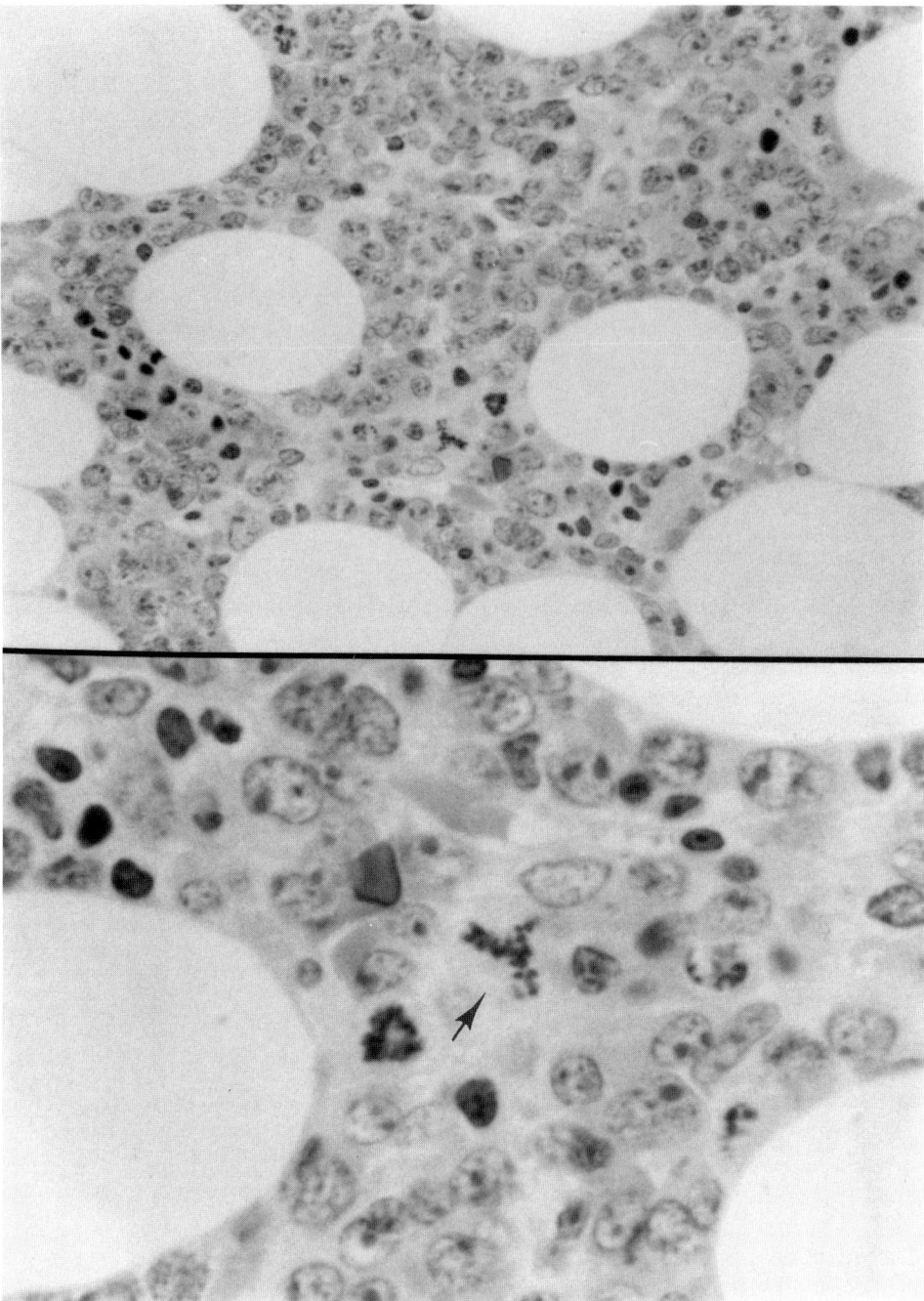

Figure 6-57. Bone marrow involvement in a large cell lymphoma with an interstitial pattern. An atypical tripolar mitotic figure is noted (arrow).

The classification introduced and recommended by an expert international panel, the Working Formulation, has proved useful for selecting treatment and reporting results, though it has some deficiencies.[477] The 10-year survival probabilities recently reported on 1153 patients with NHL were 45, 26 and 23% for patients with low-, intermediate-, and high-grade lymphomas, respectively.[478] The same study also demonstrated that the diffuse small cleaved cell category had a relatively favorable early survival but an

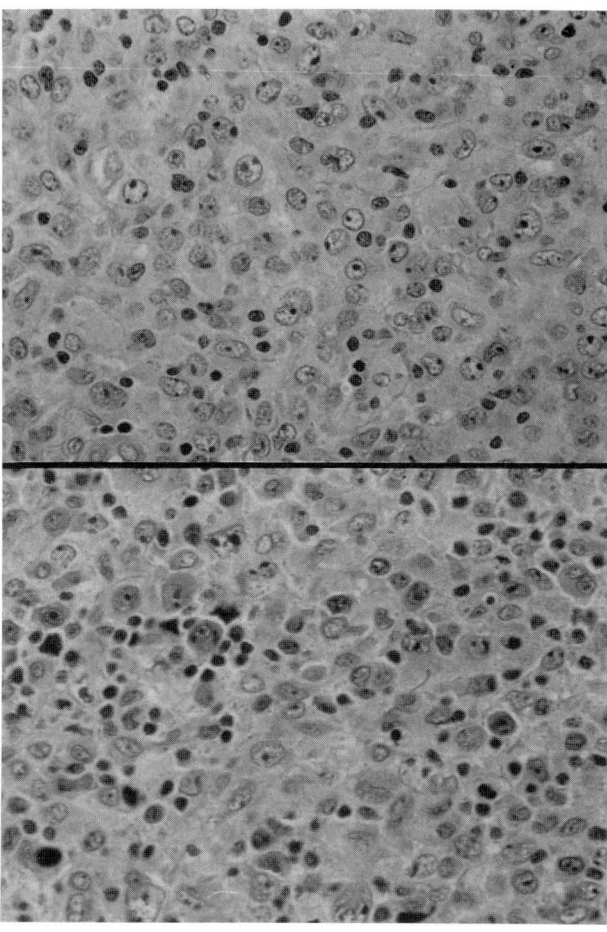

Figure 6-58. Lymph node biopsy sections demonstrating immunoblastic lymphoma composed of large cells with abundant cytoplasm and prominent nucleoli.

unfavorable late survival. The 10-year survival probabilities for follicular lymphomas, both small cleaved and mixed, were 83, 48 and 37% for stage I, stage III and stage IV, respectively. Patients with stage II disease did as poor as patients with stage III or IV disease. No significant differences were detected between patients with diffuse large cell and immunoblastic lymphomas with 10-year survival probabilities of 53, 27 and 15% for stage I, stage II, and stages III or IV, respectively.

Immunohistopathological Categories Not Included in the Working Formulation

Lymphomas of mantle zone origin fall into the category of low-grade lymphomas and are characterized by immunophenotypic features similar to those of mantle zone lymphocytes.[479-482] They express SmIgM/D, CD5, CD19, CD20, CD22, CD24, LN2, L26 and HLA-DR. The neoplasms are composed of a mixture of small round and cleaved lymphocytes arranged in a follicular or diffuse pattern (Figure 6-63). The follicular pattern is often called "mantle zone lymphoma," and the diffuse pattern is usually referred to as "intermediate lymphocytic lymphoma." The clinical course of the follicular type appears to be more favorable than that of the diffuse type, as demonstrated by a median survival of 88 and 33 months, respectively.[479] The incidence of bone marrow involvement is high and, according to one report, accounts for up to 76% of the cases.[480]

Monocytoid B-cell lymphoma is a recently described entity.[483a,483b,484a,484b] The neoplastic cells are of B-cell origin but have a monocytoid morphology demonstrated by an abundant cytoplasm and a folded nucleus (Figure 6-64). They are cytologically similar to HCL cells (see page 175), except that they are TRAP negative. The tumor cells are SmIg, CD19, CD20 and CD22 positive and may express CD11c. This entity may be closely related to the recently described CD11c+ CLL (see page 177). Most of the patients with monocytoid B-cell lymphoma have a localized disease. Bone marrow studies have been limited, but there are reports of marrow involvement.[483b] There is a strong association between monocytoid B-cell lymphoma and Sjögren's syndrome.[484a,484b]

Ki-1+ anaplastic large cell lymphoma is a newly recognized clinicopathologic entity characterized by large anaplastic lymphocytes with abundant cytoplasm and riniform nuclei, sinus infiltration of lymph nodes, and frequent (40%) extranodal involvement affecting particularly the skin and gastrointestinal tract.[485-487] Two morphologic subtypes have been described: monomorphic and pleomorphic. The pleomorphic variant often contains multinucleated RS-like cells and may be misdiagnosed as Hodgkin's disease (see Figure 6-64). The most prominent immunophenotypic characteristic of the tumor cells in anaplastic large cell lymphomas is their strong positivity for ki-1 (CD30) antigen. In addition, the tumor cells are mostly of T-cell phenotype, and often express CD25, CD71 and HLA-DR. Bone marrow involvement is infrequent. An association between this lymphoma and chromosomal translocation involving 5q35 has been demonstrated.[486b]

"Angiocentric T-cell lymphoma" is a term used to describe lymphomas with marked perivascular and vascular infiltration (Figure 6-65). These tumors are

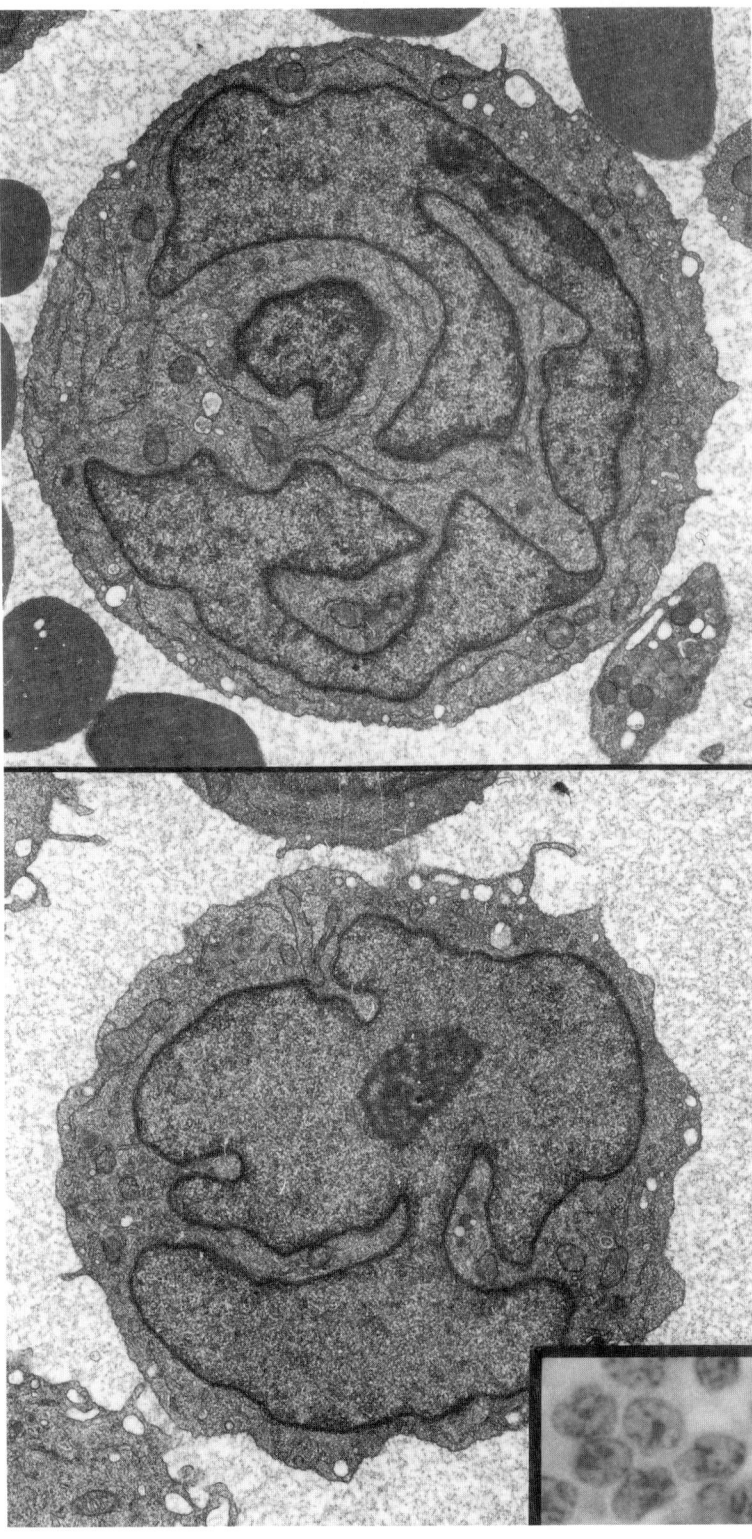

Figure 6-59. Electron microscopic characteristics of lymphoblastic lymphoma, convoluted cell type. Light microscopic features are demonstrated in the insert.

Figure 6-60. Bone marrow involvement in Burkitt's lymphoma and lymphoblastic lymphoma. (a and b): Burkitt's cells are small, monomorphous, and immature and show scanty, often vacuolated cytoplasm, round nuclei and prominent nucleoli (similar to L3-ALL; see Figures 6-1 and 6-3). Scattered macrophages create a "starry sky" pattern. (c and d): Lymphoblastic lymphoma, nonconvoluted type; morphologically similar to ALL, L1 or L2 categories (see Figures 6-1 and 6-2).

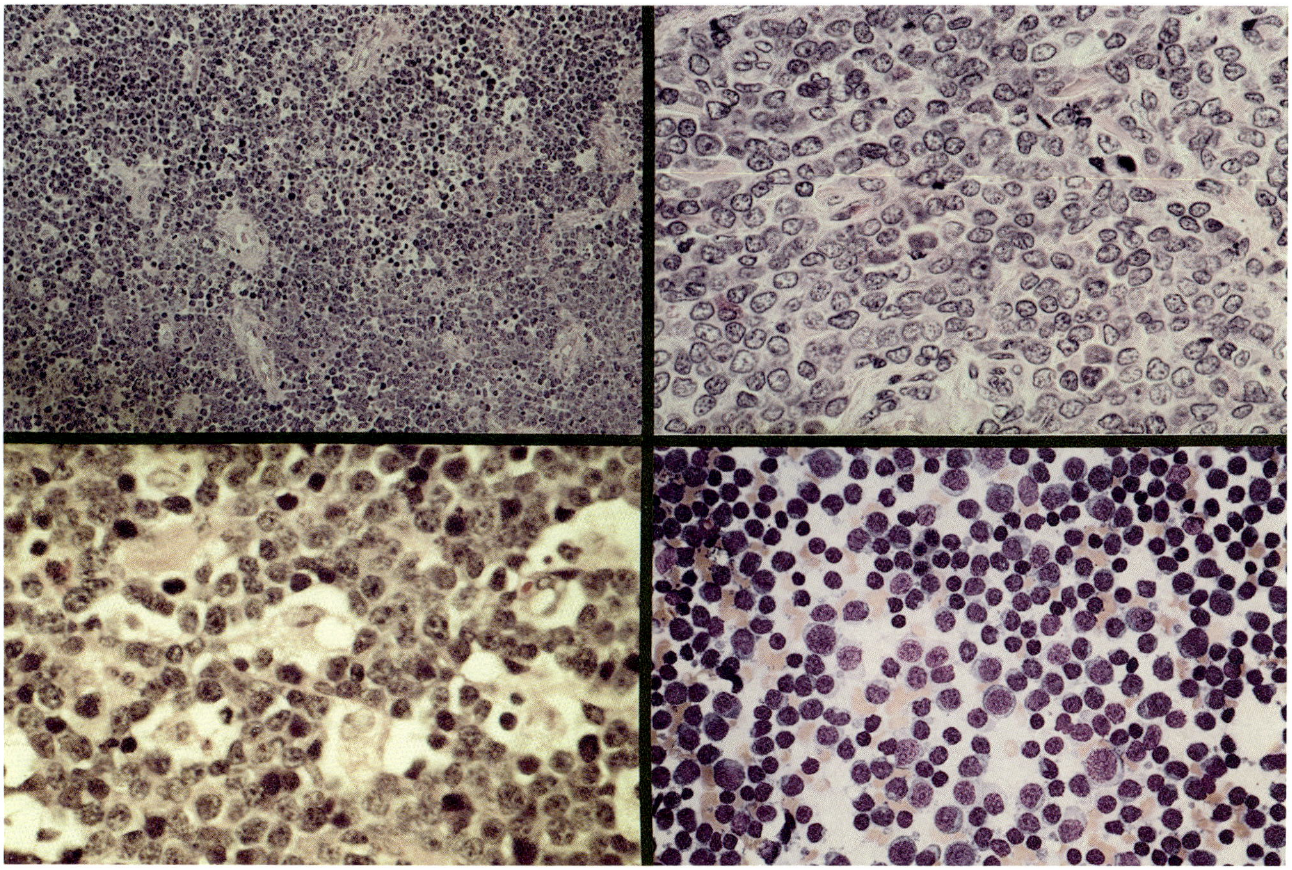

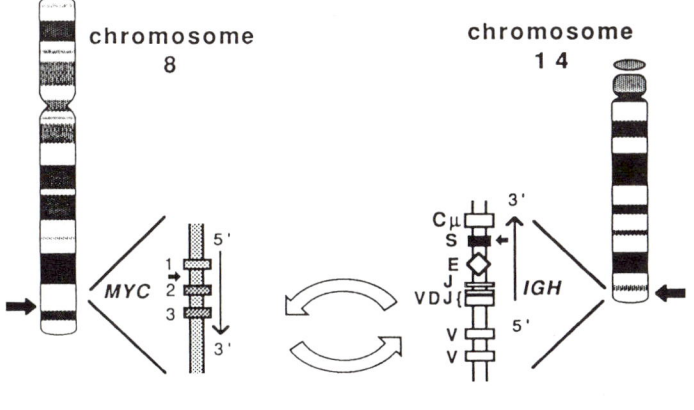

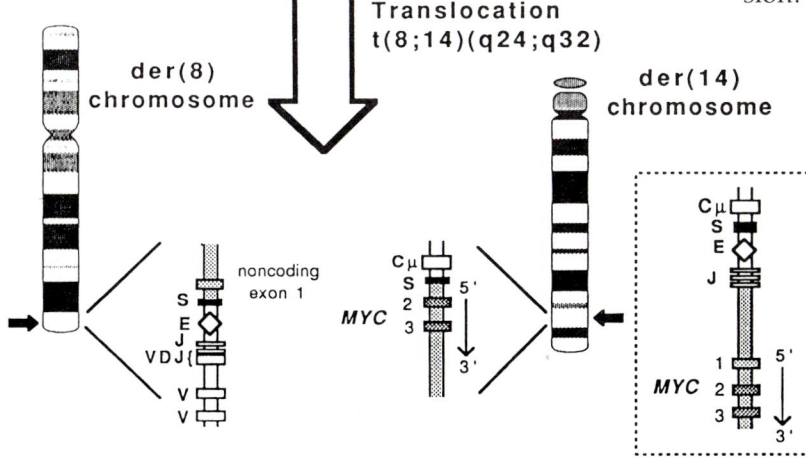

Figure 6-61. Schematic illustration of a common form of 8;14 translocation resulting in a *myc*-IGH rearrangement. Breaks often occur in the first *myc* intron and in the μ switch region (S) of IGH. The dotted box shows the result of another common form of 8;14 translocation. From McKeithan TW: Molecular biology of non-Hodgkin's lymphomas. *Semin Oncol* 17:30, 1990, with permission.

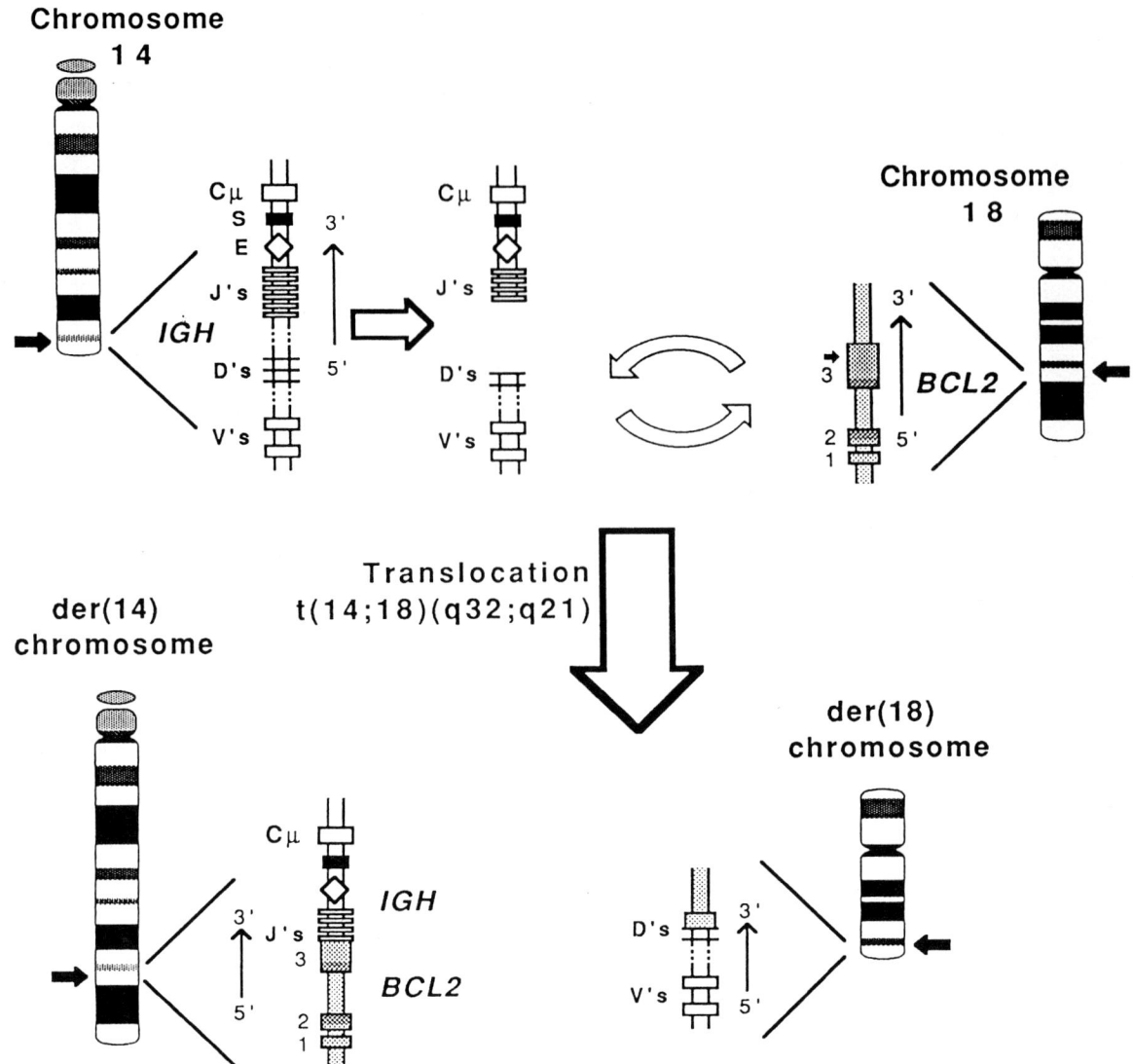

Figure 6-62. Schematic illustration of the 14;18 translocation. As a result of the translocation, BCL2 is brought into proximity with the IGH enhancer (E). From McKeithan TW: Molecular biology of non-Hodgkin's lymphomas. *Semin Oncol* 17:30, 1990, with permission.

predominantly extranodal, involving mainly the lung, upper respiratory tract and skin, and express CD2, CD3, CD5, CD7 and often CD4 antigens.[488] Angiocentric T-cell lymphomas are probably the result of malignant transformation of premalignant angiocentric and angiodestructive lymphoproliferative lesions known as "lymphomatoid granulomatosis" and "polymorphic reticulosis." Angiocentric lymphomas are diffuse large or mixed small and large cell lymphomas which often show areas of necrosis. They have an aggressive clinical course with infrequent bone marrow involvement.

A large cell lymphoma of the B-cell type with intravascular proliferation has been also reported as *"angiotropic large cell lymphoma"* or *"malignant angioendotheliomatosis."*[489,490]

HISTIOCYTIC MALIGNANCIES

Except for the acute monocytic and myelomonocytic leukemias, other malignancies of monocyte/histiocyte origin are rare. Malignant histiocytic tumors are tu-

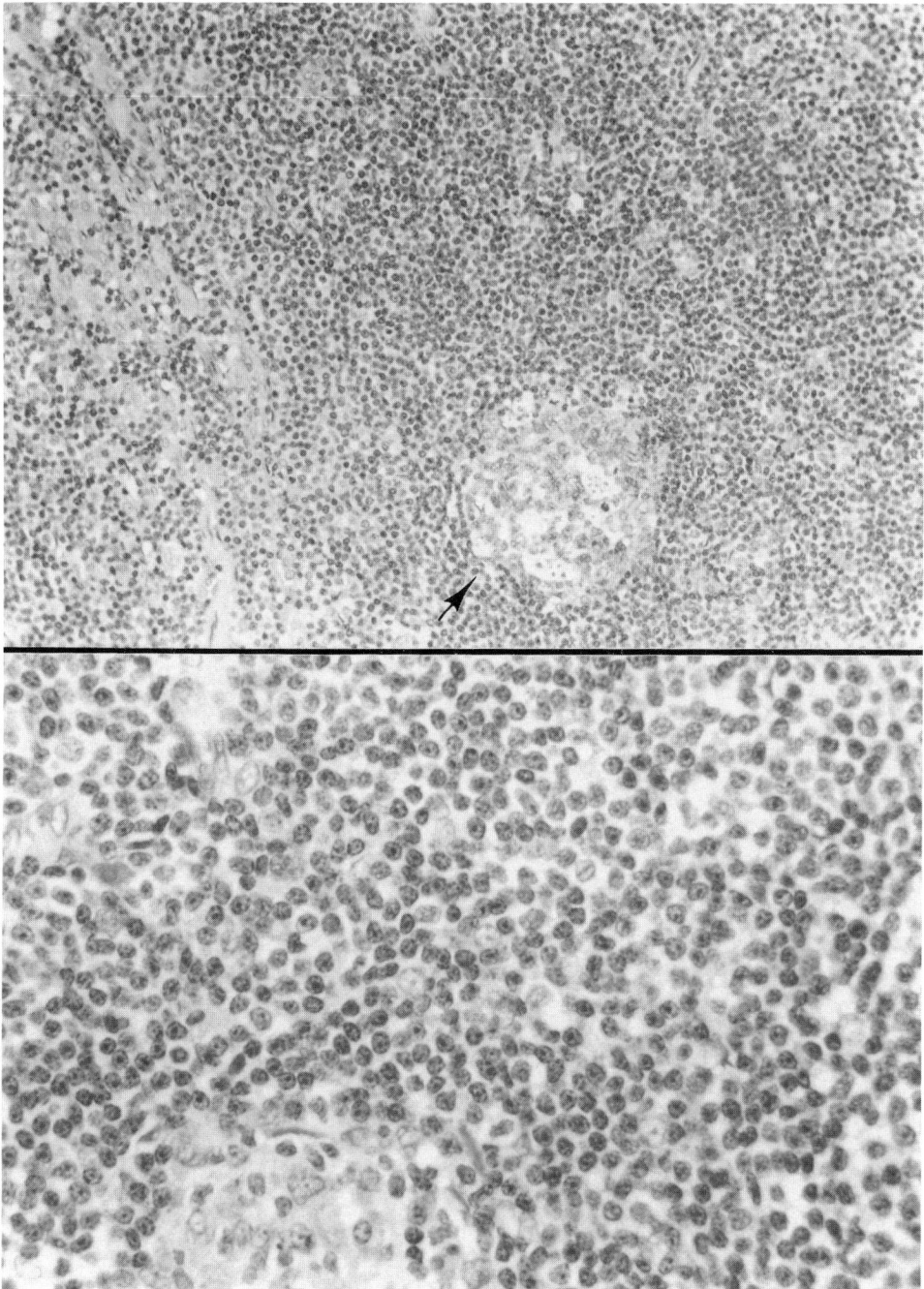

Figure 6-63. Lymph node biopsy section demonstrating mantle zone lymphoma. A remnant of the follicular structure is present (arrow), with the expansion of mantle zone lymphocytes.

mors which arise from tissue histiocytes and are clinically manifested in two major ways: (1) as tumors of the lymphoid tissues (histiocytic lymphoma) or (2) as disseminated neoplasms involving the reticuloendothelial system (malignant histiocytosis).

Histiocytic Lymphomas

True histiocytic lymphomas are extremely rare. The vast majority of large cell lymphomas that were origi-

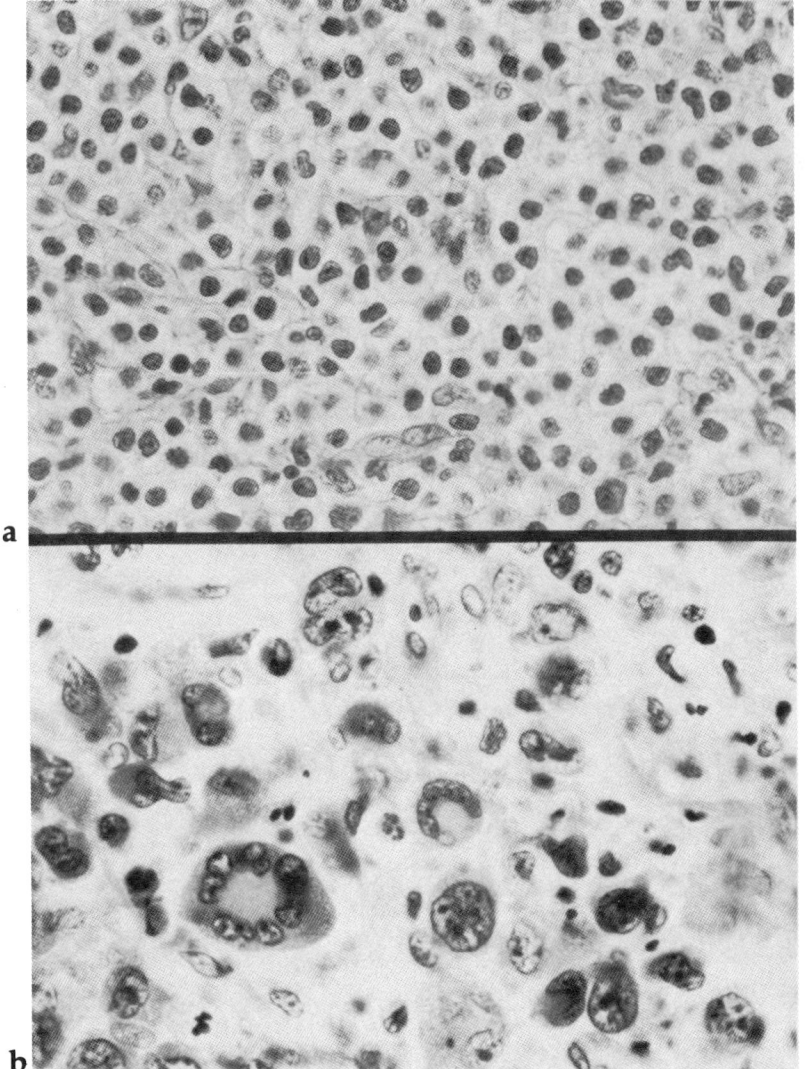

Figure 6-64. (a) Lymph node biopsy section demonstrating a monocytoid B-cell lymphoma. The tumor cells have abundant clear cytoplasm with well-defined cell borders and bland nuclei. From Sheibani K, Traweek T, Ben-Ezra J, et al: Monocytoid B-cell lymphoma (letter to the editor). *Am J Surg Pathol* 13:902, 1989, with permission. (b) Lymph node biopsy section demonstrating a large cell anaplastic lymphoma (Ki-1 Positive). Several binucleated and multinucleated RS-like cells are present. From Kadin ME: Lymphomatoid papulosis and Ki-1+ large cell lymphomas of the skin: Pathology, immunology, natural history and relevance to Hodgkin's disease, in Hanaoka M, Kadin ME, Nanba K, Watanabe S (eds), *International Colloquium on Lymphoid Malignancy. Immunocytology and Cytogenetics.* Philadelphia, Field and Woods, 1990, p 189, with permission.

nally thought to be of histiocytic origin were later demonstrated to be derived from lymphocytes.[491-495] Histiocytic lymphoma is now the diagnosis of exclusion and is used when the tumor cells in addition to the morphologic "histiocytic" characteristics, react negatively with all B- and T-cell markers and show immunophenotypic, cytochemical and electron microscopic features that are consistent with histiocytes. Morphologically, histiocytic lymphomas consist of large cells with abundant cytoplasm, with or without cytoplasmic vacuoles, granules or phagocytic particles, a round or irregular nucleus with finely dispersed chromatin and one or several nucleoli (Figure 6-66). These morphologic criteria are also observed in the nonhistiocytic large cell lymphomas, particularly malignant lymphomas of the T-cell type. Histiocytic-associated markers such as fluoride-sensitive nonspecific esterases, alpha-1 antitrypsin, alpha-1 antichymotrypsin, lysozyme and CD68 are helpful in establishing the diagnosis of a true histiocytic lymphoma.[496] Histiocytic lesions are also HLA-DR+ and show strong diffuse positivity for acid phosphatase and beta-glucuronidase, though none of these enzymes are histiocyte restricted. Electron microscopic features include cytoplasmic processes with microvilli and the presence of lysosomes and residual bodies.

Malignant Histiocytosis

Malignant histiocytosis (histiocytic medullary reticulosis) is a rare condition which involves the reticuloendothelial system, including bone marrow,

Leukemias and Lymphomas

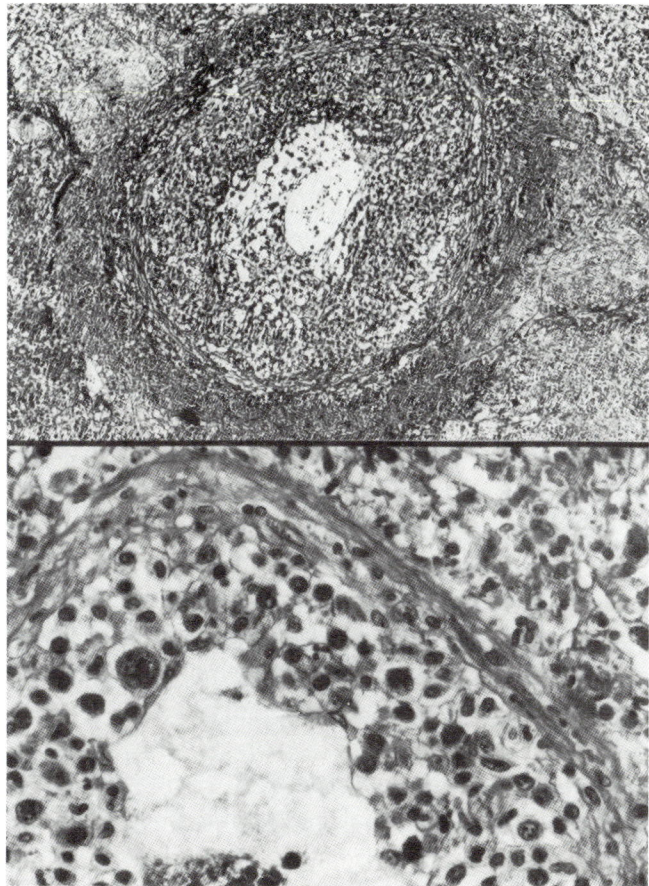

Figure 6-65. Lung biopsy section demonstrating an angiocentric lymphoma with marked vascular infiltration by atypical small and large lymphoid cells. From Lipford EH, Margolick JB, Longo DL, et al: Angiocentric immunoproliferative lesions: A clinicopathologic spectrum of post-thymic T-cell proliferations. *Blood* 72:1674, 1988, with permission.

hepatic sinusoids, splenic red pulp and lymph node sinuses.[497-502] The neoplastic histiocytes may also invade peripheral blood or other tissues. This disorder is closely related to acute monocytic leukemia, and in many instances the distinction may be arbitrary.[498,499] The neoplastic cells in malignant histiocytosis, unlike those in reactive histiocytosis, are atypical and demonstrate malignant features such as a high nuclear/cytoplasmic ratio, nuclear pleomorphism and hyperchromasia, prominent nucleoli, and sometimes atypical mitotic figures (see Figure 6-66). Tumor cells usually show strong positivity with histiocyte-associated markers such as nonspecific esterase and lysozyme stains and may also demonstrate erythrophagocytosis. However, erythrophagocytosis

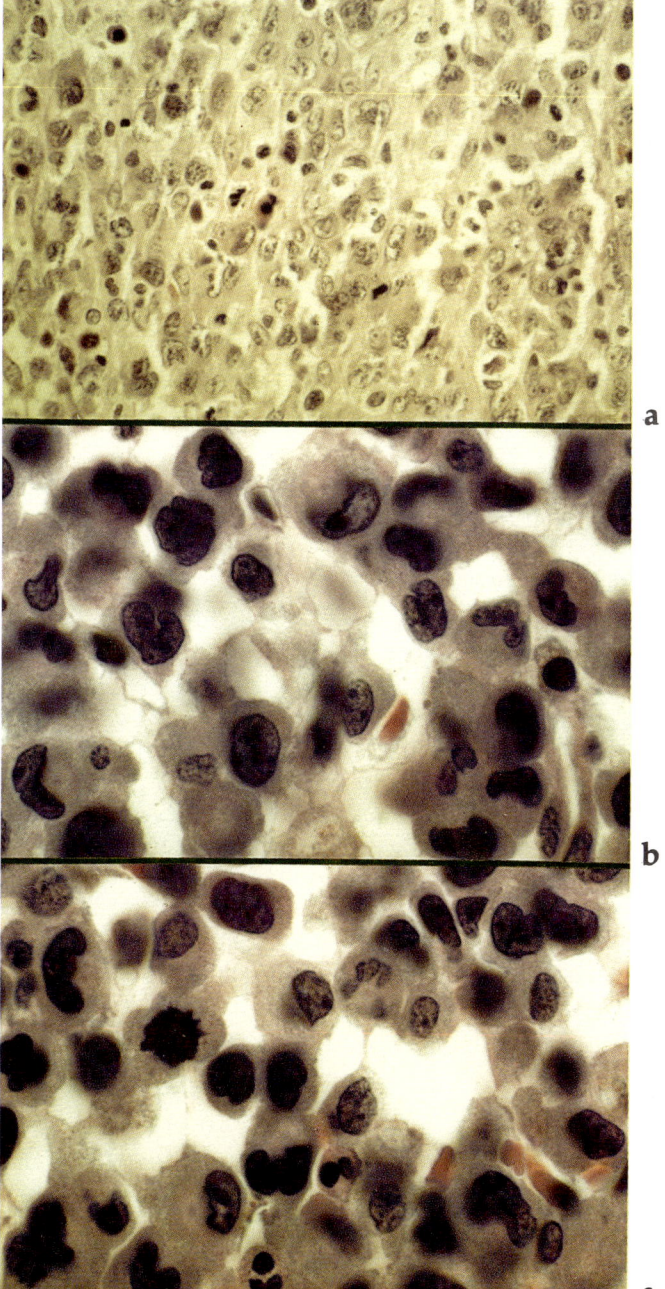

Figure 6-66. (a) Lymph node biopsy section demonstrating large, atypical cells with abundant cytoplasm and pleomorphic nuclei. The cells were muramidase (lysozyme) positive and did not react with B- and T-cell markers, suggesting a true histiocytic lymphoma. (b and c) Bone marrow biopsy section from a patient with malignant histiocytosis demonstrating large, atypical cells with abundant cytoplasm, marked nuclear polymorphism and nuclear hyperchromasia.

is not pathognomonic for malignant histiocytosis. In a number of nonhistiocytic neoplasms, particularly T-cell malignancies, there is evidence of erythrophagocytosis by tumor cells and/or by reactive macrophages present in association with tumor cells.[504,505] Malignant histiocytosis should also be differentiated from infection-associated hemophagocytosis and familial erythrophagocytic lymphohistiocytosis, which are characterized by the proliferation of reactive nonneoplastic histiocytes (see Chapter 9). Majority of the cases that were originally referred to as malignant histiocytosis now appear to be either T-cell malignancies or examples of infection-associated hemophagocytosis.[503-505]

Malignant Tumors of the Dendritic Histiocytes

Malignant tumors of the dendritic histiocytes are extremely rare.[507–510] They may arise from the Langerhans cells of the skin (malignant histiocytosis X), from interdigitating reticulum cells of the paracortical (T-cell) zones, or from dendritic reticulum cells of the follicular structures in the lymphoid tissues.

A recent report on malignant histiocytosis X (Langerhans cell sarcoma) demonstrates frequent involvement of both nodal and extranodal tissues and introduces a number of distinguishing features for malignant histiocytosis X, including noncohesive atypical cells, sparsity of eosinophils, and an aggressive clinical course.[507] Morphologically, Langerhans cells are characterized by large size, abundant cytoplasm, a folded nucleus with a central longitudinal groove, the presence of Birbeck granules and sparse lysosomal granules by electron microscopy. Langerhans cells express CD1 antigen and S-100 protein (see Table 8-8, page 266). Neoplasms of the interdigitating and dendritic reticulum cells are morphologically similar to those of Langerhans cells, except that they do not contain Birbeck granules. They primarily involve lymph nodes and are S-100$^+$ and CD1$^+$.

References

1. Molony WC, Lange RD: Leukemia in atomic bomb survivors. II. Observation on early phase of leukemia. *Blood* 9:663, 1954.
2. Ishimaru T, Hoshino T, Ichimaru M, et al: Leukemia in atomic bomb survivors, Hiroshima and Nagasaki, 1 October 1950–30 September 1966. *Radiat Res* 45:216, 1971.
3. Kamada N: The effects of radiation on chromosomes of bone marrow cells. III. Cytogenetic studies on leukemia in atomic bomb survivors. *Acta Haematol Jpn* 32:249, 1969.
4. Lilienfeld AM: *Foundations of Epidemiology*. New York, Oxford University Press, 1976.
5. Court-Brown W, Doll R: Mortality from cancer and other causes after radiotherapy for ankylosing spondylitis. *Br Med J* 2:1327, 1965.
6. Evans JS, Wennberg JE, McNeil BJ: The influence of diagnostic radiography on the incidence of breast cancer and leukemia. *N Engl J Med* 315:810, 1986.
7. Boice JD Jr: The danger of X-rays—real or apparent? *N Engl J Med* 315:828, 1986.
8. Linos A, Gray GE, Orvis AL, et al: Low-dose radiation and leukemia. *N Engl J Med* 302:1101, 1980.
9. Okada S, Hamilton HB, Egami N, et al: A review of thirty years study of Hiroshima and Nakasaki atomic bomb survivors. *J Radiat Res* 16(suppl):1, 1975.
10. Auxier JA: Dosiometry. A. Physical dose estimates for A-bomb survivors—studies at Oak Ridge, USA. *J Radiat Res* 16(suppl):1, 1975.
11. Smith PG, Doll R: Age- and time-dependent changes in the rates of radiation-induced cancers in patients with ankylosing spondylitis following a single course of X-ray treatment, In: *Late Biological Effects of Ionizing Radiation*. Vol. 1, Vienna, International Atomic Energy Agency, 1978, pp 205–18.
12. Bergsagel DE, Bailey AJ, Langley GR, et al: The chemotherapy of plasma cell myeloma and the incidence of acute leukemia. *N Engl J Med* 301:743, 1979.
13. Greene MH, Boice JD Jr, Greer BE, et al: Acute non-lymphocytic leukemia after therapy with alkylating agents for ovarian cancer: A study of five randomized clinical trials. *N Engl J Med* 307:1416, 1982.
14. Pederson-Bjergaard J, Larsen SO: Incidence of acute nonlymphocytic leukemia, preleukemia, and acute myeloproliferative syndrome up to 10 years after treatment of Hodgkin's disease. *N Engl J Med* 307:965, 1982.
15. Zarrabi MH, Rosner F, Bennett JM: Non-Hodgkin's lymphoma and acute myeloblastic leukemia: A report of 12 cases and review of the literature. *Cancer* 44:1070, 1979.
16. Rosner F, Grunwald HW, Zarrabi MH: Acute leukemia as a complication of cytotoxic chemotherapy. *Int J Radiat Oncol Biol Phys* 5:1705, 1979.
17. Zarrabi MH, Grünwald HW, Rosner F: Chronic lymphocytic leukemia terminating in acute leukemia. *Arch Intern Med* 137:1059, 1977.

18. Rosner F, Garey RW, Zarrabi MH: Breast cancer and acute leukemia: Report of 24 cases and review of the literature. *Am J Hematol* 4:151, 1978.
19. Stott H, Fox W, Girling DJ, et al: Acute leukemia after busulphan. *Br Med J* 2:1513, 1977.
20. Grunwald HW, Rosner F: Acute leukemia and immunosuppressive drug use: A review of patients undergoing immunosuppressive therapy for non-neoplastic diseases. *Arch Intern Med* 139:461, 1979.
21. Kinlen LJ, Sheil AG, Peto J, et al: Collaborative United Kingdom–Australasia study of cancer in patients with immunosuppressive drugs. *Br J Med* 2:1461, 1979.
22. Anderson JL, Fowles RE, Bieber CP, et al: Idiopathic cardiomyopathy, age, and suppressor-cell dysfunction as risk determinants of lymphoma after cardiac transplantation. *Lancet* 2:1174, 1978.
23. Louie S, Daoust PR, Schwartz RS: Immunodeficiency and the pathogenesis of non-Hodgkin's lymphoma. *Semin Oncol* 7:267, 1980.
24. Ioachim HL: Neoplasms associated with immune deficiency. *Pathol Ann* 22:177, 1987.
25. Kim JH, Durack DT: Manifestations on human T-lymphotropic virus type 1 infection. *Am J Med* 84:919, 1988.
26. Ehrlich GD, Poiez BJ: Clinical and molecular parameters of HTLV-1 infection. *Clin Lab Med* 8:65, 1988.
27. Kalyanaraman VS, Sarngadharan MG, Guroff M, et al: A new subtype of human T-cell leukemia virus (HTLV-II) associated with a T-cell variant of hairy cell leukemia. *Science* 218:571, 1982.
28. Linet MS: *The Leukemias: Epidemiologic Aspects.* New York, Oxford University Press, 1985.
29. Snyder AL, Henderson ES, Li FP, et al: Possible inherited leukemogenic factors in familial acute myelogenous leukemia. *Lancet* 1:586, 1970.
30. Chaganti RSK, Miller DR, Meyers PA, et al: Cytogenetic evidence of the intrauterine origin of acute leukemia in monozygotic twins. *N Engl J Med* 300:1032, 1979.
31. Van den Berghe D, Petit P, Van Drshoven AB, et al: Simultaneous occurrence of 5q⁻ and 21q⁻ in refractory anemia with thrombocytosis. *Cancer Genet Cytogenet* 1:63, 1979.
32. Tinegate H, Gaunt L, Hamilton PJ: The 5q⁻ syndrome: An underdiagnosed form of macrocytic anemia. *Br J Haematol* 54:103, 1983.
33. Nimer SD, Golde DW: The 5q⁻ abnormality. *Blood* 70:1705, 1987.
34. Mitelman F, Nilsson PG, Brandt L, et al: Chromosome pattern, occupation, and clinical features in patients with acute nonlymphocytic leukemia. *Cancer Genet Cytogenet* 1:197, 1981.
35. Golomb HM, Alimena G, Rowley JD, et al: Correlation of occupation and karyotype in adults with acute nonlymphocytic leukemia. *Blood* 60:404, 1982.
36. Dewald GW, Davis MP, Pierre RV, et al: Clinical characteristics of 50 patients with myeloproliferative syndrome and deletion of part of the long arm of chromosome 5. *Blood* 66:189, 1985.
37. Heubner K, Isobe M, Croce CM, et al: The human gene encoding GM-CSF is a 5q21–q32, the chromosome region deleted in the 5q⁻ anomaly. *Science* 230:1282, 1985.
38. Le Beau MM, Westbrook CA, Diaz MO, et al: Evidence for the involvement of GM-CSF and FMS in the deletion (5q) in myeloid disorders. *Science* 231:984, 1986.
39. Ishii S, Merlino GT, Pastan I: Promoter region of the human Harevy *ras* protooncogene promoter. *Science* 230:1378, 1985.
40. Nienhuis AW, Bunn HF, Turner PH, et al: Expression of the human *c-fms* proto-oncogene in hematopoietic cells and its deletion in the 5q⁻ syndrome. *Cell* 42:421, 1985.
41. Committee on Leukemia and Working Party on Leukemia in Childhood: Duration of survival of children with acute leukemia. *Br Med J* 4:7, 1971.
42. Miller RW: Epidemiology of leukemia, *Haematol Blutransfus* 1979; 23:37–41.
43. Fraumeni JF, Jr, Wagoner JK: Changing sex differentials in leukemia. *Public Health Rep* 79:1093, 1974.
44. Bennett JM, Catovsky D, Daniel MT, et al: French-American-British (FAB) Cooperative Group proposal for the classification of acute leukemias. *Br J Haematol* 33:451, 1976.
45. Bennett JM, Catovsky D, Daniel MT, et al: French-American-British (FAB) Cooperative Group: The morphological classification of acute leukemia—concordance among observers and clinical correlation. *Br J Haematol* 33:451, 1976.
46. Bennett JM, Catovsky D, Daniel MT, et al: The morphological classification of acute lymphoblastic leukemia: Concordance among observers and clinical correlations. *Br J Haematol* 47:553, 1981.
47. Palmer MK, Hann IM, Jones PM, et al: A score at diagnosis for predicting length of remission in childhood acute lymphoblastic leukemia. *Br J Cancer* 42:841, 1980.
48. Reid MM, Proctor SJ: Failure of FAB classification to predict relapse-free survival in acute leukemia. *Lancet* 2:153, 1982.
49. Lilleyman JS, Hamm IM, Stevens RF, et al: French-American-British (FAB) morphological classification of childhood lymphoblastic leukemia and its clinical importance. *J Clin Pathol* 39:998, 1986.
50. First MIC Cooperative Study Group: Morphologic, im-

munologic, and cytogenetic (MIC) working classification of acute lymphoblastic leukemia. *Cancer Genet Cytogenet* 23:189, 1986.
51. Miller DR, Krailo M, Bleyer WA, et al: Prognostic implications of blast cell morphology in childhood acute lymphoblastic leukemia: A report from the Childrens Cancer Study Group. *Cancer Treat Rep* 69:1211, 1985.
52. Wagner VM, Baehner RL: Correlation of the FAB morphologic criteria and prognosis in acute lymphocytic leukemia of childhood. *Am J Pediatr Hematol Oncol* 1:103, 1979.
53. Wolff LJ, Richardson ST, Neiburger JB, et al: Poor prognosis of children with acute lymphocytic leukemia and increased B cell markers. *J Pediatr* 89:956, 1976.
54. Sallan SE, Ritz J, Pesandro J, et al: Cell surface antigens: Prognostic implications in childhood acute lymphoblastic leukemia. *Blood* 55:395, 1980.
55. Poplack DG: Acute lymphoblastic leukemia, in Pizzo PA, Poplack DG (eds), *Principles and Practice of Pediatric Oncology*. Philadelphia, JB Lippincott, 1989, p 323.
56. Link M, Warnke R, Finlay J, et al: Monoclonal antibody characterization of surface antigens in childhood lymphoid malignancies. *Blood* 62:722, 1983.
57. Foon KA, Herzog P, Billing RJ, et al: Immunologic classification of childhood acute lymphocytic leukemia. *Cancer* 47:280, 1981.
58. Reinherz EL, Schlossmann SF: The differentiation and function of human T lymphocytes. *Cell* 19:821, 1980.
59. Roper M, Crist WM, Metzgar R, et al: Monoclonal antibody characterization of surface antigens in childhood T-cell lymphoid malignancies. *Blood* 61:830, 1983.
60. Haynes BF, Metzgar RS, Minna JD, et al: Phenotypic characterization of cutaneous T-cell lymphoma: Use of monoclonal antibodies to compare with other malignant T-cells. *N Engl J Med* 304:1319, 1981.
61. Link M, Warnke R, Finlay J, et al: A single monoclonal antibody identifies T-cell lineage of childhood lymphoid malignancies. *Blood* 62:722, 1983.
62. Thiel E, Rodt H, Huhn D, et al: Multimarker classification of acute lymphoblastic leukemia: Evidence for further T subgroups and evaluation of their clinical significance. *Blood* 56:359, 1980.
63. Madler LM, Reinherz EL, Weinstein HJ, et al: Heterogeneity of T cell lymphoblastic malignancies. *Blood* 55:805, 1980.
64. Sobol RE, Royston I, Tucker W, et al: Adult acute lymphoblastic leukemia phenotypes defined by monoclonal antibodies. *Blood* 65:730, 1985.
65. Pullen DJ, Crist WM, Falleta JM: A Pediatric Oncology Group classification protocol for acute lymphocytic leukemia (ALinC13): Immunologic phenotypes and correlation with treatment results, in Murphy SB, Gilbert JR (eds), *Leukemia Research: Advances in Cell Biology and Treatment*. Amsterdam, Elsevier, 1983, p 221.
66. Borowitz MJ, Dowell BL, Boyett JM, et al: Monoclonal antibody definition of T cell acute leukemia. A Pediatric Oncology Group Study. *Blood* 65:785, 1985.
67. Fey MF, Wainscoat JS: Molecular diagnosis of hematological neoplasms. *Blood Rev* 2:78, 1988.
68. Korsmeyer SJ: Antigen receptor genes as molecular markers of lymphoid neoplasms. *J Clin Invest* 79:1291, 1987.
69. Pesando JM, Ritz J, Lazarus H, et al: Leukemia associated-antigens in ALL. *Blood* 54:1240, 1979.
70. Ritz, J, Pesando JM, Notis-McConarty J, et al: A monoclonal antibody to human acute lymphoblastic leukemia antigen. *Nature* 283:583, 1980.
71. Greaves MF, Brown G, Rapson NT, et al: Antisera to acute lymphoblastic leukemia cells. *Clin Immunol Immunopathol* 4:67, 1975.
72. Childs GC, Stass SA, Bennett JM: The morpohologic classification of acute lymphoblastic leukemia in childhood. *Am J Clin Path* 86:503, 1986.
73. Greaves MF, Hariri G, Newman RA, et al: Selective expression of the common acute lymphoblastic leukemia (gp 100) antigen on immature lymphoid cells and their malignant counterparts. *Blood* 61:628, 1983.
74. Chessels JM, Hardisty RM, Rapson NT, et al: Acute lymphoblastic leukemia in children: Classification and prognosis. *Lancet* 2:1307, 1977.
75. Korsmeyer SJ, Hieter PA, Ravetch JV, et al: Developmental hierarchy of immunoglobulin gene rearrangements in human leukemic pre-B-cells. *Proc Natl Acad Sci USA* 78:7096, 1981.
76. Nadler LM, Korsmeyer SJ, Anderson KC, et al: B-cell origin of non-T cell acute lymphoblastic leukemia. A model for discrete stages of neoplastic and normal pre-B cell differentiation. *J Clin Invest* 74:332, 1984.
77. Korsmeyer SJ, Arnold A, Bakhshi A, et al: Immunoglobin gene rearrangement and cell surface antigen expression in acute lymphocytic leukemias of T and B cell precursor origins. *J Clin Invest* 71:301, 1983.
78. Nadler LM, Korsmeyer SJ, Anderson KC, et al: B cell origin of non-T cell acute lymphoblastic leukemia. *J Clin Invest* 74:332, 1984.
79. Foon AK, Todd RF: Immunologic classification of leukemia and lymphoma. *Blood* 68:1, 1986.
80. Flandrin G, Brouet JC, Daniel MT, et al: Acute leukemia with Burkitt's tumor cells: A study of six cases with special reference to lymphocyte surface markers. *Blood* 45:813, 1975.
81. Gordon DS, Hutton JJ, Smalley RS, et al: Terminal deoxynucleotidyl transferase (TdT), cytochemistry, and membrane receptors in adult acute leukemias. *Blood* 52:1079, 1978.

82. LeBien TW, McCormack RT: The common lymphoblastic antigen (CD10)—emancipation from a functional enigma. *Blood* 73:625, 1989.
83. Bradstock KF, Hoffbrand AV, Ganeshaguru K, et al: Terminal deoxynucleotidyl transferase expression in acute non-lymphoid leukemia: An analysis by immunofluorescence. *Br J Haematol* 47:133, 1981.
84. Jani P, Verbi W, Greaves MF, et al: Terminal deoxynucleotidyl transferase in acute myeloid leukemia. *Leuk Res* 7:17, 1983.
85. Lanham GA, Bollum FG, Williams DL, et al: Simultaneous occurrence of terminal deoxynucleotidyl transferase and myeloperoxidase in individual leukemia blasts. *Blood* 64:318, 1984.
86. Chan LC, Pegram SM, Greaves MF: Contribution of immunophenotype to the classification and differential diagnosis of acute leukemia. *Lancet* 1:475, 1985.
87. Bettelheim P, Paietta E, Majdic O, et al: Expression of a myeloid marker on TdT positive acute lymphocytic leukemia cells: Evidence by double-fluorescence staining. *Blood* 60:1392, 1982.
88. Pui CH, Dahl GV, Melvin S, et al: Acute leukemia with mixed lymphoid and myeloid phenotype. *Br J Haematol* 56:121, 1984.
89. Smith LJ, Curtis JE, Messner HA, et al: Lineage infidelity in acute leukemia. *Blood* 61:1138, 1983.
90. Weiner M, Borowitz M, Boyett J, et al: Clinical pathologic aspects of myeloid antigen positivity in pediatric patients with acute lymphoblastic leukemia (ALL). *Proc ASCO* 5:172, 1985.
91a. Sobol RE, Mick R, Royston I, et al: Clinical importance of myeloid antigen expression in adult acute lymphoblastic leukemia. *N Engl J Med* 316:1111, 1987.
91b. Drexler HG, Theil E, Ludwig W-D: Review of the incidence and clinical relevance of myeloid antigen-positive acute lymphoblastic leukemia. *Leukemia* 5:637, 1991.
92. Van den Berghe H, David G, Broeckaert-Van OS, et al: A new chromosome anomaly in acute lymphoblastic leukemia (ALL). *Hum Genet* 46:172, 1979.
93a. Third International Workshop on Chromosomes in Leukemia: Chromosomal abnormalities in acute lymphoid leukemia. *Cancer Genet Cytogenet* 4:101, 1981.
93b. Berger R, Bernheim A: Cytogenetic studies on Burkitt's lymphoma-leukemia. *Cancer Genet Cytogenet* 7:231, 1982.
94a. Kowalczyk J, Sandberg AA: A possible subgroup of ALL with 9p. *Cancer Genet Cytogenet* 9:383, 1983.
94b. Williams DL, Look AT, Melvin SL, et al: New chromosomal translocations variable with specific immunophenotypes of childhood acute lymphoblastic leukemia. *Cell* 36:101, 1984.
95a. Pui C-H, Frankel LS, Carroll AJ, et al: Clinical characteristics and treatment outcome of childhood acute lymphoblastic leukemia with t(4;11)(q21;q23): A collaborative study of 40 cases. *Blood* 77:440, 1991.
95b. Pui C-H, Crist WM, Look T: Biology and clinical significance of cytogenetic abnormalities in childhood acute lymphoblastic leukemia. *Blood* 76:1449, 1990.
95c. Heisterkamp N, Groffen J: Molecular insights into the Philadelphia translocation. *Hematol Pathol* 5:1, 1991.
96a. Fletcher JA, Lynch EA, Kimball VM, et al: Translocation (9;22) is associated with extremely poor prognosis in intensively treated children with acute lymphoblastic leukemia. *Blood* 77:435, 1991.
96b. Suryanarayan K, Hunger SP, Kohler S, et al: Consistent involvement of the *bcr* gene by 9;22 breakpoints in pediatric acute leukemias. *Blood* 77:324, 1991.
97a. Hunger SP, Galili N, Carroll AJ, et al: The t(l;19)(q23;p13) Results in Consistent Fusion of E2A and PBX1 Coding Sequences in Acute Lymphoblastic Leukemia. *Blood* 77:687, 1991.
97b. First MIC Cooperative Study Group: Morphologic, Immunologic, and Cytogenetic (MIC) working classification of acute lymphoblastic leukemias. Report of the workshop held in Leuven, Belgium, April 22–23, 1985. *Cancer Genet Cytogenet* 23:189, 1986.
98a. Fishel RS, Farnen JP, Hanson CA, et al: Acute lymphoblastic leukemia with eosinophilia. *Medicine* 69:232, 1990.
98b. Jandl JH: *Blood. Textbook of Hematology*, Boston, Little, Brown, 1987, p 629.
99. Grier HE, Weinstein HJ: Acute nonlymphoid leukemia, in Pizzo PA, Poplack DG (eds), *Principles and Practice of Pediatric Oncology*. Philadelphia, JB Lippincott, 1989, p 367.
100. Bennet JM, Catovsky D, Daniel M-T, et al: Proposed revised criteria for the classification of acute myeloid leukemia. A report of the French-American British Cooperative Group. *Ann Intern Med* 103:626, 1985.
101. Bennet JM, Catovsky D, Daniel M-T, et al: Characterization of megakaryoblastic leukemia (M7). *Ann Intern Med* 103:460, 1985.
102. Fourth International Workshop on Chromosomes in Leukemia: A prospective study of acute non-lymphocytic leukemia. *Cancer Genet Cytogenet* 11:251, 1984.
103. Second MIC Cooperative Study Group: Morphologic Immunologic, and Cytogenetic (MIC) working classification of the acute myeloid leukemias. Report of the workshop held in Leuven, Belgium, September 15–17, 1986. *Cancer Genet Cytogenet* 30:1, 1988.
104. Mertelsmann R, Thaler HT, To L, et al: Morphological classification, response to therapy, and survival in 263 adult patients with acute non-lymphoblastic leukemia. *Blood* 56:773, 1980.
105. LeMaistre A, Childs CC, Hirsch-Ginsberg C, et al:

Heterogeneity in acute undifferentiated leukemia. *Hematol Pathol* 2:79, 1988.

106a. Nguyen D, Brynes RK, Macaulay L, et al: Acute myeloid leukemia, FAB M-1 microgranular variant: A multiparameter study. *Hematol Pathol* 3:11, 1989.

106b. Smith LJ, Curtis JE, Messner HA, et al: Lineage infidelity in acute leukemia. *Blood* 61:1138, 1983.

107. Bennett JM, Daniel MT, Galton DA, et al: A variant form of hypergranular promyelocytic leukemia (M3). *Br J Haematol* 44:169, 1980.

108. Golomb HM, Rowley JD, Vardiman JW, et al: "Microgranular" acute promyelocytic leukemia: A distinct clinical, ultrastructural, and cytogenetic entity. *Blood* 55:253, 1980.

109. Edelman BB, Grossman NJ: Microgranular acute promyelocytic leukemia. A case with multiple Auer rods demonstrable only after staining for chloroacetate esterase. *Am J Clin Pathol* 79:621, 1983.

110. Longo L, Pendolfi PP, Biondi A, et al: Rearrangement and aberrant expression of the RARa gene in acute promyalocytic leukemias. *J Exp Med* 172:1571, 1990.

111. Biondi A, Rambaldi A, Alcalay M, et al: RAR-α gene rearrangements as a genetic marker for diagnosis and monitoring in acute promyelocytic leukemia. *Blood* 77:1418, 1991.

112. Longo L, Donti E, Mencaralli A, et al; Mapping of chromosome 17 breakpoints in acute myeloid leukemia. *Oncogene* 5:1557, 1991.

113. Staven P: Hypergranular acute promyelocytic leukemia with intravascular coagulation. *Scand J Haematol* 11:249, 1973.

114. Cassileth PA, Begg CB, Bennett JM, et al: A randomized study of the efficacy of consolidation therapy in adult acute nonlymphocytic leukemia. *Blood* 63:843, 1984.

115. Catovsky D: Symposium: Classification of leukemia. The classification of acute leukemia. *Pathology* 14:277, 1982.

116. Arthur DC, Bloomfield CD: Partial deletion of the long arm of chromosome 16 and bone marrow eosinophilia in acute nonlymphocytic leukemia: A new association. *Blood* 61:994, 1983.

117. Larson RA, Williams SF, LeBeau MM, et al: Acute myelomonocytic leukemia with abnormal eosinophils and *inv*(16) or t(16,16) has a favorable prognosis. *Blood* 68:1242, 1986.

118. Ferraris AM, Broccia G, Meloni T, et al: Clonal origin of cells restricted to monocytic differentiation in acute nonlymphocytic leukemia. *Blood* 64:817, 1984.

119. Tobelem G, Jacquillat C, Chastang E, et al: Acute monoblastic leukemia: A clinical and biologic study of 74 cases. *Blood* 56:481, 1980.

120. Shaw MT: The distinctive features of acute monocytic leukemia. *Am J Hematol* 4:97, 1978.

121. Straus DJ: The acute monocytic leukemia: Multidisciplinary studies in 45 patients. *Medicine* 59:409, 1980.

122. Cuttner J, Conjalka MS, Reilly M, et al: Association of monocytic leukemia in patients with extreme leukocytosis. *Am J Med* 69:555, 1980.

123. Scott RB, Ellison RR, Ley AB: A clinical study of twenty cases of erythroleukemia (di Guglielmo's syndrome). *Am J Med* 37:162, 1964.

124. Hetzel P, Gee TS: A new observation in the clinical spectrums of erythroleukemia. A report of 46 cases. *Am J Med* 64:765, 1978.

125. Reiffers J, Bernard P, Larrue J, et al: Acute erythroblastic leukemia presenting as acute undifferentiated leukemia. A report of two cases with ultrastructural features. *Leuk Res* 9:413, 1985.

126a. Chan WC, Brynes RK, Kim TH, et al: Acute megakaryoblastic leukemia in early childhood. *Blood* 62:92, 1983.

126b. Kojima S, Matsuyama T, Sato T, et al: Down's syndrome and acute leukemia in children: An analysis of phenotype by use of monoclonal antibodies and electron microscopic platelet peroxidase reaction. *Blood* 76:2348, 1990.

126c. Windebank KP, Tefferi A, Smithson AW, et al: Acute megakaryocytic leukemia (M7) in children. *Mayo Clin Proc* 64:1339, 1989.

127a. Nichols CR, Hoffman R, Einhorn LH, et al: Hematologic malignancies associated with primary mediastinal germ-cell tumors. *Ann Intern Med* 102:603, 1985.

127b. Wang SE, Fligiel S, Naeim F: Acute megakaryocytic leukemia following chemotherapy for a malignant teratoma. *Arch Pathol Lab Med* 108:202, 1984.

128a. Koike T: Megakaryoblastic leukemia: The characterization and identification of megakaryocytes. *Blood* 64:682, 1984.

128b. Ruiz-Argiielles GJ, Marin-Lopez A, Lobato-Mendizábal E, et al: Acute megakaryoblastic leukemia: A prospective study of its identification and treatment. *Br J Haematol* 62:55, 1986.

129a. Pantazis CG, Allsbrook WC Jr, Ades E, et al: Acute megakaryocytic leukemia: Flow cytometric analysis of DNA content at diagnosis and during the course of therapy. *Cancer* 60:2443, 1987.

129b. Bregsman K, Van Slyck EJ: Acute myelofibrosis. An accelerated variant of agnogenic myeloid metaplasia. *Ann Intern Med* 74:232, 1971.

130. Bird T, Proctor SJ: Malignant myelosclerosis: Myeloproliferative disorder or leukemia? *Am J Clin Pathol* 67:512, 1977.

131. Estevez JM, Urueta EE, Moran TJ: Acute megakaryocytic myelofibrosis. Case report of an unusual myeloproliferative syndrome. *Am J Clin Pathol* 62:52, 1974.
132. Hurban RH, Kuhajda FP, Mann RB: Acute myelofibrosis: Immunohistochemical study of four cases and comparison with acute megakaryocytic leukemia. *Am J Clin Pathol* 88:578, 1987.
133. Lewis SM, Szur L: Malignant myelosclerosis. *Br J Med* 2:472, 1963.
134. den Ottolander GJ, te Velde J, Brederoo P, et al: Megakaryoblastic leukemia (acute myelofibrosis): A report of three cases. *Br J Haematol* 42:9, 1979.
135. Weisenburger DW: Acute myelofibrosis terminating as acute myeloblastic leukemia. *Am J Clin Pathol* 73:182, 1980.
136. Bearman RA, Pangalis GA, Rappaport H: Acute (malignant) myelosclerosis. *Cancer* 43:279, 1979.
137. Rowly JD: Recurring chromosome abnormalities in leukemia and lymphoma. *Semin Hematol* 27:122, 1990.
138. Greaves MF: The contribution of molecular genetics to the study of leukemia. *Cancer Genet Cytogenet* 40:217, 1989.
139. Lemons RS, Eilender D, Waldman R, et al: Cloning and characterization of the t(15;17) translocation breakpoint region in acute promyelocytic leukemia. *Genes Chrom Cancer* 2:79, 1990.
140. Schiller G, Naeim F, Champlin RE: Bone marrow aplasia associated with proliferation of large granular lymphocytes and subsequent transformation to acute lymphoblastic leukemia. *Am J Hematol* 32:153, 1989.
141a. Warzynski JM, Rosen MH, Golightly MG: Acute natural killer lymphocytic leukemia in an adult presenting with massive splenomegaly. Fifth Annual Meeting, Clinical Application of Cytometry, Charleston, South Carolina, September 1990.
141b. Naeim F, Schiller G: Acute lymphoblastic leukemia of NK type: *Lab Invest* 66:84A, 1992.
142. Cerezo I, Shuster JJ, Pullen J, et al: Laboratory correlates and prognostic significance of granular acute lymphoblastic leukemia in children. A Pediatric Oncology Group study. *Am J Clin Pathol* 95:526, 1991.
143a. Simpkins H, Shoaf F, Katz J: An acute granular lymphoid leukemia with unusual cytochemistry and immunologic phenotype. *Hum Pathol* 18:93, 1987.
143b. Yanagihara E, Naeim F, Gale R, et al: Acute lymphoblastic leukemia with giant intracytoplasmic inclusions. *Am J Clin Pathol* 74:345, 1980.
144. Peterson CL, Parkin JL, Arthur DC, et al: Acute basophilic leukemia. A clinical, morphological, and cytogenetic study of eight cases. *Am J Clin Pathol* 96:160, 1991.
145. Beard MEJ, Batemen JT, Crowther DC, et al: Hypoplastic acute myelogenous leukemia. *Br J Haematol* 31:167, 1975.
146. Needleman SW, Burns PC, Dick FR, et al: Hypoplastic acute leukemia. *Cancer* 48:1410, 1981.
147. Howe RB, Bloomfield CD, Mckenna RW: Hypocellular acute leukemia. *Am J Med* 172:391, 1982.
148. Gladson CL, Naeim F: Hypocellular bone marrow with increased blasts. *Am J Hematol* 21:15, 1986.
149. Schumacher HR, Perlin E, Klos JR, et al: Hand mirror cell leukemia, a new clinical and morphologic variant. *Am J Clin Pathol* 68:531, 1977.
150. Schumacher HR: *Acute Leukemia*. New York, Igaku-Shoin, 1990, p 233.
151. Sjogren U, Norberg H, Rydgren L: Ameboid movement configuration in tumor cells of bone marrow smears from patients with leukemia. *Acta Med Scand* 201:381, 1977.
152. Glassy EF, Sun NCJ, Okun DB: Hand-mirror cell leukemia. *Am J Clin Pathol* 74:651, 1980.
153. Stass SA, Perlin E, Jaffe ES, et al: Acute lymphoblastic leukemia—hand mirror cell variant: A detailed cytological and ultrastructural study with an analysis of the immunologic surface markers. *Am J Hematol* 4:67, 1978.
154. Schumacher HR, Raineg T, Davidson L, et al: American Burkitt's lymphoma—hand-mirror variant. *Am J Clin Pathol* 70:937, 1978.
155. Schumacher HR, Clapp WL, Thomas WJ, et al: Acute lymphoblastic leukemia, hand mirror variant. *Arch Pathol Lab Med* 104:134, 1980.
156. Schumacher HR, Champion JE, Thomas WJ, et al: Acute lymphoblastic leukemia—hand mirror variant. An analysis of a large group of patients. *Am J Hematol* 7:11, 1979.
157. Marie JP, Izaguirre CA, Civin CL, et al: The presence within a single K562 cell of erythropoietic and granulopoietic differentiation markers. *Blood* 58:708, 1981.
158. Greaves MF, Mizutani S, Furley AJW, et al: Lineage promiscuity in hemopoietic differentiation and leukemia. *Blood* 67:1, 1986.
159. Gale R, Ben Bassat I: Hybrid acute leukemia. *Br J Med* 65:261, 1987.
160. Ben Bassat I, Gale RP: Hybrid acute leukemia. *Leuk Res* 8:929, 1984.
161. Kantarjian HM, Hirsch-Ginsberg C, Yee G, et al: Mixed-lineage leukemia revisited: Acute lymphoblastic leukemia with myeloperoxidase-positive blasts by electron microscopy. *Blood* 76:808, 1990.
162. Sulak LE, Clare CN, Morale BA, et al: Biphenotypic acute leukemia in adults. *Am J Clin Pathol* 94:54, 1990.
163. Bittelheim P, Paietta E, Majdic O, et al: Expression of a myeloid marker on TdT-positive acute lymphocytic leukemia cells. *Blood* 60:1392, 1982.

164. Mirro J, Zipf TF, Pui CH, et al: Acute mixed lineage leukemia. Clinicopathologic correlations and prognostic significance. *Blood* 66:1115, 1985.
165. Hoffbrand AV, Leber BF, Browett PJ, et al: Mixed acute leukemias. *Blood Rev* 2:9, 1988.
166. Pui CH, Dahl GU, Melvin S, et al: Acute leukemia with mixed lymphoid and myeloid phenotype. *Br J Haematol* 56:121, 1984.
167. Bradstock KF, Hoffbrand AV, Ganeshaguru K, et al: Terminal deoxynucleotidyl transferase expression in acute non-lymphoid leukemia. *Br J Haematol* 47:133, 1981.
168. Stass SA, Mirro J: Unexpected heterogeneity in acute leukemia: Mixed lineages and lineage switch. *Hum Pathol* 16:864, 1985.
169. Pui CH, Raimondi SC, Head DR, et al: Characterization of childhood acute leukemia with multiple myeloid and lymphoid markers at diagnosis and at relapse. *Blood* 78:1327, 1991.
170. Ferrara F, De Rosa C, Fasanaro A, et al: Myeloid antigen expression in adult lymphoblastic leukemia: Clinicohematological correlations and prognostic relevance. *Hematol Pathol* 4:93, 1990.
171. Arthur DC, Bloomfield CD, Lindquist LL, et al: Translocation 4;11 in lymphoblastic leukemia: Clinical characteristics and prognostic significance. *Blood* 59:96, 1982.
172. Childs CC, Hirsch-Ginsberg C, Culbert SJ, et al: Lineage heterogeneity in acute leukemia with the t(4;11) abnormality: Implications for acute mixed lineage leukemia. *Hematol Pathol* 2:145, 1988.
173a. Sun G, Sparkes RS, Wormsley S, et al: Are some acute leukemia with t(8;21) hybrid leukemias? *Cancer Genet cytogenet* 49:177–184, 1990.
173b. Sun G, Wormsley S, Sparkes RS, et al: Hybrid leukemia and the 5q− abnormality. *Leuk Res* 15:351, 1991.
174. Hanson C, Abaza M, Ross C, et al: Acute biphenotypic leukemia (ABL): Immunophenotyping (IPH), morphology, and cytogenetics. *Lab Invest* 64:73A, 1991.
175. Gunz FW, Dameshek W: Chronic lymphocytic leukemia in a family, including twin brothers and a son. *JAMA* 164:1323, 1957.
176. Gunz FW, Gunz JP, Veale AM, et al: Familial leukemia: A study of 909 families. *Scand J Haematol* 15:117, 1975.
177. Fraumeni JF Jr, Wertelecki W, Blattner, WA, et al: Varied manifestations of a familial lymphoproliferative disorder. *Am J Med* 59:145, 1975.
178. Culter SJ, Axtell L, Heise H, et al: Ten thousand cases of leukemia: 1940–62. *J Natl Cancer Inst* 39:993, 1967.
179. Sweet DL Jr, Golomb HM, Uttmann JE, et al: The clinical features of chronic lymphocytic leukemia. *Clin Haematol* 6:185, 1977.
180a. Bennett JM, Catovsky D, Daniel MT, et al: Proposals for the classification of chronic (mature) B and T lymphoid leukemias. *J Clin Pathol* 42:567, 1989.
180b. Dighiero G, Travade P, Cheveret S, et al: B-cell chronic lymphocytic leukemia: Present status and future directions. *Blood* 78:1901, 1991.
181. Gearhart PJ, Sigal NH, Klinman NR: Production of antibodies of identical idiotype but diverse immunoglobin classes by cells derived from a single stimulated B cell. *Proc Natl Acad Sci USA* 72:1707, 1975.
182. Brouet JC, Seligmann M: Chronic lymphocytic leukemia as an immunoproliferative disorder. *Clin Haematol* 6:169, 1977.
183. Luzzatto L, Foroni L: DNA rearrangements of cell lineage specific genes in lymphoproliferative disorders. *Prog Hematol* 14:303, 1986.
184. Ralfklaer E, Geisler C, Hansen MM, et al: Nuclear clefts in chronic lymphocytic leukemia. A light microscopic and ultrastructural study of a new prognostic parameter. *Scand J Haematol* 30:5, 1983.
185. Melo JV, Catovsky D, Gregory WM, et al: The relationship between chronic lymphocytic leukemia and prolymphocytic leukemia. IV. Analysis of survival and prognostic features. *Br J Haematol* 65:23, 1987.
186. Vallespi T, Torrabadella M, Julia A, et al: Chronic lymphocytic leukemia: A multivariate survival analysis including morphological types of lymphoid cells in peripheral blood, in Gale RP, Rai KR (eds), *Chronic Lymphocytic Leukemia. Recent Progress and Future Directions.* New York, Alan R. Liss, 1987, p 277.
187. Pangalis GA, Roussou PA, Kittas C, et al: Patterns of bone marrow involvement in chronic lymphocytic leukemia and small lymphocytic (well-differentiated) non-Hodgkin's lymphoma. Its clinical significance in relation to their differential diagnosis and prognosis. *Cancer* 54:702, 1984.
188. Getaz EP, Miller GJ: Spinal cord involvement in chronic lymphocytic leukemia. *Cancer* 43:1858, 1979.
189. Liepman MK, Votaw ML: Meningeal leukemia complicating chronic lymphocytic leukemia. *Cancer* 47:2482, 1981.
190a. Terynck T, Dighiero G, Follezou J, et al: Comparison of normal and CLL lymphocyte surface Ig determinants using peroxidase labeled antibodies. I. Detection and quantitation of light chain determinants. *Blood* 43:79, 1974.
190b. Molica S, Dattilo A, Alberti A: myelomonocytic associated antigens in B-chronic lymphocytic leukemia: Analysis of clinical significance. *Leuk Lymph* 5:139, 1991.
191a. Geisler CH, Larsen JK, Hansen NE, et al: Prognostic importance of flow cytometric immunophenotyping of 540 consecutive patients with B-cell chronic lymphocytic leukemia. *Blood* 78:1795, 1991.

191b. Naeim F. Bergmann K, Gatti RA: Membrane receptors and their redistribution in lymphoproliferative disorders. *Blood* 54:648, 1979.

192. Hannam-Harris AC, Gordon J, Smith JL: Immunoglobulin synthesis by neoplastic B lymphocytes: Free light chain synthesis as a marker of B cell differentiation. *J Immunol* 125:2177, 1980.

193. Gordon J, Melstedt H, Aman P, et al: Phenotypes in chronic B-lymphocytic leukemia probed by monoclonal antibodies and immunoglobulin secretion studies: Identification of stages of maturation arrest and the relation to clinical findings. *Blood* 62:910, 1983.

194a. Zimmerman TS, Godwin HA, Perry S: Studies of leukocyte kinetics in chronic lymphocytic leukemia. *Blood* 31:277, 1968.

194b. Theml H, Trepel F, Schick P, et al: Kinetics of lymphocytes in chronic lymphocytic leukemia: Studies using continuous 3H-thymidine infusion in two patients. *Blood* 42:623, 1973.

195. Hanson CA, Gribbin TE, Schnitzer B, et al: CD11c (Leu M5) expression characterized a B-cell lymphoproliferative disorder with features of both chronic lymphocytic leukemia and hairy cell leukemia. *Blood* 76:2360, 1990.

196. Stryckmans PA, Debusscher L, Collard E: Cell kinetics in chronic lymphocytic leukemia. *Clin Haematol* 6:159, 1977.

197. Jandl JH: Chronic lymphocytic leukemia, in Jandl JH (ed), *Blood. Textbook of Hematology.* Boston, Little, Brown, 1987, p 751.

198. Kawamura N, Muraguchi A, Hori A, et al: A case of human B cell leukemia that implicates an autocrine mechanism in the abnormal growth of leu 1 B cells. *J Clin Invest* 78:1331, 1986.

199. Abeloff MD, Waterbury L: Pure red cell aplasia and chronic lymphocytic leukemia. *Arch Intern Med* 134:721, 1974.

200. Yoo D, Pierce LE, Lessin LS: Acquired pure red cell aplasia associated with chronic lymphocytic leukemia. *Cancer* 51:844, 1983.

201. Mangan KF, Chikkappa G, Scharfman WB, et al: Evidence for reduced erythroid burst (BFU-E) promoting function of T lymphocytes in pure red cell aplasia of chronic lymphocytic leukemia. *Exp Hematol* 9:489, 1981.

202. Mangan KF, Chikkappa G, Farley F, et al: T gamma (Tγ) cells suppress growth of erythroid colony forming units in vitro in pure red cell aplasia of B-cell chronic lymphocytic leukemia. *J Clin Invest* 70:1148, 1982.

203. Sikora K, Krikorian J, Levy R: Monoclonal immunoglobulin rescue from a patient with chronic lymphocytic leukemia and autoimmune hemolytic anemia. *Blood* 54:513, 1979.

204. Oshimi K: Granular lymphocyte proliferative disorders: Report of 12 cases and review of the literature. *Leukemia* 2:617, 1988.

205. Reynolds CW, Foon KA: Tγ- lymphoproliferative disease and related disorders in man and experimental animals: A review of the clinical, cellular and functional characteristics. *Blood* 64:1146, 1984.

206. Loughran TP Jr, Draves KE, Starkebaum G, et al: Leukemia of large granular lymphocytes: Association of clonal chromosomal abnormalities and autoimmune neutropenia, thrombocytopenia and hemolytic anemia. *Ann Intern Med* 102:169, 1985.

207. Loughran TP Jr, Draves KE, Starkebaum G, et al: Induction of NK activity in large granular lymphocyte leukemia: Activation with anti-CD3 monoclonal antibody and interleukin-2. *Blood* 69:72, 1987.

208. Loughran TP Jr, Starkebaum G, Aprile JA: Rearrangement and expression of T-cell receptor genes in large granular lymphocytic leukemia. *Blood* 71:822, 1988.

209. Loughran TP, Lanier LL, Phillips JH, et al: Natural killer cells: Definition of a cell type rather than a function. *J Immunol* 137:2735, 1986.

210. Geisler C, Ralfkiaer E, Astrup L, et al: Chronic lymphocytic leukemia of T cell origin. Clinical variation possibly due to involvement of different T lymphocyte subpopulations. *Scand J Haematol* 31:109, 1983.

211. Aisenberg AC, Wilkes MB, Harris NL, et al: T-cell chronic lymphocytic leukemia. Report of a case studies with monoclonal antibody. *Am J Med* 72:695, 1982.

212. Knowles DM 2nd, Halper JP: Human T-cell malignancies. Correlative clinical, histopathologic, immunologic, and cytochemical analysis of 23 cases. *Am J Pathol* 106:187, 1982.

213. Pizzolo G, Chilosi M, Getto GL, et al: Immuno-histological analysis of bone marrow involvement in lymphoproliferative disorders. *Br J Haematol* 50:95, 1982.

214. Foon KA, Naeim F, Saxon A, et al: Leukemia of T-helper lymphocytes: Study of clinical and functional features. *Leuk Res* 5:1, 1981.

215. Gahrton G, Robert K-H: Chromosomal abnormalities in chronic B-cell lymphocytic leukemia. *Cancer Genet Cytogenet* 6:171, 1982.

216. Morita M, Minowada J, Sandberg AA: Chromosomes and causation of human cancer and leukemia. XLV. Chromosome patterns in stimulated lymphocytes of chronic lymphocytic leukemia. *Cancer Genet Cytogenet* 3:293, 1981.

217. Gahrton G, Robert K-H, Friberg K, et al: Extra chromosome 12 in chronic lymphocytic leukemia. *Lancet* 1:146, 1980.

218. Han T, Sadamore N, Ozer H, et al: Cytogenetic studies in 77 patients with chronic lymphocytic leukemia:

Correlations with clinical, immunologic, and phenotypic data. *J Clin Oncol* 2:1121, 1984.
219. Schroder J, Vuopio P, Autio K: Chromosome changes in human chronic lymphocytic leukemia. *Cancer Genet Cytogenet* 4:11, 1981.
220. Gahrton G, Juliusson G, Robert K-H, et al: Role of chromosomal abnormalities in chronic lymphocytic leukemia. *Blood Rev* 1:183, 1987.
221. Tsujimoto Y, Yunis J, Onorato-Showe L, et al: Molecular cloning of the chromosomal breakpoint of B-cell lymphomas and leukemias with the t(11;14) chromosome translocation. *Science* 224:1403, 1984.
222a. Haluska FG, Tsujimoto Y, Russo G, et al: Molecular genetics of lymphoid tumorigenesis. *Prod Nucl Acid Res Mol Biol* 36:269, 1989.
222b. Rai KR, Sawitsky A, Cronkite EP, et al: Clinical staging of chronic lymphocytic leukemia. *Blood* 46:219, 1975.
223a. Binet J-L, Catovsky D, Chandra P, et al: Chronic lymphocytic leukemia: Proposals for a revised prognostic staging system. Report from the International Workshop on CLL The Writing Committee. *Br J Haematol* 48:365, 1981.
223b. Peller S, Kaufman S: Decreased CD45RA T cells in B-cell chronic lymphocytic leukemia patients: Correlation with disease stage. *Blood* 78:1569, 1991.
223c. Hanson CA, Bockenstedt PL, Schnitzer B, et al: S-100 positive T-cell chronic lymphoproliferative disease: An aggressive disorder or an uncommon T-cell subset. *Blood* 78:1803, 1991.
224. Foucar K, Rydell RE: Richter's syndrome in chronic lymphocytic leukemia. *Cancer* 46:118, 1980.
225. Harousseau JL, Flandrin G, Tricot G, et al: Malignant lymphoma supervening in chronic lymphocytic leukemia and related disorders. Richter's syndrome: A study of 25 cases. *Cancer* 48:1302, 1981.
226. Dick FR, Maca RD: The lymph node in chronic lymphocytic leukemia. *Cancer* 41:283, 1973.
227. Splinter TA, Noorloos BV, Van Heerde P: CLL and diffuse histiocytic lymphoma in one patient: Clonal proliferation of two different B cells. *Scand J Haematol* 20:29, 1978.
228. Fitzgerald PH: Richter's syndrome with identification of marker chromosomes. *Cancer* 46:135, 1980.
229. Galton DAG, Goldman JM, Wiltshaw E, et al: Prolymphocytic leukemia. *Br J Haematol* 27:7, 1974.
230. Catovsky D: Hairy-cell leukemia and prolymphocytic leukemia. *Clin Haematol* 6:245, 1977.
231. Bearman RM, Pangalis GA, Rappaport H: Prolymphocytic leukemia. Clinical, histopathological and cytochemical observations. *Cancer* 42:2360, 1978.
232. Catovsky D, Wechsler A, Matutes E, et al: The membrane phenotype of T-prolymphocytic leukemia. *Scand J Haematol* 29:398, 1982.
233. Chan WC, Check IJ, Heffner LT, et al: Prolymphocytic leukemia of helper cell phenotype. Report of a case and review of the scientific literature. *Am J Clin Pathol* 78:437, 1982.
234. Crown DJ, Kadin ME, Anders TL: T-cell prolymphocytic leukemia. Two cases having a postthymic helper phenotype with complement receptors and 14q+ chromosome activity. *Acta Haematol* 70:43, 1983.
235. Planas AT: T-cell prolymphocytic leukemia with a suppressor phenotype. *Ann Clin Lab Sci* 13:193, 1983.
236. Pittman S, Catovsky D: Chromosome abnormalities in B-cell prolymphocytic leukemia: A study of nine cases. *Cancer Genet Cytogenet* 9:355, 1983.
237. Sadamori N, Hamm T, Monawada J, et al: Possible specific chromosome changes in prolymphocytic leukemia. *Blood* 62:729, 1983.
238. Matutes E, Brito-Babapulle V, Swansbury J, et al: Clinical and laboratory features of 78 cases of T-Prolymphocytic leukemia. *Blood* 78:3269, 1991.
239. Thiel E, Bauchinger M, Rodt H, et al: Evidence for monoclonal proliferation in prolymphocytic leukemia of T-cell origin. A cytogenetic and quantitative immunoautoradiographic analysis. *Blut* 35:427, 1977.
240. Pittman S, Morilla R, Catovsky D: Chronic T-cell leukemias. II. Cytogenetic studies. *Leuk Res* 6:33, 1982.
241. Burke JS: The value of the bone marrow biopsy in the diagnosis of hairy cell leukemia. *Am J Clinical Pathol* 70:876, 1978.
242. Flandrin G, Sigaux F, Sebahoun G, et al: Hairy cell leukemia: Clinical presentation and follow-up of 211 patients. *Semin Oncol* 11:458, 1984.
243. Golomb HM, Catovsky D, Golde DW: Hairy cell leukemia: A clinical review of 71 cases. *Ann Intern Med* 89:677, 1978.
244. Naeim F: Clinicopathological subtypes in hairy cell leukemia. *Am J Clin Pathol* 78:80, 1982.
245. Jansen J, Hermans H: Clinical staging system for hairy cell leukemia. *Blood* 69:571, 1982.
246. Damasio EE, Spirano M, Repetto M, et al: Hairy cell leukemia: A restrospective study of 235 cases by the Italian Cooperative Group (ICG-HCL) according to Jansen's clinical staging system. *Acta Haematol* 72:326, 1984.
247. Westbrook CA, Groopman JE, Golde DW: Hairy cell leukemia. Disease pattern and prognosis. *Cancer* 54:500, 1984.
248. Turner A, Kjeldsberg CR: Hairy cell leukemia: A review. *Medicine* 57:477, 1978.
249. Golomb HM, Catovsky D, Golde DW: Hairy cell leukemia: A 5 year update on 71 patients. *Ann Intern Med* 99:485, 1983.
250. Silingardi V, Federico M, Barbieri F, et al: Hairy cell

leukemia: A reversible disease? A report of two cases of spontaneous remission. *Haematologica* 70:437, 1985.
251. Naeim F: Hairy cell leukemia: Characteristics of the neoplastic cells. *Hum Pathol* 19:375, 1988.
252. Hamilton RM, De Meester S, Golomb HM: Scanning electron microscopic study of hairy cells from 15 patients with hairy cell leukemia: Morphologic subtypes. *Dev Oncol* 14:435, 1984.
253. Katayama I, Schnider G: Further ultrastructural characterization of hairy cells of leukemic reticuloendotheliosis. *Am J Pathol* 86:163, 1977.
254. Flandrin G, Daniel MT: Hairy cell leukemia: Cytochemistry and ultrastructure (TEM) in diagnosis. *Dev Oncol* 14:331, 1984.
255. Rosner MC, Golomb HM: Ribosome-lamella complex in hairy cell leukemia: Ultrastructure and distribution. *Lab Invest* 42:236, 1980.
256. Anday GJ, Goodman JR, Tishkoff GH: An unusual cytoplasmic ribosomal structure in pathologic lymphocytes. *Blood* 41:439, 1973.
257. Bartl R, Frisch B, Hill W, et al: Bone marrow histology in hairy cell leukemia: Identification of subtypes and their prognostic significance. *Am J Clin Pathol* 79:531, 1983.
258. Bouroncle BA: Leukemia reticuloendotheliosis (hairy cell leukemia). *Blood* 53:412, 1979.
259. Lee WM, Beckstead JH: Hairy cell leukemia with bone hypoplasia. *Cancer* 50:2207, 1982.
260. Naeim F, Smith G: Leukemic reticuloendotheliosis. *Cancer* 34:1813, 1974.
261. Vykoupil KF, Thiele J, Geargii A: Hairy cell leukemia. Bone marrow findings in 24 patients. *Virchows Arch (A)* 370:273, 1976.
262. Quesada JR, Reuben J, Manning JT, et al: Alpha-interferon for remission in hairy cell leukemia. *N Engl J Med* 310:15, 1984.
263. Naeim F, Jacobs AD: Bone marrow changes in patients with hairy cell leukemia treated by recombinant alpha-2 interferon. *Hum Pathol* 16:1200, 1985.
264. Jacobs AD, Champlin RE, Golde DW: Recombinant alpha-2 interferon for hairy cell leukemia. *Blood* 65:1017, 1985.
265. Golomb HM, Jacobs A, Fefer A, et al: Alpha-2 interferon therapy of hairy cell leukemia: A multicenter study of 64 patients. *J Clin Oncol* 4:900, 1986.
266. Golomb HM: Hairy cell leukemia: The importance of accurate diagnosis and sequential management. *Adv Intern Med* 29:245, 1984.
267. Golomb HM, Vardiman JW: Response to splenectomy in 65 patients with hairy cell leukemia: An evaluation of splenic weight and bone marrow involvement. *Blood* 61:349, 1983.
268. Ingoldby CJ, Ackryd N, Catovsky D, et al: Splenectomy for hairy cell leukemia. *Clin Oncol* 7:325, 1981.
269. Jansen J, Hermans H: Splenectomy in hairy cell leukemia: A retrospective multicenter analysis. *Cancer* 47:2066, 1981.
270. Ratain MJ, Vardiman JW, Golomb HM: Prognostic variables in hairy cell leukemia following splenomegaly. *Blood* 68:205a, 1986.
271. Finan MC, Su WP, LI CY: Cutaneous findings in hairy cell leukemia. *J Am Acad Dermatol* 11:788, 1984.
272. Vardiman JW, Golomb HM: Autopsy findings in hairy cell leukemia. *Semin Oncol* 11:370, 1984.
273. Yam LT, Li CY, Lam KW: Tartrate-resistant acid phosphatase isoenzyme in the reticulum cells of leukemic reticuloendotheliosis. *N Engl J Med* 284:351, 1971.
274. Katayama I, Yang JPS: Reassessment of a cytochemical test for differential diagnosis of leukemic reticuloendotheliosis. *Am J Clin Pathol* 68:268, 1977.
275. Katayama I, Li CI, Yam LT: Histochemical study of acid phosphatase isoenzyme in leukemic reticuloendotheliosis. *Cancer* 29:157, 1972.
276. Loffler H, Graubner M, Desega JF: Prolymphocytic leukemia with T-cell properties and tartrate resistant acid phosphatase. *Hamatol Bluttransfus* 20:175, 1976.
277. Naeim F, Capastagno VJ, Johnson CE JR, et al: Sezary syndrome: Tartrate-resistant acid phosphatase in the neoplastic cells. *Am J Clin Pathol* 71:528, 1979.
278. Van der Planken M, Peetermens M: Acid alpha naphthyl acetate esterase and beta-glucuronidase in hairy cell leukemia. *Blut* 41:137, 1980.
279. Variakojis D, Vardiman JW, Golomb HM: Cytochemistry of hairy cells. *Cancer* 45:72, 1980.
280. Naeim F, Hoon DS, Cheng L, et al: Reactivity of neoplastic cells in hairy cell leukemia with antisera to S-100 protein. *Am J Clin Pathol* 88:86, 1087.
281. Sansoni P, Rowden G, Manara GC, et al: Immunoelectron microscopic demonstration of S-100 protein in hairy cell leukemia cells. *Am J Clin Pathol* 89:374, 1988.
282. Burns GFM, Cawley JC, Higgy KE, et al: Hairy cell leukemia: A B-cell neoplasm with severe deficiency of circulating normal B-lymphocytes. *Leuk Res* 2:33, 1978.
283. Golomb HM, Davis S, Wilson C, et al: Surface immunoglobulins on hairy cells of 55 patients with hairy cell leukemia. *Am J Hematol* 12:397, 1982.
284. Hsu SM, Yang K, Jaffe ES: Hairy cell leukemia: A B-cell neoplasm with unique antigenic phenotype. *Am J Clin Pathol* 80:421, 1983.
285. Jansen J, Bien TW, Kersey JH: The phenotype of the neoplastic cells of hairy cell leukemia studied by monoclonal antibodies. *Blood* 59:609, 1982.
286. Jansen J, Ottolander GJ, Schuit HR, et al: Hairy cell leukemia: Its place among the chronic B cell leukemias. *Semin Oncol* 11:386, 1984.

287. Anderson KC, Boyd AW, Fisher DC, et al: Hairy cell leukemia: A tumor of preplasma cells. *Blood* 65:620, 1985.
288. Arkels YS, Lade-Lewin D, Savopous D, et al: Bone lesions in hairy cell leukemia. *Cancer* 53:2401, 1984.
289. Catovsky D, Costello C, Loukopoulos D, et al: Hairy cell leukemia and myelomatosis: Chance association or clinical manifestation of the same B-cell disease spectrum. *Blood* 57:7, 1981.
290. Quesada JR, Keating MJ, Lisshitz HL, et al: Bone involvement in hairy cell leukemia. *Am J Med* 74:228, 1983.
291. Korsmeyer J, Green WC, Cossman J, et al: Rearrangement and expression of immunoglobulin genes and expression of Tac antigens in hairy cell leukemia. *Proc Natl Acad Sci USA* 80:4522, 1983.
292a. Cleary ML, Wood GS, Warnke R, et al: Immunoglobulin gene rearrangement in hairy cell leukemia. *Blood* 64:99, 1984.
292b. Kluin-Nelemans HC, Krouels MM, Jansen JH, et al: Hairy cell leukemia preferentially expresses the IgG3-subclass. *Blood* 75:972, 1990.
293. Naeim F, Bergman K, Gatti RA: Membrane receptors and their redistribution in lymphoproliferative disorders. *Blood* 54:648, 1979.
294. Naeim F: Cytoskeletal control of redistribution of surface membrane receptors in hairy cells. *Am J Clin Pathol* 74:660, 1980.
295. Cawley JC, Burns GF, Nash TA, et al: Hairy cell leukemia with T-cell features. *Blood* 51:61, 1987.
296. Naeim F, Gatti, RA, Johnson CE, et al: Hairy cell leukemia, a heterogeneous chronic lymphoproliferative disorder. *Am J Med* 65:479, 1978.
297. Saxon A, Stevens RH, Golde DW: T-lymphocyte variant of hairy cell leukemia. *Ann Intern Med* 88:322, 1978.
298. Semenzato G, Basso G, Cartei G, et al: Hairy cell leukemia with T cell features. *Br J Haematol* 46:491, 1980.
299. Chen ISY, Laughlin J, Gasson JC, et al: Molecular characterization of the genome of a novel human T-cell leukemia virus. *Nature* 305:502, 1983.
300. Foon KA, Naeim F, Saxon A, et al: Leukemia of T-helper lymphocytes: Study of clinical and functional features. *Leuk Res* 5:1, 1981.
301. Rosenblatt DJ, Golde DW, Wacksman W, et al: A second isolate of HTLV-II associated with atypical hairy cell leukemia. *N Engl J Med* 315:372, 1986.
302. Rosenblatt DJ, Gieogi JV, Glaspy J, et al: Oligoclonal integration of HTLV-II in OKT8+ T-cells in a patient with "atypical" hairy cell leukemia: Evidence for two malignancies. *J Cell Biol Biochem [Suppl]* 11A:206, 1987.
303. Sohn CC, Blayney DW, Misset JL, et al: Leukopenic chronic T cell leukemia mimicking hairy cell leukemia: Association with human retroviruses. *Blood* 67:46, 1986.
304. Naeim F, Jensen L, Susi E, et al: Use of deoxyribonucleic acid probes in the identification of cell origin and detection of cellular contamination in human lymphoblastoid cell lines. *Lab Invest* 60:347, 1989.
305. Burns GF, Worman CP, Cawley JC: Fluctuations in the T and B characteristics of two cases of T-cell hairy-cell leukemia. *Clin Exp Immunol* 39:76, 1980.
306. Worman CP, Beverly PC, Cawley JC: Alterations in the phenotype of hairy cells during culture in the presence of PHA: Requirement for T cells. *Blood* 59:895, 1982.
307. Armitage RJ, Worman CP, Galvin MC, et al: Hairy cell leukemia with B-T hybrid features: A study with a panel of monoclonal antibodies. *Am J Hematol* 18:335, 1985.
308. Khalid G, Li Y-S, Flemans RJ, et al: Chromosomal abnormalities in a case of hairy cell leukemia. *Leuk Res* 5:431, 1971.
309. Lele KP, Fillippa DA, Chaganti RSK: Cytogenetic studies of hairy cell leukemia. *Cancer Genet Cytogenet* 4:325, 1970.
310. Sadamori N, Sandberg AA: 14q and 6q anomalies in a case with hairy cell leukemia. *Cancer Genet Cytogenet* 8:899, 1983.
311. Ueshima Y, Alimena G, Rowley JD: et al: Cytogenetic studies in patients with hairy cell leukemia. *Hematol Oncol* 1:215, 1983.
312. Knight RA, Worman CP, Cawley JCL: Defective autologous and allogeneic mixed lymphocyte reactions in hairy cell leukemia. *Clin Exp Immunol* 53:600, 1983.
313. Mackowiak PA, Demian SE, Sutker WL, et al: Infections of hairy cell leukemia: Clinical evidence of pronounced cell-mediated immunity. *Am J Med* 68:718, 1980.
314. Ruco LP, Procopio A, Macclallini V, et al: Severe deficiency of natural killer activity in the peripheral blood of patients with hairy cell leukemia. *Blood* 61:1132, 1983.
315. Ruco LP, Stoppacciaro A, Valtieri M, et al: Hairy cell leukemia: Absence of natural killer activity and of interleukin 1 release on OKM-1+ spleen hairy cells. *Clin Immunol Immunopathol* 26:47, 1983.
316. Smith BR, Rosenthal DS, Ault KA: Natural killer lymphocytes in hairy cell leukemia: Presence of phenotypically identifiable cells with defective functional activity. *Exp Hematol* 13:139, 1985.
317. Ruben JM, Ip S, Quesada JR: Effect of IFN-α therapy on cellular and plasma IL-2 in hairy cell leukemia, abstracted. *Blood* 68:231a, 1986.

318. Pizzolo G, Chilosi M, Semenzato G: The soluble interleukin-2 receptor in haematological disorders. *Br J Haematol* 67:377, 1987.
319. Steis RG, Marcon L, Clark J, et al: Serum soluble IL-2R receptor as a tumor marker in patients with hairy cell leukemia. *Blood* 71:1304, 1988.
320a. Cawley JC, Burns GF, Hayhoe RGH: A chronic lymphoproliferative disorder with distinctive features: A distinct variant of hairy-cell leukemia. *Leuk Res* 4:547, 1980.
320b. Catovsky D, O'Brien M, Melo JV, et al: Hairy cell leukemia (HCL) variant: An intermediate disease between HCL and B-prolymphocytic leukemia. *Semin Oncol* 11:362, 1984.
321. Hanson CA, Ward PCJ, Schnitzer B: A multilobular variant of hairy cell leukemia with morphologic similarities to T-cell lymphoma. *Am J Surg Pathol* 13:679, 1989.
322. Uchiyama T, Yodoi J, Sagawa K, et al: Adult T-cell leukemia: Clinical and hematologic features of 16 cases. *Blood* 50:481, 1977.
323. Broder S, Bunn PA, Jaffe ES, et al: T-cell lymphoproliferative syndrome associated with human T-cell leukemia/lymphoma virus. *Ann Intern Med* 100:546, 1984.
324. Kim JH, Durack DT: Manifestation of human T-lymphotropic virus type 1 infection. *Am J Med* 84:919, 1988.
325. Yasuda K, Sei Y, Yokoyama MM, et al: Healthy HTLV-1 carriers in Japan: The hematological and immunological characteristics. *Br J Haematol* 64:195, 1986.
326. Kawano F, Yamaguchi K, Nishimura H, et al: Variation in the clinical courses of adult T-cell leukemia. *Cancer* 55:851, 1985.
327. Yamaguchi K, Nishimura H, Kohrogi H, et al: A proposal for smoldering adult T-cell leukemia: A clinicopathologic study of five cases. *Blood* 62:758, 1983.
328. Kinoshita K, Kamihira S, Yamada Y, et al: Clinical, hematological and pathological features of T-cell leukemia-lymphoma in the Nagasaki district. *Acta Hematol Jpn* 44:1431, 1981.
329. Catovsky D, Greaves MF, Rose M, et al: Adult T-cell lymphoma-leukemia in blacks from the West Indies. *Lancet* 1:639, 1982.
330. Blayney DW, Jaffe ES, Blattner WA, et al: The human T-cell leukemia/lymphoma virus associated with American adult T-cell leukemia/lymphoma. *Blood* 62:401, 1983.
331. Bunn PA, Schechter GP, Jaffe E, et al: Clinical course of retrovirus-associated adult T-cell lymphoma in the United States. *N Engl J Med* 309:257, 1983.
332. Grossman B, Schechter GP, Horton JE, et al: Hypercalcemia associated with T-cell lymphoma-leukemia. *Am J Clin Pathol* 75:149, 1981.
333. Jaffe ES, Blattner WA, Blayney DW, et al: The pathologic spectrum of adult T-cell leukemia/lymphoma in the United States. *Am J Surg Pathol* 8:263, 1984.
334. Kuefler PR, Bunn PA: Adult T-cell leukemia/lymphoma. *Clin Haematol* 15:695, 1986.
335. Wascman W, Golde DW, Chen ISY: HTLV and human leukemia: Perspectives 1986. *Semin Hematol* 23:245, 1986.
336. Brouet JC, Flandrin G, Seligmann M: Indications of the thymus-derived nature of the proliferating cells in six patients with Sezary syndrome. *N Engl J Med* 289:341, 1973.
337. Lutzner M, Edelson R, Schein P, et al: Cutaneous T-cell lymphomas. The Sezary syndrome, mycosis fungoides, and related disorders. *Ann Intern Med* 83:534, 1975.
338. Kung PC, Berger CL, Goldstein G, et al: Cutaneous T-cell lymphomas: Characterization by monoclonal antibodies. *Blood* 57:261, 1981.
339. Boumsell L, Bernard A, Reinherz EL, et al: Surface antigens on malignant Sezary and T-CLL cells correspond to the mature T cells. *Blood* 57:526, 1981.
340. Saal F, Gessain A, Lasneret J, et al: Detection of retrovirus particles and reverse transcriptase activity in mid-term cultured peripheral blood and lymph node cells from a French woman with Sezary syndrome. *Nouv Rev Fr Hematol* 31:333, 1989.
341. Kaltoft K, Bisballe S, Rasmussen HF, et al: C-type particles are inducible in SE-Ax, a continuous T-cell line from a patient with Sezary syndrome. *Arch Dermatol Res* 280:264, 1988.
342. Fine RM: HTLV-V: A new human retrovirus associated with cutaneous T-cell lymphoma (mycosis fungoides). *Int J Dermatol* 27:473, 1988.
343. Greene MH, Dalager NA, Lamberg SI, et al: Mycosis fungoides: Epidemiologic observations. *Cancer Treat Rep* 62:597, 1979.
344. Fischmann AB, Bunn PA, Guccion JG, et al: Exposure to chemicals, physical agents, and biologic agents in mycosis fungoides and Sezary syndrome. *Cancer Treat Rep* 63:591, 1979.
345. Meijer CJLM, van Leeuwen AWFM, van der Loo EM, et al: Cerebriform (Sezary-like) mononuclear cells in healthy individuals. A morphologically distinct population of T cells. *Virchows Arch [B]* 25:95, 1977.
346. Matutes E, Robinson D, O'Brien M, et al: Candidate counterpart of Sezary cells and adult T-cell lymphoma-leukemia cells in normal peripheral blood: An ultrastructural study with the immuno-gold method and monoclonal antibodies. *Leuk Res* 7:787, 1983.

347. Slotz W, Schmoeckel C, Burg G, et al: Circulating Sezary cells in the diagnosis of Sezary syndrome (quantitative and morphological analyses). *J Invest Dermatol* 81:314, 1983.
348. Chu AC, Morris JF: Sezary cell morphology induced in peripheral blood lymphocytes: Re-evaluation. *Blood* 73:1603, 1989.
349. Duncan SC, Winklemann RK: Circulating Sezary cells in hospitalized dermatology patients. *Br J Dermatol* 99:171, 1978.
350. Flaxman BA, Zelazny G, van Scott EJ: Nonspecificity of characteristic cells in mycosis fungoides. *Arch Dermatol* 104:141, 1971.
351. Lutzner MA, Hobbs JW, Horvath P: Ultrastructure of abnormal cells in Sezary syndrome, mycosis fungoides and parapsoriasis en plaque. *Arch Dermatol* 103:375, 1971.
352. Chu AC, Robinson D, Hawk JLM, et al: Immunologic differentiation of the Sezary syndrome due to cutaneous T cell lymphoma and chronic actinic dermatitis. *J Invest Dermatol* 86:134, 1986.
353. Janier M, Katlama C, Flaguel B, et al: The pseudo-Sezary syndrome with CD8 in a patient with acquired immunodeficiency syndrome (AIDS). *Ann Intern Med* 110:738, 1989.
354. Edelson RL: Cutaneous T cell lymphoma: Mycosis fungoides, Sezary syndrome, and other variants. *J Am Acad Dermatol* 2:89, 1980.
355. Scheffer E, Meijer CJLM, van Volten WA, et al: A histologic study of lymph nodes from patients with the Sezary syndrome. *Cancer* 57:2375, 1986.
356. Schein PS, MacDonald JS, Edelson R: Cutaneous T-cell lymphoma. *Cancer* 38:1859, 1976.
357. Salhany KE, Greer JP, Cousar JB, et al: Marrow involvement in cutaneous T-cell lymphoma. A clinicopathologic study of 60 cases. *Am J Clin Pathol* 92:747, 1989.
358. Berger R, Baranger L, Berheimm A, et al: Cytogenetics of T-cell malignant lymphoma. Report of 17 cases and review of the chromosomal breakpoints. *Cancer Genet Cytogenet* 36:123, 1988.
359. Ralfkiaer E, Larsen JK, Christensen IBJ, et al: DNA analysis by flow cytometry in cutaneous T-cell lymphomas. *Br J Dermatol* 120:597, 1989.
360. Mecucci C, Louwagie A, Thomas J, et al: Cytogenetic studies in T-cell malignancies. *Cancer Genet Cytogenet* 30:63, 1988.
361. Melo JV, Hegde U, Parreira A, et al: Splenic B cell lymphoma with circulating villous lymphocytes: Differential diagnosis of B cell leukemias with large spleens. *J Clin Pathol* 40:642, 1987.
362. Nieman RS, Sullivan AF, Jaffe R: Malignant lymphoma simulating leukemic reticuloendotheliosis. A clinicopathologic study of ten cases. *Cancer* 43:329, 1979.
363. Isaacs R: Lymphosarcoma cell leukemia. *Ann Intern Med* 11:657, 1937.
364. Spiro S, Galton DAG, Wiltshaw E, et al: Follicular lymphoma: a survey of 75 cases with special reference to the syndrome resembling chronic lymphocytic leukemia. *Br J Cancer* 31(suppl II): 60, 1975.
365. Come SE, Jaffe ES, Anderson JC, et al: Non-Hodgkin's lymphomas in leukemic phase: Clinicopathologic correlations. *Am J Med* 69:667, 1980.
366. Melo JV, Robinson DSF, de Oliveira MP, et al: Morphology and immunology of circulating cells in the leukemic phase of follicular lymphoma. *J Clin Pathol* 41:951, 1988.
367. Barr RD, Fialkow PJ: Clonal origin of chronic myelocytic leukemia. *N Engl J Med* 289:307, 1973.
368. Fialkow PJ, Jacobson RJ, Papayannopoulou T: Chronic myelocytic leukemia. Clonal origin in a stem cell common to the granulocyte, erythrocyte, platelet and monocyte/macrophage. *Am J Med* 63:125, 1977.
369. Martin PJ, Najfeld V, Hansen JA, et al: Involvement of the B-lymphoid system in chronic myelogenous leukemia. *Nature* 287:49, 1980.
370. Koeffler HP, Levine AM, Sparkes M, et al: Chronic myelocytic leukemia: Eosinophils involved in the malignant clone. *Blood* 55:1063, 1980.
371. Nowell PC, Hungerford DA: A minute chromosome in human chronic granulocytic leukemia. *Science* 132:1497, 1960.
372. Rowley JD: A new consistent chromosomal abnormality in chronic myelogenous leukemia identified by quinacrine fluorescence and Geimsa staining. *Nature* 243:290, 1973.
373. Gupta CM, Kalousek DK, Eaves CJ, et al: Cytogenetic studies of early myeloid progenitor compartments in Ph positive chronic myeloid leukemia. 1. Persistence of Ph negative committed progenitors that are suppressed from differentiating in vivo. *Br J Haematol* 56:633, 1984.
374. Lisker R, Caras L, Mutchinik O, et al: Late appearing Philadelphia chromosome in two patients with chronic myelogenous leukemia. *Blood* 56:812, 1980.
375. Kantarjian HM, Talpaz M, Gutterman JU: Chronic myelogenous leukemia—past, present, and future. *Hematol Pathol* 2:91, 1988.
376. Rowley JD: Ph-positive leukemia, including chronic myelogenous leukemia. *Clin Haematol* 9:55, 1978.
377. Lawler SD: The cytogenetics of chronic granulocytic leukemia. *Clin Haematol* 6:55, 1977.
378. Yunis JJ: Genes and chromosomes in the pathogenesis and prognosis of human cancers. *Adv Pathol* 2:143, 1989.
379. Kerman SL, Miller RB, Heritage DW: Translocation (1;17) in accelerating and blast phases of chronic myelogenous leukemia. *Cancer Genet Cytogenet* 20:269, 1986.

380. Gunz FW: Ionizing radiation and human leukemia, in Gunz FW, Henderson ES (eds), *Leukemia*, ed 4. New York, Grune and Stratton, 1983, p 359.
381. Gunz FW, Gunz JP, Veale AMO: Familial leukemia: A study of 909 families. *Scand J Haematol* 15:117, 1975.
382. Coulombel L, Kalousek DK, Evans CJ, et al: Long term marrow culture reveals chromosomally normal hematopoietic progenitor cells in patients with Philadelphia chromosome-positive chronic myelogenous leukemia. *N Engl J Med* 308:1493, 1983.
383. Hogge DE, Coulombel L, Kalousek DK, et al: Nonclonal hemopoietic progenitor cells detected in a G6PD heterozygote with chronic myelogenous leukemia revealed after long-term marrow cultures. *Am J Hematol* 24:389, 1987.
384. Koduro P, Goh JC, Allen SL, et al: Different patterns of chromosome and molecular brakage in classic Ph^1 chronic myelogenous leukemia (CML) and variant Ph^1 CML. *Hematol Pathol* 5:57, 1991.
385. Heisterkamp N, Stephenson JR, Groffen J, et al: Localization of the *c-abl* oncogene adjacent to a translocation breakpoint in chronic myelogenous leukemia. *Nature* 306:239, 1983.
386. Groffen J, Stephenson JR, Heisterkamp N, et al: Philadelphia chromosomal breakpoints are clustered within a limited region, *bcr*, on chromosome 22. *Cell* 36:93, 1984.
387. Shtivelman E, Lipshitz B, Gale RP, et al: Fused transcription of *abl* and *bcr* genes in chronic myelogenous leukemia. *Nature* 315:550, 1985.
388. Marcelle C, Gale RP, Prokocimer M, et al: Analysis of *bcr-abl* mRNA in chronic myelogenous leukemia patients and identification of a new *bcr*-related sequence in human DNA. *Genes Chrom Cancer* 1:172, 1989.
389. Chen SJ, Flandrin G, Daniel MT, et al: Philadelphia-positive acute leukemia: Lineage promiscuity and inconsistently rearranged breaking cluster region. *Leukemia* 2:261, 1988.
390. Kantajian HM, Dixon D, Keating MJ, et al: Characteristics of accelerated disease in chronic myelogenous leukemia. *Cancer* 61:1441, 1988.
391. Schilling RF, Crowley JJ: Prognostic signs in chronic myelogenous leukemia. *Am J Hematol* 7:1, 1979.
392. Theologides A: Unfavorable signs in patients with chronic myelogenous leukemia. *Ann Intern Med* 76:95, 1972.
393. Breton-Gorius J, Reyes F, Vernevt JP, et al: The blast crisis of chronic granulocytic leukemia. Megakaryocytic nature of cells revealed by presence of platelet-peroxidase: A cytochemical ultrastructural study. *Br J Haematol* 39:295, 1978.
394. Ekblom M, Borgstrom G, Willebrand E, et al: Erythroid blast crisis in chronic myelogenous leukemia. *Blood* 62:591, 1983.
395. Allen SL, Coleman M: Terminal-phase chronic myelogenous leukemia: Approaches to treatment. *Cancer Invest* 3:491, 1985.
396. Kantarjian HM, Keating MJ, Talpaz M, et al: Chronic myelogenous leukemia in blast crisis. Analysis of 242 patients. *Am J Med* 83:445, 1987.
397. Gralnick HR, Harbor J, Vogel C: Myelofibrosis in chronic granulocytic leukemia. *Blood* 37:152, 1971.
398. Castro-Malaspina H, Schaison G, Passe S, et al: Subacute and chronic myelomonocytic leukemia in children (juvenile CML). *Cancer* 54:675, 1984.
399. Altman AJ, Baehner RL: In vitro colony forming characteristics of chronic granulocytic leukemia in childhood. *J Pediatr* 86:221, 1975.
400. Grier HE: Chronic myeloproliferative disorders and myelodysplasia, in Nathan DG, Oski FA (eds), *Hematology of Infancy and Childhood*, ed 3. Philadelphia, WB Saunders, 1987, p 1064.
401. Altman AJ: Chronic leukemia of childhood, in Pizzo PA, Poplack DG (eds), *Principles and Practice of Pediatric Oncology*. Philadelphia, JB Lippincott, 1989, p 383.
402. Mays JA, Neerhout RC, Baby GC, et al: Juvenile chronic granulocytic leukemia. Emphasis on cutaneous manifestation and underlying neurofibromatosis. *Am J Dis Child* 134:654, 1980.
403. Herrod HG, Dow LW, Sullivan JL: Persistent Epstein-Barr infection mimicking juvenile chronic myelogenous leukemia: Immunologic and hematologic studies. *Blood* 61:1098, 1983.
404. Palmer CG, Provisor AJ, Weaver DD, et al: Juvenile chronic granulocytic leukemia in a patient with trisomy 8, neurofibromatosis, and prolonged Epstein-Barr virus infection. *J Pediatr* 102:888, 1983.
405. Maurer HC, Vida LN, Hong GR: Similarities of the erythrocytes in juvenile chronic myelogenous leukemia to fetal erythrocytes. *Blood* 39:778, 1972.
406. Travis SF: Fetal erythropoiesis in juvenile chronic myelocytic leukemia. *Blood* 62:602, 1983.
407. Ghione F, Merucci C, Symann M: Cytogenetic investigation in childhood chronic myelocytic leukemia. *Cancer Genet Cytogenet* 20:317, 1986.
408. You W, Weisbrot IM: Chronic neutrophilic leukemia. Report of two cases and review of the literature. *Am J Clin Pathol* 72:233, 1979.
409. Jakson IMD, Clark RM: A case of neutrophilic leukemia. *Am J Clin Sci* 249:72, 1965.
410. Silverstein CB, Zellner DC, Shivakumar BN, et al: Neutrophilic leukemia. *Ann Intern Med* 80:110, 1974.
411. Berman RM, Kjeldsberg CR, Pangalis GA, et al: Chronic monocytic leukemia in adults. *Cancer* 48:2239, 1981.
412. Benvenisti DS, Ultmann JE: Eosinophilic leukemia. Report of five cases and review of the literature. *Ann Intern Med* 71:731, 1969.

413. Stockdill G, Hartley SE, Allan NC: Eosinophilic leukemia in association with a double Philadelphia chromosome. *Postgrad Med J* 56:268, 1980.
414. Weinfeld A, Westin J, Swolin B: Ph¹ negative eosinophilic leukemia with trisomy 8. *Scand J Haematol* 18:413, 1977.
415a. Travis WD, Li CY, Hoagland HC, et al: Mast cell leukemia: Report of a case and review of the literature. *Mayo Clin Proc* 61:957, 1986.
415b. Metcalfe DD: Classification and diagnosis of mastocytosis: Current status. *J Invest Dermatol* 96:2S, 1991.
416. van Kammen E: Generalized mastocytosis. *Acta Haematol* 52:129, 1974.
417. Lennert K, Parwaresch MR: Mast cells and mast cell neoplasia: A review. *Histopathology* 3:349, 1979.
418. Fine JD: Mastocytosis. *Int J Dermatol* 19:117, 1980.
419. Jane SM, Sutherland R, Salem HH: Malignant systemic mastocytosis. *Aust NZ J Med* 18:610, 1988.
420. Travis WD, Li CY, Yam LT, et al: Significance of systemic mast cell disease with associated hematologic disorders. *Cancer* 62:965, 1988.
421. Kyle RA, Pease GL: Basophilic leukemia. *Arch Intern Med* 118:205, 1966.
422. Jones SE, Rosenberg SA, Kaplan HS: Non-Hodgkin's lymphomas: 1. Bone marrow involvement. *Cancer* 29:954, 1972.
423. Dick F, Bloomfield CD, Brunning RD: Incidence, cytology and histopathology of non-Hodgkin's lymphomas in the bone marrow. *Cancer* 33:1382, 1974.
424. Coller BS, Chabner BA, Gralnick HR: Frequencies and patterns of bone marrow biopsies in non-Hodgkin's lymphomas: Observations on the value of bilateral biopsies. *Am J Hematol* 3:105, 1977.
425. Bennett JM, Cain KC, Glick JH, et al: The significance of bone marrow involvement in non-Hodgkin's lymphomas: The Eastern Cooperative Oncology Group experience. *J Clin Oncol* 4:1462, 1986.
426. Mckenna RW, Hernandez JA: Bone marrow in malignant lymphoma. *Hematol Oncol Clin North Am* 2:617, 1988.
427. Ebie N, Loew JM, Gregory SA: Bilateral trephine bone marrow biopsy for staging non-Hodgkin's lymphoma—a second look. *Hematol Pathol* 3:29, 1989.
428. Brunning RD, Bloomfield CD, McKenna RW, et al: Bilateral trephine bone marrow biopsies in lymphoma and other neoplastic diseases. *Ann Intern Med* 82:365, 1975.
429. Kadin ME: Possible origin of the Reed-Sternberg cell from an interdigitating cell. *Cancer Treat Rep* 66:601, 1982.
430. Strauchen JA, Dimitriu-Bona A: Immunopathology of Hodgkin's disease: Characterization of Reed-Sternberg cells with monoclonal antibodies. *Am J Pathol* 123:293, 1986.
431. Knowel DM, Neri A, Pelicci PG, et al: Immunoglobulin and T-cell receptor beta-chain gene rearrangement analysis of Hodgkin's disease: Implications for lineage determination and differential diagnosis. *Proc Natl Acad Sci USA* 83:7942, 1986.
432. Stein H, Mason DY, Gerdes J, et al: The expression of the Hodgkin's disease associated antigen Ki-1 in reactive and neoplastic lymphoid tissue: Evidence that Reed-Sternberg cells and histiocytic malignancies are derived from activated lymphoid cells. *Blood* 66:848, 1985.
433. Anastasi J, Variakojis D: Heterogeneity in Hodgkin's disease: No simple answer for a complex disorder. *Hum Pathol* 19:1251, 1988.
434. Bartl R, Frisch B, Burkhardt R, et al: Assessment of bone marrow histology in Hodgkin's disease. Correlation with clinical factors. *Br J Haematol* 51:345, 1982.
435. Myers CE, Chabner BA, DeVita VT, et al: Bone marrow involvement in Hodgkin's disease: Pathology and response to MOPP chemotherapy. *Blood* 44:197, 1974.
436. O'Carroll DI, McKenna RW, Brunning RD: Bone marrow manifestations of Hodgkin's disease. *Cancer* 38:1717, 1976.
437. Rosenberg SA: Hodgkin's disease of the bone marrow. *Cancer Res* 31:1733, 1971.
438. Rappaport H, Berard CW, Butler JJ, et al: Report of the Committee on Histopathological Criteria Contributing to Staging of Hodgkin's Disease. *Cancer Res* 31:1864, 1971.
439. Pinkus GS, Said JW: Hodgkin's disease, lymphocyte predominant type—a distinct entity? Unique staining profile for L+H variants for Reed-Sternberg cells defined by monoclonal antibodies to leukocyte common antigen, granulocyte specific antigen, and B cell specific antigen. *Am J Pathol* 118:1, 1985.
440. Hsu SM, Yang K, Jaffe ES: Phenotypic expression of Hodgkin's and Reed-Sternberg cells in Hodgkin's disease. *Am J Pathol* 118:209, 1985.
441. Thangavelu M, le Beau MM: Chromosomal abnormalities in Hodgkin's disease. *Hematol Oncol Clin North Am* 3:221, 1989.
442. Kristofferssen U, Heim S, Mandahl N, et al: Cytogenetic studies in Hodgkin's disease. *Acta Pathol Microbiol Immunol Scand* 95:289, 1987.
443. Rowley JD: Chromosomes in Hodgkin's disease. *Cancer Treat Rep* 66:639, 1982.
444. Schouten HC, Sanger WG, Armitage JO: Chromosomal abnormalities in malignant lymphoma and Hodgkin's disease. *Leuk Lymph* 5:93, 1991.

445. Schouten HC, Sanger WA, Duggan M, et al: Chromosomal abnormalities in Hodgkin's disease. *Blood* 73:2149, 1989.
446. Henry-Amar M, Somers R: Survival outcome after Hodgkin's disease: A report from the international data base on Hodgkin's disease. *Semin Oncol* 17:758, 1990.
447. National Cancer Institute sponsored study of classifications of non-Hodgkin's lymphoma. Summary and description of a working formulation for clinical usage. The non-Hodgkin's lymphoma pathologic classification project. *Cancer* 49:2112, 1982.
448. Kluin PM, Krieken JH, Kleiverda K, et al: Discordant morphologic characteristics of B-cell lymphomas in bone marrow and lymph node biopsies. *Am J Clin Pathol* 94:59, 1990.
449. Freeman C, Berg JW, Culter SJ: Occurrence and prognosis of extranodal lymphomas. *Cancer* 29:252, 1972.
450. Clayton F, Butler JJ, Ayala AG, et al: Non-Hodgkin's lymphoma in bone. Pathology and radiologic features with clinical correlates. *Cancer* 60:2494, 1987.
451. Pangalis GA, Nathwani BN, Rappaport H: Malignant lymphoma, well differentiated lymphocytic: Its relationship with chronic lymphocytic leukemia and macroglobulinemia of Waldenstrom. *Cancer* 39:999, 1977.
452. Bartl R, Frisch B, Mahl G, et al: Bone marrow histology in Waldenstrom's macroglobulinemia. Clinical relevance and subtype recognition. *Scand J Haematol* 31:359, 1983.
453. Reed M, McKenna RW, Bridges R, et al: morphologic manifestations of monoclonal gammopathies. *Am J Clin Pathol* 76:8, 1981.
454. Brunning RD, McKenna RW: Bone marrow manifestations of malignant lymphoma and lymphoma-like conditions, in Sommers C, Rosen PP (eds), *Pathology Annual*, Part 1. New York, Appleton-Century-Crofts, 1979, p 59.
455. Bartl R, Frisch B, Burkhardt R, et al: Lymphoproliferations in the bone marrow: Identification and evaluation, classification and staging. *J Clin Pathol* 37:233, 1984.
456. Stein H, Lennert K, Feller AC, et al: Immunohistological analysis of human lymphoma: Correlation of histological and immunological categories. *Adv Cancer Res* 42:67, 1984.
457. Picker LJ, Weiss LM, Mediros LM, et al: Immunophenotypic criteria for the diagnosis of non-Hodgkin's lymphomas. *Am J Pathol* 128:181, 1987.
458. Ritz J, Nadler LM, Bhan AK, et al: Expression of common acute lymphoblastic leukemia antigen (CALLA) by lymphomas of B-cell and T-cell lineage. *Blood* 58:648, 1981.
459. Deegan MJ: Membrane antigen analysis in the diagnosis of lymphoid leukemias and lymphomas. *Arch Pathol Lab Med* 113:606, 1989.
460. Swerdlow SH, Murray LJ, Habeshaw JA, et al: Lymphocytic lymphoma B-chronic lymphocytic leukemia—an immunohistopathological study of peripheral B lymphocyte neoplasia. *Br J Cancer* 50:587, 1984.
461. Spier CM, Grogan TM, Fielder K, et al: Immunophenotypes in "well-differentiated" lymphoproliferative disorders, with emphasis on small lymphocytic lymphoma. *Hum Pathol* 17:1126, 1986.
462. Farhi DC: Germinal centers in the bone marrow. *Hematol Pathol* 3:133, 1989.
463. Hanson CA, Brunning RD, Gajl-Peczalka KJ, et al: Bone marrow manifestations of peripheral T-cell lymphoma. *Am J Clin Pathol* 86:449, 1986.
464. Auger MJ, Nash JRG, Mackie MJ: Marrow involvement with T cell lymphoma initially presenting as abnormal myelosis. *J Clin Pathol* 39:134, 1986.
465. Pangalis GA, Moran EM, Rappaport H: Blood and bone marrow findings in angioimmunoblastic lymphadenopathy. *Blood* 51:71, 1978.
466. Guarda LA, Butler JJ: Lymphoma versus AIDS. *Am J Clin Pathol* 80:546, 1983.
467. Duggan MJ, Weisenburger DD, Sun NC, et al: Bone marrow findings in immunodeficiency syndromes. *Hematol Oncol Clin North Am* 2:637, 1988.
468. Nathwani BN, Rappaport H, Moran EM, et al: Malignant lymphoma arising in angioimmunoblastic lymphadenopathy. *Cancer* 41:578, 1978.
469. Nathwani BN, Winberg CD, Bearman RM: Angioimmunoblastic lymphadenopathy with dysproteinemia and its progression to malignant lymphoma, in Jaffe ES (ed), *Surgical Pathology of the Lymph Nodes and Related Organs*. Philadelphia, WB Saunders, 1985, p 57.
470. Nathwani BN, Kim H, Rappaport H: Malignant lymphoma, lymphoblastic. *Cancer* 38:964, 1976.
471. McKenna RW, Parkin J, Brunning R: Morphological and ultrastructural characteristics of T-cell acute lymphoblastic leukemia. *Cancer* 44:1290, 1979.
472. Yunis JJ: Genes and chromosomes in the pathogenesis and prognosis of human cancers. *Adv Pathol* 2:147, 1989.
473. Magrath IT: Malignant non-Hodgkin's lymphoma, in Pizzo PA, Poplack DG (eds), *Principles and Practice of Pediatric Oncology*. Philadelphia, JB Lippincott, 1989, p 415.
474. Taub R, Kirsch I, Morton C, et al: Translocation of the c-myc gene into the immunoglobulin heavy chain locus in human Burkitt lymphoma and murine plasmacytoma cell. *Proc Natl Acad Sci USA* 79:7837, 1982.
475. Dall-Favera R, Bergni M, Erikson J, et al: Human

c-myc oncogene is located on the region of chromosome 8 that is translocated in Burkitt lymphoma cells. *Proc Natl Acad Sci USA* 79:7824, 1982.

476. Fifth International Workshop on Chromosomes in Leukemia-Lymphoma: Correlation of chromosome abnormalities with histologic and immunologic characteristics in non-Hodgkin's lymphoma and adult T cell leukemia-lymphoma. *Blood* 70:1554, 1987.

477. Burke JS: The histopathologic classification of non-Hodgkin's lymphomas: Ambiguities in the Working Formulation and two newly reported categories. *Semin Oncol* 17:3, 1990.

478. Simon R, Durrleman S, Hoppe RT, et al: The non-Hodgkin lymphoma pathologic classification project. Long-term follow-up of 1153 patients with non-Hodgkin lymphomas. *Ann Intern Med* 109:939, 1988.

479. Weisenburger DD, Duggan MJ, Perry DA, et al: Non-Hodgkin's lymphomas of mantle zone origin. *Pathol Annu* 26:139, 1991.

480. Weisenburger DD, Nathwani BN, Diamond LW, et al: Malignant lymphoma, intermediate lymphocytic type: A clinicopathologic study of 42 cases. *Cancer* 48:1415, 1981.

481. Weisenburger DD, Linder J, Daley DT, et al: Intermediate lymphocytic lymphoma: An immunohistologic study with comparison to other lymphocytic lymphomas. *Hum Pathol* 18:781, 1987.

482. Mori N, Oka K, Kojima M: Immunohistochemical study of mantle zone lymphoma. *Am J Clin Pathol* 89:143, 1988.

483a. Sheibani K, Sohn CC, Burke JS, et al: Monocytoid B-cell lymphoma: A novel B-cell neoplasm. *Am J Pathol* 124:310, 1986.

483b. Sheibani K, Burke JB, Swartz WG, et al: Monocytoid B-cell lymphoma. Clinicopathologic study of 21 cases of a unique type of low-grade lymphoma. *Cancer* 62:1531, 1988.

484a. Ngan B-Y, Warnke RA, Wilson M, et al: Monocytoid B-cell lymphoma: A study of 36 cases. *Hum Pathol* 22:409, 1991.

484b. Shin SS, Sheibani K, Fishleder A, et al: Monocytoid B-cell lymphoma in patients with Sjogren's syndrome: A clinicopathologic study of 13 patients. *Hum Pathol* 22:422, 1991.

485. Agnarsson BA, Kadin ME: Ki-1 positive large cell lymphoma. A morphologic and immunologic study of 19 cases. *Am J Surg Pathol* 12:264, 1988.

486a. Mason DY, Bastard C, Rimokh R, et al: CD30-positive large cell lymphomas associated with chromosomal translocation involving 5q35. *Br J Haematol* 74:161, 1990.

486b. Kinney MC, Geer JP, Glik AD, et al: Anaplastic large-cell Ki-1 malignant lymphomas. Recognition, biological and clinical implications. *Pathol Ann* 26:1, 1991.

487. Kadin ME, Said JW: Pathology of malignant lymphoma. *Curr Op Oncol* 2:822, 1990.

488. Lipford EH, Margolick JB, Longo DL, et al: Angiocentric immunoproliferative lesions: A clinicopathologic spectrum of post-thymic T-cell proliferations. *Blood* 72:1674, 1988.

489. Sheibani K, Battifora H, Winberg CD, et al: Further evidence that "malignant angioendotheliomatosis" is an angiotropic large cell lymphoma. *N Engl J Med* 314:943, 1986.

490. Stroup RM, Sheibani K, Moncada A, et al: Angiotropic (intravascular) large cell lymphoma. A clinicopathologic study of seven cases with unique clinical presentations. *Cancer* 66:1781, 1990.

491. Warnke R, Miller R, Grogan T, et al: Immunologic phenotype in 30 patients with diffuse large cell lymphoma. *N Engl J Med* 303:293, 1980.

492. Isaacson P, Wright DH, Jones DB: Malignant lymphoma of true histiocytic (monocyte/macrophage) origin. *Cancer* 51:80, 1983.

493. Thomas P, Said JW, Rosenfelt FP, et al: True histiocytic lymphoma: An immunohistochemical and ultrastructural study of two cases. *Am J Clin Pathol* 81:243, 1984.

494. Mirchandani I, Shah I, Palutke M, et al: True histiocytic lymphoma. A report of four cases. *Cancer* 52:1911, 1983.

495. Levine EG, Hanson CA, Jaszcs W, et al: True histiocytic lymphoma. *Semin Oncol* 18:39, 1991.

496. Hsu S-M, Ho Y-S, Hsu P-L: Lymphoma of true histiocytic origin. Expression of differential phenotypes in so-called true histiocytic lymphoma and malignant histiocytosis. *Am J Pathol* 138:1389, 1991.

497. Ladish S, Jaffe ES: The histiocytoses in Pizzo AP, Poplack DG (eds), *Principles and Practice of Pediatric Oncology*, Philadelphia, JB Lippincott, 1989, p 491.

498. Lampert IA, Catovsky D, Bergier N: Malignant histiocytosis: A clinicopathological study of 12 cases. *Am J Clin Pathol* 40:65, 1978.

499. DiSant'-Agnese PA, Ettinger LJ, Ryan CK, et al: Histiomonocytic malignancy—a spectrum of disease in an 11-month-old infant. *Cancer* 52:1417, 1983.

500. Ducaman BS, Wick MR, Morgan TW, et al: Malignant histiocytosis: A clinical, histologic, and immunohistochemical study of 20 cases. *Hum Pathol* 15:368, 1984.

501. Esseltine DW, Leeuw NKM, Berry GR: Malignant histiocytosis. *Cancer* 52:1904, 1983.

502. Huhn D, Meister R: Malignant histiocytosis: Morphologic and cytochemical findings. *Cancer* 42:1349, 1978.

503. Falini B, Pileri S, De Solas I, et al: Peripheral T-cell lymphoma associated with hemophagocytic syndrome. *Blood* 75:434, 1990.

504. Chan EYT, Chan GTC, Todd D, et al: Peripheral T-cell lymphoma presenting as hemophagocytic syndrome. *Hematol Oncol* 7:275, 1989.
505. Robb-Smith AHT: Before our time: Half a century of histiocytic medullary reticulosis: A T-cell teaser? *Histopathology* 17:279, 1990.
506. Abe R, Akaike Y, Yokoyama A, et al: High incidence of 17p13 chromosomal abnormalities in malignant histiocytosis. *Cancer* 65:2689, 1990.
507. Ben-Ezra J, Bailey A, Azumi N, et al: Malignant histiocytosis X—a distinct clinicopathologic entity. *Cancer* 68:1050, 1991.
508. Chan WC, Zaatai G: Lymph node interdigitating reticulum cell sarcoma. *Am J Clin Pathol* 85:739, 1986.
509. Monda L, Warnke R, Rosai J: A primary lymph node malignancy with features suggestive of dendritic reticulum cell differentiation: A report of four cases. *Am J Pathol* 122:562, 1986.
510. Rabkin MS, Kjeldsberg CR, Hammond ME, et al: Clinical, ultrastructural, immunohistochemical and DNA content of lymphomas having features of interdigitating reticulum cells. *Cancer* 61:1594, 1988.

7 PLASMA CELL DYSCRASIA

Plasma cells are the end products of the B-lymphocyte lineage. They account for about 1–2% of the cells in normal bone marrow and are increased in a variety of pathologic conditions, such as viral and bacterial infections; hemolytic, megaloblastic and iron deficiency anemias; marrow hypoplasia; collagen vascular disorders; idiopathic thrombocytopenic purpura; diabetes mellitus; cardiovascular diseases and malignancies (carcinomas, lymphomas, CML).[1-3] This reactive plasmacytosis is polyclonal and usually does not exceed 15% of the bone marrow cells, though occasionally it may reach up to 50% or even more[2,3] (Figure 7-1). Morphologic distinction between a reactive and a malignant process is at times difficult. Overall, in reactive plasmacytosis, plasma cells are mostly mature, nucleocytoplasmic asynchrony is usually not a prominent feature, nucleoli are infrequent and plasma cells rarely appear in clusters.

"Plasma cell dyscrasia" and "monoclonal gammopathy" are terms used to imply a monoclonal proliferation of plasma cells and/or of Ig-secreting B lymphocytes. The monoclonal cells in each patient express identical Ig properties such as a single light chain (kappa or lambda), and demonstrate identical heavy and light chain Ig gene rearrangements.

ETIOLOGY AND PATHOGENESIS

The etiology and pathogenesis of monoclonal gammopathies are not known. Studies on experimental animals strongly suggest that deregulation in immune function may play a role in the pathogenesis of these disorders. For example, evidence of an increased incidence of monoclonal gammopathies in thymectomized aging C57BL/KalwRij and CBA/BrARij mice was reported by Radl et al.[4,5] These investigators proposed following events for the development of monoclonal gammopathies in the experimental animals: (1) impairment of T-cell function and lack of B-cell suppression by T cells and (2) a spontaneous or virus-induced mutation resulting in monoclonal proliferation of a B-cell clone.

An inverted helper/suppressor ratio has been reported in the peripheral blood lymphocytes of patients with plasma cell myeloma and in monoclonal gammopathies of undetermined significance in humans.[6-8] There is also a report of the development of IgA multiple myeloma in a patient with aplastic anemia 10 months after being treated with antithymocyte globulin.[9]

Radiation appears to be one of the contributing factors in the development of monoclonal gammopathies. An increased incidence of multiple myeloma has been reported in atomic bomb survivors, in radiation workers at the Sellafield nuclear power plant in England, and in patients who received more than 50 rads.[10-12]

Genetic factors may also play a role in the development of monoclonal gammopathies in some patients. There are several reports of familial clusters of two or more first-degree relatives with multiple myeloma.[13-15]

CLINICOPATHOLOGIC FEATURES

The incidence of monoclonal gammopathies increases with age and is extremely rare under the age of 40. Monoclonal gammopathies are divided into five major clinicopathologic subtypes: (1) monoclonal gammopathy of undetermined significance ("benign" monoclonal gammopathy), (2) plasma cell myeloma (multiple myeloma) and plasmacytoma, (3) Waldenstrom's macroglobulinemia and plasmacytoid

Plasma Cell Dyscrasia

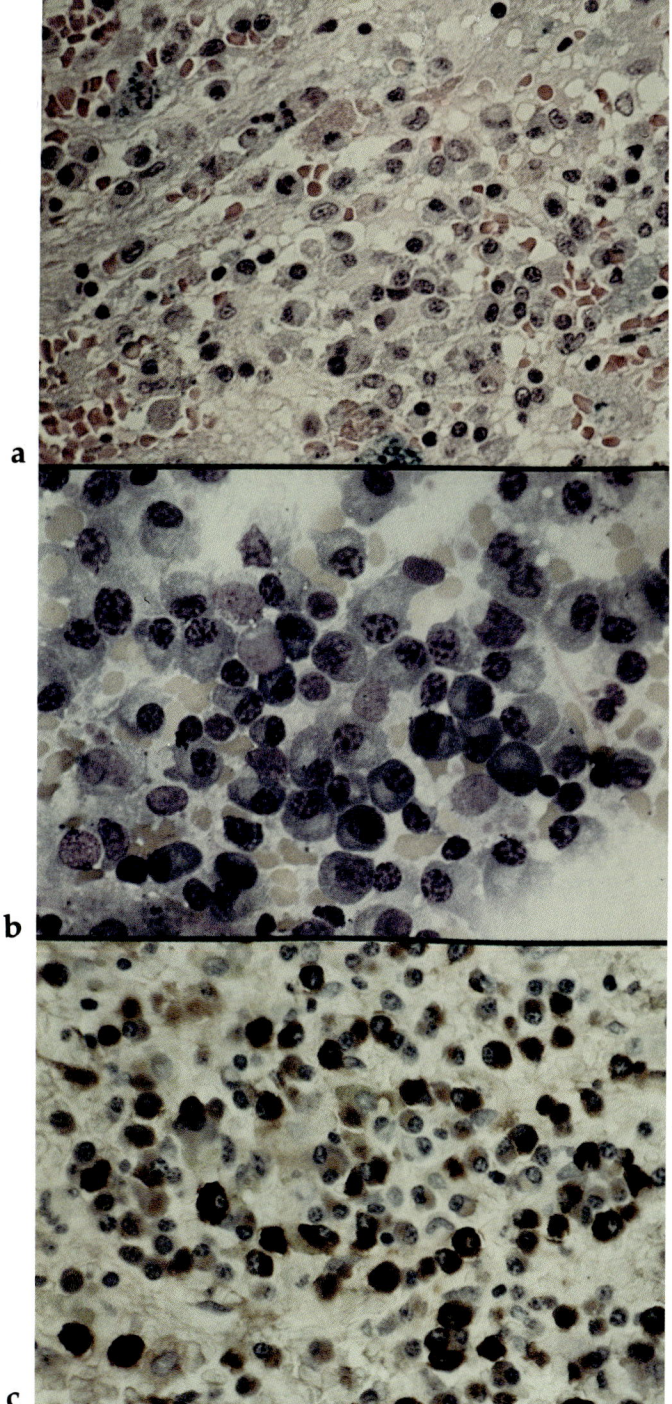

Figure 7-1. Marked reactive plasmacytosis in a patient who recently had chemotherapy for AML. (a) Bone marrow clot section; (b) bone marrow smear; (c) marrow clot section stained for Ig kappa light chain by immunoperoxidase technique. Some of the plasma cells are positive and some are negative. The negative ones express Ig lambda light chain (not shown), indicating a ployclonal reactive process.

B-cell lymphomas, (4) heavychain disorders and (5) amyloidosis and amyloidomas associated with light chain Ig. Overall, the incidence of each Ig class in monoclonal gammopathies correlates well with the level of that particular Ig in normal serum. For example, the highest concentration of serum Ig in normal conditions belongs to the IgG class, and IgG gammopathy is the most frequent (60%) form of gammopathy. Monoclonal gammopathies of IgA, IgM, IgD and IgE account for about 20, 9, <1 and <1% of gammopathies, respectively.[16]

Monoclonal Gammopathy of Undetermined Significance

Monoclonal gammopathy of undetermined significance (MGUS) is a clinically indolent and stable condition characterized by <5% plasma cells in the bone marrow, <3 g/dl monoclonal Ig in the serum, lack or trace amounts of Bence Jones protein in the urine, and lack of anemia, hypercalcemia, renal insufficiency or osteolytic lesions.[17] Other terms applied to this clinical entity include "benign," "idiopathic," "asymptomatic" and "nonmyelomatous" gammopathies. MGUS is a disorder of old age, affecting about 3% of persons aged over 70 years.[18-20] Approximately 10% of MGUS patients develop a malignant course at 5 years,[21] and the rate almost doubles at 10 years.[17] The presence of Bence Jones (light chain) proteinuria, an elevated level of serum beta-2-microglobulin, increased acid phosphatase activity, reduced numbers of CD4+ T cells and increased numbers of Ig-secreting cells and idiotype-bearing lymphocytes in the peripheral blood are strongly suggestive of a malignant process in borderline cases.[22-28] Although Bence Jones proteinuria has been recognized as a feature of malignant monoclonal gammopathies, a number of patients with Bence Jones proteinuria show a benign course with a long-standing, stable condition (idiopathic Bence Jones proteinuria).[23,29] According to Kyle and associates, the most reliable mean of differentiating a benign course from a malignant one is the serial measurement of monoclonal protein in the serum and urine and periodic evaluation of clinical and laboratory features to determine whether progression to malignancy has occurred.[17,29] Since MGUS behaves as a premalignant condition in a significant proportion of patients, the use of the term "benign" monoclonal gammopathy for this condition is inappropriate.

Multiple Myeloma and Plasmacytoma

Plasma cell neoplasms may develop as multifocal lesions in the bone marrow (multiple myeloma) or as a solitary mass in the bone or soft tissues (plasmacytoma).

Multiple Myeloma

Multiple myeloma (MM), or plasma cell myeloma or myelomatosis, is a multifocal plasma cell neoplasm of the bone marrow with overproduction of monoclonal Ig (paraprotein, M component) or Ig light-chains (Bence Jones protein) often associated with anemia, multiple osteolytic lesions, hypercalcemia, abnormal renal function and increased susceptibility to infections. The peak period of incidence is between 50 and 60 years, with no sex predilection. Involvement below age 40 is extremely rare.

The associated destructive bone lesions in MM are responsible for the most distressing clinical features, such as intractable bone pain, fractures and hypercalcemia. The available data suggest that osteoclastic activation is the primary mechanism of osteolysis in this disorder.[30,31] The increased osteoclastic activity is probably due to the release of a local osteoclastic activating factor by MM cells.[32,33] A combination of bone resorption and impairment of renal function leads to hypercalcemia.

PATHOLOGY: Bone marrow examination is one of the key factors in the diagnosis of MM. However, because of the multifocal nature of the disease and random sampling of the bone marrow, marrow examination may sometimes not yield the diagnosis of MM. This happens in approximately 6% of patients with clinical and laboratory evidence of MM.[34,35] In addition, reactive plasmacytosis may resemble MM. Thus, the bone marrow examination should always be correlated with clinical, laboratory and radiologic findings. Based on the criteria established by the National Cancer Institute (NCI) and the Eastern Cooperative Oncology Group (ECOG), the requirements for the diagnosis of MM are the presence of monoclonal serum and/or urine protein and evidence of plasmacytoma (bone or soft tissue) or marrow plasmacytosis of >5% (NCI) to 10% (ECOG).[36,37]

Morphologic diagnosis of MM is relatively easy in classical cases. In such cases, bone marrow sections and smears show increased numbers of plasma cells, which may vary from small, patchy clusters to extensive marrow infiltration, with virtually complete replacement of normal hematopoietic cells (Figures 7-2 to 7-6). The presence of homogeneous nodules of plasma cells equal to or greater than one-half of a high-power microscopic field in marrow sections is considered one of the most reliable morphologic findings in the diagnosis of MM.[38] Increased osteoclastic activity is often evident when plasma cell clusters are

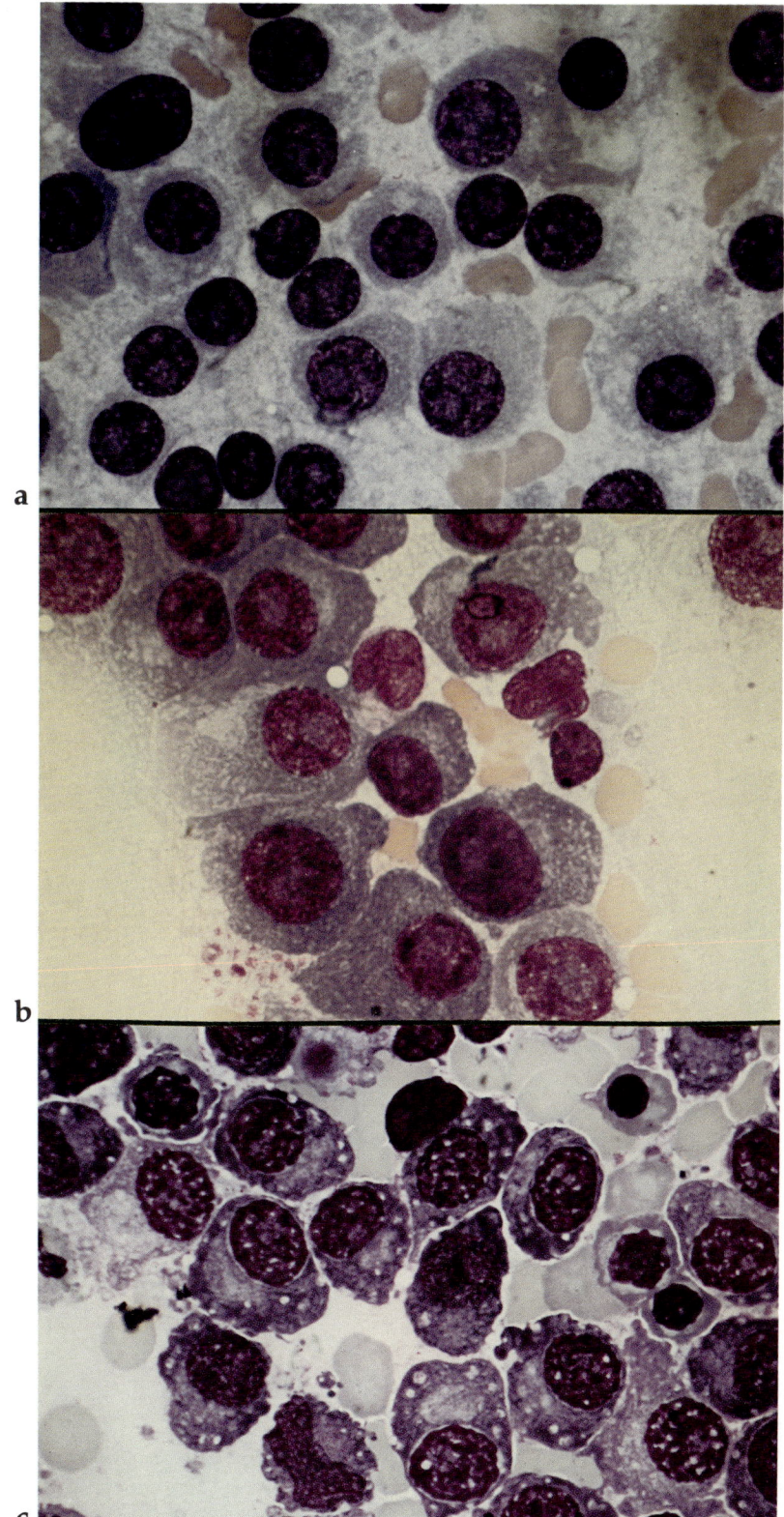

Figure 7-2. Bone marrow smears from patients with MM demonstrating plasma cells in immature (a), intermediate (b), and more mature (c) forms.

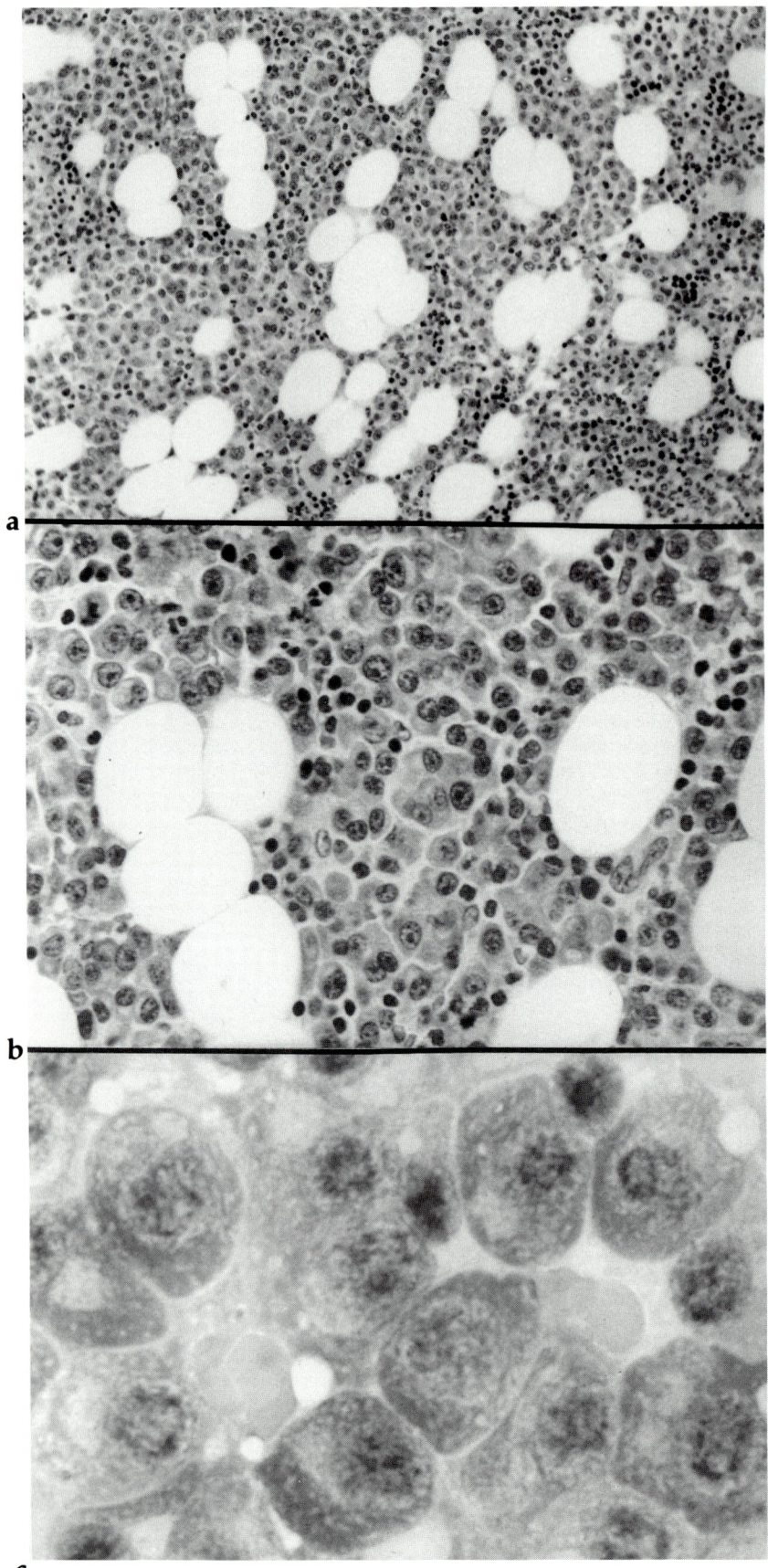

Figure 7-3. Bone marrow biopsy section (a, b) and smear (c) from a patient with MM exhibiting interstitial marrow infiltration by immature plasma cells.

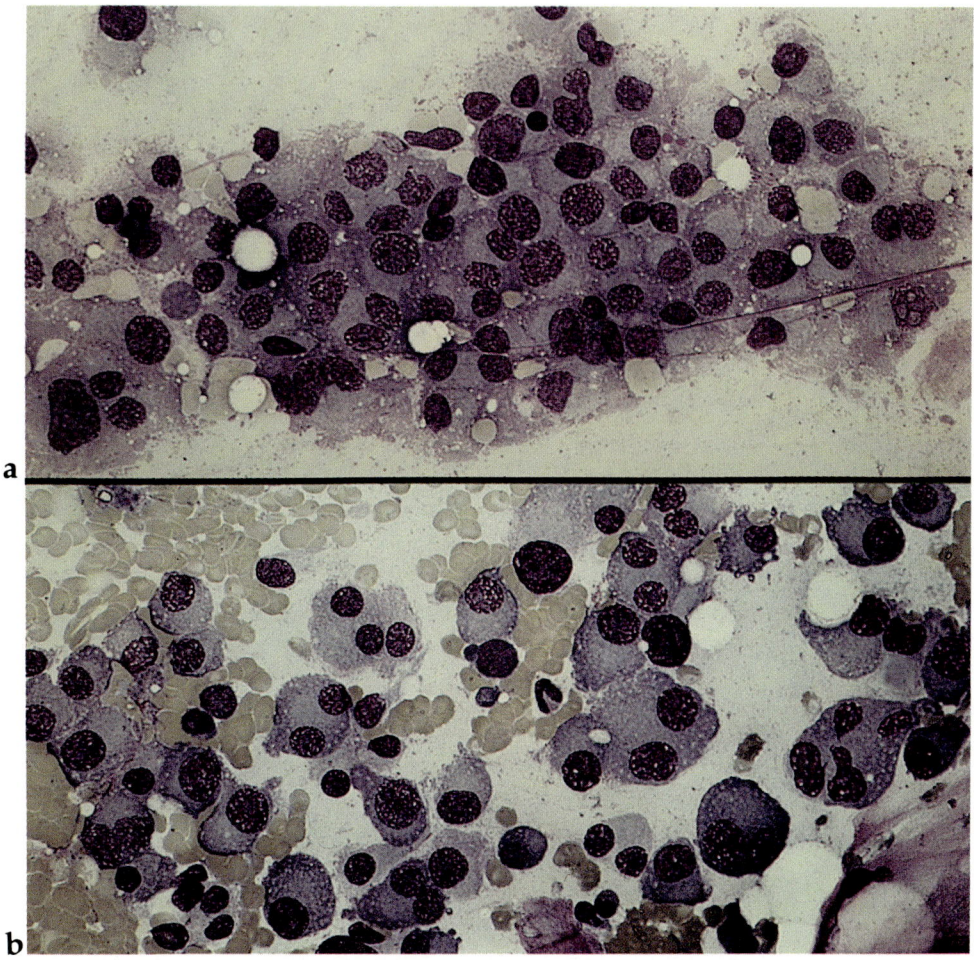

Figure 7-4. Bone marrow smears from two patients with MM demonstrating immature (a) and bi- and multinucleated (b) plasma cells.

in close proximity to bone trabeculae. Approximately 10% of the patients with MM show significant marrow fibrosis, which may lead to unsuccessful marrow aspiration and inadequate marrow smears.[39]

The neoplastic cells display a wide spectrum of morphology (see Figures 7-2 to 7-6). Some tumors are predominantly composed of mature plasma cells with minimal atypical changes, and others are composed of markedly pleomorphic cells with nuclear/cytoplasm asynchronism, finely dispersed nuclear chromatin, prominent nucleoli and pronounced multinuclearity (four or more nuclei per cell) (see Figures 7-2 and 7-4). A small proportion of MMs (2–15%) consists predominantly of plasmablasts.[40,41a] Plasma blasts are characterized by a large nucleus, a very prominent centrally located nucleolus and a moderate rim of basophilic cytoplasm with a faint perinuclear paler area (see Figures 7-2 and 7-6). Mott cells and Dutcher bodies (nuclear inclusions) may be present but are not pathognomonic features of MM (see Figures 7-5 and 7-6). MM cells express a monotypic cytoplasmic Ig (kappa or lambda) and are positive for PCA-1, PC-1 and CD38 (OKT 10) surface antigens.[41b] In addition, some MM cells may express CD10 (CALLA), myelomonocytic-associated antigens (such as CD13 and CD14), T-cell-associated antigens (such as CD2, CD3 and CD4),[42-44a] or NK-associated antigen CD56.[44b]

Several investigators have studied the correlation between MM morphology and prognosis.[38,39,45,46] In a clinicopathologic study of 676 cases, MM was classified into three major types: low-grade, intermediate-grade and high-grade.[39] Low-grade MM was the most frequent type, accounting for 71% of the

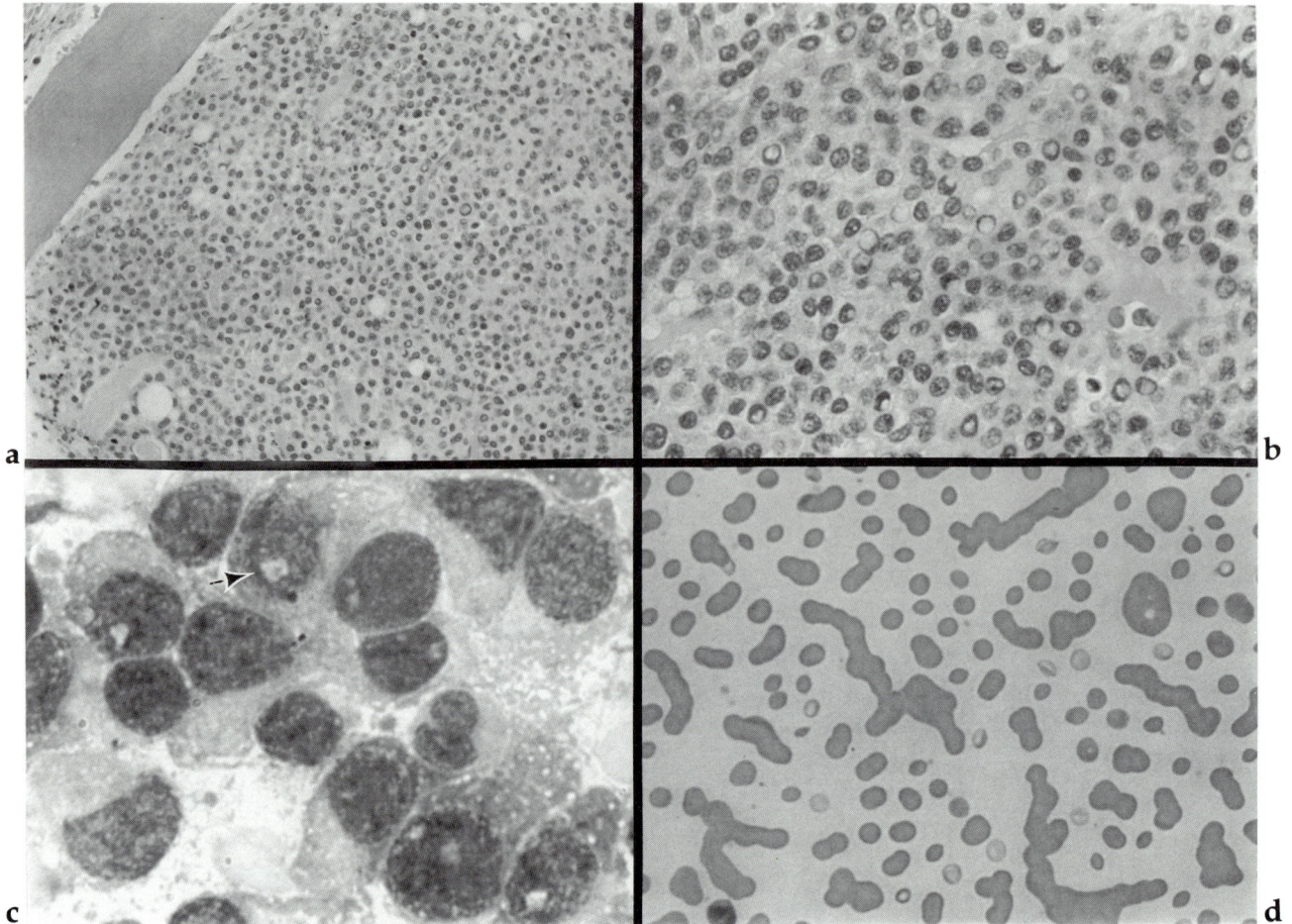

Figure 7-5. Multiple myeloma. (a, b) Bone marrow biopsy sections demonstrating diffuse infiltration with plasma cells, many with nuclear inclusions (Dutcher bodies); (c) bone marrow smear showing several immature plasma cells, some with nuclear inclusions (arrow); (d) peripheral blood smear exhibiting red blood cell rouleaux formation.

cases, with a median survival of 51 months from the onset of symptoms. This group consisted of either small, mature plasma cells (mean size, 13 μm) or mature plasma cells of normal size (mean size, 21 μm) (Marschalko type).

Intermediate-grade MM (28%) had a median survival of 23 months from the onset of symptoms. The tumors were composed of cleaved, polymorphous and asynchronous cell types (see Figure 7-4).

High-grade MM accounted for 20% of the cases, with a median survival of 9 months from the onset of symptoms. High-grade tumors were predominantly composed of plasmablasts. The association between poor prognosis and plasmablastic subtype has been confirmed by other investigators. In a report by Greipp and associates,[40] the plasmablastic group had an estimated survival of 10 months compared to 35 months for other groups. The cells of the plasmablastic subtype often express CD10 (CALLA) antigen.[42] Other frequent findings in patients with plasmablastic MM are elevated levels of Bence Jones protein (>1 g/24 hours), serum creatinine >2 g/dl, lambda light chain phenotype and labeling index >1.0%.[40]

Plasma cells are the predominant but not the only cell type involved in MM. Several investigators have shown the presence of a subpopulation of peripheral blood B lymphocytes expressing the same idiotype found in myeloma cells.[28,47-49a] In addition, Ig gene rearrangement studies by Southern blot analysis have shown identical rearranged Ig genes in the peripheral blood lymphocytes and myeloma cells in MM pa-

Plasma Cell Dyscrasia

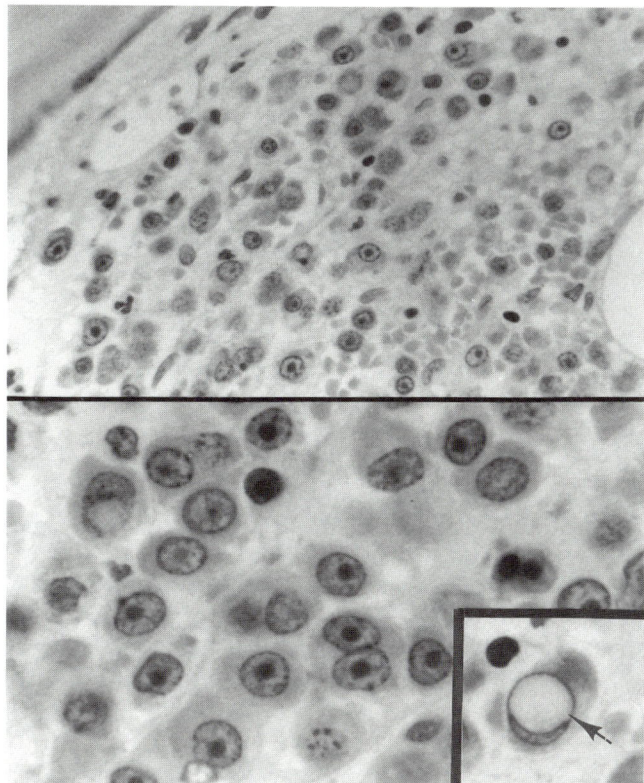

Figure 7-6. Bone marrow biopsy section from a patient with MM demonstrating immature plasma cells with prominent nucleoli (plasmablasts). The insert shows a Dutcher body (arrow).

tients.[49b] A pre-B-like myeloma has been reported by Grogan et al., characterized by the coexpression of cytoplasmic μ, CD10, TdT (pre-B phenotype), and PCA-1 and PC-1 (plasma cell antigens).[50] According to the authors, the pre-B myeloma cells may represent the stem cell population in MM.

CYTOGENETICS AND DNA ALTERATIONS: Approximately 50% of MM patients have an abnormal karyotype. The most common chromosomal abnormalities are trisomy 3, 5, 9 and 15 and monosomy 13 and 16.[51] Chromosomal translocations have also been reported in MM and include t(8;14)(q24;q32) and t(8;14)(q13;q32).[51] 8q24 and 11q13 are the sites of the *c-myc* and *bcl-1* proto-oncogenes, respectively, and 14q32 is the locus of the Ig heavy chain gene. Molecular changes suggestive of *c-myc* translocation and *bcl-1* rearrangement have been demonstrated.[52,53] Elevated levels of H-ras p21 protein have been reported in bone marrow cells of MM patients with active disease.[54] An inverse relationship has been found between the presence of trisomy 11 and H-ras p21 levels (H-ras is located on chromosome 11). DNA content analysis by flow cytometry demonstrates DNA aneuploidy in the majority of MM cases, with hyperdiploidy being the most common form.[55] An association between aneuploidy and advanced stage, shorter remission duration, and shorter patient survival has been reported by several investigators.[56-58]

OTHER PROGNOSTIC FACTORS: A number of staging systems have been developed for the identification of subsets of patients with a poor prognosis.[59,60] The most popular staging system is the one proposed by Durei et al., in which tumor mass is correlated with clinical features, response to therapy and survival.[59] This system has three stages:

Stage I (low tumor mass; $<0.6 \times 10^{12}$ myeloma cells/m^2) with the presence of all of the following:
Hemoglobin >10 g/dl
Serum calcium <12 mg/dl
Normal bone X-ray or solitary lytic lesion
Serum IgG value <5 mg/dl or IgA value <3 mg/dl
Urine light chain (Bence Jones) M component <4 g/24 hours

Stage II (intermediate tumor mass; $0.6–1.2 \times 10^{12}$ myeloma cells/m^2) with laboratory parameters fitting neither low nor high tumor mass criteria

Stage III (high tumor mass; $>1.2 \times 10^{12}$ myeloma cells/m^2) with one or more of the following:
Hemoglobin <8.5 g/dl
Serum calcium >12 mg/dl
Advanced lytic bone lesions
Serum IgG value >7 g/dl or IgA value >5 g/dl
Urine light chain (Bence Jones) M component >12 g/24 hours

Other factors associated with a poor prognosis include elevated serum creatinine (>2 mg/dl), presence of extramedullary disease, plasma cell leukemia, systemic amyloidosis, increased plasma cell acid phosphatase activity and a high plasma cell labeling index.[61-63] The CD10 (CALLA)-positive myeloma has been considered to be an aggressive subtype with a poor prognosis.[40] Multiple expression of myelomonocytic antigens, such as coexpression of CD13 and CD14, has been associated with more aggressive disease and a shorter survival duration.[41] In a recent study by Spier et al.[44] T-cell antigen-positive MMs demonstrated a very short survival, with 80% of patients dying within 5 months.

Solitary Plasmacytomas

Solitary plasmacytomas of bone and soft tissues are relatively rare and account for <10% of plasma cell neoplasms.[64,65] The upper respiratory tract and the oral cavity (nasal fossa, maxillary sinus, nasopharynx, base of the tongue and epiglottis) are the most frequent sites for extramedullary plasmacytomas, and flat and short bones (vertebral bodies, scapula, rib, ilium, and skull) are the predominant sites for bone plasmacytomas. Solitary plasmacytomas are morphologically indistinguishable from MM and show monotypic staining for kappa or lambda light chains by immunoenzyme techniques. In some patients who appear to have a solitary plasmacytoma, additional studies (bone survey and/or bone marrow examination) may disclose evidence of multifocal lesions (MM). However, a considerable proportion of patients with solitary plasmacytomas eventually develop MM. In one study, >55% of bone and >15% of extramedullary tumors progressed to MM within 10 years.[66] Tumors which consist predominantly of immature plasma cells have a higher incidence of progression to MM.[66] Up to 25% of solitary plasmacytomas may secrete a monoclonal Ig which is detectable in the serum and/or urine.[64] The prognosis of solitary plasmacytoma is significantly better than that of MM.

Other Variants of Monoclonal Plasma Cell Lesions

SMOLDERING MULTIPLE MYELOMA: Smoldering MM is an asymptomatic disorder with elevated monoclonal serum Ig (>3 g/dl) and bone marrow plasmacytosis ($\geq$10%), but with no evidence of osteolytic lesions (negative radiologic studies), hypercalcemia, anemia or renal failure.[39,67] Plasma cells are well differentiated and are diffusely intermixed with the normal hematopoietic cells. The clinical behavior of smoldering MM is very similar to that of MGUS.

NONSECRETORY MULTIPLE MYELOMA: Nonsecretory MM is a variant of MM in whcih all the clinicopathologic features of classical MM are present except detectable serum monoclonal protein or Bence Jones proteinuria.[68] Patients with nonsecretory MM have extensive osteolytic lesions and occasionally may show evidence of generalized amyloidosis. It is postulated that nonsecretory myeloma cells may produce small amounts of protein fragments not detectable by available techniques.[68]

PLASMA CELL LEUKEMIA: Plasma cell leukemia is a form of MM in which a large number of plasma cells are present in the peripheral blood. Criteria suggested for the diagnosis of plasma cell leukemia include an absolute plasma cell count of 2000/μl and/or >20% plasma cells in the peripheral blood differential count.[69] Plasma cell leukemia occurs in about 1–2% of patients with MM.[69,70] A significant proportion of plasma cell leukemias are of the IgD or IgE type.[71,72]

OSTEOSCLEROTIC MYELOMA (POEMS SYNDROME): POEMS syndrome is a chronic inflammatory demyelinating polyneuropathy associated with single or multiple osteosclerotic plasma cell lesions.[73,74] The term "POEMS" stands for polyneuropathy, organomegaly, endocrinopathy, monoclonal protein and skin alterations.[75] Bone marrow biopsy samples show evidence of osteosclerosis and plasmacytosis. Monoclonal proteins are almost always of the lambda light chain class and usually measure less than 3 g/dl in serum. The presence of Bence Jones protein is infrequent.

IGM Monoclonal Gammopathy

Approximately 10% of monoclonal gammopathies are of the IgM class.[16] IgM gammopathies are characterized by their tendency to involve extramedullary lymphoid tissues and are composed of lymphocytes, plasmacytoid lymphocytes and/or a mixture of plasma cells and lymphocytes. Because of these features, they are considered a variant of NHL (IgM-secreting lymphoma). IgM monoclonal gammopathies may be arbitrarily divided into two overlapping groups: (1) Waldenstrom's macroglobulinemia and (2) other IgM-associated lymphoproliferative disorders.

Waldenstrom's Macroglobulinemia

Waldenstrom's macroglobulinemia (WM) is considered a variant of small lymphocytic lymphoma with plasmacytic features. It is usually manifested by lymphadenopathy, hepatomegaly, splenomegaly and bone marrow involvement. Other organs such as the respiratory system (lungs, pleura) and kidneys may also be involved. WM is a disease of old age, usually affecting patients over 60.[76,77] Anemia, leukopenia and thrombocytopenia may be present. Approximately 20% of the patients show symptoms of hyperviscosity, and cryoglobulinemia (Raynaud's phenomenon) occurs in about 15% of patients.[78] Circulating IgM may coat platelets and cause platelet dysfunction and bleeding. Osteolytic lesions and hypercalcemia are uncommon. The monoclonal Ig in about 75% of the cases is IgM kappa. A light chain proteinuria can be detected in up to 80% of the patients if the urine is concentrated before electrophoresis.[76]

Bone marrow examination usually reveals a focal or diffuse infiltration of the marrow space by small lymphoplasmacytoid cells. These cells have smaller amounts of cytoplasm than plasma cells but, similar to plasma cells, show an eccentric nucleus and a perinuclear clear zone (Figures 7-7 to 7-9). The nuclear chromatin pattern is closer to that of a lymphocyte than to that of a plasma cell nucleus.[79] Nuclear inclusins (Dutcher bodies) are frequent, and there may be evidence of marrow mastocytosis. However, the morphologic features described above are not pathognomonic for WM and have occasionally been observed in monoclonal gammopathies of other Ig classes.

Other IgM-Associated Lymphoproliferative Disorders

The association between monoclonal IgM gammopathies and lymphoid malignancies has been known for a long time.[80-82] This association is most frequently demonstrated in CLL and in diffuse NHLs.[28,83-86] In a report by Alexanian,[83] monoclonal gammopathy was found in 4.5% of the 640 patients with diffuse lymphoproliferative disorders (CLL, diffuse lymphomas) and in none of the 292 patients with nodular lymphoma. In a similar report by Hobbs and associates, >60% of the lymphoma patients with IgM gammopathy had diffuse lymphoma compared to only 13% with follicular lymphoma.[87] Angioimmunoblastic lymphadenopathy and angiofollicular lymphadenopathy (Castleman's disease) are infrequently associated with monoclonal gammopathies.[88,89]

Heavy Chain Disease

Heavy chain diseases are monoclonal proliferations of lymphoplasmacytic cells that synthesize and secrete defective Ig heavy chains. These heavy chains (gamma, alpha, mu and delta) have a deletion of the amino terminal end of the Fd region, but their Fc region is intact.[90-95]

Alpha heavy chain disease is the most common form of heavy chain gammopathies. The peak incidence is between 20 and 30 years, and the disease occurs in two clinical forms: an intestinal form, which is prevalent in Mediterranean, Asian and South American countries, and a less common respiratory form reported in the United States and the Netherlands. The clinical spectrum ranges from a stable, benign course to the development of lymphoma.[96]

Gamma heavy-chain disease is often associated with lymphadenopathy and hepatosplenomegaly. Anemia or pancytopenia may occur. Bone marrow findings are nondiagnostic, but a bone marrow lymphoplasmacytosis may be present which is often associated with eosinophilia.

Almost all patients with *mu heavy-chain* disease have CLL. Most patients also excrete large amounts of kappa light chains in the urine, frequently demonstrate lymphadenopathy, and often display vacuolated plasma cells in the bone marrow.[92,97,98]

Delta chain-disease has been described in a 70-year-old man with osteolytic lesions, infiltration of the bone marrow with atypical plasma cells and progressively fatal renal failure.[94]

Light Chain-Associated Amyloidosis

Primary or light chain amyloidosis (AL) is a systemic disorder associated with plasma cell dyscrasia and is the most common form of AL in the United States.[99] The great majority of patients with AL do not demonstrate overt MM or any other lymphoplasmacytic neoplasm. However, 5–15% of the patients with MM may show evidence of systemic AL. In a report by Gretz and Kyle,[100] approximately two-thirds of the 153 AL patients demonstrated a low level of monoclonal protein (median, 0.85 g/dl) in their serum. The predominant Ig light chain was lambda, accounting for 62% of the patients. Screening of the urine for Bence Jones protein increased the detection of monoclonal protein from 65% (serum only) to 85% (both serum and urine). Five-year survival was close to 20%.

Microscopic examination of bone marrow biopsy and clot sections reveals an eosinophilic extracellular deposit of amyloid. The deposit is found predominantly within and around the vessel walls and is usually

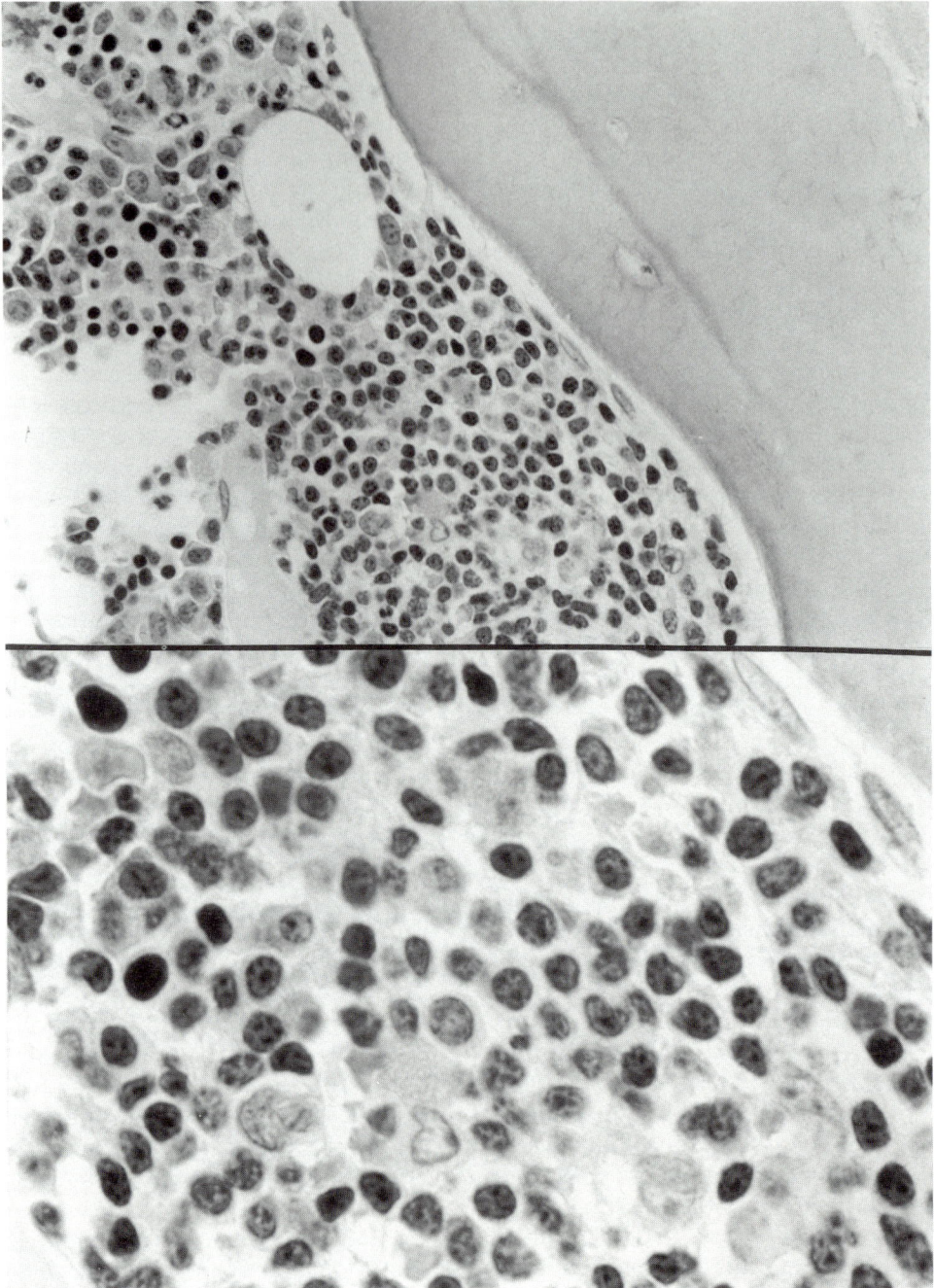

Figure 7-7. Bone marrow biopsy section from a patient with Waldenstrom's macroglobulinema demonstrating aggregates of lymphoplasmacytic cells adjacent to the bone trabeculae.

stained with Congo red dye. The Congo red-stained amyloid is birefringent under polarized light and appears apple green in color. This reaction is due to the binding of the Congo red to the beta-pleated sheet structures of the amyloid fibers.[101a] The immunoenzyme staining preparations may demonstrate monoclonal plasma cells in the bone marrow samples involved with AL.[101b]

Plasma Cell Dyscrasia

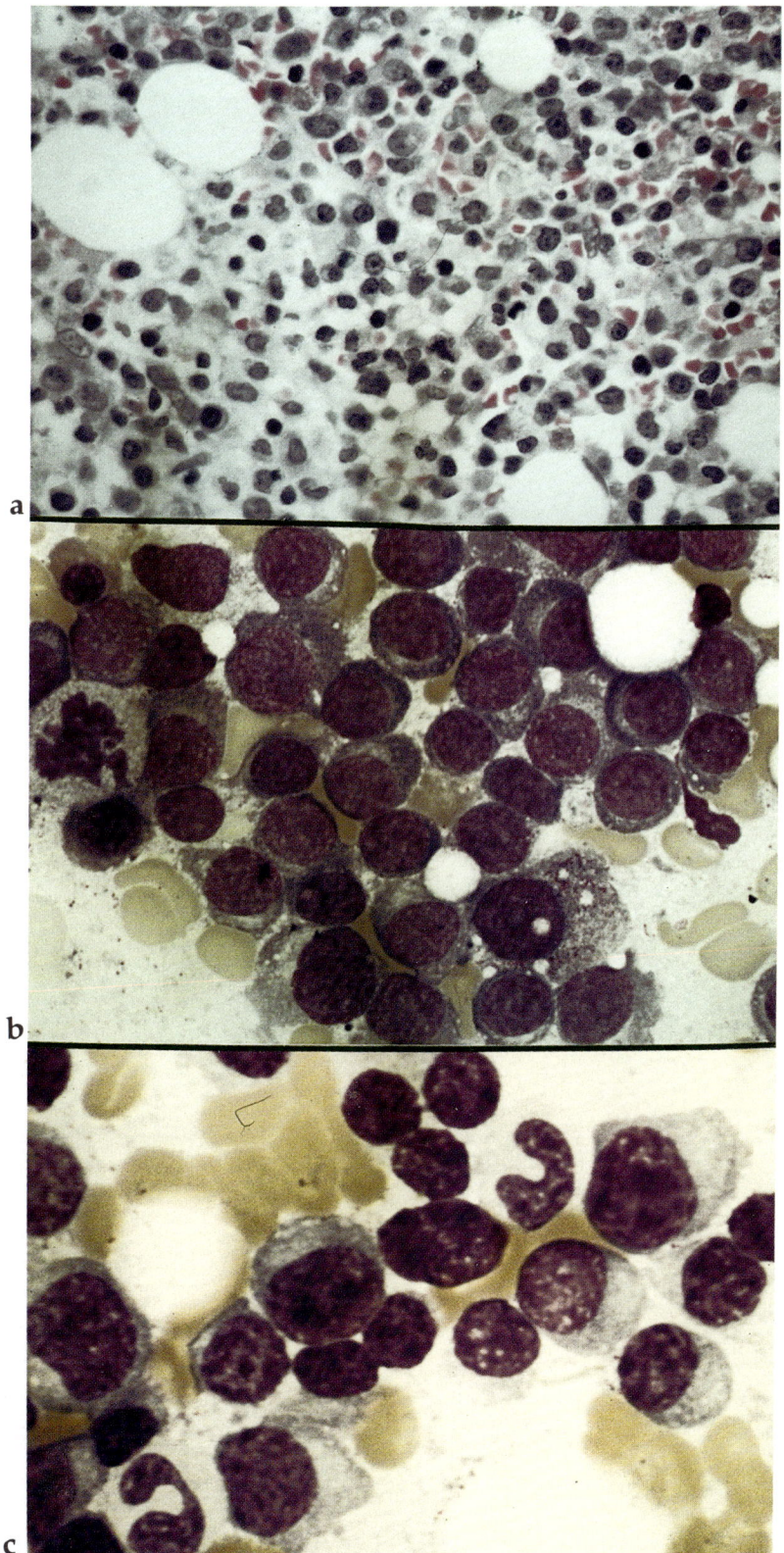

Figure 7-8. Waldenstrom's macroglobulinemia. (a) Bone marrow biopsy section demonstrating lymphoplasma cell infiltration; (b, c) bone marrow smears showing clusters of lymphoplasmacytic cells.

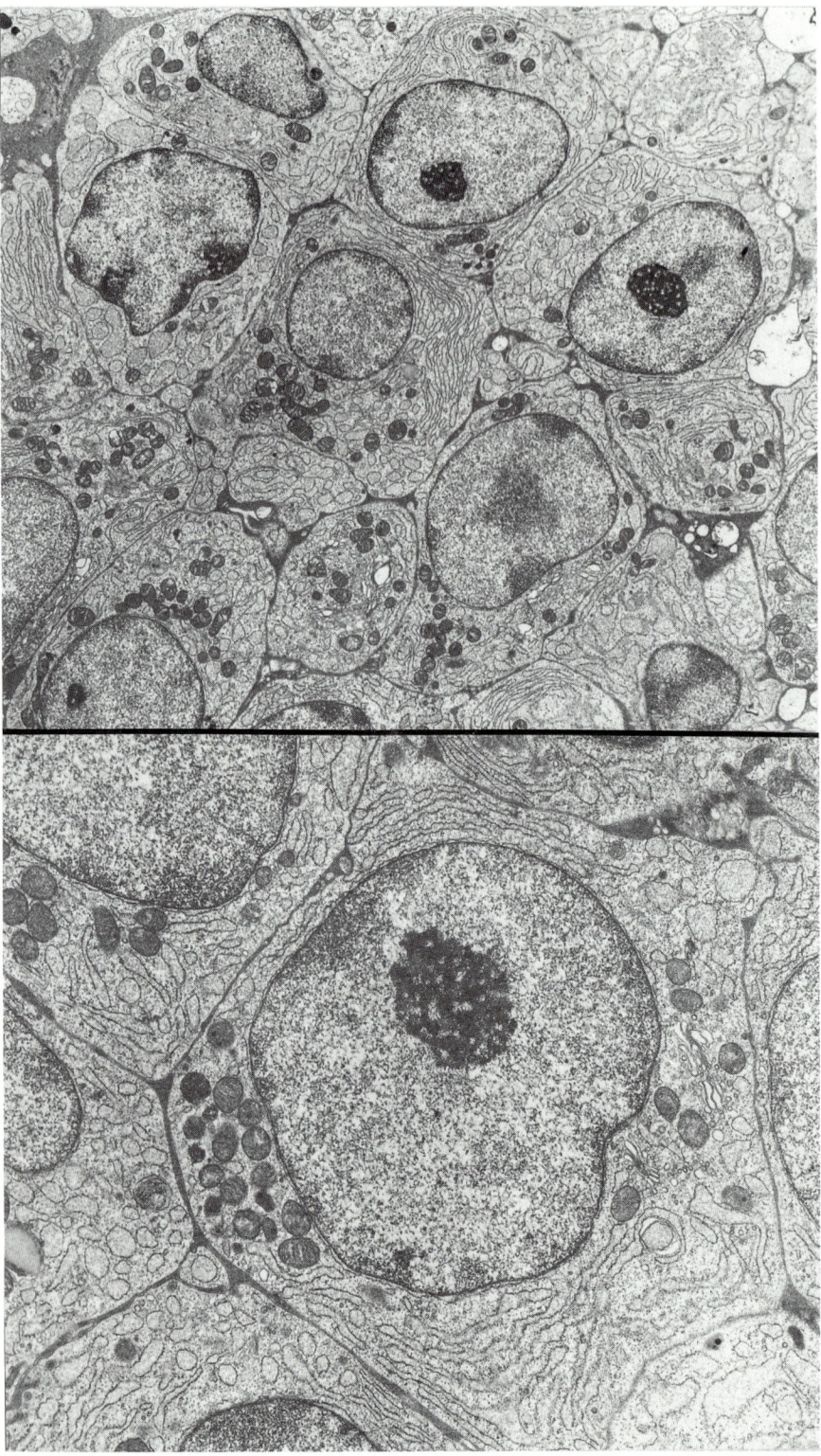

Figure 7-9. Electron microscopic features of the neoplastic cells in a patient with Waldenstrom's macroglobulinemia. The cells show variable amounts of cytoplasm with abundant rough endoplasmic reticulum and numerous mitochondria.

Other Gammopathies

Biclonal and Triclonal Gammopathies

Biclonal gammopathies have been reported by several investigators.[102-105] The majority of the patients have a benign clinical course. The two monoclonal serum proteins may arise from one plasma cell clone due to a defect ("freeze") in the Ig switching process[103] or from two separate plasma cell clones.

Triclonal gammopathies have been reported in a patient with NHL and in a patient with plasma cell dyscrasia who subsequently developed AIDS.[106]

Association of Monoclonal Gammopathies with Diseases Other Than Lymphoproliferative Disorders

Elevation of monoclonal Ig has been reported in association with a number of hematologic and nonhematologic disorders. Pernicious anemia, Gaucher's disease, acquired von Willebrand's disease, pure red blood cell aplasia, myeloproliferative disorders and myelodysplastic syndromes are among the hematologic disorders in which the presence of monoclonal protein has been reported.[107-113]

Approximately 5–6% of the patients with peripheral neuropathy or myopathy demonstrate monoclonal proteinemia.[114,115] A variety of connective tissue diseases and dermatology disorders such as rheumatoid arthritis, lupus erythematosus, papular mucinosis, pyoderma gangrenosum, diffuse plane xanthomatosis and necrobiotic xanthogranuloma have been reported in association with monoclonal Ig.[116-121] Monoclonal gammopathy has also been reported in patients with chronic active hepatitis, primary biliary cirrhosis, Henoch-Schonlein purpura and AIDS.[122-125] Prolonged or transient monoclonal gammopathy has been observed in a number of patients with acute myelomonocytic leukemia, CML and CML in monocytic blast crisis.[28,126,127] A significant number of bone marrow transplant patients may develop transient monoclonal gammopathies which may last for periods ranging from a couple of weeks to several months.[128] There is a strong correlation between the development of graft-versus-host disease and the appearance of M components. M components have also been detected in patients with renal or liver transplants.[28,129]

In some of these disorders, such as acquired von Willebrand's disease, pure red blood cell aplasia and Henoch-Schonlein purpura, the monoclonal protein may play an etiologic role. For example, monoclonal proteins with anti-vWF activities have been reported in some patients with monoclonal gammopathies.[130,131] Blocking effects of monoclonal protein in the maturation of the erythroid burst-forming unit (BFU-E) has been demonstrated in some cases of pure red blood cell aplasia,[109] and a clonal IgM antibody against peripheral nerve myelin was detected in a patient with peripheral neuropathy.[132]

References

1. Wickramasighe SN: Blood and bone marrow, in Symers W st C (ed), *Systemic Pathology*, ed 3, Vol 2. Edinburgh, Churchill Livingstone, 1986, p 73.
2. Hyun BH, Kwa D, Gabaldon H, et al: Reactive plasmacytic lesions of the bone marrow. *Am J Clin Pathol* 65:921, 1976.
3. Canale DD, Collins RD: Use of bone marrow particle sections in the diagnosis of multiple myeloma. *Am J Clin Pathol* 61:382, 1974.
4. Radl J, De Glopper E, van Den Berg P, et al: Idiopathic paraproteinemia. 1. Studies in animal model—the aging C57BL/KaLwRij mouse. *Clin Exp Immunol* 33:395, 1978.
5. Radl J, De Glopper E, van Den Berg P, et al: Idiopathic paraproteinemia. III. Increased frequency of paraproteinemia in thymectomized aging C57BL/KalwRij and CBA/BrARij mice. *J Immunol* 125:31, 1980.
6. De Rossi G, De Sanctis G, Bottari B, et al: Surface markers and cytotoxic activities of lymphocytes in monoclonal gammopathy of undetermined significance and untreated multiple myeloma: Increased phytohemagglutinin-induced cellular cytotoxicity and inverted helper/suppressor cell ratio are features common to both diseases. *Cancer Immunol Immunother* 25:133, 1987.
7. Levinson AI, Hoxie JA, Mathews DM, et al: Analysis of the relationship between T cell subsets and in vitro responses in multiple myeloma. *J Clin Lab Immunol* 16:23, 1985.
8. San Miguel JF, Caballero MD, Gonzalez M: T-cell subpopulations in patients with monoclonal gammopathies: Essential monoclonal gammopathy, multiple myeloma, and Waldenstrom macroglobulinemia. *Am J Hematol* 20:267, 1985.
9. Beyer GS, Glant MD, Hoffman R: Development of IgA multiple myeloma in a patient with aplastic anemia treated with antithymocyte globulin, letter. *N Engl J Med* 314:247, 1986.
10. Ichimaru M, Ishimaru T, Mikami M, et al: Multiple

myeloma among atomic bomb survivors in Hiroshima and Nagasaki, 1950–76: Relationship to radiation dose absorbed by marrow. *J Natl Cancer Inst* 69:323, 1982.
11. Smith PG, Douglas AJ: Mortality of workers at the Sellafield of British Nuclear Fuels. *Br Med J* 293:845, 1986.
12. Darby SC, Doll R, Gill SK, et al: Long-term mortality after a single treatment course with X-rays in patients treated for ankylosing spondylitis. *Br J Cancer* 55:179, 1987.
13. Grosbois B, Gueguen M, Fauchet R, et al: Multiple myeloma in two brothers: An immunochemical and immunogenetic familial study. *Cancer* 58:2417, 1986.
14. Judson IR, Wiltshaw E, Newland AC: Multiple myeloma in a pair of monozygotic twins: The first reported case. *Br J Haematol* 60:551, 1985.
15. Maldonado JE, Kyle RA: Familial myeloma: Report of eight families and study of serum proteins in their relatives. *Am J Med* 57:875, 1974.
16. Osterland KC: Monoclonal gammopathies—their identification and biological significance. *Clin Chim Acta* 180:1, 1989.
17. Kyle RA: "Benign" monoclonal gammopathy. *JAMA* 251:1849, 1984.
18. Hallen J: Frequency of "abnormal" serum globulins (M-components) in the aged. *Acta Med Scand* 173:737, 1963.
19. Axelsson U, Bachmann R, Hallen J: Frequency of pathological proteins (M-components) in 6,995 sera from an adult population. *Acta Med Scand* 179:235, 1966.
20. Kyle RA, Finkelstein S, Elveback, et al: Incidence of monoclonal proteins in a Minnesota community with a cluster of multiple myeloma. *Blood* 40:719, 1972.
21. Kyle RA: Monoclonal gammopathy of undetermined significance: Natural history in 241 cases. *Am J Med* 64:814, 1978.
22. Hobbs JR: Paraproteins, benign or malignant? *Br Med J* 3:699, 1967.
23. Dammacco F, Waldenstrom J: Bence Jones proteinuria in benign monoclonal gammopathies: Incidence and characteristics. *Acta Med Scand* 184:403, 1968.
24. Morell A, Riesen W; Serum β2-microglobulin, serum creatinine and bone marrow plasma cells in benign and malignant monoclonal gammopathy. *Acta Haematol* 64:87, 1980.
25. Spira G, Carter A, Tatarsky I, et al: Lymphocyte subpopulations in benign monoclonal gammopathy. *Scand J Haematol* 31:78, 1983.
26. Shimizu K, Ohnishi K, Kunii A: Differentiation of benign monoclonal gammopathy and smouldering multiple myeloma from frank myeloma. *Clin Exp Immunol* 50:569, 1982.
27. Carmagnola AL, Boccadoro M, Massaia M, et al: The idiotypic specificities of lymphocytes in human monoclonal gammopathies: Analysis with the fluorescence activated cell sorter. *Clin Exp Immunol* 51:173, 1983.
28. Kyle RA, Lust JA: Monoclonal gammopathies of undetermined significance. *Semin Hematol* 26:176, 1989.
29. Kyle RA, Greipp PR: "Idiopathic" Bence Jones proteinuria: Long-term follow-up in seven patients. *N Engl J Med* 306:564, 1982.
30. Mundy GR, Raisz LG, Cooper RA, et al: Evidence for the secretion of an osteoclast stimulating factor in myeloma. *N Engl J Med* 291:1041, 1974.
31. Valentin-Opran A, Chardon SA, Meunier PJ, et al: Quantitative histology of myeloma induced bone changes. *Br J Haematol* 52:601, 1982.
32. Mundy GR, Bertolini DR: Bone destruction and hypercalcemia in plasma cell myeloma. *Semin Oncol* 13:291, 1986.
33. Osse RG, Murray TM, Mundy GR, et al: Observations on the mechanism of bone resorption induced by multiple myeloma marrow culture fluids and partially purified osteoclast-activity factor. *J Clin Invest* 67:1472, 1981.
34. Kyle RA: Multiple myeloma: Review of 869 cases. *Mayo Clin Proc* 50:29, 1975.
35. Buss DH, Prichard RW, Hartz JW, et al: Comparison of the usefulness of bone marrow sections and smears in diagnosis of multiple myeloma. *Hematol Pathol* 1:35, 1987.
36. Committee of the Chronic Leukemia-Myeloma Task Force, National Cancer Institute: Proposed guidelines for protocol studies. II. Plasma cell myeloma. *Cancer Chemother Rep* 4:145, 1973.
37. Costa G, Engle RL Jr, Schilling A, et al: Melphelan and prednisone: An effective combination for treatment of multiple myeloma. *Am J Med* 54:589, 1973.
38. Canale DD, Collins RD: Use of bone marrow particle sections in the diagnosis of multiple myeloma. *Am J Clin Pathol* 61:382, 1974.
39. Krzyzaniak RL, Buss DH, Cooper MR, et al: Marrow fibrosis and multiple myeloma. *Am J Clin Pathol* 89:63, 1988.
40. Greipp PR, Raymond NM, Kyle RA, et al: Multiple myeloma: Significance of plasmablastic subtype in morphological classification. *Blood* 65:305, 1985.
41a. Bartl R, Frisch B, Fatewh-Moghadam A, et al: Histologic classification and staging of multiple myeloma. A retrospective and prospective study of 674 cases. *Am J Clin Pathol* 87:342, 1987.
41b. Anderson K, Cochran M, Barut B: Phenotypic and

functional characterization of normal and malignant plasma cells. *Eur J Haematol* 43:19, 1990.
42. Durie BGM, Grogan TM: CALLA-positive myeloma: An aggressive subtype with poor survival. *Blood* 66:229, 1985.
43. Grogan TM, Durie BMG, Spier CM, et al: Myelomonocytic antigen positive multiple myeloma. *Blood* 73:763, 1989.
44a. Spier CM, Grogan TM, Durie BGM, et al: T-cell antigen-positive multiple myeloma. *Mod Pathol* 3:302, 1990.
44b. Van Camp B, Durie BGM, Spier C, et al: Plasma cells in multiple myeloma express a natural killer cell-associated antigen: CD56(NKH-1; Leu 19). *Blood* 76:377, 1990.
45. Wukke K, Varbiro M, Rudiger KD, et al: Cytological and histological classification of multiple myeloma. *Hematologica* 14:315, 1981.
46. Bartl R, Frisch B, Burkhardt R, et al: Bone marrow histology in myeloma: Its importance in diagnosis, prognosis, classification and staging. *Br J Haematol* 51:361, 1982.
47. Bast EJE, van Camp B, Reynaert P, et al: Idiotypic peripheral blood lymphocytes in monoclonal gammopathy. *Clin Exp Immunol* 47:677, 1982.
48. Sugai S, Takiguchi T, Hirose Y, et al: B-cell malignancy and monoclonal gammopathy, and idiotype of cell surface and serum immunoglobulin. *Jpn J Clin Oncol* 13:533, 1983.
49a. Warburton P. Joshua DE, Gibson J, et al: CD10-(CALLA)-positive lymphocytes in myeloma: Evidence that they are a malignant precursor population and are of germinal center origin. *Leuk Lymph* 1:11, 1991.
49b. Berensen, J. Wong R, Kim K, et al: Evidence for peripheral blood B lymphocyte but not T lymphocyte involvement in multiple myeloma. *Blood* 70:1550, 1987.
50. Grogan TM, Durei BGM, Lomen C, et al: Delineation of a novel pre-B cell component in plasma cell myeloma: Immunological, immunophenotypic, genotypic, cytologic, cell culture, and kinetic features. *Blood* 70:932, 1987.
51. Gould J, Alexanian R, Goodacre A, et al: Plasma cell karyotype in multiple myeloma. *Blood* 71:453, 1988.
52. Sevanayagam P, Blick M, Narni F, et al: Alteration and abnormal expression of the *c-myc* oncogene in human multiple myeloma. *Blood* 71:30, 1988.
53. Sevanayagam P, Goodacre A, Strong L, et al: Alterations of *bcl-1* oncogene in human multiple myeloma, abstracted. *Proc Annu Meet Am Assoc Cancer Res* 28:19, 1987.
54. Tsuchiya H, Epstein J, Sevanayagam P, et al: Correlated flow cytometric analysis of *H-ras p21* and nuclear DNA in multiple myeloma. *Blood* 72:796, 1988.

55. Latrielle J, Balogie B, Johnston D, et al: Ploidy and proliferative characteristics in monoclonal gammopathies. *Blood* 59:43, 1982.
56. Balogie B, Alexanian R, Dixon D, et al: Prognostic implications of tumor cell DNA content in multiple myeloma. *Blood* 66:338, 1985.
57. Bunn PA, Krasnow S, Makuch RW, et al: Flow cytometric analysis of DNA content of bone marrow cells in patients with plasma cell myeloma: Clinical implications. *Blood* 59:528, 1982.
58. Balogie B, Alexanian R, Gehan EA, et al: Marrow cytometry and prognosis in myeloma. *J Clin Invest* 72:853, 1982.
59. Durei BGM, Salmon SE: A clinical staging system for myeloma: Correlation of measured myeloma cell mass with presenting clinical features, response to treatment, and survival. *Cancer* 36:842, 1975.
60. Gassmann W, Pralle H, Haferlich S: Staging systems for multiple myeloma: A comparison. *Br J Haematol* 59:703, 1985.
61. Greipp PR, Witzig TE, Gonchoroff NJ, et al: Immunofluorescence labeling indices in myeloma and related monoclonal gammopathies. *Mayo Clin Proc* 62:969, 1987.
62a. Durie BGM, Salmon SE, Moon TE: Pretreatment tumor mass, cell kinetics, and prognosis in multiple myeloma. *Blood* 55:367, 1980.
62b. Saeed SM, Stock-Novack D, Pohlod R, et al: Prognostic correlation of plasma cell acid phosphatase and b-glucuronidase in multiple myeloma: A Southwest Oncology Group Study. *Blood* 78:3281, 1991.
63. Monteccuco C, Riccardi A, Ucci G: Analysis of human myeloma cell kinetics. *Acta Haematol* 75:153, 1986.
64. Bataille R: Localized plasmacytomas. *Clin Hematol* 11:113, 1982.
65. Wiltshaw E: The natural history of extramedullary plasmacytoma and its relation to solitary plasmacytoma of bone and myelomatosis. *Medicine* 55:217, 1976.
66. Meis JM, Butler JJ, Osborne BM, et al: Solitary plasmacytoma of bone and extramedullary plasmacytomas. A clinicopathologic and immunohistochemical study. *Cancer* 59:1475, 1987.
67. Kyle RA, Greipp PR: Smoldering multiple myeloma. *N Engl J Med* 302:1347, 1980.
68. Azar HA, Zaino EC, Pham TD, et al: "Nonsecretory" plasma cell myeloma: Observation on seven cases with electron microscopic studies. *Am J Clin Pathol* 58:618, 1972.
69. Kyle RA, Maldonado JE, Bayrd ED: Plasma cell leukemia. Report of 17 cases. *Arch Intern Med* 133:813, 1974.
70. Azwadzki ZA, Kapadia S, Barnes AE: Leukemic my-

elomatosis (plasma cell leukemia). *Am J Clin Pathol* 70:605, 1978.
71. Ben-Basset I, Frand UI, Isersky C, et al: Plasma cell leukemia with IgD paraprotein. *Arch Intern Med* 121:361, 1968.
72. Endo T, Okumura H, Kikuchi K, et al: Immunoglobin E (IgE) multiple myeloma. A case report and review of the literature. *Am J Med* 70:1127, 1981.
73. Driedger H, Prizanski W: Plasma cell neoplasia with osteosclerotic lesions. *Arch Intern Med* 139:892, 1979.
74. Katatsuki K, Sanada I: Plasma cell dyscrasia with polyneuropathy and endocrine disorder: Clinical and laboratory features of 109 cases. *Jpn J Clin Oncol* 13:543, 1983.
75. Bardwick PA, Zvaifler NJ, Gill GN, et al: Plasma cell discrasia with polyneuropathy, organomegaly, endocrinopathy, M protein, and skin changes: The POEMS syndrome: Report of two cases and review of the literature. *Medicine* 59:311, 1980.
76. Kyle RA, Garton JP: The spectrum of IgM monoclonal gammopathy in 430 cases. *Mayo Clin Proc* 62:719, 1987.
77. MacKenzie MR, Fudenbeg HM: Macroglobulinemia: An analysis of forty patients. *Blood* 39:874, 1972.
78. Somer T: Rheology of paraproteinemias and the plasma hyperviscosity syndrome. *Bailliere's Clin Haematol* 1:695, 1987.
79. Rywlin AM, Civantos F, Ortega RS, et al: Bone marrow histology in monoclonal macroglobulinemia. *Am J Clin Pathol* 63:769, 1975.
80. Azar HA, Hill WT, Osserman EF: Malignant lymphoma and lymphocytic leukemia associated with myeloma-type serum proteins. *Am J Med* 23:239, 1957.
81. Krauss S, Sokal JE: Paraproteinemia in the lymphomas. *Am J Med* 40:400, 1966.
82. Kim H, Heller P, Rappaport H: Monoclonal gammopathies associated with lymphoproliferative disorders: A morphologic study. *Am J Clin Pathol* 59:282, 1973.
83. Alexanian R: Monoclonal gammopathy in lymphoma. *Arch Intern Med* 135:62, 1975.
84. Moore DF, Migliore PJ, Shullenberger CC, et al: Monoclonal macroglobulinemia in malignant lymphoma. *Ann Intern Med* 72:43, 1970.
85. Magrath I, Benjamin D, Papadopoulos S: Serum monoclonal immunoglobulin bands in undifferentiated lymphomas of Burkitt types. *Blood* 61:726, 1983.
86. Sinclair D, Dagg JH, Dwar AE, et al: The incidence, clonal origin and secretory nature of serum paraproteins in chronic lymphocytic leukemia. *Br J Haematol* 64:725, 1986.
87. Hobbs JR, Carter PM, Cooke KB, et al: IgM paraproteins. *J Clin Pathol* 28 (suppl 6):54, 1974.

88. Steinberg AD, Seldin MF, Jafffe ES, et al: Angioimmunoblastic lymphadenopathy with disproteinemia. *Ann Intern Med* 108:575, 1988.
89. Heineman VL, Phyliky RL, Banks PM: Angiofollicular lymph node hyperplasia and peripheral neuropathy: Association with monoclonal gammopathy. *Mayo Clin Proc* 57:379, 1982.
90. Franklin EG, Lowenstein J, Bigelow B, et al: Heavy chain (7S gamma globulin) disease. A new clinical entity. *Am J Med* 37:332, 1964.
91. Seligmann M, Danon F, Hurez D, et al: Alpha chain disease: A new immunoglobulin abnormality. *Science* 162:1396, 1968.
92. Seligmann M, Mihaesco E, Preud'homme JL, et al: Heavy chain disease: Current findings and concepts. *Immunol Rev* 48:145, 1979.
93. Forte FA, Prelli F, Yount WJ, et al: Heavy-chain disease of the μ (γM) type: Report of the first case. *Blood* 36:137, 1970.
94. Vilpo JA, Irjala K, Vilijanen MK, et al: δ-Heavy chain disease: A study of a case. *Clin Immunol Immunopathol* 17:584, 1980.
95. Kyle RA, Greipp PR, Banks PM: The diverse picture of gamma heavy-chain disease. Report of seven cases and review of the literature. *Mayo Clin Proc* 56:439, 1981.
96. Gilinsky NH, Novis BH, Wright JP, et al: Immunoproliferative small intestine disease: Clinical features and outcome in 30 cases. *Medicine* 66:438, 1987.
97. Franklin EC: The heavy chain diseases. *Harvey Lect* 78:1, 1984.
98. Franklin EC: μ-Chain disease. *Arch Intern Med* 135:71, 1975.
99. Kyle RA, Greipp PR: Amyloidosis (AL): Clinical and laboratory features of 229 cases. *Mayo Clin Proc* 58:665, 1983.
100. Gretz MA, Kyle RA: Primary systemic amyloidosis—a diagnostic primer. *Mayo Clin Proc* 64:1505, 1989.
101a. Glenner GG: Amyloid deposit and amyloidosis. The β-fibrillosis. *N Engl J Med* 52:148, 1980.
101b. Wu S S-H, Brady K, Anderson JJ, et al: The predictive value of bone marrow morphologic characteristics and immunostaining in primary (AL) amyloidosis. *Am J Clin Pathol* 96:95, 1991.
102. Kyle RA, Robinson RA, Katzmann JA: The clinical aspects of biclonal gammopathies. Review of 57 cases. *Am J Med* 71:999, 1981.
103. Lucivero G, Miglietta A, dell'Osso A, et al: Double (IgAk + IgGk) paraproteinemia in a single patient: Immunofluorescence evidence for a common plasma cell clone "frozen" at the switch phase. *Acta Hematol* 75:224, 1986.
104. Nilsson T, Norberg B, Rudolphi O, et al: Double

gammopathies: Incidence and clinical course of 20 patients. *Scand J Haematol* 36:103, 1986.
105. Riddell S, Traczyk Z, Paraskevas F, et al: The double gammopathies: Clinical and immunological studies. *Medicine* 65:135, 1986.
106. Berg AR, Weisenburger DD, Linder J, et al: Lymphoplasmacytic lymphoma: Report of a case with three monoclonal proteins derived from a single neoplastic clone. *Cancer* 57:1797, 1986.
107. Selroos O, von Knorring J: Immunoglobulins in pernicious anemia: Including a report on a patient with pernicious anemia, IgA deficiency and an M component of kappa-type IgG. *Acta Med Scand* 194:571, 1973.
108. Shoenfeld Y, Berliner S, Pinkhas J, et al: The association of Gaucher's disease and dysproteinemias. *Acta Haematol* 59:99, 1978.
109. Mant MJ, Hirsh J, Gauldie J, et al: Von Willebrand's syndrome presenting as an acquired bleeding disorder in association with a monoclonal gammopathy. *Blood* 42:429, 1973.
110. Resegotti L, Dolci C, Palestro G, et al: Paraproteinemic variety of pure red cell aplasia: Immunological studies in 1 patient. *Acta Haematol* 60:227, 1978.
111. Balducci L, Hardy C, Dreiling B, et al: Pure red cell aplasia associated with paraproteinemia: In vitro studies of erythropoiesis. *Haematologica* 17:353, 1984.
112. Berner Y, Berrebi A: Myeloproliferative disorders and nonmyelomatous paraprotein: A study of five patients and review of the literature. *Isr J Med Sci* 22:109, 1986.
113. Economopoulos T, Economidou J, Giannopoulos G, et al: Immune abnormalities in myelodysplastic syndromes. *J Clin Pathol* 38:908, 1985.
114. Isobe T, Osserman EF: Pathologic conditions associated with plasma cell dyscrasias: A study of 806 cases. *Ann NY Acad Sci* 190:507, 1971.
115. Kelly JJ Jr, Kyle RA, O'Brien PC, et al: prevalence of monoclonal protein in peripheral neuropathy. *Neurology* 31:1480, 1981.
116. Zawadzki ZA, Benedek TG: Rheumatoid arthritis, dysproteinemic arthropathy, and paraproteinemia. *Arthritis Rheum* 12:555, 1969.
117. Michaux JL, Hermans JF: Thirty cases of monoclonal immunoglobulin disorders other than myeloma or macroglobulinemia: A classification of diseases associated with the production of monoclonal-type immunoglobulins. *Am J Med* 46:562, 1969.
118. James K, Fudenberg H, Epstein WL, et al: Studies on a unique diagnostic serum globulin in papular mucinosis (lichen myxedematosus). *Clin Exp Immunol* 2:153, 1967.
119. Powell FC, Schoeter AL, Su WPD, et al: Pyoderma gangrenosum and monoclonal gammopathy. *Arch Dermatol* 119:468, 1983.
120. Jones RR, Baughan ASJ, Cream JJ, et al: Complement abnormalities in diffuse plane xanthomatosis with paraproteinemia. *Br J Dermatol* 101:711, 1979.
121. Finan MC, Winkelmann RK: Necrobiotic xanthogranuloma with paraproteinemia: A review of 22 cases. *Medicine* 65:376, 1986.
122. Heer M, Joller-Jemelka H, Fontana A, et al: Monoclonal gammopathy in chronic active hepatitis. *Liver* 4:255, 1984.
123. Hendrick AM, Mitchison HC, Bird AG, et al: Paraproteins in primary biliary cirrhosis. *Q J Med* 60:681, 1986.
124. Dosa S, Cairns SA, Mallick NP, et al: Relapsing Henoch-Schonlein syndrome with renal involvement in a patient with IgA monoclonal gammopathy. A study of the results of immunosuppressant and cytotoxic therapy. *Nephron* 26:145, 1980.
125. Herito K, Hallquist AE, Tamor RH: Paraproteinemia in a patient with acquired immunodeficiency syndrome (AIDS) or lymphadenopathy syndrome (LAS). *Clin Chem* 31:1224, 1985.
126. Raz I, Polliack A: Coexistence of myelomonocytic leukemia and monoclonal gammopathy or myeloma: Simultaneous presentation in three patients. *Cancer* 53:83, 1984.
127. Van Camp B, Reynaerts N, Naets JP, et al: Transient IgA-λ paraproteinemia during treatment of acute myelomonoblastic leukemia. *Blood* 55:21, 1980.
128. Mitus AJ, Stein R, Rappeport JM, et al: Monoclonal and oligoclonal gammopathy after bone marrow transplantation. *Blood* 74:2764, 1989.
129. Randl J, Valentijin RM, Haaijman JJ, et al: Monoclonal gammopathies in patients undergoing immunosuppressive treatment after renal transplantation. *Clin Immunol Immunopathol* 37:98, 1985.
130. Bovill EG, Ershler WB, Golden EA, et al: A human myeloma-produced monoclonal protein directed against the active subpopulation of von Willebrand factor. *Am J Clin Pathol* 85:115, 1986.
131. Mohri H, Noguchi T, Kodama F, et al: Acquired von Willebrand disease due to inhibitor of human myeloma protein specific for von Willebrand factor. *Am J Clin Pathol* 87:663, 1987.
132. Latov N, Sherman WH, Nemni R, et al: Plasma-cell dyscrasia and peripheral neuropathy with monoclonal antibody to peripheral nerve myelin. *N Engl J Med* 303:618, 1980.

8 WHITE BLOOD CELL DISORDERS

DISORDERS OF THE GRANULOCYTES

Functional Abnormalities

Functional abnormalities of granulocytes may be the result of either intrinsic defects (such as degranulation abnormalities, chemotactic disorders, and myeloperoxidase deficiency) or extrinsic disorders (such as abnormalities of opsinizing systems due to antibody and/or complement defects).[1] The qualitative granulocytic defects are relatively rare; the most prominent forms are listed in Table 8-1. Chediac-Higashi syndrome, chronic granulomatous disease, myeloperoxidase deficiency, and leukocyte adhesion deficiency are discussed in this chapter.

Chediak-Higashi Syndrome

Chediak-Higashi syndrome (CHS) is a rare autosomal recessive disease characterized by the presence of giant cytoplasmic granules in all types of peripheral blood leukocytes, particularly neutrophils. The giant granules result from deregulation of lysosomal membrane activities, leading to continuous fusion of the primary and secondary lysosomal granules. This fusion process is associated with leakage of the hydrolytic enzymes into the cytoplasm and structural damage.[2,3] The giant granules in CHS leukocytes can fuse with bacteria-containing phagosomes, but they are not able to destroy the bacteria due to the inadequate concentration of the hydrolytic enzymes.[2] Evidence of deregulation of membrane activities is also demonstrated in neutrophil surface membranes, with spontaneous capping of the surface molecules, impaired adherence to surfaces, and a reduced chemotactic response.[4] Membrane-associated functional alterations have also been demonstrated in other cells of CHS patients, such as NK cells, erythrocytes, platelets and melanocytes.[4-7] Other features of the disease include neutropenia, thrombocytopenia and peripheral neuropathy. The accelerated phase of CHS is sometimes associated with lymphohistiocytic hemophagocytosis.[8] Albinism occurs due to pathologic aggregation of melanosomes in melanocytes.

Chronic Granulomatous Disease

Chronic granulomatous disease (CGD) is characterized by the deficiency of respiratory burst oxidase and by the inability of the phagocytes to manufacture microbicidal oxidants such as hydrogen peroxide. The respiratory burst oxidase is an NADPH oxidase which is dormant in resting leukocytes but becomes active in stimulated cells.[9] The oxidase-activating system is complex, and consists of a mixture of cytosol and plasma membrane components. Only one plasma membrane component has been identified so far: a unique heme protein called *cytochrome* b_{558}. Cytochrome b is an oligomer consisting of two subunits: a 91-kD glycoprotein (gp91-phox) and a 22-kD protein (p22-phox). Other oxidase components include a cytosolic G protein and 47-kD (p47-phox) and 67-kD(p67-phox) proteins[10-14] (Figure 8-1).

CDG is an inherited disorder with either an X-linked or an autosomal recessive mode of transmission.[14-17] X-linked CGD almost exclusively involves men. In rare conditions women are affected. These conditions include CDG homozygosity, heterozygosity with a coexistent inactivated normal chromosome and Turner's syndrome (the presence of a single X chromosome).[18,19] Autosomal recessive CGD occurs with equal frequency in both sexes.[20]

CGD is classified into three major inherited forms: X-linked cytochrome b-negative (type I), autosomal recessive cytochrome b-positive (type II) and autosomal recessive cytochrome b-negative (type III), which account for approximately 65%, 30% and less than 5% of the cases, respectively.[1] Other types of CGD are extremely rare.

White Blood Cell Disorders

Table 8-1 Neutrophil Dysfunction*

Disorder	Etiology	Impaired function
I. Intrinsic		
Degranulation abnormalities CHS	Unknown; pathologically activated membrane (?)	Neutropenia; decreased chemotaxis; defective degranulation; delayed microbial killing
Specific granule deficiency	Missing transfactor gene expression (?)	Impaired chemotaxis and bacterial killing
Adhesion abnormalities Congenital leukocyte adherence deficiency	Absence of CD11/CD18 surface adhesive glycoproteins	Decreased adherence to surfaces and particles
Neutrophil actin dysfunction	Defective polymerization of neutrophil cytoplasmic actin	Impaired chemotactic responsiveness ingestion, regulation of granule fusion
Cytomatrix disorders Developmental immaturity in neonatal neutrophils	Immature membrane—cytoskeletal	Immature chemotactic responsiveness
Energy (ATP) generation	Hyperalimentation without phosphate supplementation	Impaired chemotactic responsiveness and ingestion
Chronic granulomatous disease	Genetic deficiency of respiratory burst oxidase	Failure to kill catalase-positive microbes
Myeloperoxidase deficiency	Failure to process precursor proteins posttranslationally	Hydrogen peroxide-dependent antimicrobial activity
Deficiencies of glutathione reductase and glutathione synthetase	Failure to detoxify hydrogen peroxidase	Excessive formation of hydrogen peroxide
II. Extrinsic		
Antibody-deficiency syndromes	Genetic Acquired idiopathic Secondary to lymphatic neoplasms	Deficiency of serum chemotactic activity and opsonic activity for encapsulated pathogens
Disorders of complement (C1r, C2, C3, C4)	Genetic absence	Alterations in serum chemotactic and opsonic activity
Depletion of multiple factors; inhibitors of activation	Autoimmune disorders, other inflammatory states, sickle cell anemia, Hodgkin's disease, sarcoidosis, renal disease	Deficient serum chemotactic and/or opsonic activity
Drug effects	Ethanol	Impaired locomotion and ingestion
	Glucocorticoids	Impaired locomotion, chemotaxis, ingestion, degranulation, and aggregation
Plasminogen proactivator deficiency	Genetic absence	Deficient serum chemotactic activity

* Adapted from Boxer LA Qualitative abnormalities of neutrophils, in Williams WJ, Beutler E, Erslev AJ, et al (eds) *Hematology*, ed 4. New York, McGraw-Hill, 1990, p 82.

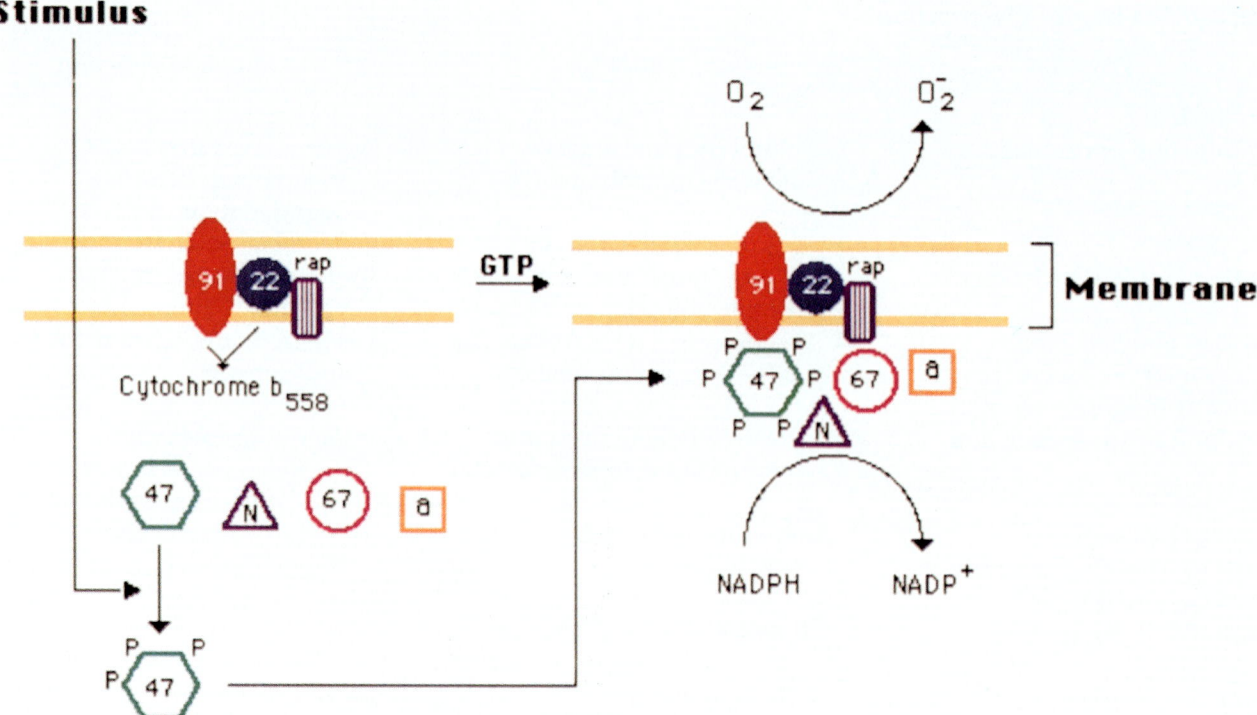

Figure 8-1. Schematic model of the NADPH oxidase in granulocytes after exposure to a stimulus. Once associated with the membrane, oxidase becomes catalytically active and p47-phox is phosphorylated further. Adapted from Smith RM, Curnutte JT: Molecular basis of chronic granulomatous disease. *Blood* 77:673, 1991.

CGD patients develop serious infections with catalase-positive bacteria but not with catalase-negative bacteria. Catalase is a hydrogen peroxidase-catabolizing enzyme. When catalase-positive microorganisms such as *Staphylococcus aureus*, most gram-negative enteric bacteria, *Candida albicans* and *Aspergillus* species enter CGD neutrophils, they are not exposed to hydrogen peroxide and the hydrogen peroxide generated by the microorganisms is inactivated by their own catalase. The inability of the neutrophils and monocytes to kill the phagocytosed, catalase-positive microorganisms leads to proliferation and spread of the germs and to the formation of abscesses and granulomas.

The severity of the infection and the recurrence rate are variable, and the onset of clinical manifestations may range from early infancy to adulthood. The most common forms of infection are pneumonia, dermatitis, lymphadenitis and liver abscess. Other less frequent forms of infection involve the musculoskeletal, gastrointestinal, genitourinary and central nervous systems.

Diagnosis of CGD is based on the demonstration of defective respiratory burst oxidase in neutrophils. The method most frequently used is the nitroblue tetrazolium (NBT) test,[18,21] in which the oxygen produced in the course of a respiratory burst reduces the yellow, water-soluble tetrazolium dye to an insoluble deep blue pigment.

Myeloperoxidase Deficiency

Myeloperoxidase (MPO) deficiency is a relatively common hereditary or acquired disorder of neutrophils and monocytes. The hereditary form is probably an autosomal recessive trait, with a prevalence of 1:2000.[22] Acquired MPO deficiency may occur in myelodysplastic syndromes and AML.

MPO plays a critical role in the microbicidal activity of neutrophils. However, in the absence of MPO, auxilliary mechanisms protect most MPO-deficient patients from severe infections, except for some patients with diabetes mellitus who may develop se-

White Blood Cell Disorders

vere candidiasis. Stimulated neutrophils release MPO into the phagolysosomes or the extracellular space, and the combination of MPO, hydrogen peroxide and chloride ion (the MPO-H_2O_2-Cl system) generates toxic mediators with cytocidal activities.[22,23] In addition, the MPO-H_2O_2-Cl system modulates the inflammatory response in a number of ways, such as inactivation of chemotaxins, some of the secreted granule contents and α1-proteinase inhibitor.[22,24-27]

Leukocyte Adhesion Deficiency

Leukocyte adhesion deficiency is an autosomal recessive trait characterized by deficiency of surface membrane adhesion molecules. Adhesion molecules (integrins) represent a family of three glycoproteins, each composed of α and β subunits. The β subunit (CD18) is identical in all three glycoproteins and the α subunit is different in each glycoprotein, designated as CD11a, CD11b, and CD11c, respectively, for glycoproteins Mac-1 (expressed on monocytes, neutrophils and NK cells), LFA-1 (found on lymphocytes) and p150,90 (expressed on monocytes and neutrophils). Adhesion deficiencies are associated with abnormal, adherence-dependent functions of leukocytes, causing recurrent bacterial infections, pus formation and delayed wound healing.[28]

Neutropenia

Neutropenia is a relatively common disorder caused by a variety of etiologic factors (Table 8-2). Three major mechanisms are involved in the development of neutropenia: (1) defective production of neutrophils, (2) increased destruction or utilization of neutrophils, and (3) a shift from the circulating to the marginal pool.[29,30] Drugs and microorganisms are the most common etiologic factors and usually cause neutropenia by more than one mechanism.

Congenital Neutropenia

Congenital neutropenia consists of a heterogeneous group of disorders which occur as an acquired phenomenon or as a genetic disorder that can be sporadic, autosomal recessive (Kostmann syndrome), autosomal dominant, or sex-linked.[31] Clinical manifestations, which usually occur in early childhood,

Table 8-2 Major Causes of Neutropenia

Congenital
　Kostmann syndrome
　Familial benign chronic neutropenia
Associated with other congenital anomalies
　CHS
　Schwachmann-Diamond syndrome
　Cartilage-hair hypoplasia
Associated with functional abnormalities
　Lazy-leukocyte syndrome
　Myelokathexis
Associated with other hematologic disorders
　Transcobalamin II deficiency
　Myelodysplastic syndrome
　Aplastic anemia
　Leukemia
　Myelofibrosis
　Bone marrow infiltration
　Hypersplenism
Cyclic neutropenia
Immune-associated
　Alloimmune neonatal neutropenia
　Neutropenia associated with autoimmune disorders
Drug-induced
Dialysis neutropenia
Neutropenia associated with infectious diseases
Others:　Neutropenia due to nutritional deficiencies and endocrine disorders

may be relatively mild, with occasional skin infections, or very grave, with repeated severe, life-threatening infections. Bone marrow examination may reveal normocellularity, with apparent "maturation arrest" at the promyelocyte, myelocyte or metamyelocyte level.[31,32a,32b] There is often a variable increase in monocytes, eosinophils and plasma cells. Granulocytic cells may show dysplastic changes that include cytoplasmic vacuolization, decreased primary and secondary granules, and nuclear abnormalities[31] (Figure 8-2).

Cyclic Neutropenia

Cyclic neutropenia is characterized by recurrent episodes of severe neutropenia at relatively regular intervals.[33] This disorder involves both children and

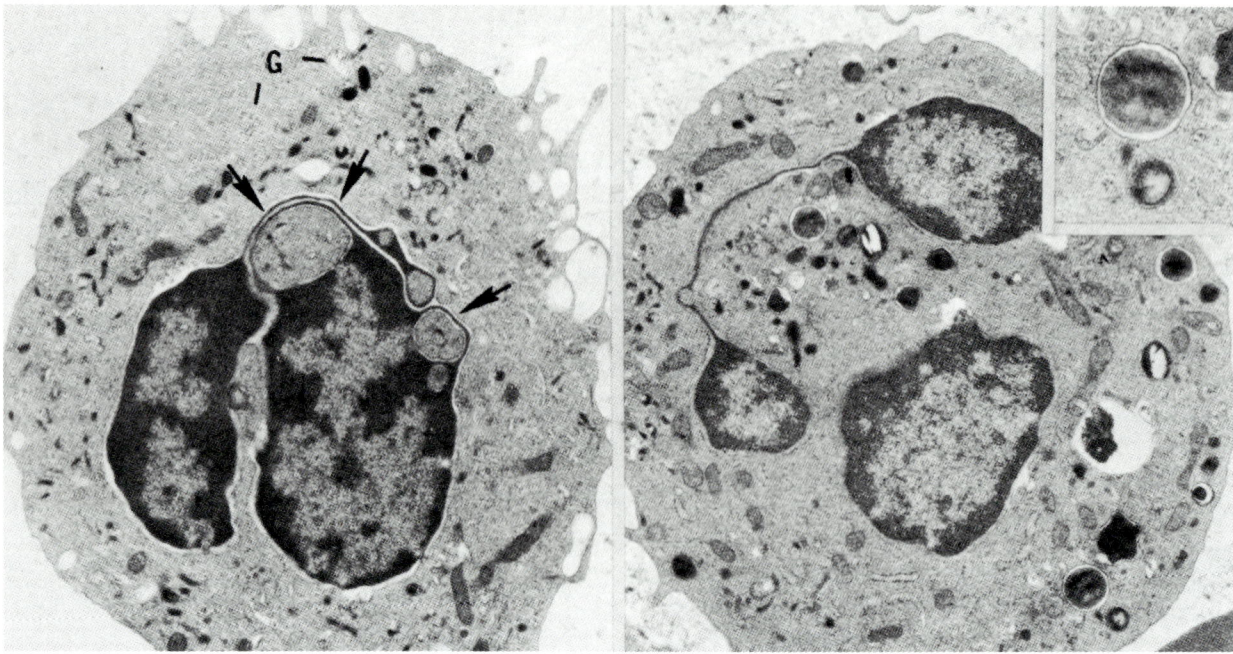

Figure 8-2. Electron microscopic photographs of segmented neutrophils from a patient with congenital neutropenia. There is evidence of nuclear envelope reduplication and cytoplasmic nuclear pockets (arrows) and the presence of a few primary and secondary granules; the insert shows a secondary granule with an electron-lucent central portion and an electron-dense rim. From Parmley RT, Crist WM, Ragab AH, et al: Congenital dysgranulopoietic neutropenia: Clinical, serologic, ultrastructural and in vivo proliferative characteristics. *Blood* 56:465, 1980, with permission.

adults, and may be associated with quantitative changes in other blood cells. The exact mechanism of neutropenic episodes, which occur approximately every 3 weeks, is not well understood but appears to be due to a defect in the regulation of hematopoietic stem cells.[33,34] Cyclic neutropenia in adults may be associated with a clonal proliferation of the large granular lymphocytes (large granular lymphocytic leukemia).[35]

Alloimmune (Isoimmune) Neonatal Neutropenia

This disorder is a relatively common neutropenia observed in approximately 3% of newborns.[36,37] There is evidence of maternal IgG antibody production against fetal neutrophils during gestation.[38] The antibody crosses the placenta and damages the infant's neutrophils. The neutropenia is usually severe and is often associated with peripheral blood monocytosis and eosinophilia. Bone marrow shows myeloid hyperplasia, with a decline in band and segmented neutrophils.

Autoimmune Neutropenia

Autoimmune disorders, such as systemic lupus erythematosus, rheumatoid arthritis, and Sjögren syndrome, may demonstrate moderate to severe neutropenia. This type of neutropenia is often associated with an increased concentration of IgG on the surface of neutrophils.[39] Approximately 1% of patients with rheumatoid arthritis may develop Felty syndrome, which is characterized by splenomegaly and neutropenia. Some patients with Felty syndrome demonstrate an increased number of large granular lymphocytes (NK cells) in their peripheral blood.[40]

Bone marrow is usually normocellular, with no diagnostic changes. Some patients may show a hypo- or hypercellular marrow. Mild lymphoplasmacytosis is a frequent finding.

Drug-Induced Neutropenia

There are two major known mechanisms of drug-induced neutropenias. One is a dose-related, drug-induced cytotoxicity affecting protein synthesis or cell replication of the granulocytic precursors. The other is a drug-induced, antibody-mediated granulocytic destruction, in which drugs or their metabolites are the source of haptens or antigens and neutropenia is the result of drug–antibody interactions with the neutrophils. A large number of drugs may cause a mild to moderate neutropenia with no clinical symptoms[41-45] (Table 8-3). Severe neutropenia (agranulocytosis) is rare and is usually associated with fever, sweating, myalgia, vomiting, sore throat and dysphagia. The rate of recovery after elimination of the offending drug is dependent on the extent of bone marrow damage. If the bone marrow precursor cells are relatively intact, recovery will occur within 4–7 days, and usually overproduction (rebound) with marked neutrophilia will follow.

Other Types of Neutropenia

MYELOKATHEXIS: This is an extremely rare form of chronic childhood granulocytopenia with an unknown etiology, characterized by bone marrow myeloid hyperplasia, peripheral neutropenia and degenerative changes in segmented neutrophils. One possible mechanism of neutropenia is defective release of neutrophils from bone marrow. The degenerative changes include nuclear hypersegmentation (with excessive length and thinness of the nuclear filaments), cytoplasmic vacuolization and hypogranularity.[46,47]

LAZY-LEUKOCYTE SYNDROME: This is an extremely rare condition characterized by severe peripheral neutropenia, poor neutrophil chemotaxis and severely impaired random motility of leukocytes.[48,49] Bone marrow is normocellular and shows an adequate number of mature neutrophils.

DIALYSIS NEUTROPENIA: Activation of the complement components due to the contact of plasma with the dialysis membrane may lead to increased neutrophil adhesiveness and aggregation in the lung and other tissues, causing neutropenia. This type of neutropenia is transient and is often followed by a rebound neutrophilia.

NEUTROPENIA ASSOCIATED WITH INFECTIONS: Infectious diseases may cause neutropenia via a variety of mechanisms, such as destruction of the precursor cells (e.g., infectious mononucleosis, viral hepatitis, Kawasaki disease, and AIDS),[50-53] endothelial cell damage (e.g., dengue fever, measles, *Rikettsia* and *Babesia*), or increased utilization at the site of infection.[42] Chronic infections which are associated with splenomegaly, such as tuberculosis, typhoid fever and malaria, may also cause neutropenia because of splenic sequestration.[54]

Eosinopenia and Basopenia

Eosinopenia (eosinophilopenia) may be associated with aplastic anemia, Cushing's syndrome, acromegaly and systemic lupus erythematosus. Exercise, emotional stress, trauma, and administration of corticosteroids, corticotrophin or adrenaline are also associated with a transient eosinopenia.[55] Acute infections may cause eosinopenia.[56]

Basopenia (basophilopenia) has been associated with urticaria and occurs immediately after anaphylaxic shocks. It has also been reported in hyperthyroidism, pregnancy, the onset of ovulation, corticosteroid therapy and in association with granulocytosis.[57] There are occasional reports of patients with total absence of eosinophils and/or basophils.[58-60]

Neutrophilia

An increased number of neutrophils in the peripheral blood (neutrophilia, neutrophilic granulocytosis) is based on the following mechanisms: (1) an acceleration of bone marrow granulocytopoiesis, (2) an increase in the release of cells from the marrow reserve pool to the peripheral blood, (3) a shift from the marginal pool to the circulating pool (demargination), (4) a decline in neutrophil utilization, or (5) a combination of (1) to (4).

Neutrophilia caused by increased granulocytopoiesis is usually associated with infections, inflammations, cancers, endocrinopathies (e.g., eclampsia, hyperthyroidism, Cushing's syndrome) and hematologic disorders.[61-63] Proliferation of the cells in the mitotic pool (stem cells, myeloblasts, promyelocytes and myelocytes) is probably induced by

Table 8-3 Drugs Which May Induce Neutropenia*

Antibacterial agents	Antimalarials
Cephalosporins	Amodiaquine
Chloramphenicol	Chloroquine
Clindamycin	Dapsone
Gentamicin	Pyrimethamine
Isoniazid	Quinine
Para-aminosalicylic acid	**Anthithyroid drugs**
Penicillins	Carbimazole
Rifampin	Methimazole
Streptomycin	Propylthiouracil
Sulfonamides	**Cardiovascular drugs**
Tetracyclines	Captopril
Vancomycin	Disopyramide
Anticonvulsants	Hydralazine
Carbamazepine	Methyldopa
Mephenytoin	Procainamide
Phenytoin	Propranolol
Antidepressants	Quinidine
Amitriptyline	Tocainide
Amoxapine	**Diuretics**
Desipramine	Acetazolamide
Doxepin	Chlorthalidone
Imipramine	Chlorothiazide
Antihistamines—H$_2$ blockers	Ethacrynic acid
Cimetidine	Hydrochlorothiazide
Ranitidine	**Hypoglycemic agents**
Anti-inflammatory agents and analgesics	Chlorpropamide
	Tolbutamide
Indomethacin	**Hypnotics and sedatives**
Gold salts	Chlordiazepoxide and
Pentazocine	other benzodiazepines
Para-aminophenol derivatives	Meprobamate
Acetaminophen	**Other Drugs**
Phenacetin	Allopurinol
Pyrazolon derivatives	Levamisole
Aminopyrine	Penicillamine
Dipyrone	Chlorpromazine
Oxyphenbutazone	Phenothiazines
Phenylbutazone	

* Adapted from Dale DC Neutrophilia, Williams WJ, Beutler E, Erslev AJ, et al (eds), *Hematology*, ed 4. New York, McGraw-Hill, 1990, p 816.

the release of some growth-promoting mediators. For example, production of a granulocytic CSF by tumor cells has been reported in a case of gastric carcinoma.[64] In CML, in addition to increased granulopoiesis, there is evidence of increased granulocyte survival in peripheral blood.

Granulocytosis due to the demargination of granulocytes is a transient condition usually caused by vigorous exercise, electric shock, emotional stress, vomiting, convulsions, paroxysmal tachycardia, or infusion of catecholamines.[65,66] Demargination neutrophilia is usually associated with lymphocytosis and monocytosis.

Neutrophilia in acute conditions is caused primarily by the release of neutrophils from the bone marrow reserve into the peripheral blood.[67] The re-

White Blood Cell Disorders

serve consists of metamyelocytes, bands and segmented neutrophils (the nonmitotic marrow pool), but usually bands and segmented cells are the only cells that are released into the peripheral blood in normal conditions. This shift of cells from the bone marrow to the peripheral blood pool is an immediate response to infections, inflammations, and certain hormones (epinephrine, corticosteroids, CSFs) and chemicals (lithium salts, endotoxin, venoms, vaccines).[68-70] The shift from marrow pool to blood pool is often associated with a higher percentage of circulating bands (left shift), which often has been used as a sign of acute infection, particularly in children.

Certain functional abnormalities of neutrophils, such as deficiency of adhesion molecules, may also be associated with neutrophilia due to decreased utilization of the neutrophils.

The term *leukemoid reaction* is often used to refer to extreme neutrophilia. The major features that are used to differentiate leukemoid reactions from CML are lack of early immature myeloid cells in the peripheral blood, elevated LAP scores and lack of Ph^1 chromosome[71] (see Chapter 6). Bone marrow biopsy sections in leukemoid reactions show a higher frequency of paratrabecular fat, and demonstrate more sinusoids and fewer capillaries than bone marrow biopsy sections in CML.[72] There are also fewer pseudo-Gaucher cells and a higher percentage of mast cells in the bone marrow of patients with leukemoid reactions compared to those with CML.

Eosinophilia

Eosinophilia (eosinophilic leukocytosis) is observed in a variety of conditions, such as allergic and inflammatory processes, protozoan and metazoan infections, immunodeficiencies and autoimmune disorders, malignancies, and hypereosinophilic syndromes (Table 8-4). In most instances, reactive eosinophilia is the result of accelerated proliferation of the eosinophils in the marrow. A number of hematpoietic growth factors and interleukins regulate eosinophilic production and maturation (Figure 8-3). Non-lineage-specific, synergistic factors act on very early progenitor cells, while lineage-specific factors regulate committed progenitors and eosinophilic precursors. Eosinophil migration from bone marrow into the circulation and tissues is influenced by several factors, such as eosinophil chemotactic factor of anaphylaxis, histamine, C5a, antigen–antibody complexes, leukotriene B4, and platelet activating factor (PAF).[73,74]

Table 8-4 Conditions Associated With Eosinophilia

Parasites
  Protozoan infections
    Pneumocystis, toxoplasmosis, amebiasis, malaria
  Metazoan infections
    Nematodes, trematodes, cestodes, arthropods

Allergic and inflammatory disorders
  Hay fever, asthma, angioneurotic edema, urticaria and angioderma, serum sickness, allergic vasculitis, Stevens-Johnson syndrome, psoriasis, eczema, dermatitis herpetiformis, pemphigus vulgaris, ichthyosis, other dermatides, eosinophilic gastroenteritis, ulcerative colitis, regional enteritis, milk precipitin disease

Malignancies and premalignancies
  Hematologic
    Hodgkin's disease, mycosis fungoides, other non-Hodgkin's lymphomas, acute lymphocytic leukemia, acute myelogenous leukemia, chronic myelogenous leukemia, eosinophilic leukemia, chronic myeloproliferative disorders, multiple myeloma, heavy chain disease
  Other malignancies
    Carcinomas, brain tumors, melanoma

Histiocytosis
  Langerhans cell histiocytosis
  Familial erythrophagocytic lymphohistiocytosis

Hypereosinophilic syndrome

Miscellaneous
  Immunodeficiency syndromes, autoimmune disorders, sarcoidosis, splenectomy, chronic renal disease, peritoneal dialysis, pleural effusion, hypoxia, radiotherapy, familial eosinophilia

Hypereosinophilic Syndromes

Marked reactive eosinophilias of unknown etiology are referred to as *idiopathic hypereosinophilic syndromes* and are characterized by (1) persistent eosinophilia equal to or greater than 1500/μl for >6 months, (2) evidence of eosinophilic tissue infiltration, and (3) no underlying cause for the eosinophilia.[75] Activated T cells appear to play a role in the mechanism of eosinophilia in hypereosinophilic syndromes. A subset of IL-2-stimulated CD4$^+$ CD8$^-$ T lymphocytes is able to produce a CFU-Eo growth-stimulating factor.[76] This production is inhibited by hydrocortisone or cyclosporine A. AIDS patients receiving IL-2 may also show hypereosinophilia.[77]

Hypereosinophilia is associated with an increased proportion of hypodense eosinophils. Hypodense

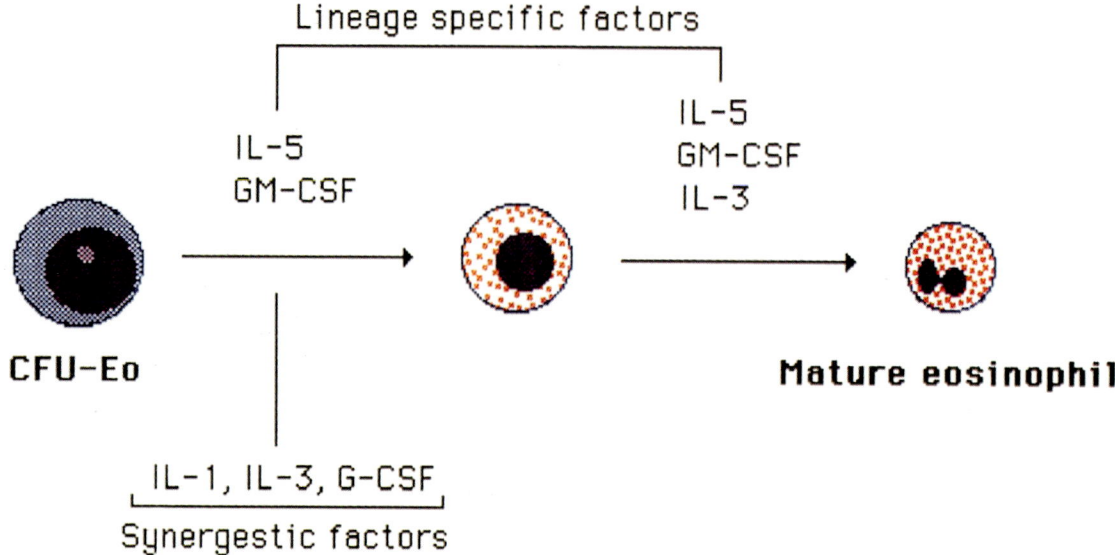

Figure 8-3. Schematic illustration of the effect of hematopoietic growth factors on eosinophil maturation. Adapted from Liesveld JL and Abboud CN: State of the art: The hypereosinophilic syndromes. *Blood Rev* 5:29, 1991.

eosinophils show higher than normal oxygen consumption; have a greater number of IgG, Fc, and complement receptors; demonstrate increased cytotoxicity for antibody-coated targets; and are degranulated with low eosinophil cationic protein levels.[78] The eosinophils in hypereosinophilic syndromes are often atypical and may show abnormal nuclear segmentation, doughnut-shaped nuclei, and hypogranulation (Figure 8-4). Bone marrow shows marked eosinophilia (usually >30%), with a shift to the left (Figure 8-5).

Hypereosinophilic syndrome has a male predominance, with a peak incidence in the fifth decade. The organs most frequently involved are the heart, lungs, skin and nervous system.[73] Patients with hypereosinophilic syndrome often have a hypercoagulable status.

Other Conditions Associated with Eosinophilia

TRYPTOPHAN-INDUCED EOSINOPHILIA-MYALGIA SYNDROME: This syndrome has been reported in association with the use of some tryptophan products and is characterized by peripheral eosinophilia and scleroderma-like features including muscle tenderness, fatigue, edema, arthralgia, neuropathy, rash, cough, and dyspnea.[79,80a,80b] Tryptophan has been used to treat insomnia, depression and other symptoms.

EOSINOPHILIA ASSOCIATED WITH MALIGNANT TUMORS: Eosinophilias observed in association with a variety of solid tumors such as bronchogenic carcinoma, medullary carcinoma of the thyroid and malignant fibrous histiocytoma are probably the result of a tumor-derived eosinophilopoietic factor.[81,82]

Eosinophilia has also been observed in association with hematopoietic malignancies such as CML, AML, ALL and multiple myeloma. A subtype of AML-M4 is associated with atypical eosinophilia and chromosomal aberrations of 16q22 (see page 151). Some of the AMLs (e.g., AML-M5) demonstrate trisomy 22 with eosinophilia. Some of the CD10-positive acute lymphoblastic leukemias are associated with (5;14)(q31;q32) translocation and hypereosinophilia.[83,84]

True eosinophilic leukemia probably represents an aggressive unresponsive spectrum of the hypereosinophilic syndromes. It is characterized by a marked eosinophilia with massive organ involvement and no response to corticosteroid therapy or even chemotherapy (see page 189). True eosinophilic leukemias may show chromosomal aberrations.[85]

White Blood Cell Disorders

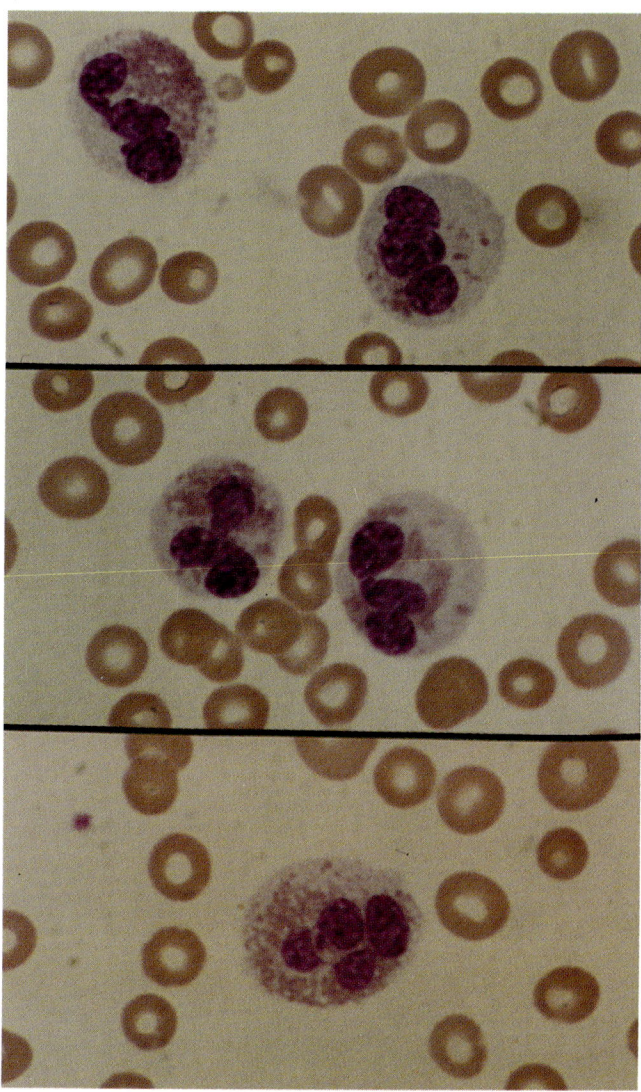

Figure 8-4. Peripheral blood smear from a patient with hypereosinophilic syndrome demonstrating large, atypical, hypersegmented eosinophils. Some of the eosinophils are hypogranular.

Basophilia

Basophilia (basophil leukocytosis) may occur in inflammations and infections such as hypersensitivity reactions, ulcerative colitis, rheumatoid arthritis, chickenpox, influenza, smallpox and tuberculosis.[86] Other conditions associated with basophilia include irradiation, iron deficiency, endocrinopathies (hypothyroidism, diabetes mellitus) and myeloproliferative disorders (particularly CML and AML). Certain subtypes of AML such as promyelocytic leukemia and AMLs with t(6;9), t(3;6) and inversion of chromosome 16 may demonstrate bone marrow basophilia.[87-89]

True basophilic leukemia is rare and is characterized by a hypercellular bone marrow with a myeloid left shift and marked basophilia (see page 191). It may demonstrate clinical symptoms that result from the release of mediators from basophils, such as flushing, palpitations, hives, pruritus and angioedema.[90,91]

Mastocytosis

Bone marrow mastocytosis is a prominent feature of primary mast cell disorders and has also been associated with a variety of hematologic and nonhematologic conditions such as chronic lymphoproliferative disorders, myelodysplastic and myeloproliferative syndromes, AML, aplastic anemia, chronic liver disease, bone marrow fibrosis, and osteoporosis.[92-96] A revised classification was proposed in the recent symposium on "Clinical Advances in Mastocytosis," in which four major categories were recognized: (1) indolent mastocytosis, (2) mastocytosis associated with hematologic disorders, (3) aggressive mastocytosis, and (4) mastocytic leukemia[97,98] (Table 8-5). Many of the conditions in category 1, such as indolent forms with cutaneous disease (urticaria pigmentosa) or with bone marrow mast cell aggregates, as well as all conditions in categories 2 through 4, are commonly associated with bone marrow mastocytosis.[99-107]

Bone marrow involvement in mast cell disorders is typically focal or nodular, with foci of spindle-shaped mast cells against a fibrotic background found in perivascular, paratrabecular, or other locations (Figure 8-5). Mast cells show fine cytoplasmic redish-purple to purplish-black granules. The cytoplasmic granules are better demonstrated with the Giemsa or toluidine blue stains. The stains may appear negative in the decalcified tissues; thus nondecalcified, plastic-embedded biopsy specimens, marrow clots and smears are preferred. Mast cell clusters are often mixed with variable amounts of eosinophils and lymphocytes. The term *"mastocytic eosinophilic fibrohistiocytic lesion of the bone marrow"* has been referred to the bone marrow lesions that are composed of spindle-shaped, fibroblast-like mast cells mixed with eosinophils.

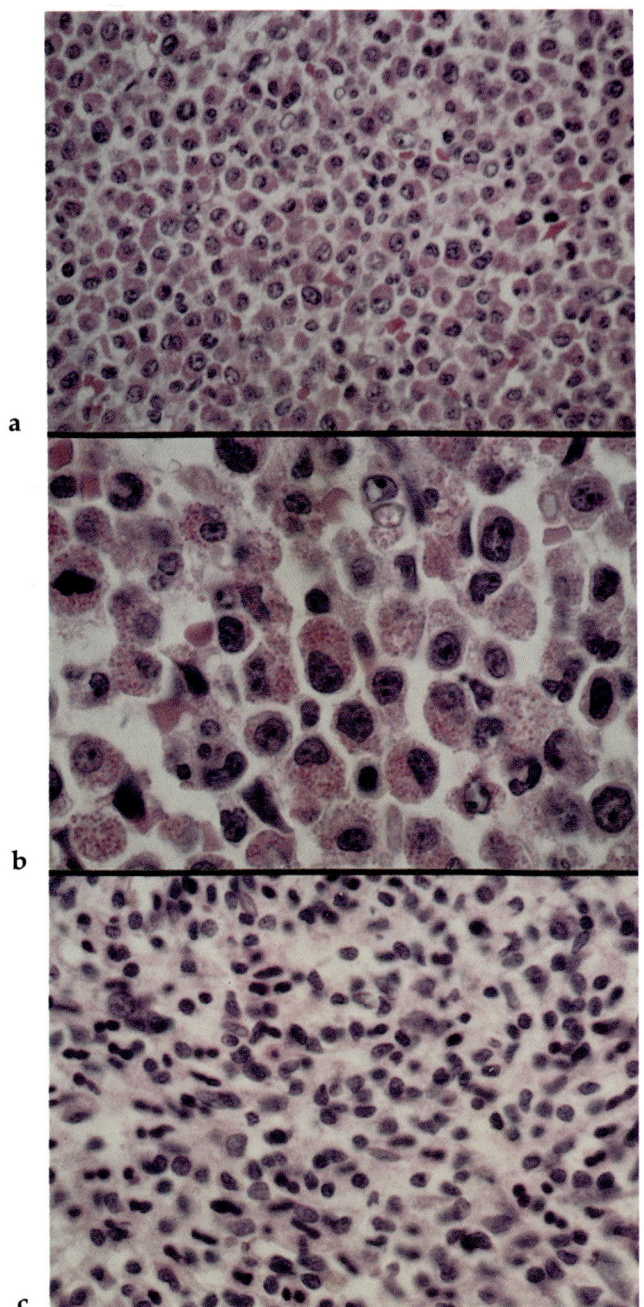

Figure 8-5. Bone marrow biopsy section from a patient with hypereosinophilic syndrome demonstrating marked eosinophilia with a shift to the left (a and b). Bone marrow biopsy section from a patient with systemic mastocytosis. Mast cells show granular cytoplasm and elongated nuclei (c).

[101-103] These lesions are often associated with osteoporosis. The extent of the lymphocytic component may vary from a few scattered lymphocytes to a predominantly lymphocytic cluster with a small number of mast cells.[100] The lymphoid component is usually a mixture of B and T lymphocytes, with virtual absence of the NK cells. Bone marrow mastocytosis may be associated with trabecular thickening. Bone marrow mast cell lesions in children are somewhat different from those in adults. They are smaller, are more frequently perivascular, do not show trabecular thickening, are often composed of

Table 8-5 Classification of Mast Cell Disorders*

  I. Indolent
    A. Syncope
    B. Cutaneous disease
    C. Ulcer disease
    D. Malabsorption
    E. Bone marrow mast cell aggregates
    F. Skeletal disease
    G. Hepatosplenomegaly
    H. Lymphadenopathy
 II. Hematologic disorder
    A. Myeloproliferative
    B. Myelodysplastic
III. Aggressive Lymphadenopathic mastocytosis with eosinophilia
IV. Mastocytic leukemia

* Revised classification proposed in the symposium on "Clinical Advances in Mastocytosis: An Interdisciplinary Roundtable Discussion," 1990 (Ref. 98).

Table 8-6 Disorders of Monocytes and Histiocytes

  I. **Qualitative disorders**
    1. Chronic granulomatous disease
    2. CHS
    3. Defective mononuclear leukocyte chemotaxis
    4. Effects of corticosteroid therapy and tobacco smoking
    5. Osteoclast deficiency (osteopetrosis)
 II. **Quantitative disorders**
    1. Reactive
        A. Monocytopenia
        B. Monocytosis
        C. Histiocytosis
            a. Langerhans cell histiocytosis (class I histiocytosis, histiocytosis X)
            b. Hemophagocytic syndromes (class II histiocytosis)
              —Familial hemophagocytic lymphohistiocytosis
              —Infection-associated hemophagocytic histiocytosis
              —Sinus histiocytosis with massive lymphadenopathy
    2. Premalignant and malignant conditions (class III histiocytosis)
        A. Chronic myelomonocytic leukemia
        B. Juvenile chronic myelogenous leukemia
        C. Chronic monocytic leukemia
        D. Acute myelomonocytic and monocytic leukemias
        E. Malignant histiocytosis
        F. True malignant histiocytic lymphoma
III. **Lysosomal storage diseases**
    1. Sphingolipidosis
    2. Glycoproteinosis
    3. Mucolipidosis
    4. Mucopolysaccharidosis
    5. Others

mast cells with round or oval nuclei, are less fibrotic, and often yield large aggregates of mast cells in marrow smears.[99]

Diagnosis of mast cell disorders is accomplished by careful clinical evaluation of patients and the use of histologic examination of key tissues together with the measurement of urinary and/or plasma levels of biochemical markers of mast cells.[108] Biochemical markers include histamine, prostaglandin D2, tryptase, and heparin.

MONOCYTIC AND HISTIOCYTIC DISORDERS

Disorders of monocytes and histiocytes (macrophages) are predominantly quantitative. Qualitative abnormalities, such as chronic granulomatous disease and CHS, are rare and are associated with similar defects in the granulocytes. A classification of monocytic and histiocytic disorders is presented in Table 8-6. The quantitative reactive disorders are as follows:

Monocytopenia and Monocytosis

Monocytopenia is a rare event and occurs in patients with aplastic anemia and hairy cell leukemia, after glucocorticoid administration, and in severe thermal injuries.[109-111] Cyclic neutropenia is also associated with intermittent periods of monocytopenia. A decreased absolute peripheral blood monocyte count has been observed in patients with rheumatoid arthritis, systemic lupus erythematosus, and AIDS.[112-114]

Monocytosis is more frequent than monocytopenia and is observed in a wide variety of conditions such as infections, inflammations, hematologic disorders and malignant conditions (Table 8-7). Certain chronic or subacute infections, such as tuberculosis, syphilis and subacute bacterial endocarditis, demonstrate monocytosis.[115-117] A number of collagen vascular disorders such as polyarteritis nodosa, temporal arteritis, systemic lupus erythematosus and rheumatoid arthritis may show mild to moderate monocytosis.[118-120] Premalignant and malignant hematologic conditions are the most frequent causes of monocytosis. They include myelodysplastic syndromes (particularly CMML), myeloproliferative disorders, CML, CMoL, AMML and AML. Hodgkin's disease, non-Hodgkin's lymphomas and multiple myeloma. Other hematologic disorders which may show monocytosis are hemolytic anemia, histiocytosis, chronic neutropenias and idiopathic thrombocytopenic purpura.[120,121]

Table 8-7 Conditions Associated with Monocytosis

I. **Infections**
   Tuberculosis, syphilis, subacute bacterial endocarditis, cytomegalovirus infection, disseminated candidiasis
II. **Inflammatory and immune-associated disorders**
   Myositis, temporal arteritis, polyarteritis nodosa, rheumatoid arthritis, systemic lupus erythematosus, sarcoidosis, ulcerative colitis, regional enteritis, alcoholic liver disease
III. **Hematologic disorders**
   1. Premalignant and malignant conditions: myelodysplastic syndromes, myeloproliferative disorders, AML, CML, CMoL, Hodgkin's disease, non-Hodgkin's lymphomas, multiple myeloma
   2. Nonneoplastic conditions: histiocytosis, hemolytic anemias, chronic neutropenias, postsplenectomy, idiopathic thrombocytopenic purpura
IV. **Nonhematopoietic malignancies**
V. **Drug-related**
   Chloropromazine, ampicillin, tetrachloroethane, glucocorticoid

Histiocytosis

Langerhans Cell Histiocytosis (Class 1 Histiocytosis)

Langerhans cell histiocytosis (LCH) is the current term for the disorders previously called *histiocytosis X*. This disorder, based on the extent of the disease and the sites of involvement, embraces a wide variety of clinical manifestations including eosinophilic granuloma, Letterer-Siwe disease, Hand-Schuller-Christian disease, Hashimoto-Pritzker syndrome, self-healing reticulohistiocytosis and pure cutaneous histiocytosis.[122-128]

ETIOLOGY AND PATHOGENESIS: The etiology and pathogenesis of LCH are not well understood. It has been suggested that Langerhans cell proliferation in LCH escapes the control mechanisms due to immunologic aberrations.[129-132] Patients with LCH may show abnormal thymic histology and may demonstrate in vitro autocytotoxicity against fibroblasts or red cells by their own effector cells.[129,130,132] Cigarette smoking may play a role in the development of pulmonary LCH in adults.[133]

PATHOLOGY: Bone is the most frequent site of involvement and is affected in about 80% of LCH cases.[134] The most commonly affected bone is the skull, followed by the femur, pelvis, tibia, scapula, vertebrae, and ribs. Bone involvement in over one-third of the cases is also associated with bone marrow involvement. Other frequently involved tissues in LCH are skin, lymph nodes, spleen, liver and lungs, followed by orbital and orodental tissues, ear, central nervous system and gastrointestinal tract.[134] Biopsy specimens from the involved areas demonstrate focal or diffuse infiltration of large histiocytes with abundant, ill-defined, finely granular or vacuolated eosinophilic cytoplasm and an oval, riniform or indented nucleus (Figures 8-6 and 8-7). Mitotic figures are absent or extremely rare, and nucleoli are inconspicuous. The histiocytic infiltrate is often mixed with various amounts of inflammatory cells, particularly eosinophils. In more chronic lesions, inflammatory cells are replaced by fibrosis (Figure 8-7). Multinucleated giant cells may be present and may appear individually or in clusters. Marrow smears show increased numbers of histiocytes, with abundant vacuolated or finely granular cytoplasm and round or irregular nuclei (Figure 8-8).

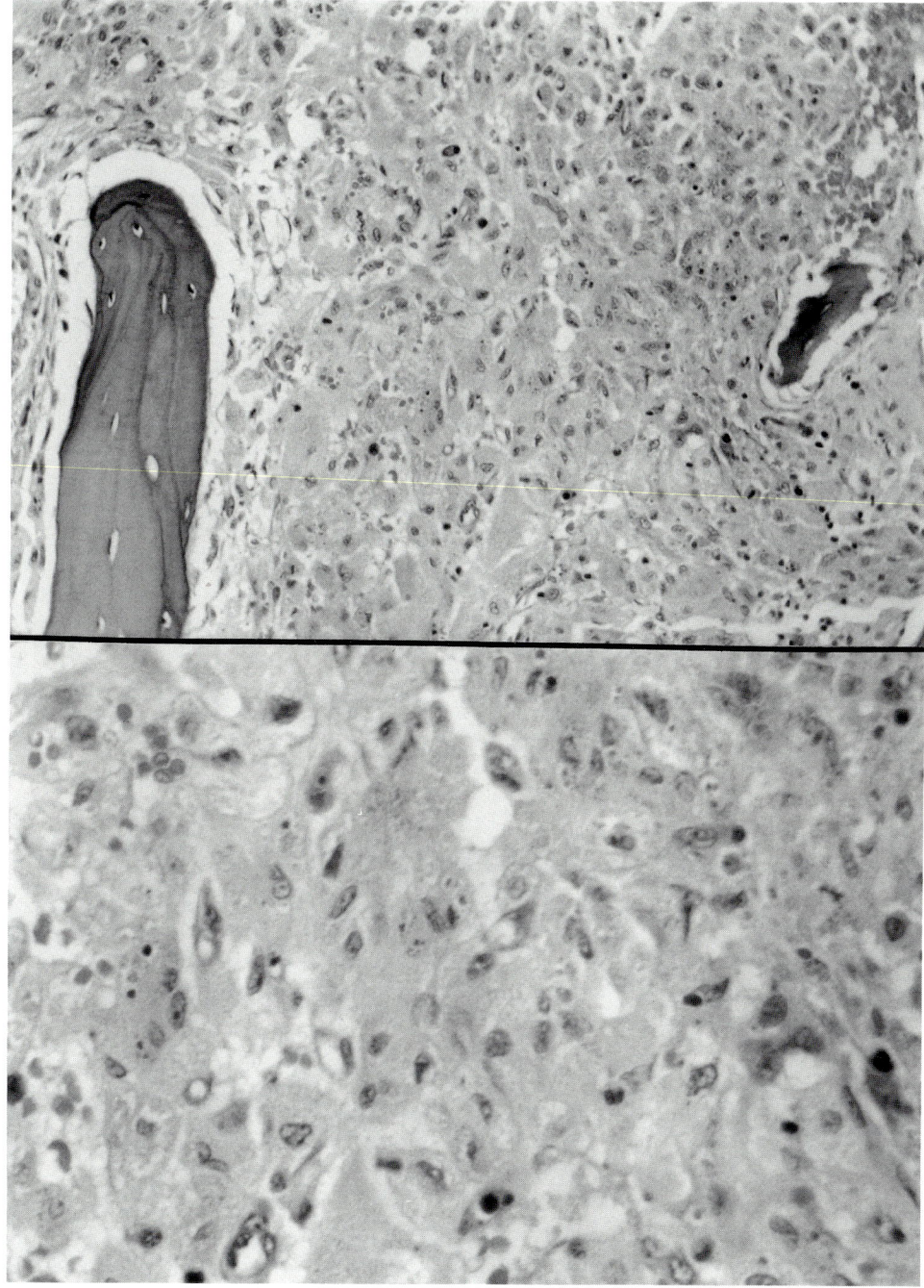

Figure 8-6. Bone marrow section from a patient with Langerhans cell histiocytosis showing diffuse marrow involvement. Langerhans cells have abundant, finely granular cytoplasm and a bland vesicular nucleus.

Electron microscopy demonstrates the characteristic cytoplasmic granules known as *Birbeck* or *Langerhans cell granules* (Figure 8-9). These granules are rod-shaped, often with an expanded end resembling a tennis racket. Langerhans cells express CD1 (T-6) antigen; are positive for ATPase, alpha-D-mannosidase, and S-100 protein; and bind to peanut lectin. Langerhans cells, unlike ordinary histiocytes, are usually negative for nonspecific esterase and alpha-1-anti-chymotrypsin (Table 8-8).

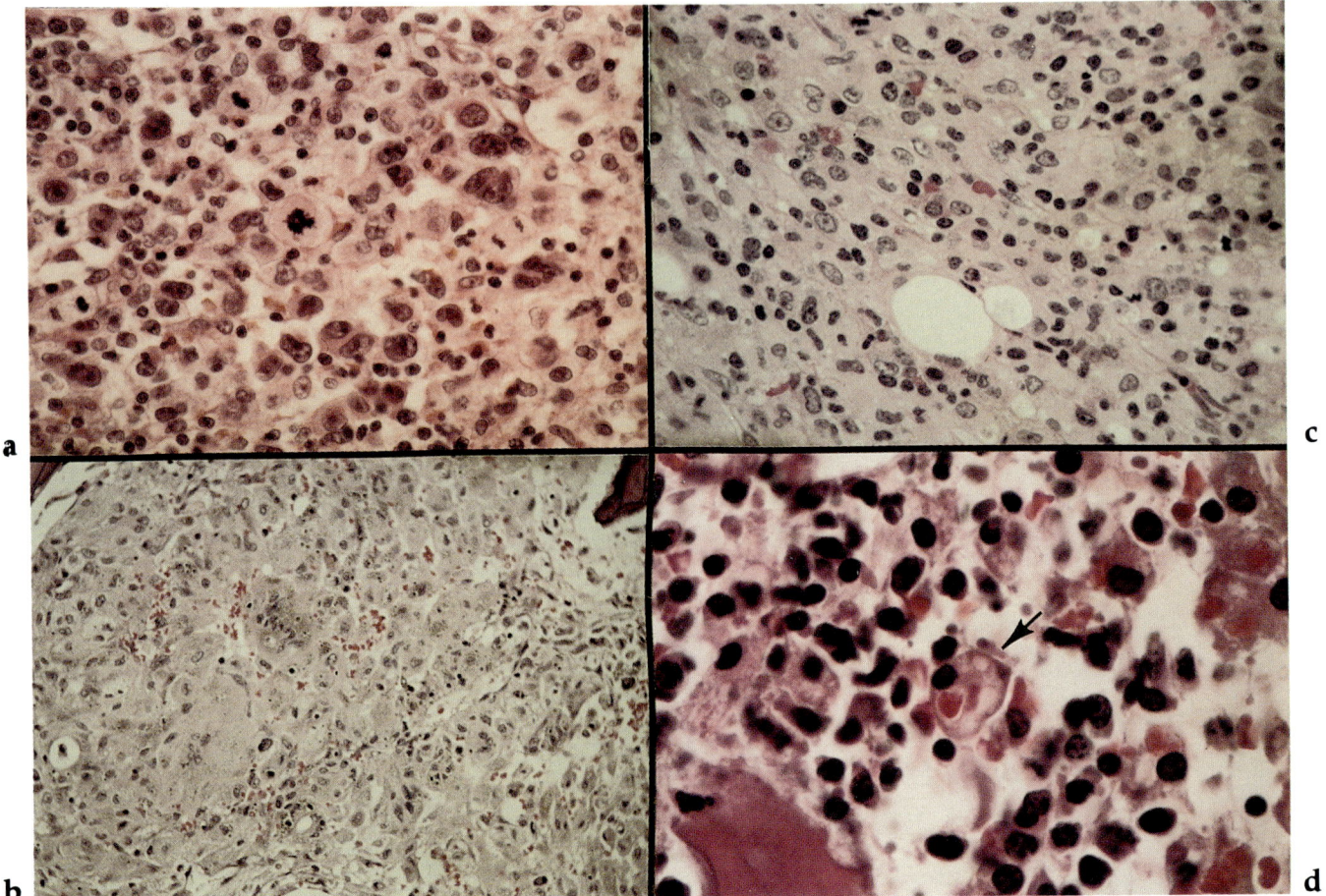

Figure 8-7. Bone marrow biopsy sections in the early stages of involvement with Langerhans cell histiocytosis are usually accompanied by inflammatory cells, particularly eosinophils (a); the inflammatory response gradually declines (b, c). A bone marrow biopsy section from a patient with hemophagocytic lymphohistiocytosis demonstrating several erythrophagocytic histiocytes (d, arrow).

According to the Writing Group of the Histiocytic Society, a "definitive diagnosis" of LCH in a histiocytic lesion requires the demonstration of Birbeck granules or expression of CD1 antigen. A "designated diagnosis" is justified when the histologic findings are supported by positivity for two or more of the following markers: ATPase, alpha-D-mannosidase, S-100 protein and binding to peanut lectin.[128]

Langerhans cell histiocytosis may be associated with neutrophilia, increased serum alkaline phosphatase and an elevated sedimentation rate.

CLINICAL ASPECTS: Langerhans cell histiocytosis is predominantly a childhood disease. Over 70% of patients are under 10 years of age, and over 90% are diagnosed before age 30.[135,136] Symptoms and signs depend on the extent of the disease. The most frequent clinical findings are fever, skin lesions, hepatosplenomegaly and lymphadenopathy. Bone pain and tenderness caused by osseous lesions occur frequently in the head (skull, ear, mastoid), leg, back or chest. Primary pulmonary involvement and isolated generalized lymphadenopathy are more common in adults.

Isolated bone lesions have a good prognosis. Poor prognostic factors are young age (<2 years), multiple organ involvement and pancytopenia.[135,137,138] A scoring system was proposed by Lahey based on the number of organs involved; the mortality rate was zero with a score of 1, 35% with a score of 3 or 4 and

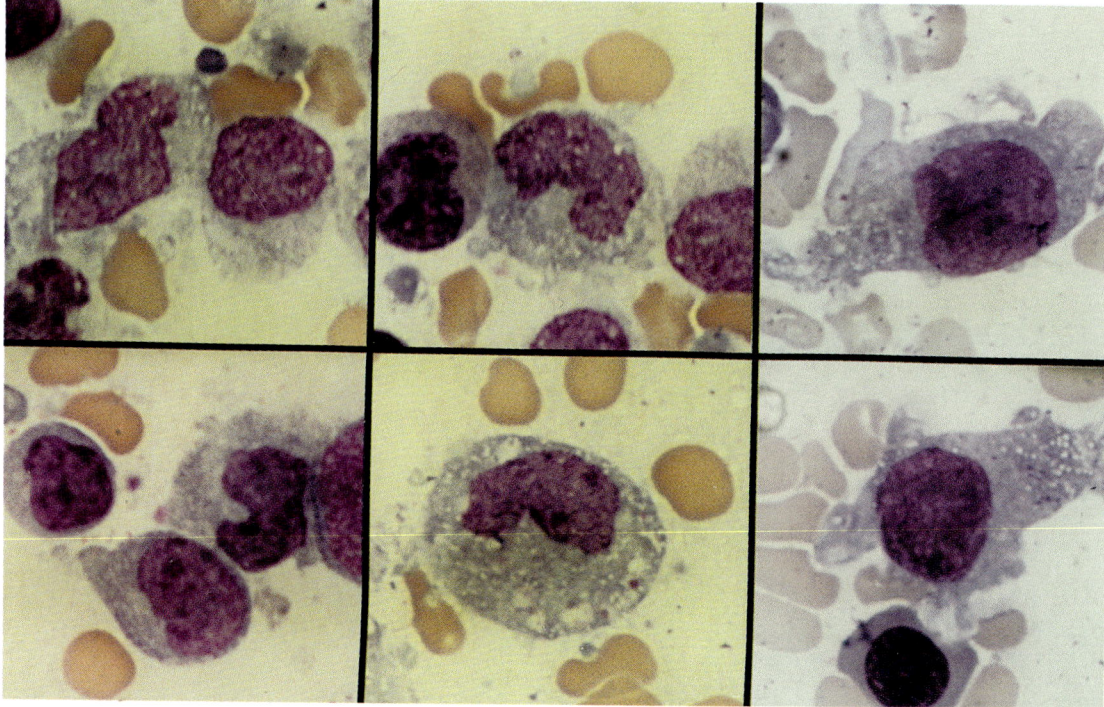

Figure 8-8. Langerhans cell histiocytosis. Bone marrow smears demonstrating large mononuclear cells with abundant cytoplasm and round, oval or folded nuclei.

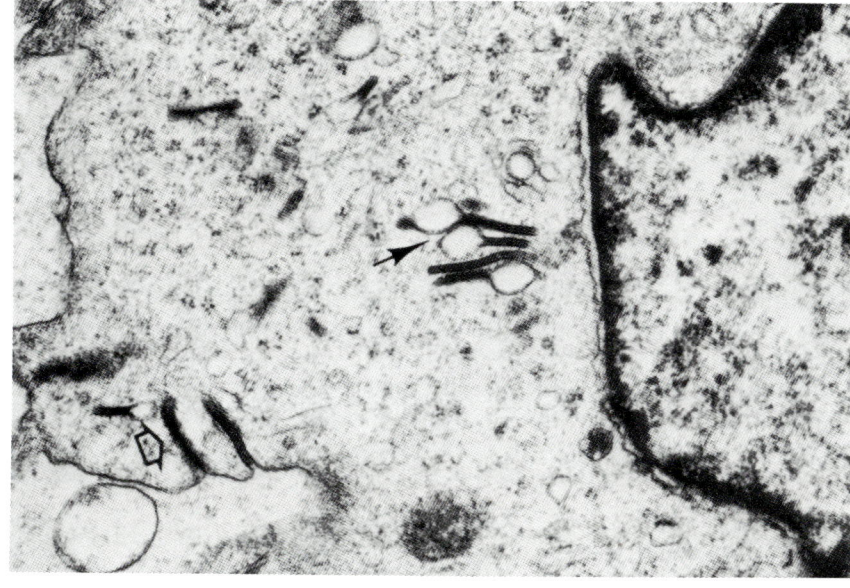

Figure 8-9. Electron microscopy of a Langerhans cell displaying Birbeck granules (arrow). From Favora BE, Jaffe R: Pathology of Langerhans cell histiocytosis. *Hematol Oncol North Am* 1:75, 1987, with permission.

Table 8-8 Features of Histiocytic Subsets

Features	Monocyte	Macrophage	LC[a]	DRC[b]	IRC[c]
Nonspecific esterase	+	+ +	±	−	±
Acid phosphatase	+	+ +	±	−	±
Alpha 1-antitrypsin	+	+	−	−	−
Lysozyme	+	+	−	−	−
Mannosidase	−	−	+	+	+
ATPase	−	−	+	+	+
S-100	−	−	+	+	+
CD1	−	−	+	±	±
CD11c	+	+	−	−	−
CD13/CD33	+	−	−	−	−
CD14	+	±	±	±	±
CD21	+	+	−	+	−
FcIgG	+	+	+	+	+
HLA-DR	+	+	+	+	+
Birbeck granules	−	−	+	−	−

[a] Langerhans cell.
[b] Dendritic reticulum cell.
[c] Interdigitating reticulum cell.

100% with a score of 8.[139] Occasional cases of *malignant histiocytosis X* have been reported (see Chapter 6).

Hemophagocytic Syndromes (Class II Histiocytosis)

This group of histiocytic disorders is characterized by proliferation of non-Langerhans reactive histiocytes, with evidence of hemophagocytic activities. The three most common types are hemophagocytic lymphohistiocytosis (familial hemophagocytic reticulosis), infection-associated hemophagocytic syndrome, and sinus histiocytosis with massive lymphadenopathy.

HEMOPHAGOCYTIC LYMPHOHISTIOCYTOSIS (FAMILIAL HEMOPHAGOCYTIC LYMPHOHISTIOCYTOSIS): The clinicopathologic features of hemophagocytic lymphohistiocytosis include evidence of a systemic disorder with lesional predilection for bone marrow, lymph nodes, spleen, liver and meninges; lack of evidence of an infectious process; and evidence of reactive lymphohistiocytosis with varying degrees of hemophagocytosis.[128]

ETIOLOGY AND PATHOGENESIS. The etiology and pathogenesis of hemophagocytic lymphohistiocytosis remain uncertain. Lymphohistiocytosis appears to be a reactive process rather than a malignancy.[140,141] Multiple immune defects have been reported in association with this disorder, such as impaired NK cell activity, decreased monocyte-dependent cytotoxicity, impaired IL-2 and interferon production, and a decreased T-cell response to mitogens.[142-145] The clinicopathologic similarities between familial erythrophagocytic lymphohistiocytosis, Infection-associated hemophagocytosis, and the accelerated phase of CHS and their association with immunodeficiency states may suggest a common pathway of an abnormal immune response, leading to marked unregulated histiocytic proliferation and activation.[142] According to Brown and associates, many of the findings in hemophagocytic syndromes such as fever, hypofibrinogenemia, thrombocytopenia and hyperlipidemia may be secondary to increased production of prostaglandins E2 and F2α by hyperactivated histiocytes.[146]

PATHOLOGY. Erythrophagocytic lymphohistiocytosis is characterized by a diffuse infiltration of lymphocytes and histiocytes into various organs, such as liver, spleen, lymph nodes, thymus, bone marrow and the central nervous system. Other sites of involvement include the lungs, gastrointestinal tract and genitourinary system. Skin involvement is extremely rare.

White Blood Cell Disorders

The histiocytes have abundant, finely granular or vacuolated cytoplasm, with a bland, oval, cleaved or folded nucleus and lack of the cytologic features of malignancy. Mitotic figures are absent or extremely rare and hemophagocytosis, particularly erythrophagocytosis, is prominent (Figures 8-7, 8-10 and 8-11). These histiocytes, unlike the Langerhans cells, are strongly positive for nonspecific esterase, acid phosphatase, alpha-1-antitrypsin and lysozyme; express CD11c and CD68 antigens; and are negative for CD1 antigen and S-100 protein (Table 8-8). They also do not demonstrate Birbeck granules by electron microscopic examination.

Bone marrow biopsy specimens and/or aspirates may show focal or diffuse involvement. Sometimes the first marrow biopsy attempt may yield nondiagnostic findings; thus, additional marrow samples are required.[147]

Laboratory findings include anemia, which is often associated with neutropenia and thrombocytopenia; hyperlipidemia with increased serum triglycerides; a low to normal cholesterol level; and hyperprostaglandinemia.[141,146,148] Hyperbilirubinemia, coagulation factor deficiencies (particularly hypofibrinogenemia) and elevated serum enzymes are frequently observed and are evidence of hepatic involvement.

CLINICAL ASPECTS. Hemophagocytic lymphohistiocytosis is predominantly a familial disease (probably autosomal recessive) but may also occur sporadically.[128] The disease affects neonates and infants, with over 80% of the cases presenting before 2 years of age,[142] and over 65% of the cases occur in siblings.[149,150] Irritability, failure to thrive, anorexia and diarrhea are frequent findings, and virtually all patients have fever and develop hepatosplenomegaly early in the course of the disease. Approximately 30% of the patients show neurologic abnormalities.[151,152]

INFECTION-ASSOCIATED HEMOPHAGOCYTIC SYNDROME: This syndrome presents a clinicopathologic picture

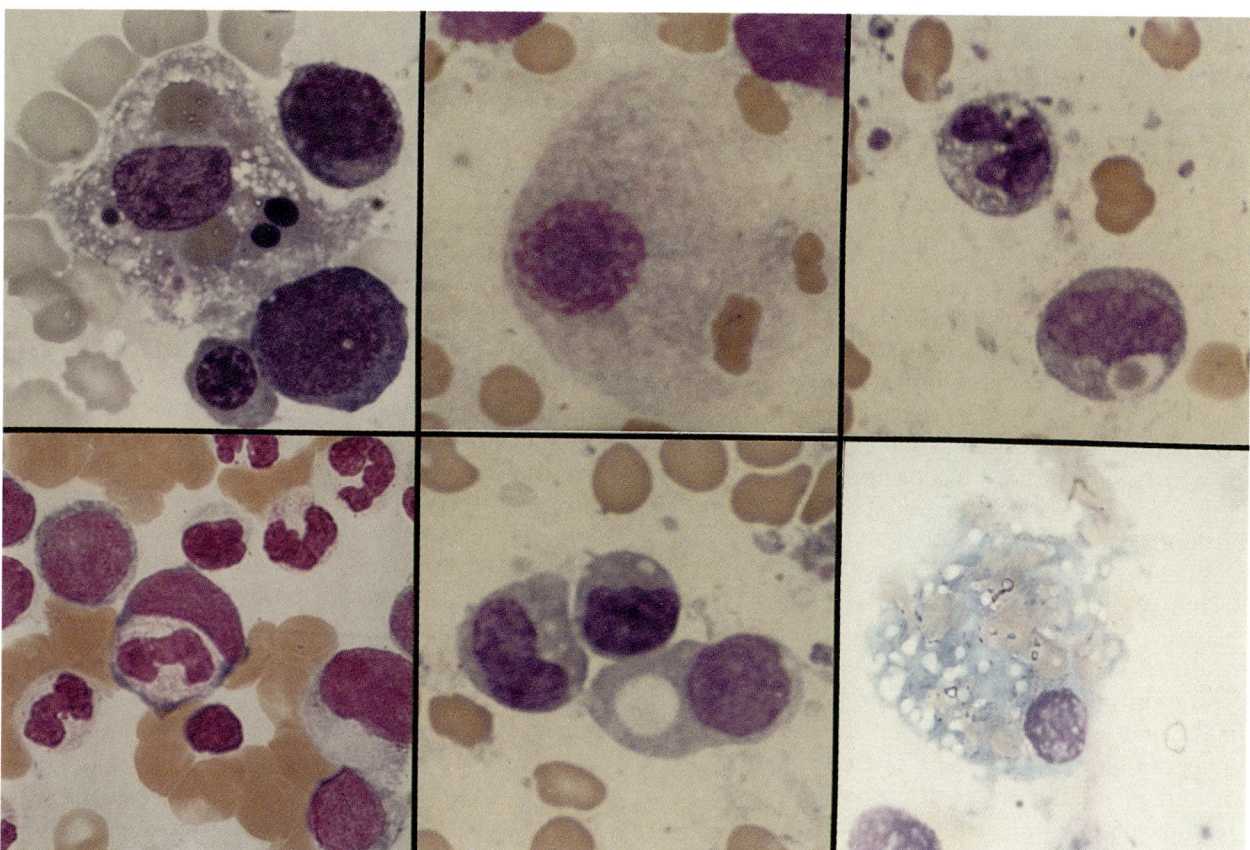

Figure 8-10. Bone marrow smears demonstrating macrophages with a variety of hemophagocytoses.

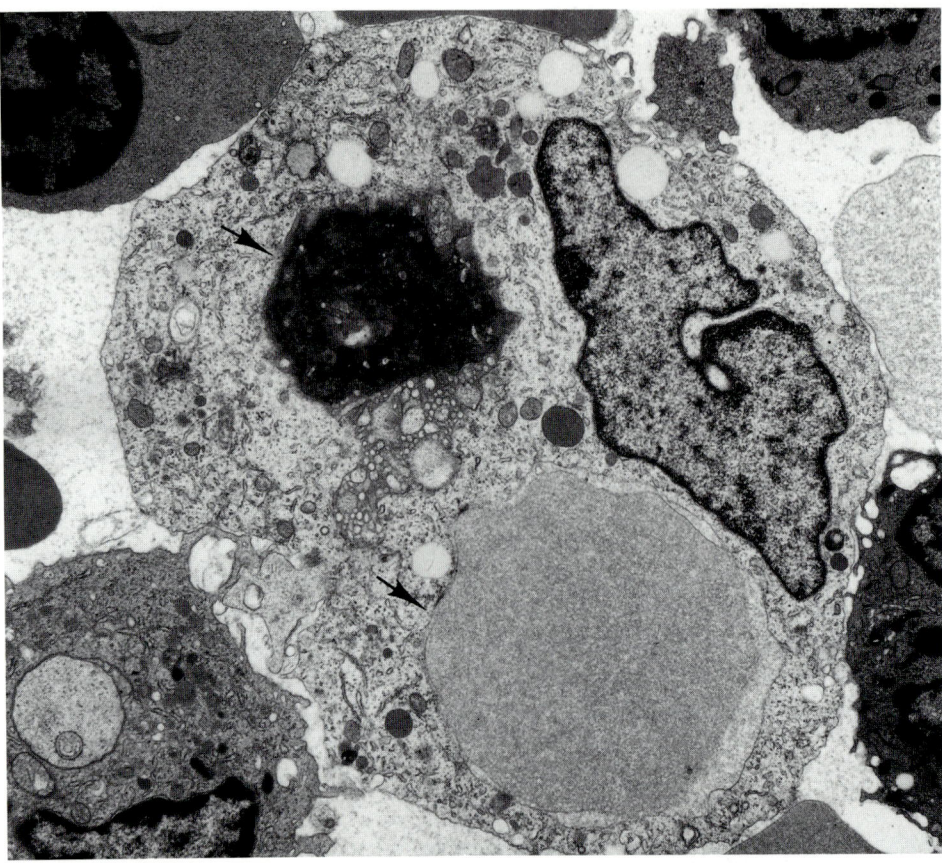

Figure 8-11. Electron microscopy of a macrophage with remnants of a phagocytosed red cell and nuclear debris.

which is almost identical to that observed in familial hemophagocytic lymphohistiocytosis, except that (1) it is not a familial disorder and (2) it is associated with infections. The syndrome generally develops in patients with preexisting immunologic abnormalities or malignancies. A wide variety of microorganisms are able to induce a hemophagocytic histiocytosis, including viruses, bacteria, mycobacteria, fungi, parasites and rickettsiae[153-164] (see Table 3-3, Chapter 3).

The hemophagocytic histiocytes are mature and bland-appearing, with no cytologically atypical features. They often contain phagocytosed red cells, but they may also show evidence of platelet or leukocyte phagocytosis. The hemophagocytic histiocytes are most commonly found in the bone marrow but may also be present in the lymph nodes, spleen and liver. Bone marrow biopsy specimens often appear hypercellular and may show areas of fibrosis.

The clinical course, in addition to anemia or pancytopenia, may be complicated by coagulation abnormalities, hepatic dysfunction and renal failure. In the majority of patients, however, the syndrome is self-limited and resolves within several weeks.[164]

SINUS HISTIOCYTOSIS WITH MASSIVE LYMPHADENOPATHY: Sinus histiocytosis with massive lymphadenopathy (Rosai-Dorfman syndrome) is a rare benign, chronic process with unknown etiology and pathogenesis which is seen most often in blacks under the age of 20.[165,166] It is characterized by massive bilateral cervical lymphadenopathy associated with fever, polyclonal hypergammaglobulinemia, neutrophilic leukocytosis and an elevated erythrocyte sedimentation rate. The lymph node sinuses are loaded with large histiocytes with abundant, finely granular or vacuolated cytoplasm, and there is evidence of marked emperipolesis (engulfed cells within histiocytic cytoplasm). The engulfed cells are predominantly lymphocytes. Extranodal involvement has been observed in about one-fourth of the cases. The most common sites are the skin, orbits, respiratory tract, salivary glands and bone.[167,168]

White Blood Cell Disorders

Histiocytic Malignancies (Class III Histiocytosis)

Histiocytic malignancies are discussed in Chapter 6. They consist of monocytic disorders (chronic myelomonocytic leukemia, juvenile chronic myelogenous leukemia, chronic monocytic leukemia, acute myelomonocytic leukemia and acute monocytic leukemia), malignant histiocytosis and true histiocytic lymphomas. Malignant histiocytosis and true histiocytic lymphomas are extremely rare. Most if not all cases that had been originally diagnosd as malignant histiocytosis later proved to be either a reactive histiocytosis (infection-associated hemophagocytic histiocytosis) or a malignancy of lymphocytic origin, particularly T-cell lymphoma. Similarly, the vast majority of the originally diagnosed histiocytic lymphomas turned out ot be of lymphocytic (immunoblastic or large cell lymphocytic lymphoma) rather than histiocytic origin.

Lysosomal Storage Diseases

Lysosomal storage diseases are the result of hereditary deficiencies of one of the lysosomal enzymes necessary for glycolipid and glycoprotein degradation. The end result is accumulation of the glycolipid or glycoprotein substrates in macrophages. These disorders, based on the accumulated substrates, have been classified into sphingolipidosis, glycoproteinosis, mucolipidosis and mucopolysaccharidosis[169] (Table 8-9). Gaucher's disease and Niemann-Pick disease, which are variants of sphingolipidosis, are associated with significant bone marrow pathology and are briefly discussed here.

GAUCHER'S DISEASE: Gaucher's disease is an autosomal recessive lysosomal storage disease due to deficiency of glucocerebrosidase.[170-172] Glucocerebrosidase catalyzes the degradation of glucocerebroside to ceramide and glucose. Deficiency of this enzyme leads to accumulation of the substrate in the tissue macrophages, particularly in the liver, spleen, lymph nodes and bone marrow (Figure 8-12). The glucocerebrosidase gene complex has been sequenced and is located at region q21 of chromosome 1.[173,174] Recent studies suggest that Gaucher's disease is the result of glucocerebroside gene mutations.[175-177]

Pathologic features are characterized by the tissue accumulation of macrophages known as *Gaucher cells*. Gaucher cells have abundant cytoplasm, with characteristic wrinkles or striations (Figure 8-13). The cytoplasmic appearance is due to the stackup of the greatly hydrophobic glucocerebroside molecules in bilayered membranous sheets.[172] The cytoplasm is PAS positive and demonstrates strong acid phosphatase activity which is usually not inhibited by tartaric acid. The nucleus is small and is often pushed to one side. Electron microscopy reveals spindle- or rod-shaped, membrane-bound cytoplasmic inclusions consisting of numerous small, tubular structures 13 to 75 nm in diameter.[178]

Bone marrow biopsy specimens reveal a cellular marrow with accumulation of the Gaucher cells in a focal, interstitial or diffuse pattern (Figures 8-12 and 8-13). This histiocytic accumulation is often associated with increased reticulin and/or dense collagen fibers. Due to the presence of fibrosis, bone marrow aspiration may not yield an adequate number of cellular elements.

Table 8-9 Lysosomal Storage Diseases

Sphingolipidoses
  Gaucher's disease
  Niemann-Pick disease
  Farber's disease
  Fabry's disease
  Krabbe's disease
  Metachromatic leukodystrophy
  GM_1 gangliosidosis
  GM_2 gangliosidosis
Glycoproteinoses
  Sialidosis
  Fucosidosis
  Mannosidosis
  Aspartyl-glycosaminuria
Mucolipidoses
  Mucolipidosis II
  Pseudo-Hurler polydystrophy
  Mucolipidosis IV
Mucopolysaccharidoses
  Mucopolysaccharidosis I
  Hunter's disease
  Sanfilippo disease
  Morquio disease
  Maroteaux-Lamy syndrome
  Sly syndrome
  Multiple sulfatase deficiency
Other lysosomal storage diseases
  Cystinosis
  Pompe's disease
  Wolman's disease

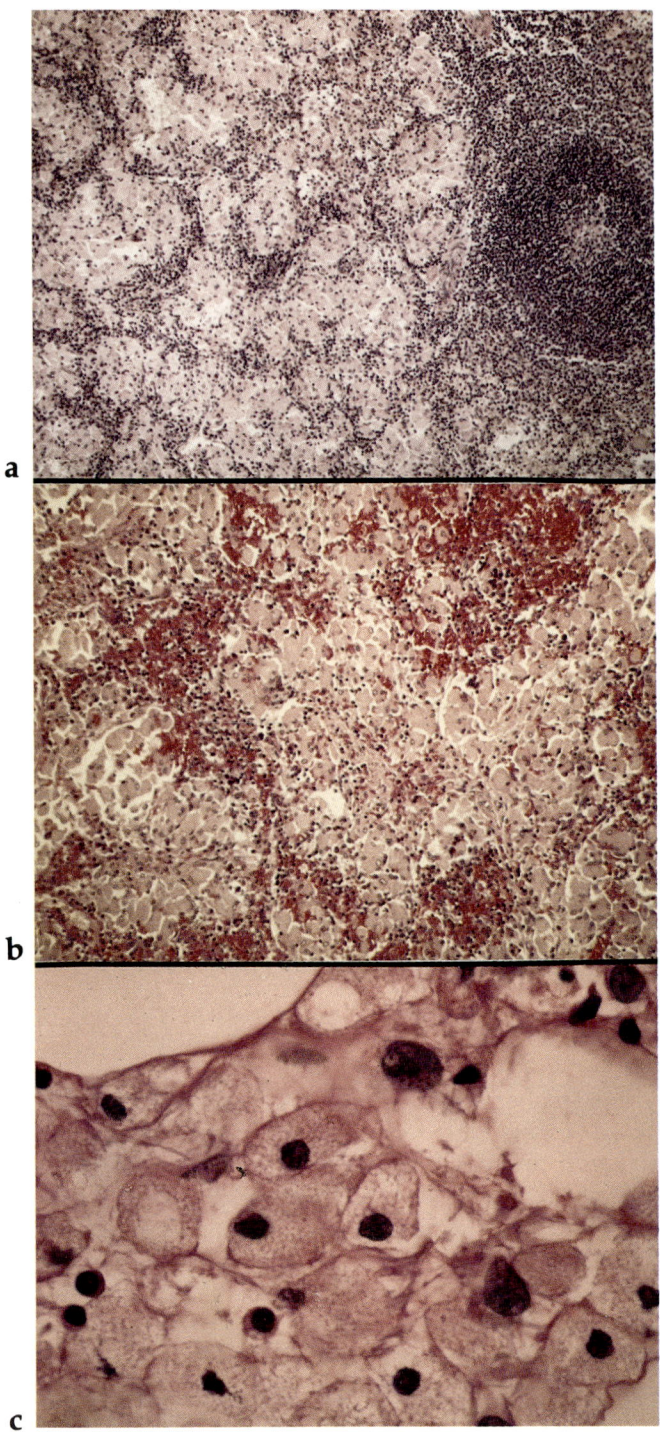

Figure 8-12. Sections of a lymph node (a), spleen (b) and bone marrow (c) from a patient with Gaucher's disease demonstrating massive accumulation of histiocytes.

Peripheral blood examination reveals a decline in leukocyte beta-glucosidase activity, an assay which is strongly recommended for the diagnosis of Gaucher's disease.[179] Other findings include a mild to moderate normochromic, normocytic anemia, with or without leukopenia and/or thrombocytopenia, and markedly elevated serum acid phosphatase activity. Activity of other hydrolases such as beta-glucuronidase, beta-hexaminidase and angiotensin-converting enzyme is also frequently increased. Patients with extensive liver involvement have abnormal liver function tests.

Based on the clinical manifestations, Gaucher's

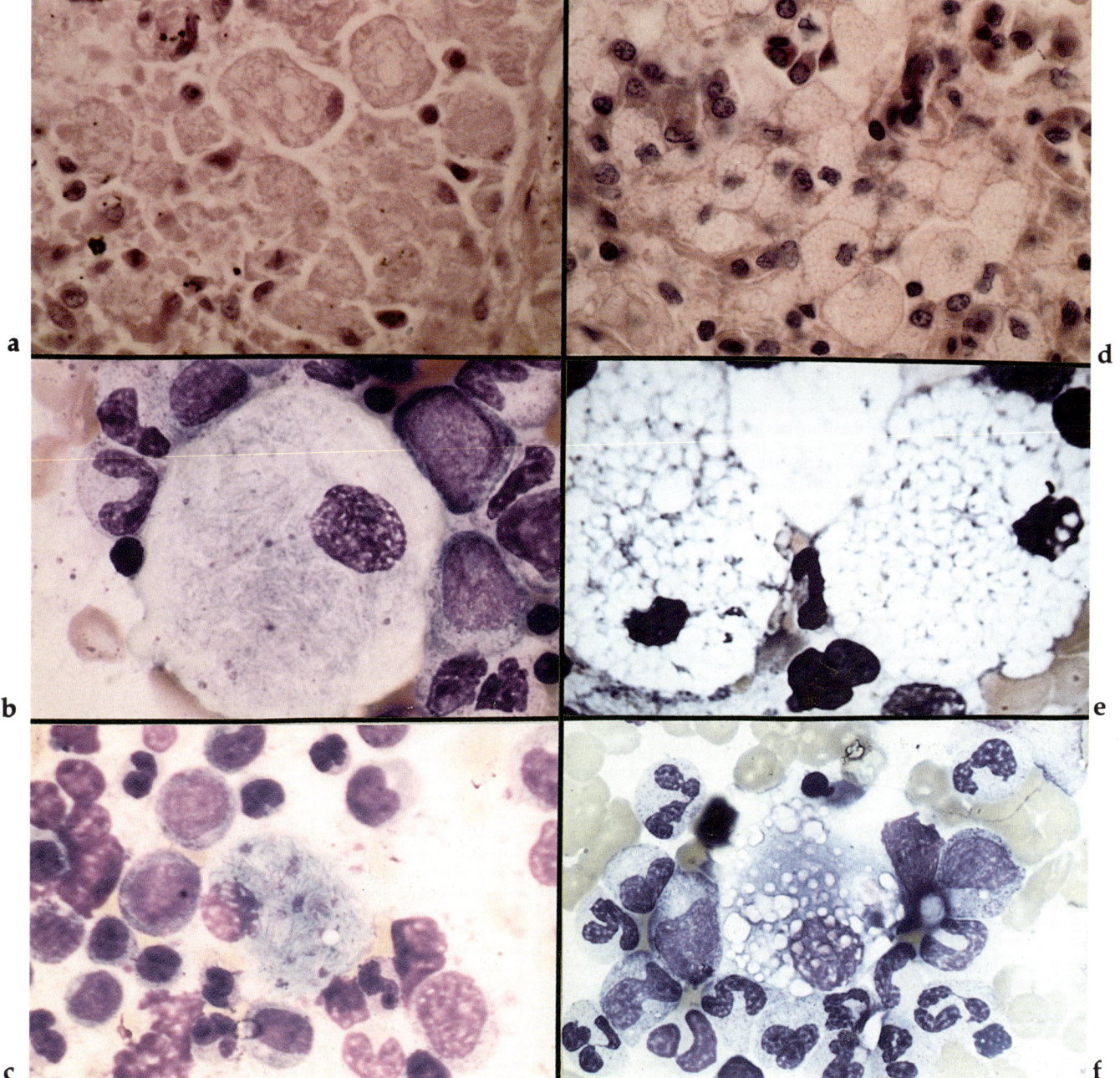

Figure 8-13. Bone marrow involvement in storage diseases. Biopsy section (a) and marrow smear (b) demonstrating Gaucher cells with abundant wrinkled cytoplasm; marrow smear from a patient with CML displaying a pseudo-Gaucher cell (c). Biopsy section (d) and marrow smear (e) demonstrating Niemann-Pick cells (type I) with evenly vacuolated cytoplasm. Vacuolated histiocyte from the bone marrow smear of a patient with hypercholesterolemia (f).

disease is divided into three major types: type 1, type 2 and type 3. All three types demonstrate involvement of the reticuloendothelial system (hepatosplenomegaly, lymphadenopathy and bone marrow infiltration) but differ in the presence and extent of neurologic abnormalities. Type 1 (nonneuropathic) Gaucher's disease, known also as the *chronic adult type*, is the most common form and is frequently observed in Ashkenazi Jews. The defect is present at conception, but clinical manifestations may range from an asymptomatic status to a severely debilitating course. However, the life expectancy of the majority of individuals with type 1 Gaucher's disease is normal.[175] Type 2 (acute neuropathic) Gaucher's disease is a rapidly progressing, fatal disease which affects children at an early age (average age at diagnosis is 2–4 months) and is associated with severe neurologic symptoms. Patients with type 3 (subacute neuropathic) Gaucher's disease share the clinical features of type 1, but, in addition, manifest neurologic symptoms.

NIEMANN-PICK DISEASE: Niemann-Pick disease is a rare autosomal recessive disorder characterized by the deficiency of lysosomal sphingomyelinase and the accumulation of the sphingomyelin in the lysosomes. Based on its biochemical characteristics, Niemann-Pick disease has been divided into two major groups: group I and group II.[180-182]

Group I, or Niemann-Pick sphingomyelinosis, is a clear-cut enzymopathy with a primary deficiency of sphingomyelinase leading to widespread deposition of lysosomal sphingomyelin crystals.

Group II, or Niemann-Pick cholesterolosis (altered cellular cholesterol homeostasis), consists of a group of disorders in which the depression of sphingomyelinase activity is a secondary phenomenon and is not as severe as in group I. The decline in sphingomyelinase activity in this group is probably due to a deficiency in the translocation of cholesterol from lysosomes to other intracellular membrane sites and to a decreased cholesterol esterification rate in lysosomes.

The characteristic histopathologic feature of Niemann-Pick disease is the presence of foamy histiocytes in various tissues (Figure 8-13). This morphologic appearance is due to the progressive dilatation and multiplication of the sphingomyelin-laden lysosomal system. Further sphingomyelin deposition and expansion of the lysosomal structure may lead to almost total obstruction of the cytoplasmic space and a uniformly foamy appearance of the affected cells (Niemann-Pick cells) (Figure 8-13). Ultrastructurally, the lysosomal deposit may appear as membranous (arranged in wavy, concentric or zebra fashion) or homogeneous ("washed out," lucent) lysosomal deposits. The Niemann-Pick cells in group I contain lipid and lipopigment and stain intensively with iron hematoxylin. The lipid is found in the form of uniform anisotropic droplets and stains moderately with Sudan black B. Cresyl violet and PAS stains are either negative or weakly positive.[183] The unstained, air-dried marrow smears are birefringent under polarized light. The Niemann-Pick cells in group II show no uniform droplet deposition, contain more cholesterol and significantly less lipopigment than the cells in group I, and show considerable variability in the intensity of vacuole staining in any given cell. Unlike group I, the unstained marrow smear in group II is not birefringent under polarized light.[182]

Peripheral blood examination may reveal a mild normocytic, normochromic anemia. The leukocytes lack sphingomyelinase activity, and lymphocytes may show cytoplasmic vacuoles containing sphingomyelin.[184,185]

Clinically, group 1 Niemann-Pick disease is divided into two subtypes: neuronopathic (type A) and visceral (type B). The neuronopathic type, also known as the *infantile type*, is a rapidly progressive disease involving the central nervous system and having an extremely poor prognosis. The visceral type has a slower clinical course, and the affected children often reach adulthood.

Group II Niemann-Pick disease is less frequent, is associated more often with a late onset, and overall has a less aggressive course than group I. This group is divided into subtypes C (chronic neuronopathic form), D (Nova Scotia variant) and E (adult non-neuronopathic form).[180,186,187]

Disorders of the Lymphocytes

Lymphocytopenia (Lymphopenia)

Lymphocytopenia is one of the hallmarks of congenital and acquired immunodeficiency syndromes and is frequently associated with collagen vascular diseases and malignancies.[188-193] Lymphocytopenia occurs in patients with aplastic anemia, zinc deficiency, tuberculosis, Hodgkin's disease, sarcoidosis and renal failure. Cancer chemotherapy and radiotherapy, administration of glucocorticoids and antilymphocyte globulin, thoracic duct drainage and surgery may also cause lymphocytopenia. Congenital and acquired immunodeficiency syndromes are briefly discussed here.

Congenital Immunodeficiency Syndromes

Congenital immunodeficiency syndromes are associated with a defect in antigen-specific T-cell function

White Blood Cell Disorders

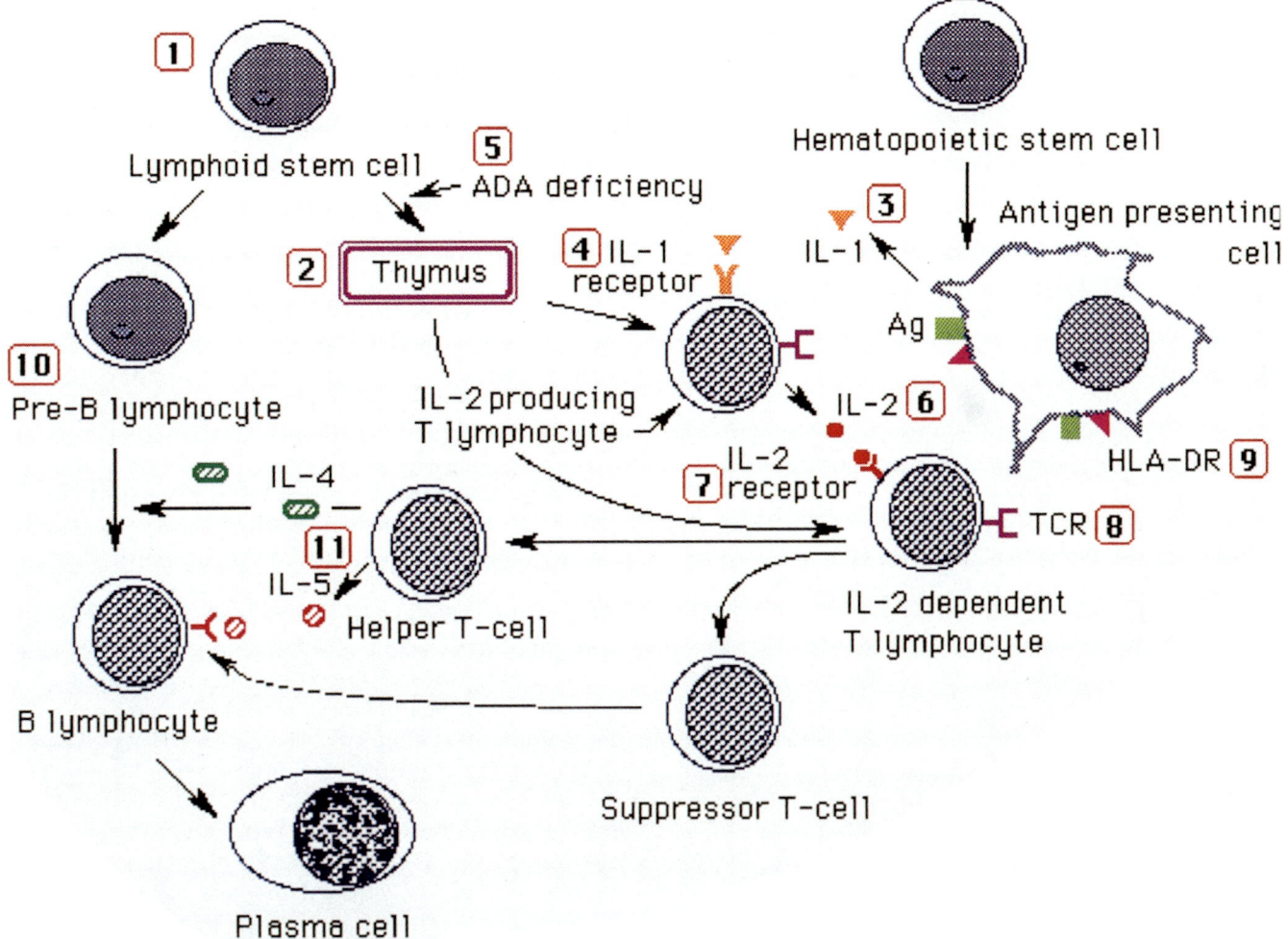

Figure 8-14. Schematic representation of the primary defects in congenital immunodeficiency syndromes:
1. Absence of lymphoid stem cells
2. Hypoplasia of thymus (Di George syndrome)
3. Absence of IL-1 production
4. Lack of expression of the IL-1 receptor
5. Absence of adenosine diaminase
6. Lack of IL-2 production
7. Lack of expression of the IL-2 receptor
8. Absence of T-cell receptor expression
9. Lack of HLA-DR expression
10. Defect in B-cell maturation (X-linked agammaglobulinemia)
11. Lack of T-cell-derived cytokines (common variable agammaglobulinemia).
Adapted from Weinberg KI, Parkman R, Congenital immunodeficiency diseases, in Williams WJ, Beutler E, Erslev AJ, et al (eds), Hematology, ed 4. New York, McGraw-Hill, 1990, p. 963.

and/or an inability to produce antibodies (Figure 8-14). The most prominent clinicopathologic variants are severe combined immune deficiency. Di George syndrome, Wiscott-Aldrich syndrome and agammaglobulinemia.

SEVERE COMBINED IMMUNE DEFICIENCY (SCID): This is characterized by defective humoral and cellular responses. The primary defects include absence of lymphoid stem cells, adenosine deaminase (ADA) deficiency, a defect in the expression of the T-cell receptor, IL-2 receptor, or HLA-DR; lack of IL-1 or IL-2 production; and a block in T-lymphocyte maturation (Figure 8-14). The affected children suffer from recurrent infections, which usually start 3 months after birth.[188,190]

DI GEORGE SYNDROME: This syndrome is associated with a quantitative T-cell deficiency caused by thymic hypoplasia due to congenital abnormalities of the third and fourth pharyngeal pouches. Affected children also show evidence of hypoparathyroidism and midline cardiac defects.[194]

WISCOTT-ALDRICH SYNDROME: This is an X-linked recessive disorder associated with progressive depletion of the T lymphocytes in the paracortical areas of the lymph nodes and peripheral blood, with a variable loss of cellular immunity (195a). The disease is also manifested with thrombocytopenia and eczema. The primary membrane defect appears to be an abnormal expression of glycoproteins sialophorin (CD43) in T lymphocytes and gp 1b in platelets;[195b,196a] degradation of these glycoproteins may result in membrane fragmentation and shortened T lymphocyte and platelet survival.[188] Serum immunoglobulin assays frequently demonstrate decreased IgM, normal IgG and elevated IgA and IgE levels. The bone marrow is usually normocellular and often shows abundant megakaryocytes, some with vacuolated cytoplasm.

Patients with Wiscott-Aldrich syndrome have a high risk of developing malignancies, particularly large cell lymphoma.[196b]

AGAMMAGLOBULINEMIA: This disease consists of two major subtypes: X-linked agammaglobulinemia and common variable agammaglobulinemia.

X-LINKED VARIANT. This is a recessive disease which affects only males and is associated with a marked decline of all Ig classes. The primary defect appears to be a block in B-cell maturation at the pre-B stage and, thus, inability of the B cells to produce antibodies.[197-199] The affected B lymphocytes are not able to translocate the variable region of the mu immunoglobin heavy chain genes.[200]

Bone marrow examination reveals lymphocytopenia, with absence of plasma cells. The B lymphocytes lack surface Ig and C3 receptors.[201,202]

COMMON VARIABLE AGAMMAGLOBULINEMIA (CVAG). This consists of a heterogeneous group of disorders that are not X-linked, and most of them do not have a defect in B-cell maturation. The failure of immunoglobulin synthesis in some patients is due to inadequate cytokine production (such as IL-4 and IL-5) by helper T cells, and in others is the result of excessive suppressor T-cell activity.[203-205] No significant changes are seen in the bone marrow of patients with CVAG.

Acquired Immunodeficiency Syndrome (AIDS)

ETIOLOGY AND PATHOGENESIS: AIDS is an HIV-induced illness with a broad spectrum of clinical manifestations. HIV (human immunodeficiency virus) is a retrovirus which binds primarily to CD4 membrane receptors expressed on T-helper lymphocytes and cells of the monocyte/macrophage lineage. There are two major types of HIV: HIV-I and HIV-II. HIV-I is widespread in the USA, Europe and other parts of the world, while HIV-II is primarily detected in West Africans.[206] HIV may actively replicate and cause cytopathicity and cell death, or it may produce a latent, chronic, low-level infection. The latent state can be transformed into an active virus-replicating phase.[207a,b] The infected $CD4^+$ T cells appear to be predominantly of the $CD29^+/CD45^+$ subset (memory cells), which in normal conditions are stimulated by recall antigens, express CD2 and CD3, and provide help to B lymphocytes for Ig production.[208] The exact mechanism of depletion and dysfunction of the infected cells is not clear. However, several mechanisms have been suggested, such as formation of syncytia (multinucleated giant cells resulted from fusion of numerous T-cells), cytotoxic effects of antiviral antibodies, release of cytokines that are toxic to helper T-cells, and inappropriate induction of programmed cell death (PCD).[209] PCD (also called *activation-induced cell death, apoptosis*) is a physiologic mechanism of cell depletion which follows incomplete signal transduction, such as cAMP increase, and is associated with endogenous endonuclease activation. PCD is characterized by degradation of the entire DNA into oligonucleosome fragments[210,211]

Similar to helper T cells, involvement of mononuclear phagocytic system with HIV is via the CD4 molecule.[215] Macrophages are more susceptible to HIV infection than monocytes, probably because they express more CD4 molecules.[207,216]

The effects of HIV on growth of hematopoietic progenitor cells in AIDS patients is still controversial, though the overwhelming majority of the reports demonstrate impaired bone marrow function, hematopoietic dysplasia and/or HIV in bone marrow cells.[217-221] It has been shown that antibodies to the viral envelope gp120 glycoprotein block the responses of hematopoietic progenitors to the growth factors such as erythropoietin and GM-CSF.[222] A positive response to GM-CSF has been reported in leukopenic AIDS patients.[223a]

The routes of transmission include: (1) sexual, both in homosexuals and heterosexuals, (2) parenteral, such as, intravenous drug use, transfusion, needle stick (rare), and invasive medical and dental procedures (rare), (3) maternal to child in perinatal period or by breast feeding, and (4) through skin or mucous membrane (very rare).[223b] Homosexuals, intravenous drug users, hemophiliacs and children born from HIV infected mothers are the prime targets of HIV infection.

PATHOLOGY: The bone marrow changes are discussed in Chapter 3. Briefly, bone marrow specimens reveal a normo- or hypercellular marrow, often with an elevated M:E ratio, a myeloid left shift, and mild to severe dysplastic changes of one or all hematopoietic lines.[217,220,224-229] A polyclonal lymphoplasmacytosis is common, sometimes with activated lymphocytes and immature plasma cells (Figure 8-15). Reticulin fibrosis and gelatinous transformation of marrow are frequent features. Azidothymidine (AZT)-treated patients may show megaloblastic changes or bone marrow hypocellularity, with reduction of the erythroid, granulocytic and/or megakaryocytic cells.[230]

Approximately 3% of patients with AIDS eventually develop lymphoma. AZT therapy may increase this rate up to 40%. About 30% of the AIDS patients with lymphoma show bone marrow involvement.[202] AIDS-associated lymphomas are mostly high-grade B-cell lymphomas, frequently of the immunoblastic or small, noncleaved lymphocytic (Burkitt's) type. Bone marrow involvement with Kaposi's sarcoma is uncommon.[231]

Evidence of opportunistic infections such as *Mycobacterium avium-intracellulare*, *Pneumocystis carinii*, and *Cryptococcus* species is frequently detected in bone marrow biopsy samples. The infected bone marrow usually shows aggregates of foamy epithelioid histiocytes (granulomas) containing microorganisms (Figure 8-15).

Peripheral blood examination reveals pancytopenia in over 50% of the cases. Anemia is common and is usually normochromic normocytic, with a decreased reticulocyte count, an increased iron and an elevated serum ferritin level. Approximately 65 to 80% of patients with AIDs demonstrate lymphopenia, which is characteristically associated with a reduction in the number of CD4$^+$ cells and a reversal of the CD4:CD8 ratio. The absolute number of peripheral blood DC4 T-cells appears to be the most reliable prognostic indicator in the HIV infected patients. There is an increase in the proportion of atypical lymphocytes. About half of the AIDS patients show a mild to moderate neutropenia, and approximately 30% demonstrate absolute monocytopenia. Thrombocytopenia is a frequent complication and, in some cases, is autoimmune-related (ITP-like syndrome).[232]

HIV antibodies are reaised against various components of the virus such as envelope glycoproteins gp 120 and gp 41, and core protein p24, and are detected by a variety of techniques, such as enzyme-linked immunoabsorbant assay (ELISA), Western blot, radioimmunoassay and immunofluorescence.[233,234] The most popular techniques are ELISA and Western blot analysis.

CLINICAL ASPECTS: The Centers for Disease Control (CDC) has classified the clinical manifestations of the HIV infection into four major groups: (I) acute infection, (II) asymptomatic infection, (III) persistent generalized lymphadenopathy and (IV) other diseases consisting of subgroups: A, constitutional disease; B, neurologic disease; C, secondary infectious disease; D, secondary cancers; and E, other conditions.[235] Acute infection is characterized by flu-like symptoms such as headache, sore throat, fever, lethargy, myalgia and arthralgia which may last for a period ranging from days to weeks. A large proportion of HIV-infected patients (an estimated 1–1.5 million in the United States) are asymptomatic. A significant number of patients in this group eventually develop symptoms within 5 to 10 years after infection.[236,237a,b] In persistent generalized lymphadenopathy (group III), the cervical, axillary and inguinal lymph nodes are frequently involved. The enlarged lymph nodes show reactive hyperplasia which in the early stages is predominantly follicular and later on is associated with the infiltration of the follicles by T cells and eventually destruction of the follicular structures. Plasmacytosis is a common feature. The advanced stage (group IV) is associated with opportunistic infections, neurologic symptoms and secondary malignancies.

Lymphocytosis

Lymphocytosis is a common hematologic abnormality observed in most viral infections, certain bacterial infections (pertussis, brucellosis, tuberculosis, syphilis), autoimmune disorders, thyrotoxicosis, cigarette smoking, X-linked lymphoproliferative syndrome,

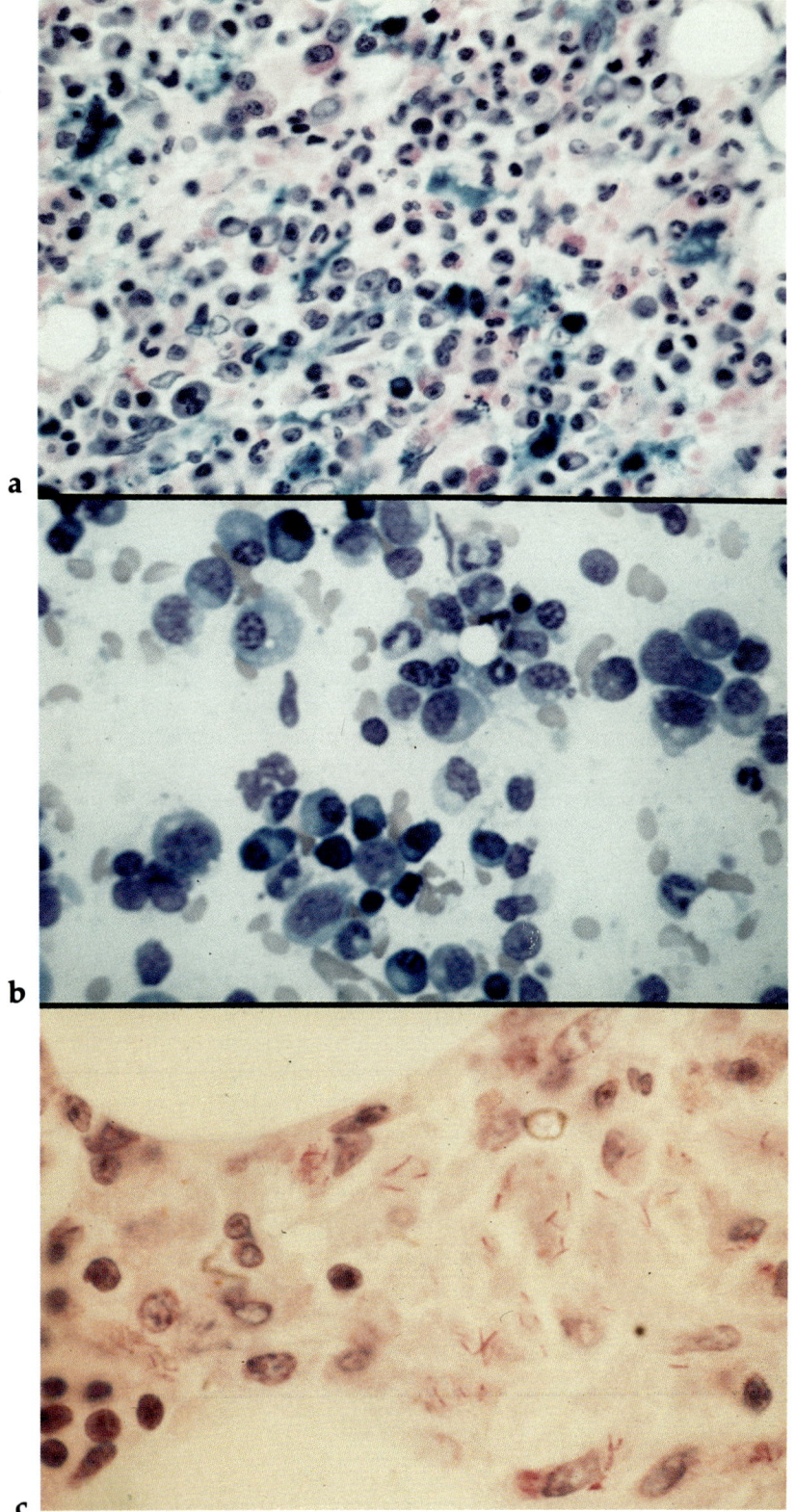

Figure 8-15. Bone marrow biopsy section (a) and smear (b) from a patient with AIDS showing marked plasmacytosis. An acid-fast stained biopsy section demonstrates numerous microbacteria in a patient with AIDS (c).

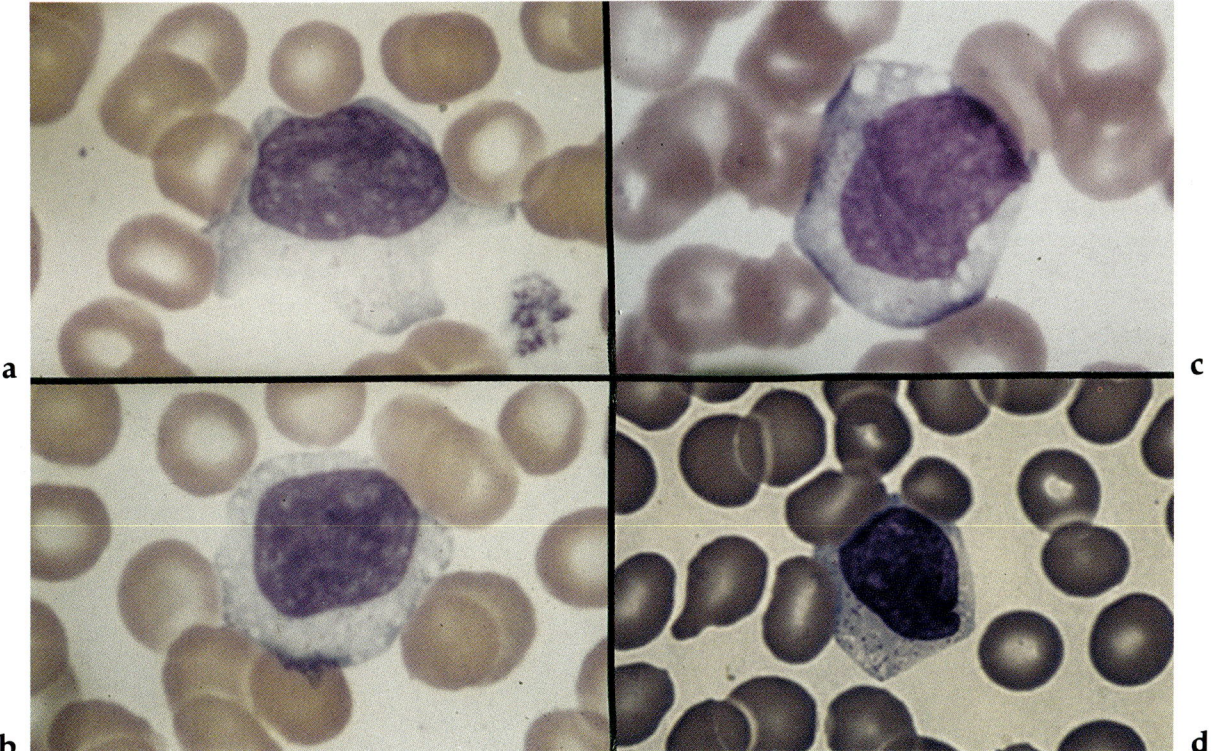

Figure 8-16. Peripheral blood smears from a patient with infectious mononucleosis demonstrating activated ("atypical") lymphocytes. These cells are pleomorphic, have abundant cytoplasm with variable degrees of basophilia, may show scalloping of the cytoplasmic membrane around red blood cells (a) and may demonstrate cytoplasmic vacuolization (b). The nucleus is round, oval or irregular, the chromatin is clumped and the nucleoli are small or inconspicuous.

acute and chronic idiopathic lymphocytosis and after splenectomy. Lymphocytosis in certain conditions, particularly viral infections, is associated with an increased number of activated lymphocytes. Activated or atypical lymphocytes are large and polymorphic and have abundant cytoplasm (Figure 8-16). Atypical lymphocytosis is one of the characteristic features of infectious mononucleosis but has also been observed in cytomegalovirus, varicella-zoster virus, rubella virus, adenovirus, and hepatitis virus infections.

Infectious Mononucleosis

Infectious mononucleosis (IM) is the clinical manifestation of a primary infection of the epithelial cells of the oropharynx and B lymphocytes with Epstein-Barr virus (EBV). B lymphocytes possess a receptor for EBV; the entry of EBV into the B cells causes polyclonal B-cell proliferation and expression of a new antigen; this new antigen, in turn, initiates a polyclonal T-cell counterresponse which leads to the suppression of B-cell proliferation (a self-limited process). Alternatively, if there is a T-cell suppressor regulatory defect, as in X-linked lymphoproliferative syndrome, B-cell proliferation continues and a B-cell malignancy may occur.[238,239]

The propensity to develop IM is closely related to the age of the infected individual. Infection during infancy or childhood generally does not result in distinctive clinical symptoms; in contrast, approximately 50% of infected persons between ages 16 and 22 develop clinical symptoms.[240,241] The most frequent symptoms and signs are malaise, sweating, sore throat, headache, anorexia, nausea, fever, lymphadenopathy, pharyngitis, splenomegaly and hepatomegaly.

Peripheral blood examination reveals lymphocytosis (>50% and >4500/µl) and often more than 20% atypical lymphocytes (Figure 8-16). The majority of the atypical lymphocytes are of CD8+ T cells with suppressor/cytotoxic activities. Anemia, granulocytopenia and thrombocytopenia may occur, and leukocyte alkaline phosphatase activity tends to be low. The heterophil antibody test is positive, indicating the presence of an antibody against sheep, horse and beef red blood cells but not reactive to guinea pig kidney cells. Specific antibodies against EBV antigens such as virus capsid antigens (VCA), EBV nuclear antigen (EBNA), and antibody to the nuclear antigens synthesized in the infected cells [early antigen (EA)-specific antibody] are also detected.

Bone marrow examination reveals lymphocytosis with the presence of large, pleomorphic lymphocytes. This abnormal morphology may occasionally lead to the misinterpretation and diagnosis of lymphoma. The lymphocytic population in IM is polyclonal, with the predominance of CD8+ cells, and in situ hybridization techniques may reveal EBV DNA in the infected cells. Small granulomas may be present, and there may be evidence of hemophagocytosis.

X-linked Lymphoproliferative Syndrome

X-linked lymphoproliferative syndrome is a recessive disorder characterized by the development of hypo- or agammaglobulinemia, fatal IM, or non-Hodgkin's lymphoma after infection with EBV.[242-244] The lymphoid proliferation is the result of a T suppressor cell regulatory defect.[245] The X-linked lymphoproliferative syndrome is manifested in young males, with the age of onset ranging from 5 month to 30 years.

Peripheral blood shows lymphocytosis in the early stage of the disease and often pancytopenia in advanced conditions. Bone marrow demonstrates granulocytosis, which is followed by lymphocytosis and eventually by hemophagocytic histiocytosis and destruction of normal bone marrow cells. Those patients who develop non-Hodgkin's lymphoma may show bone marrow or peripheral blood involvement. The lymphomas are extranodal, high grade, and of B-cell type.

Idiopathic Lymphocytosis

Occasionally, the primary cause of lymphocytosis is not known, though a viral etiology is always presumed. Lymphocytosis may be clinically acute or chronic. Acute lymphocytosis (*acute infectious lymphocytosis*) is a self-limited disorder in young children (<10 years old) characterized by a moderate (20,000–30,000/µl) to severe (100,000/µl) lymphocytosis. It may persist for several weeks and is usually not associated with lymphadenopathy or splenomegaly. Fever, abdominal pain and diarrhea may occur. The lymphoproliferation is predominantly of the T lymphocyte, helper phenotype, though a case with the B-cell variant has been reported.[246,247] Bone marrow lymphocytosis may be minimal or extensive.

Chronic B-cell lymphocytosis is a rare condition of unknown etiology which has been reported in young to middle-aged women. It is characterized by a persistent polyclonal peripheral blood B lymphocytosis (4000 to 14,000/µl), the presence of atypical binucleated lymphocytes in the peripheral blood and normal bone marrow histology.[248,249]

References

1. Boxer LA: Qualitative abnormalities of neutrophils, in Williams WJ, Beutler E, Erslev AJ, et al (eds), *Hematology*, ed 4. New York, McGraw-Hill, 1990, p 821.
2. White JG, Clawson CC: The Chediak-Higashi syndrome: The nature of the giant neutrophil granules and their interaction with cytoplasm and foreign particles. *Am J Pathol* 98:151, 1980.
3. Hosli P, Griscelli C, Good RA: Chediak-Higashi syndrome: 1. Biological abnormality and prospects for prenatal diagnosis. *Monogr Hum Genet* 9:126, 1978.
4. Boxer LA, Clark RA, Kimball HR: Defective granulocyte chemotaxis in the Chediak-Higashi syndrome. *J Clin Invest* 50:2645, 1971.
5. Haliots T, Roder J, Klein M, et al: Chediak-Higashi gene in humans. 1. Impairment of natural-killer function. *J Exp Med* 151:1039, 1980.
6. Ingraham LM, Burns PC, Boxer LA, et al: Fluidity properties and lipid composition of erythrocyte membranes in Chediak-Higashi syndrome. *J Cell Biol* 89:510, 1981.
7. Boxer GL, Holmsen H, Robkin L, et al: Abnormal platelet function in Chediak-Higashi syndrome. *Br J Haematol* 35:521, 1977.
8. Bejaoui M, Veber F, Girault D, et al: Phase acceleree de la malade Chediak-Higashi. *Arch Fr Pediatr* 46:733, 1989.
9. Babior B, Woodman RC: Chronic granulomatous disease. *Semin Hematol* 27:427, 1990.
10. Ligeti E, Doussiere J, Vignais PV: Activation of the O_2-generating oxidase in plasma membrane from bovine polymorphonuclear neutrophils by arachidonic acid, a cytosolic factor of protein nature, and nonhydrolyzable analogues of GTP. *Biochemistry* 27:193, 1988.

11. Borregaard N, Heiple JM, Simons ER, et al: Subcellular localization of the b-cytochrome component of the human neutrophil microbicidal oxidase: Translocation during activation. *J Cell Biol* 97:52, 1983.
12. Borregaard N, Tauber AI: Subcellular localization of the human neutrophil NADPH-oxidase: B-cytochrome and associated flavoprotein. *J Biol Chem* 259:47, 1984.
13. Segal AW, Jones OTG: Novel cytochrome b system in phagocytic vacuoles of human granulocytes. *Nature* 276:515, 1978.
14. Smith RM, Curnutte JT: Molecular basis of chronic granulomatous disease. *Blood* 77:673, 1991.
15. Battat L, Franke U: Nsi 1 RFLP at the X-linked chronic granulomatous disease locus (CYBB). *Nucleic Acids Res* 17:361, 1989.
16. Biggar WD, Buron S, Holmes B: Chronic granulomatous disease in an adult male: A proposed X-linked defect. *J Pediatr* 88:63, 1976.
17. Dinauer MC, Pierce EA, Bruns GA, et al: Human neutrophil cytochrome b light chain (p22-phox). Gene structure, chromosomal location, and mutations in cytochrome-negative autosomal recessive chronic granulomatousdisease. *J Clin Invest* 86:1729, 1990.
18. Curnutte JT, Babior BM: Chronic granulomatous disease, in Harris H, Hirschhorn K (eds), *Advances in Human Genetics*. New York, Plenum, 1987, p 229.
19. Mille EL, Rholl KS, Quie PG: X-linked inheritance in females with chronic granulomatous disease. *J Clin Invest* 66:332, 1980.
20. Clark RA, Malech HL, Gallin JI, et al: Genetic variants of chronic granulomatous disease: Prevalence of two discrete cytosolic components of the NADPH oxidase system. *N Engl J Med* 321:647, 1989.
21. Baehner RL, Nathan DG: Quantitative nitroblue tetrazolium test in chronic granulomatous disease. *N Engl J Med* 278:971, 1968.
22. Nauseef WM: Myeloperoxidase deficiency. *Hematol Oncol Clin North Am* 2:135, 1988.
23. Klebanoff SJ: Oxygen-dependent cytotoxic mechanisms of phagocytes. *Adv Host Defense Mechanisms* 1:111, 1982.
24. Clark RA, Borregaard N: Neutrophils autoinactivate secretory products by myeloperoxidase-catalysed oxidation. *Blood* 65:913, 1985.
25. Clark RA, Klebanoff SJ: Chemotactic factor inactivation by the myeloperoxidase-hydrogen peroxide-halide system. *J Clin Invest* 64:913, 1979.
26. Clark RA, Stone P, El-Hag A, et al: Myeloperoxidase-catalyzed inactivation of α1-protease inhibitor by human neutrophils. *J Biol Chem* 256:3348, 1981.
27. Clark RA, Szot S: Chemotactic factor inactivation by stimulated human neutrophils mediated by myeloperoxidase-catalyzed methionine oxidation. *J Immunol* 128:1507, 1982.
28. Anderson DC, Springer TA: Leukocyte adhesion deficiency: An inherited defect in the Mac-1, LFA-1, and p150,95 glycoproteins. *Annu Rev Med* 38:175, 1987.
29. Dale DC: Neutropenia, in Williams WJ, Beutler E, Erslev AJ, et al, (eds), *Hematology*, ed 4. New York, McGraw-Hill, 1990, p 807.
30. Bishop CR, Rothstein G, Ashenbrucker HE, et al: Leukokinetic studies. XIV. Blood neutrophil kinetics in chronic, steady-state neutropenia. *J Clin Invest* 50:1678, 1971.
31. Parmley RT, Crist WM, Ragab AH, et al: Congenital dysgranulopoietic neutropenia: Clinical, serologic, ultrastructural and in vivo proliferative characteristics. *Blood* 56:465, 1980.
32a. Kostman R: Infantile genetic agranulocytosis. *Acta Pediatr Scand* 64:362, 1975.
32b. Rosen RB, Kang S-J: Congenital agranulocytosis terminating in acute myelomonocytic leukemia. *J Pediatr* 94:406, 1979.
33. Dale DC, Hammond WP: Cyclic neutropenia: A clinical review. *Blood Rev* 2:1, 1988.
34. Krance RA, Spurce WE, Forman SJ, et al: Human cyclic neutropenia transferred by allogeneic bone marrow grafting. *Blood* 60:1263, 1982.
35. Loughran TP, Clark EA, Price TH, et al: Adult-onset cyclic neutropenia is associated with increased large granular lymphocytes. *Blood* 68:1082, 1986.
36. Verheugt FWA, Noord-Bokhurst JC, et al: A family with allo-immune neonatal neutropenia: Group-specific pathogenicity of maternal antibodies. *Vox Sang* 36:1, 1979.
37. Minchinton RM, McGrath KM: Alloimmune neonatal neutropenia—a neglected diagnosis? *Med J Aust* 147:139, 1987.
38. Lalezari P, Murphy GB, Allen FH Jr: A new neutrophil-specific antigen involved in the pathogenesis of neonatal neutropenia. *J Clin Invest* 50:1108, 1971.
39. Logue GL, Shimm DS: Autoimmune granulocytopenia. *Annu Rev Med* 31:191, 1980.
40. Wallis WJ, Loughran TP, Kadin ME, et al: Polyarthritis and neutropenia associated with circulating large lymphocytes. *Ann Intern Med* 103:357, 1985.
41. Dale DC: Neutropenia, in Williams WJ, Beutler E, Erslev AJ, et al (eds), *Hematology*, ed 4. New York, McGraw-Hill, 1990, p 807.
42. Pisciotta AV: Drug-induced agranulocytosis. Peripheral destruction of polymorphonuclear leukocytes and their marrow precursors. *Blood Rev* 4:226, 1990.
43. The International Agranulocytosis and Aplastic Anemia Study: Risks of agranulocytosis and aplastic anemia. *JAMA* 256:1749, 1986.
44. Vincent PC: Drug-induced aplastic anemia and agranulocytosis. Incidence and mechanisms. *Drugs* 31:52, 1986.

45. Roeser HP: Drug–bone marrow interactions. *Med J Aust* 146:145, 1987.
46. Zuelzer WW: "Myelokathexis"—A new form of chronic granulocytopenia. *N Engl J Med* 270:699, 1964.
47. Bassan R, Viero P, Minetti B, et al: Myelokathexis: A rare form of chronic benign granulocytopenia. *Br J Haematol* 58:115, 1984.
48. Miller ME, Oski FA, Harris MB: Lazy-leukocyte syndrome. A new disorder of neutrophil function. *Lancet* 1:665, 1971.
49. Constantopoulos A, Karpathios T, Nicolaidou P, et al: Lazy-leukocyte syndrome. A case report. *J Pediatr* 87:945, 1975.
50. Habib MA, Babka JC, Burningham RA: Profound granulocytopenia associated with infectious mononucleosis. *Am J Med Sci* 265:339, 1973.
51. Nagaraju M, Weitzman S, Baumann G: Viral hepatitis and agranulocytosis. *Am J Dig Dis* 18:247, 1973.
52. Calabro JJ, Williamson P, Love ES, et al: Kawasaki syndrome. *N Engl J Med* 306:237, 1982.
53. Murphy MF, Metcalfe P, Waters AH, et al: Incidence and mechanism of neutropenia and thrombocytopenia in patients with human immunodeficiency virus infection. *Br J Haematol* 66:337, 1987.
54. Amorosi EL: Hypersplenism. *Semin Hematol* 2:249, 1965.
55. Beeson PB, Bass DA: *The Eosinophil*. Philadelphia, WB Saunders, 1977.
56. Bass DA: Eosinopenia of acute infection. Production of eosinopenia by chemotactic factors of acute infection. *J Clin Invest* 65:1265, 1980.
57. Juhlin L: The effects of corticotropin and corticosteroids on the basophil and eosinophil granulocytes. *Acta Haematol* 29:157, 1963.
58. Franklin W, Goetzl EJ: Total absence of eosinophils in a patient with an allergic disorder. *Ann Intern Med* 94:352, 1981.
59. Juhlin L, Michaelsson G: A new syndrome characterized by absence of eosinophils and basophils. *Lancet* 1:1233, 1977.
60. Galli SJ, Colvin RB, Orenstein NS, et al: Patients without basophils. *Lancet* 2:409, 1977.
61. Twomey JJ, Leavell BS: Leukemoid reaction to tuberculosis. *Arch Intern Med* 116:21, 1965.
62. Shoenfeld Y, Tal A, Berliner S, et al: Leukocytosis in nonhematological malignancies—a possible tumor-associated marker. *J Cancer Res Clin Oncol* 111:54, 1986.
63. Riddle PE, Dincsoy HP: Primary squamous cell carcinoma of the thyroid associated with leukocytosis and hypercalcemia. *Arch Pathol Lab Med* 111:373, 1987.
64. Obara T, Ito Y, Kodama T, et al: A case of gastric carcinoma associated with excessive granulocytosis. Production of a colony-stimulating factor by the tumor. *Cancer* 56:782, 1985.
65. Foster NK, Martyn JB, Rangna RE, et al: Leukocytosis of exercise: Role of cardiac output and catecholamines. *J Appl Physiol* 61:2218, 1986.
66. Muir AL, Cruz M, Martin BA, et al: Leukocyte kinetics in the human lung: Role of exercise and catecholamines. *J Appl Physiol* 57:711, 1984.
67. Dale DC, Fauci AS, Guerry D, et al: Comparison of agents producing a neutrophilic leukocytosis in man. *J Clin Invest* 56:808, 1975.
68. Dale DC: Neutrophilia, in Williams WJ, Beutler E, Erslev AJ, et al (eds), *Hematology*, ed 4. New York, McGraw-Hill, 1990, p 816.
69. Kreger BE, Craven DE, McCabe WR: Gram-negative bacteremia, IV. Reevaluation of clinical features and treatment in 612 patients. *Am J Med* 68:344, 1980.
70. Effect of lithium on neutrophil mass and production. *N Engl J Med* 298:178, 1978.
71. Ramos FJ, Zamora F, Perez-Sicillia M, et al: Chronic granulocytic leukemia versus neutrophilic leukemoid reaction. *Am J Med* 88:83, 1990.
72. Schmid C, Frisch B, Beham A, et al: Comparison of bone marrow histology in early chronic granulocytic leukemia and in leukemoid reaction. *Eur J Haematol* 44:154, 1990.
73. Liesveld JL, Abboud CN: State of the art: The hypereosinophilic syndromes. *Blood Rev* 5:29, 1991.
74. Silberstein DS, Austen KF, Owen WF: Hemopoietins for eosinophils: Glycoprotein hormones that regulate the development of inflammation in eosinophilia-associated disease. *Hematol Oncol Clin North Am* 3:511, 1989.
75. Chusid MJ, Dale DC, West BC, et al: Hypereosinophilic syndrome: Analysis of 14 cases with review of the literature. *Medicine* 54:1, 1975.
76. Enokihara H, Furusawa S, Kajitani H, et al: Interleukin 2 stimulates the T cells from patients with eosinophilia to produce CFU-Eo growth stimulating factor. *BR J Haematol* 69:431, 1988.
77. Kern P, Dietrich M: Eosinophil differentiating activity in sera of patients with AIDS under recombinant IL-2 substitution. *Blut* 52:249, 1986.
78. Wingvist I, Olofsson T, Olsson I, et al: Altered density, metabolism and surface receptors of eosinophils in eosinophilia. *Immunology* 47:531, 1982.
79. Hertzman PA, Belvins WL, Mayer J, et al: Association of the eosinophilia-myalgia syndrome with the ingestion of tryptophan. *N Engl J Med* 322:869, 1990.
80a. Winkelmann RK, Connolly SM, Quimby SR: Histologic features of the l-tryptophan-related eosinophiliamyalgia (faciitis) syndrome. *Mayo Clin Proc* 66:457, 1991.

80b. Martin RW, Duffy J: Eosinophilic faciitis associated with the use of l-tryptophan: A case-control study and comparison of clinical and histopathologic features. *Mayo Clin Proc* 66:892, 2992.

81. Slungaard A, Ascensao J, Zanjani E, et al: Pulmonary carcinoma with eosinophilia: Demonstration of a tumor-derived eosinophilopoietic factor. *N Engl J Med* 309:778, 1983.

82. Balducci L, Chapman SW, Little DD, et al: Paraneoplastic eosinophilia: Report of a case with in vitro studies of hemopoiesis. *Cancer* 64:2250, 1989.

83. Baumgarten E, Wegner RD, Fengler R, et al: Calla-positive acute leukemia with t(5q;14q) translocation and hypereosinophilia—a unique entity? *Acta Haematol* 82:85, 1989.

84. Fishel RS, Farnen JP, Hanson, CA, et al: Acute lymphoblastic leukemia with eosinophilia. *Medicine* 69:232, 1990.

85. Stockdill G, Hartley SE, Alen NC: Eosinophilic leukemia in association with a double Philadelphia chromosome. *Postgrad Med J* 56:268, 1980.

86. Lichtman MA: Basophilopenia, basophilia and mastocytosis, in Williams WJ, Beutler E, Erslev AJ, et al (eds), *Hematology*, ed 4. New York, McGraw-Hill, 1990, p 849.

87. Pearson MG, Vardiman JW, Le Beau MM, et al: Increased numbers of marrow basophils may be associated with t(6;9) in ANLL. *Am J Hematol* 18:393, 1985.

88. Hoyle CF, Sherrington P, Hayhoe FG: Translocation (3;6)(q21;p21) in acute myeloid leukemia with abnormal thrombopoiesis and basophilia. *Cancer Genet Cytogenet* 30:261, 1988.

89. Matsuura Y, Sato N, Kimura F, et al: An increase in basophils in a case of acute myelomonocytic leukemia associated with marrow eosinophilia and inversion of chromosome 16. *Eur J Haematol* 39:457, 1987.

90. Dvorak Am, Dickersin GR, Connell AB, et al: Degranulation mechanisms in human leukemic basophils. *Clin Immunol Immunopathol* 5:235, 1976.

91. Lewis RA, Goetzl EJ, Wasserman SI, et al: The release of four mediators of immediate hypersensitivity from human leukemic basophils. *J Immunol* 114:87, 1975.

92. Yoo D, Lessin LS, Jensen WN: Bone marrow mast cells in lymphoproliferative disorders. *Ann Intern Med* 88:753, 1978.

93. Yoo D, Lessin LS: Bone marrow mast cell content in preleukemic syndrome. *Am J Med* 73:539, 1982.

94. Fohlmeister I, Reber T, Fischer R: Bone marrow mast cell reaction in preleukemia and in aplastic anemia. *Virchows Arch [A]* 405:503, 1985.

95. Lennert K, Parwaresh MR: Mast cells and mast cell neoplasia—a review. *Histopathology* 3:349, 1979.

96. Frame B, Nixon RK: Bone marrow mast cells in osteoporosis of aging. *N Engl J Med* 279:626, 1968.

97. Metcalfe DD: Classification and diagnosis of mastocytosis: Current status. *J Invest Dermatol* 96:2S, 1991.

98. Metcalfe DD: Conclusions—clinical advances in mastocytosis: An interdisciplinary roundtable discussion. *J Invest Dermatol* 96:64S, 1991.

99. Parker RI: Hematologic aspects of mastocytosis: 1: Bone marrow pathology in adult and pediatric systemic mast cell disease. *J Invest Dermatol* 96:47S, 1991.

100. Horny H-P, Kaiserling E: Lymphoid cells and tissue mast cells of bone marrow lesions in systemic mastocytosis: A histological and immunohistological study. *Br J Haematol* 69:449, 1988.

101. Rywlin AM, Hoffman EP, Ortega RS: Eosinophilic fibrohistiocytic lesion of bone marrow: A distinctive new morphologic finding, probably related to drug hypersensitivity. *Blood* 40:464, 1972.

102. Te Velde J, Vismans FJFE, Leenheers-Binnendijk L, et al: The eosinophilic fibrohistiocytic lesion of the bone marrow. A mastocellular lesion in bone disease. *Virchows Arch* (Pathol Anat) 377:277, 1978.

103. Rywlin AM: Mastocytic eosinophilic fibrohistiocytic lesion of the bone marrow. American Society of Clinical Pathologists-check sample. *Hematology* 24:1, 1982.

104. Tharp MD: The spectrum of mastocytosis. *Am J Med Sci* 289:117, 1985.

105. Ridell B, Olafsson JH, Roupe G, et al: The bone marrow finding in systemic mastocytosis. *Hum Pathol* 16:808, 1985.

106. Webb TA, Lin CY, Yam LT: Systemic mast cell disease: A clinical and hematopathological study of 26 cases. *Cancer* 49:927, 1982.

107. Travis WD, Li C-Y, Yam LT, et al: Significance of systemic mast cell disease with associated hematologic disorders. *Cancer* 62:965, 1988.

108. Roberts JL, II, Oates JA: Biochemical diagnosis of systemic mast cell disorders. *J Invest Dermatol* 96:19S, 1991.

109. Twomey JJ, Douglas CC, Sharkey O Jr: The monocytopenia of aplastic anemia. *Blood* 41:187, 1973.

110. Jankila AJ, Wallace JH, Yam LT: Generalized monocyte deficiency in leukemic reticuloendotheliosis. *Scand J Haematol* 29:153, 1982.

111. Peterson V, Hensbrough J, Buerk C, et al: Regulation of granulopoiesis following severe thermal injury. *J Trauma* 23:19, 1983.

112. Isenberg DA, Martin P, Hajirousou V, et al: Haematologic reassessment of rheumatoid arthritis using automated methods. *Br J Rheumatol* 25:152, 1986.

113. Isenberg DA, Patterson KG, Todd-Pokropek A, et al: Haematological aspects of systemic lupus erythematosus; a reappraisal using automated methods. *Acta Haematol* 67:242, 1982.

114. Treacy M, Lai L, Costello C, et al: Peripheral blood and

bone marrow abnormalities in patients with HIV related disease. *Br J Haematol* 65:289, 1987.
115. Flinn JW: A study of differential blood count in 1000 cases of active pulmonary tuberculosis. *Ann Intern Med* 2:622, 1929.
116. Daland GA, Gottlieb L, Wallerstein RO, et al: Hematologic observation in bacterial endocarditis. *J Lab Clin Med* 48:827, 1956.
117. Rosahn PD, Pearce L: The blood cytology in untreated and treated syphilis. *Am J Med Sci* 187:88, 1934.
118. Buchan GS, Palmer DG, Gibbins BL: The response of human peripheral blood mononuclear phagocytes to rheumatoid arthritis. *J Leukocyte Biol* 37:221, 1985.
119. Budman DR, Steinberg AD: Hematologic aspects of systemic lupus erythematosus. Current concepts. *Am Intern Med* 86:220, 1977.
120. Maldonado JE, Hanlon DG: Monocytosis: A current appraisal. *Mayo Clin Proc* 40:248, 1965.
121. Cutting HO, Lang JE: Familial benign chronic neutropenia. *Ann Intern Med* 61:876, 1964.
122. Lichtenstein L: Histiocytosis X, integration of eosinophilic granuloma of bone, Letterer-Siwe disease and Hand-Schuller-Christian disease and related manifestations of a single nosologic entity. *Arch Pathol* 56:84, 1953.
123. Hashimoto K, Griffin D, Kohsbaki M: Self-healing reticulohistiocytosis. A clinical, histologic, and ultrastructural study of the fourth case in the literature. *Cancer* 49:331, 1982.
124. Wolfson SL, Botero F, Hurwitz S, et al: Pure cutaneous histiocytosis X. *Cancer* 48:2236, 1981.
125. Newton WA Jr, Hamoudi AB: Histiocytosis: A histologic classification with clinical correlation. *Perspect Pediatr Pathol* 1:251, 1973.
126. Broadbent V, Pritchard J, Davies EG, et al: Spontaneous remission of multisystem histiocytosis X. *Lancet* 1:253, 1984.
127. Nezelof C, Frileux-Herbet F, Cronier-Sachot J: Disseminated histiocytosis X, analysis of prognostic factors based on a retrospective study of 50 cases. *Cancer* 44:1824, 1979.
128. Writing Group of the Histiocytic Society: Histiocytosis syndromes in children. *Lancet* 1:208, 1987.
129. Osband ME, Lipton JM, Lavin P, et al: Histiocytosis X: Demonstration of abnormal immunity, T-cell histamine H2 receptor deficiency, and successful treatment with thymic extracts. *N Engl J Med* 304:146, 1981.
130. Hamoudi AB, Newton WA Jr, Mancer K, et al: Thymic changes in histiocytosis. *Am J Clin Pathol* 77:169, 1982.
131. Nesbit ME, O'Leary M, Dehner LP: The immune system and histiocytosis syndromes. *Am J Pediatr Hematol Oncol* 3:141, 1981.
132. Kraballe K, Zachraiae H, Herlin T, et al: Histiocytosis-X: An autoimmune disease? Studies on antibody-dependent monocyte-mediated cytotoxicity. *Br J Dermatol* 105:13, 1981.
133. Hance AJ: Smoking and interstitial lung disease: The effect of cigarette smoking on the incidence of pulmonary histiocytosis X and sarcoidosis. *Ann NY Acad Sci* 465:643, 1986.
134. Callihan TR: The surgical pathology of the differentiated histiocytoses, in Jaffe ES (ed), *Surgical Pathology of the Lymph Node and Related Organs*. Philadelphia, WB Saunders, 1985, p 357.
135. Komp DM: Langerhans cell histiocytosis. *N Engl J Med* 316:747, 1987.
136. Dolezal JF, Thompson ST: Hand-Schuller-Christian disease in a septuagenarian. *Arch Dermatol* 114:85, 1978.
137. Berry DH, Gersnik MV, Humphrey GB, et al: Natural history of histiocytosis X: A Pediatric Oncology Group study. *Med Pediatr Oncol* 14:1, 1986.
138. McLelland J, Pritchard J, Chu AC: Current controversies. *Hematol Oncol Clin North Am* 1:147, 1987.
139. Lahey ME: Prognosis in reticuloendotheliosis in children. *J Pediatr* 60:664, 1962.
140. Perry MC, Harrison EG, Burgert EO, et al: Familial erythrophagocytic lymphohistiocytosis—report of two cases and clinicopathologic review. *Cancer* 38:209, 1976.
141. Goldberg J, Nezelof C: Lymphohistiocytosis: A multifactorial syndrome of macrophage activation. Clinicopathological study of 38 cases. *Hematol Oncol* 4:275, 1986.
142. Loy TS, Diaz-Arias AA, Perry MC: Familial erythrophagocytic lymphohistiocytosis. *Semin Oncol* 18:34, 1991.
143. Ladish S, Poplack DG, Holiman B, et al: Immunodeficiency in familial erythrophagocytic lymphohistiocytosis. *Lancet* 1:581, 1978.
144. Kataoka Y, Todo S, Morioka Y, et al: Impaired natural killer activity and expression of IL-2 receptor antigen in familial erythrophagocytic lymphohistiocytosis. *Cancer* 65:1937, 1990.
145. McClain K, Gehrz R, Grieson H, et al: Virus-associated histiocytic proliferation in children—Frequent association with Epstein-Barr virus and congenital or acquired immunodeficiencies. *Am J Pediatr Hematol Oncol* 10:196, 1988.
146. Brown RE, Bowman WP, D'Cruz CA, et al: Endoperoxidation, hyperprostaglandinemia, and hyperlipidemia in a case of erythrophagocytic hemophagocytosis—Reversal with VP-16 and indomethacin. *Cancer* 60:2388, 1987.
147. Weiss CZ, Norris DG: Familial erythrophagocytic lymphohistiocytosis. *J Med Soc NJ*: 74:539, 1977.

148. Ansbacher LE, Singsen BH, Hosler MW, et al: Familial erythrophagocytic lymphohistiocytosis: An association with serum lipid abnormalities. *J Pediatr* 102:270, 1983.
149. Hsu TS, Komp DM: Clinical features of familial histiocytosis. *Am J Hematol Oncol* 3:61, 1981.
150. Janka GE: Familial hemophagocytic lymphohistiocytosis. *Eur J Pediatr* 140:221, 1981.
151. Martin JJ, Cras P: Familial erythrophagocytic lymphohistiocytosis—A neuropathologic study. *Acta Neuropathol (Ber)* 66:140, 1985.
152. Retwitz W, Saver O, Burrow HM, et al: Neurological and neuropathological findings in familial erythrophagocytic lymphohistiocytosis. *Brain Dev* 5:322, 1983.
153. Risdall RJ, McKenna RW, Nesbit ME, et al: Virus-associated hemophagocytic syndrome: A benign histiocytic proliferation distinct from malignant histiocytosis. *Cancer* 44:993, 1979.
154. Auerbach M, Haubenstock A, Soloman G: Systemic babesiosis: Another cause of the hemophagocytic syndrome. *Am J Med* 80:301, 1986.
155. Gill K, Marrie TJ: Hemophagocytosis secondary to *Mycoplasma pneumoniae* infection. *Am J Med* 82:668, 1987.
156. Kokkini G, Giotaki HG, Moutsopoulos HM: Transient hemophagocytosis in *Brucella melitensis* infection. *Arch Pathol Lab Med* 108:213, 1984.
157. Martin-Moreno S, Soto-Guzman O, Bernaldo-de-Quiros J, et al: Pancytopenia due to hemophagocytosis in patients with brucellosis: A report of four cases. *J Infect Dis* 147:445, 1983.
158. Risdall RJ, Brunning RD, Hernandez JI, et al: Bacteria-associated hemophagocytic syndrome. *Cancer* 54:2968, 1984.
159. Udden MM, Banez E, Sears DA: Bone marrow histiocytic hyperplasia and hemophagocytosis with pancytopenia in typhoid fever. *Am J Med Sci* 291:396, 1986.
160. Barnes N, Bellamy D, Ireland R, et al: Pulmonary tuberculosis complicated by haemophagocytic syndrome and rifampicin-induced tubulointerstitial nephritis. *Br J Dis Chest* 78:395, 1984.
161. Campo E, Condom E, Miro MJ, et al: Tuberculosis-associated hemophagocytic syndrome. *Cancer* 58:2640, 1986.
162. Matzner Y, Behar A, Berri E, et al: Systemic leishmaniasis mimicking malignant histiocytosis. *Cancer* 43:398, 1979.
163. Estrove Z, Bruck R, Shtalrid M, et al: Histiocytic hemophagocytosis in Q fever. *Arch Pathol Lab Med* 108:7, 1984.
164. Reiner AP, Spivak JL: Hemophagocytic histiocytosis—A report of 23 new patients and a review of the literature. *Medicine* 67:369, 1988.
165. Rosai J, Dorfman RF: Sinus histiocytosis with massive lymphadenopathy: A newly recognized benign clinicopathologic entity. *Arch Pathol* 87:63, 1969.
166. Rosai J, Dorfman RF: Sinus histiocytosis with massive lymphadenopathy—a pseudolymphomatous benign disorder: Analysis of 34 cases. *Cancer* 30:1188, 1972.
167. Foucar E, Rosai J, Dorfman RF: The ophthalmologic manifestations of sinus histiocytosis with massive lymphadenopathy. *Am J Ophthalmol* 87:354, 1979.
168. Heidelberger K, Schnitzer B, Tilford D, et al: Sinus histiocytosis with massive lymphadenopathy and gross skeletal involvement. *Skeletal Radiol* 5:42, 1980.
169. Glew RH, Basu A, Prence EM, et al: Lysosomal storage diseases. *Lab Invest* 53:250, 1985.
170. Brady RO, Kanfer JN, Shapiro D: Metabolism of glucocerebrosides. II. Evidence of an enzyme deficiency in Gaucher's disease. *Biochem Biophys Res Commun* 18:221, 1965.
171. Patrick AD: A deficiency of glucocerebrosidase in Gaucher's disease. *Biochem J* 97:17, 1965.
172. Glew RH, Basu A, LaMarco KL, et al: Mammalian glucocerebrosidase: Implications for Gaucher's disease. *Lab Invest* 58:5, 1988.
173. Horowitz M, Wilder S, Horowitz Z, et al: The human glucocerebrosidase gene and pseudogene: Structure and evolution. *Genomics* 4:87, 1989.
174. Ginns EI, Choudary PV, Martin BM, et al: Isolation of cDNA clones from human β-glucocerebrosidase using the λgtll expression system. *Biochem Biophys Res Commun* 123:574, 1984.
175. Martin BM, Sidransky E, Ginns EI: Gaucher's disease: Advances and challenges. *Adv Pediatr* 36:277, 1989.
176. Tsuji S, Choudary PV, Martin BM, et al: A mutation in the human glucocerebrosidase gene in neuropathic Gaucher disease. *N Engl J Med* 316:570, 1987.
177. Tsuji S, Martin BM, Barranger JA, et al: Genetic heterogeneity in the type 1 Gaucher disease: Multiple genotypes in Ashkenazic and non-Ashkenazic individuals. *Proc Natl Acad Sci USA* 85:2349, 1988.
178. Brady RO, King FM: Gaucher's disease, in Hers HG, van Hoof F (eds), *Lysosomes and Storage Diseases*. New York, Academic Press, 1973, p 381.
179. Beutler E, Saven A: Misuse of marrow examination in the diagnosis of Gaucher disease. *Blood* 76:646, 1990.
180. Elleder M: Niemann-Pick disease. *Pathol Res Pract* 185:293, 1989.
181. Philiprat M: Revised classification of Neimann-Pick disease. Quoted in Elledre M, Jirasek A: Niemann-Pick disease. Report of a symposium. *Acta Univer Carolina Med* 29:259, 1983.
182. Elleder M: Classification of Niemann-Pick disease. Quoted in Eddeler M, Jirasek A: Niemann-Pick disease. Report of a symposium. *Acta Univer Carolina Med* 29:259, 1983.

183. Elleder M, Hrodek J, Cihula J: Niemann-Pick disease: Lipid storage in bone marrow macrophages. *Histochem J* 15:1065, 1983.
184. Snyder RA, Brady RO: The use of white cells as a source of diagnostic material for lipid storage disease. *Clin Chim Acta* 25:331, 1969.
185. Lazarus SS, Vethamany VG, Schneck L, et al: Fine structure and histochemistry of peripheral blood cells in Niemann-Pick disease. *Lab Invest* 17:155, 1967.
186. Brady RO, Filling-Katz MR, Barton NW, et al: Niemann-Pick types C and D. *Neurogenet Dis* 7:75, 1989.
187. Butler JB, Comly ME, Kruth HS, et al: Niemann-Pick variant disorders: Comparison of errors of cellular cholesterol homostasis in groups D and C fibroblasts. *Proc Natl Acad Sci USA* 84:556, 1987.
188. Weinberg KI, Parkman R: Congenital immunodeficiency diseases, in Williams WJ, Beutler E, Erslev AJ, et al (eds), *Hematology*, ed 4. New York, McGraw-Hill, 1990, p 963.
189. Edwards KM, Cooper MD, Lawton AR, et al: Severe combined immunodeficiency associated with T4+ helper cells. *J Pediatr* 105:70, 1984.
190. Gelfand EW, Dosch H-M: Diagnosis and classification of severe combined immunodeficiency disease. *Birth Defects* 19:65, 1983.
191. Gatti RA, Meuwissen HJ, Allen HD, et al: Immunologic reconstitution of X-linked lymphopenic immunologic deficiency. *Lancet* 2:1366, 1968.
192. Cooper MD, Chase HP, Lowman JT, et al: Wiskott-Aldrich syndrome: An immunologic deficiency disease involving the afferent limb of immunity. *Am J Med* 44:499, 1968.
193. Zachareski LR, Linman JW: Lymphocytopenia: Its causes and significance. *Mayo Clin Proc* 46:168, 1971.
194. Di George AM: Congenital absence of thymus and its immunologic consequences: Coocurrence with congenital hypoparathyroidism. *Birth Defects* 4:116, 1968.
195a. Kwan SP, Lehner T, Hagemenn T, et al: Localization of the Wiscott-Aldrich syndrome between two flanking markers, TIMP and DXS255, on Xp11.22-Xp11.3 *Genomics* 10:29, 1991.
195b. Parkmen R, Remold-O'Donnell E, Kenney DM, et al: Surface protein abnormalities in the lymphocytes and platelets from patients with Wiscott-Aldrich syndrome. *Lancet* 2:1387, 1981.
196a. Park JK, Rosenstein YJ, Remold-O'Donell E, et al: Enhancement of T-cell activation by the CD43 molecule whose expression is defective in Wiscott-Aldrich syndrome. *Nature* 350: 706, 1991.
196b. Perry GS III, Spector BD, Schuman LM, et al: The Wiscott-Aldrich syndrome in the United States and Canada (1892–1979). *J Pediatr* 97:72, 1980.
197. Rosen FS, Cooper MD, Wedgwood RJP: The primary immunodeficiencies. Part 1. *N Engl J Med* 311:235, 1984.
198. Rosen FS, Cooper MD, Wedgwood RJP: The primary immunodeficiencies. Part II. *N Engl J Med* 311:300, 1984.
199. Rosen FS, Wedgwood RJ, Eibl M: Primary immunodeficiency diseases. Report of a World Health Organization Scientific Group. *Clin Immunol Immunopathol* 40:166, 1986.
200. Schwaber J, Molgaard H, Orkin SH, et al: Early pre-B cells from normal and X-linked agammaglobulinemia produce Cmu without an attached VH region. *Nature* 304:355, 1983.
201. Good RA: Studies on agammaglobulinemia. II. Failure of plasma cell formation in the bone marrow and lymph nodes of patients with agammaglobulinemia. *J Lab Clin Med* 46:167, 1955.
202. Duggan MJ, Weisenburger D, Sun NCJ, et al: Bone marrow findings in immunodeficiency syndromes. *Hematol Oncol North Am* 2:637, 1988.
203. Geha RS, Schneeberger E, Merler E, et al: Heterogeneity of common variable agammaglobulinemia. *N Engl J Med* 291:1, 1974.
204. Reinherz EL, Rubinstein A, Geha RS, et al: Abnormalities of immunoregulatory T cells in disorders of immune function. *N Engl J Med* 301:1018, 1979.
205. Waldman TA, Durm M, Border S, et al: Role of suppressor T cells in pathogenesis of common variable hypogammaglobulinemia. *Lancet* 2:609, 1974.
206. Essex M, Kanki PJ: The origin of the AIDS virus. *Sci Am* (October) 259:64, 1988.
207a. Fauci AS, Schnittman SM, Poli G, et al: Immunopathogenic mechanisms in human immunodeficiency virus (HIV) infection. *Ann Intern Med* 114:678, 1991.
207b. Haseltine WA: Molecular biology of the human immunodeficiency virus type 1. *FASEB J* 5:2349, 1991.
208. Schnittman SM, Lane HC, Greenhouse J, et al: Preferential infection of CD4+ memory T cells by human immunodeficiency virus type I: Evidence for a role in the selective T-cell functional defects observed in infected individuals. *Proc Natl Acad Sci USA* 87:6058, 1990.
209. Ameisen JC, Capron A: Cell dysfunction and depletion in AIDS: The programmed cell death hypothesis. *Immunol Today* 12:102, 1991.
210. Duvall E, Wyllie AH: Death and the cell. *Immunol Today* 7:115, 1986.
211. McConkey DJ, Orrenius S, Jondal M: Cellular signalling in programmed cell death (apoptosis). *Immunol Today* 11:120, 1990.
212. Margolick JB, Volkman DJ, Lane HC, et al: Clonal

analysis of T lymphocytes in the acquired immunodeficiency syndrome. Evidence for an abnormality affecting helper and suppressor T cells. *J Lab Invest* 76:709, 1985.
213. Offenbach A, Langlade-Demoyen P, Dadaglio G, et al: Unusually high frequencies of HIV-specific cytotoxic T lymphocytes in humans. *J Immunol* 142:452, 1989.
214. Pantaleo G, De Maria A, Koenig S, et al: CD8+ T lymphocytes of patients with AIDS maintain broad cytolytic function despite the loss of human immunodeficiency virus-specific cytotoxicity. *Proc Natl Acad Sci USA* 87:4818, 1990.
215. Perno CF, Baseler MV, Broder S, et al: Infection of monocytes by human immunodeficiency virus type I blocked by inhibitors of CD4-gp 120 binding, even in the presence of enhancing antibodies. *J Exp Med* 171:1043, 1990.
216. Potts BJ, Maury W, Martin MA: Replication of HIV-I in primary monocyte cultures. *Virology* 175:465, 1990.
217. Mehta KU, Gascon P, Tannir N, et al: Impaired bone marrow in AIDS. *N Engl J Med* 86:623, 1989.
218. Candido A, Rossi P, Menichella G, et al: Indicative morphological myelodysplastic alterations of bone marrow in overt AIDS. *Haematologica* 75:327, 1990.
219. Lunardi-Iskanar Y, Georgoulias V, Bertoli AM, et al: Impaired in vitro proliferation of hemopoietic precursors in HIV-1-infected subjects. *Leuk Res* 13:573, 1989.
220. Sun NCJ, Shapshak P, Lachant NA, et al: Bone marrow examination in patients with AIDS and AIDS-related complex (ARC)—Morphologic and in situ hybridization studies. *Am J Clin Pathol* 92:589, 1989.
221. Molina JM, Scadden DT, Sakaguchi M, et al: Lack of evidence for infection of or effect on growth of hematopoietic progenitor cells after in vivo or in vitro exposure to human immunodeficiency virus. *Blood* 76:2476, 1990.
222. Donahue RE, Johnson MM, Zon LI, et al: Suppression of in vitro haematopoiesis following human immunodeficiency virus infection. *Nature* 326:200, 1987.
223a. Groopman JE, Mitsuyasu RT, DeLeo MJ, et al: Effects of recombinant human granulocyte-macrophage colony-stimulating factor on myelopoiesis in the acquired immunodeficiency syndrome. *N Engl J Med* 317:593, 1987.
223b. Blattner WA: HIV epidemiology: Past, present, and future. *FASEB J* 5:2340, 1991.
224. Harris CE, Biggs JC, Concannon AJ, et al: Peripheral and bone marrow findings in patients with acquired immune deficiency syndrome. *Pathology* 22:206, 1990.
225. Berstein ZP, Gworek MA, Small BM: Hematologic abnormalities in patients with the acquired immunodeficiency syndrome. *J Med* 20:177, 1989.
226. Castella A, Croxon TS, Mildvan D, et al: The bone marrow in AIDS—a histologic, hematologic, and microbiologic study. *Am J Clin Pathol* 84:425, 1985.
227. Shenoy CM, Lin JH: Bone marrow findings in acquired immunodeficiency syndrome (AIDS). *Am J Med Sci* 292:372, 1986.
228. Geller SA, Muller R, Greenberg ML, et al: Acquired immunodeficiency syndrome—distinctive features of bone marrow biopsies. *Arch Pathol Lab Med* 109:138, 1985.
229. Schnider DR, Picker LJ: Myelodysplasia in the acquired immunodeficiency syndrome. *Am J Clin Pathol* 84:144, 1985.
230. Richman DD, Fischl MA, Grieco MH, et al: The toxicity of azidothymidine (ATZ) in the treatment of patients with AIDS and AIDS-related complex. *N Engl J Med* 317:192, 1987.
231. Conran RM, Granger E, Reddy VB: Kaposi's sarcoma of bone marrow. *Arch Pathol Lab Med* 110:1083, 1986.
232. Ratner L: Human immunodeficiency virus-associated autoimmune thrombocytopenic purpura: A review. *Am J Med* 86:194, 1989.
233. Jackson JB, Balfour HH: Practical diagnostic testing for human immunodeficiency virus. *Clin Microbiol Rev* 1:124, 1988.
234. Smith RD: The pathology of HIV infection. *Arch Pathol Lab Med* 114:235, 1990.
235. Centers for Disease Control: Revision of the CDC surveillance case definition for acquired immunodeficiency syndrome. *MMWR* 36 (suppl 15):35, 1987.
236. Lui KJ, Lawrence DN, Morgan WM, et al: A model-based approach for estimating the mean incubation period of transfusion-associated acquired immunodeficiency syndrome. *Proc Natl Acad Sci USA* 83:3051, 1986.
237a. World Health Organization Global Statistics. *AIDS* 4:1173, 1990.
237b. Palca J: The sobering geography of AIDS. *Science* 252:372, 1991.
238. Hanto DW, Frizzera G, Gajl-Peczaska KJ, et al: Epstein-Barr virus, immunodeficiency and B-cell lymphoproliferation. *Transplantation* 39:461, 1985.
239. Harrington DS, Weisenburg DD, Purtilo DT: Malignant lymphoma in the X-linked lymphoproliferative syndrome. *Cancer* 59:1419, 1987.
240. Sawyer RN, Evans AS, Niederman JC, et al: Prospective studies of a group of Yale University freshmen. 1. Occurrence of infectious mononucleosis. *J Infect Dis* 123:263, 1971.
241. Giller RH, Grose C: Epstein-Barr virus: The hematologic and oncologic consequences of virus–host interaction. *Crit Rev Oncol* 9:149, 1989.

242. Purtilo DT, Cassel CK, Yang JPS, et al: X-linked recessive progressive combined variable immunodeficiency (Duncan's disease). *Lancet* 1:935, 1975.
243. Purtilo DT, DeFlorio D, Hutt LM, et al: Variable phenotype expression of an X-linked recessive lymphoproliferative syndrome. *N Engl J Med* 297:1077, 1977.
244. Purtilo DT, Sakamoto K, Barnabei V, et al: Epstein-Barr virus-induced diseases in boys with the X-linked lymphoproliferative syndrome. *Am J Med* 73:49, 1982.
245. Harada S, Bechtold T, Seeley JK, et al: Cell-mediated immunity to Epstein-Barr virus (EBV) and natural killer cell (NK-cell) activity in the X-linked lymphoproliferative syndrome. *Int J Cancer* 30:739, 1982.
246. Bertotto A, De Felicis-Arcangeli C, Spinozzi F, et al: Acute infectious lymphocytosis: Phenotype of the proliferating cell. *Acta Paediatr Scand* 74:633, 1985.
247. Saulsbury FK: B cell proliferation in acute infectious lymphocytosis. *Pediatr Infect Dis J* 6:1127, 1987.
248. Gordon DS, Jones BM, Browning SW, et al: Persistent polyclonal lymphocytosis of B lymphocytes. *N Engl J Med* 307:232, 1982.
249. Perreault C, Boileau J, Gyger M, et al: Chronic B-cell lymphocytosis. *Eur J Haematol* 42:361, 1989.

9 DISORDERS OF RED BLOOD CELLS: ANEMIAS

Anemia, a decline in blood hemoglobin (Hb) level, is caused by blood loss, deficient erythropoiesis or increaswed red blood cell (RBC) destruction, and is characterized on the basis of the size (normocytic, microcytic or macrocytic) and the Hb content of the RBCs (normochromic, hypochromic or hyperchromic). Biochemical analyses of the blood provide valuable information regarding the cause of anemia. These analyses include measurement of serum iron and iron-binding capacity; ferritin, folate and vitamin B_{12} levels; durg and antibody levels; RBC enzyme assays; and Hb electrophoresis.

Peripheral blood examination plays a key role in the diagnosis and classification of anemias and usually

Table 9-1 RBC and Related Parameters in Healthy Adults

	Men	Women
RBC count (x 10^{12}/l)	4.7–6.1	4.2–5.4
Hb (g/dl)	14–18	12–16
Hematocrit (%)	42–52	37–47
Mean corpuscular volume (MCV) (fl)	80–94	81–99
Mean corpuscular Hb (MCH) (pg)	27–31	27–31
Mean corpuscular Hb concentration (MCHC) (%)	32–36	32–36
RBC distribution width (RDW) (%)	11.5–14.5	11.5–14.5

Table 9-2 Age-dependent Changes for RBC Parameters in Healthy Individuals*

Age	Hb (g/dl) Mean (Average)	RBC (x 10^{12}/l) Mean (Average)	MCV (fl) Mean (Average)
Cord blood	17.1 (13.5–20.7)	4.6 (3.6–5.6)	113 (101–125)
1 day	19.4 (15.1–23.7)	5.3 (4.2–6.4)	110 (99–121)
1 month	13.9 (10.7–17.1)	4.3 (3.3–5.3)	101 (91–112)
6 months	12.6 (11.1–14.1)	4.7 (3.9–5.5)	76 (68–85)
12 months	12.7 (11.3–14.1)	4.7 (4.1–5.3)	78 (71–84)
3 years	12.4 (10.4–14.7)	4.7 (3.9–5.5)	78 (68–88)
5 years	12.7 (10.7–14.7)	4.7 (3.7–5.6)	80 (72–88)
10 years	13.2 (10.8–15.6)	4.8 (3.9–5.7)	81 (68–94)
20 years			
Male	15.9 (13.7–18.3)	5.3 (4.6–6.2)	89 (78–99)
Female	13.8 (11.7–15.8)	4.6 (4.0–5.4)	89 (76–99)
60 years			
Male	15.9 (13.8–18.4)	5.0 (4.3–5.9)	93 (82–103)
Female	13.9 (11.8–15.9)	4.6 (3.9–5.3)	90 (77–100)

* Adapted from Wickramasinghe SN, (Blood and Bone Marrow. Churchill Livingstone, London, 1986, pp 5)

shows a significant change in RBC indices and RBC morphology (Table 9-1). The normal range of the RBC count, HB and Hematocrit (Hct, percentage of the packed RBC volume in blood) depends on the age and sex of the individual (Table 9-2).

Although peripheral blood is the most informative sample in the diagnosis and classification of anemias, bone marrow examination provides additional valuable information including bone marrow cellularity, estimation of stored iron and presence or lack of marrow replacement by a primary or metastatic neoplasm, fibrosis or an inflammatory process. In general, anemia caused by blood loss or RBC destruction is associated with erythroid hyperplasia of the bone marrow and reticulocytosis, while anemia due to ineffective erythropoiesis is characterized by reticulocytopenia with a bone marrow which may be hypo-, normo- or hypercellular.

CLASSIFICATION

There are two different approaches in the classification of anemias. One is based on RBC morphology, in which anemias are divided into three major groups: microcytic, normocytic and macrocytic. This approach is simple and practical; the necessary information is obtained by routine microscopic examination of the peripheral blood smear and the results of a complete blood count (CBC) analysis. This information is used in the management and treatment of common forms of anemia such as iron, folate and vitamin B_{12} deficiency anemias. In this classification the underlying mechanism of the anemia is not taken into consideration.

The second classification is based on a pathophysiologic approach in which anemias are classified based on their underlying mechanisms. In this classification anemias are divided into two major categories: (1) anemia caused by decreased RBC production and (2) anemia caused by increased RBC destruction or loss (Table 9-3).

In this chapter, most anemias, especially those associated with significant bone marrow changes, are discussed. Disorders which result from disturbance of proliferation and differentiation of the pleuripotent stem cells such as aplastic anemia, polycythemia rubra vera, myelodysplastic syndromes and erythroleukemia are discussed in other chapters.

Table 9-3 Pathophysiologic Classification of Anemia*

1. Anemia caused predominantly by decreased RBC production
   A. Disturbance of proliferation and differentiation of pleuripotent stem cells
      (1) Aplastic anemia
      (2) Myelodysplastic anemia
   B. Disturbance of proliferation and differentiation of erythroid progenitor cells
      (1) Pure red cell aplasia
      (2) Congenital dyserythropoietic anemia
      (3) Anemia of chronic renal failure
      (4) Anemia of endocrine disorders
   C. Disturbance of DNA synthesis
      (1) Vitamin B_{12} deficiency
      (2) Folate deficiency
      (3) Defects in purine and pyrimidine metabolism
   D. Disturbance of Hb synthesis
      (1) Iron deficiency
      (2) Thalassemia
      (3) Congenital atransferrinemia
      (4) Idiopathic pulmonary hemosiderosis
   E. Unknown or multiple mechanisms
      (1) Anemia of chronic disorders
      (2) Anemia associated with marrow infiltration
      (3) Sideroblastic anemia
2. Anemia caused predominantly by increased erythrocyte destruction or loss
   A. RBC intrinsic abnormality
      (1) Globin abnormality
         Sickle cell disease and related disorders, unstable Hbs, low oxygen-affinity hemoglobinopathies
      (2) Membrane defect
         Hereditary spherocytosis, elliptocytosis, acanthocytosis, stomatocytosis
      (3) Enzyme deficiency
         Porphyria, deficiency of glucose-6-phosphatase dehydrogenase, Pyruvate kinase and other enzymes
      (4) Paroxysmal nocturnal hemoglobinuria
   B. Extrinsic abnormality
      (1) Blood loss
      (2) Mechanical
      (3) Chemical
      (4) Infections
      (5) Antibody mediated
      (6) Hyperactivity of the monocyte/macrophage system

* Adapted from Erslev AJ, Classification and manifestations. In Hematology, Williams WJ, Beutler E, Erslev AJ and Lichtman MA (eds), 4th Ed., McGraw-Hill Publishing Co., New York, 1990, pp 423.

DISTURBANCE OF PROLIFERATION AND DIFFERENTIATION OF ERYTHROID PROGENITOR CELLS

Pure Red Cell Aplasia

Etiology and Pathogenesis

Pure red cell aplasia, a term used to express bone marrow erythroid hypoplasia, is divided into two major types: acute and chronic.

Acute pure red cell aplasia (aplastic crisis) is a self-limited process which has been observed in a variety of hemolytic disorders such as sickle cell anemia, hereditary spherocytosis, and acquired hemolytic anemia.[3-6] The aplastic crisis is usually preceded by an infection such as gastroenteritis, mumps, viral hepatitis or interstitial pneumonia. Parvovirus infection appears to play an important role in its pathogenesis, particularly in patients with an underlying hemolytic anemia.[4-9] Parvovirus infects the erythroid progenitor cells, leading to erythroid hypoplasia. The hypoplastic state is transient and disappears by the termination of the parvovirus infection. Other reported contributing factors include immunologic suppression of the erythroid progenitor cells and drug toxicity.[10-12]

Chronic pure red cell aplasia is either congenital or acquired. The congenital form (Diamond-Blackfan anemia) is demonstrated in early childhood, usually between the ages of 2 weeks and 1 year, and appears to be the result of defective erythroid-committed stem cells. The defective stem cells show a slow growth rate in culture, are insensitive to erythropoietin or burst- promoting factors, and display abnormal maturation.[13,14]

Acquired pure red cell aplasia is a rare disease affecting predominantly adult patients. It has been reported in association with thymoma, systemic lupus erythematosus, rheumatoid arthritis, chronic active hepatitis and chronic lymphoid leukemias.[15-20] The association of pure red cell aplasia with lymphoproliferative disorders (especially those with a decreased T-helper:T-suppressor ratio) and with collagen-vascular disorders strongly supports an autoimmune etiology. Approximately 50% of the patients with pure red cell aplasia demonstrate antibodies with suppressor effects on the in vitro growth of both allogeneic and autologous erythroid progenitor cells.[21-23]

Pathology

In general, bone marrow specimens of patients with pure red cell aplasia show normo- to hypercellularity, with a markedly elevated M:E ratio due to severe erythroid depletion and rare late erythroid progenitor cells (Figure 9-1). The erythroid cells may show vari-

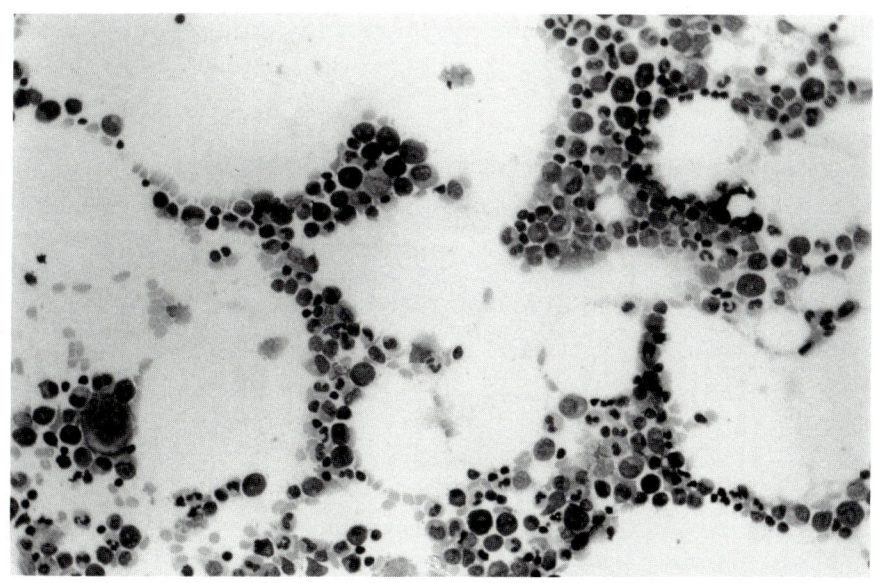

Figure 9-1. Bone marrow smear from a patient with pure red cell aplasia demonstrating a markedly elevated M:E ratio and rare late erythroid progenitor cells.

ous degrees of dysplastic changes. Parovirus-induced aplasia is often associated with prominent megaloblastic changes and the presence of giant rubriblasts displaying an intensely basophilic cytoplasm. The granulocytic and megakaryocytic lines show progressive, normal maturation, and the lymphocytes and plasma cells are unremarkable. The erythroid progenies in the chronic variants are macrocytic, and in most cases show increased expression of the i surface antigen and fetal Hb.[24] There is absolute reticulocytopenia, and the serum erythropoietin titer is elevated. Serum iron is normal or elevated, with increased saturation of iron-binding protein. Serum folic acid and vitamin B_{12} levels are normal.

Clinical Aspects

Aplastic crisis is a transient acute suppression of erythropoiesis usually found in patients with underlying hemolytic disorders. This transient suppression is followed by a rapid recovery phase which may be associated with bone pain (probably due to rapid bone marrow expansion), reticulocytosis, granulocytosis and thrombocytosis.

A variety of congenital abnormalities, such as strabismus, inverted nipples, webbed neck and bone deformities, have been reported in association with the congenital form of chronic pure red cell aplasia. Chronic pure red cell aplasia may eventually lead to congestive heart failure with hepatosplenomegaly.

Congenital Dyserythropoietic Anemias

Congenital dyserythropoietic anemias (CDAs) are a group of hereditary refractory anemias characterized by ineffective and dysplastic erythropoiesis. Three major types are distinguished: type I, type II and type III[25] (Table 9-4).

Congenital Dyserythropoietic Anemia Type I

CDA type I is a rare autosomal recessive hereditary disorder manifested in infancy or adolescence and characterized by a moderate macrocytic anemia, slight hyperbilirubinemia and often splenomegaly.[26] The exact mechanism of dyserythropoiesis in this hereditary disorder is not known, though the defect appears to be at the stem cell level.[27]

The bone marrow is hypercellar, with marked erythroid hyperplasia and dysplasia. Dysplastic changes are mostly confined to the middle and late stages of erythroid maturation (polychromatic and orthochromatic nucleated RBCs) and include cells with nuclear irregularity; double segmented nuclei; binucleation with nuclei of different sizes, textures and stainability; and pairs of nucleated RBCs attached by a chromatin bridge. There are also mild to moderate megaloblastic changes. Electron microscopy reveals widening of the nuclear membrane pores, with vacuolization and disintegration of nuclear chromatin.[28]

Peripheral blood shows anisocytosis, poikilocytosis, macrocytosis and a normal to slightly elevated reticulocyte count (1-5%). The serum haptoglobulin level is low, and the serum iron level is normal to elevated.

Congenital Dyserythropoietic Anemia Type II

CDA type II, also known as HEMPAS (hereditary erythroblastic multinuclearity with a positive acid-

Table 9-4 Most Prominent Pathologic Features of Three Types of Congenital Dyserythropoietic anemia

Features	Type I	Type II	Type III
Genetics	Recessive	Recessive	Dominant
Anemia	Mild to moderate, macrocytic	Mild to severe, normocytic	Mild, macrocytic
Reaction with			
Anti-i	±	+ + +	±
Anti-I	+	+ + +	+
Acid serum test	−	+	−
Marrow erythroid line	Megaloblastic, bilobulated nuclei, chromatin bridges	Bi- and multi-lobulated nuclei	Gigantoblasts

Disorders of Red Blood Cells: Anemias

ified serum test), is a hereditary recessive anemia which has been reported more frequently than the two other types.[29] The age of onset varies from infancy to late adulthood, and the degree of anemia ranges from slight to severe. Hepatomegaly, jaundice and gallstone formation are common in the severe forms.

The primary defect in HEMPAS appears to be a deficiency of *N*-acetylglucosaminyltransferase II, which leads to a reduction in the glycosylation of several red cell membrane proteins.[30]

Bone marrow examination in HEMPAS shows erythroid hyperplasia with a marked abnormality of the nucleated RBCs in the middle to late stages of maturation. A significant proportion of these cells (10–35%) show bi- or multilobated nuclei, and many are binucleated (Figure 9-2). Because of overdestruction of the erythroid precursor cells, cell debris and membrane lipoproteins are accumulated in the macrophages, and many macrophages may resemble Gaucher cells (pseudo-Gaucher cells). Electron microscopic examination of the nucleated RBCs reveals an excess of endoplasmic reticulum parallel to the cell membrane ("double membrane" appearance).[31] The pathognomonic feature of HEMPAS is red cell lysis by acidified (pH 6.8) normal sera, but not by the pa-

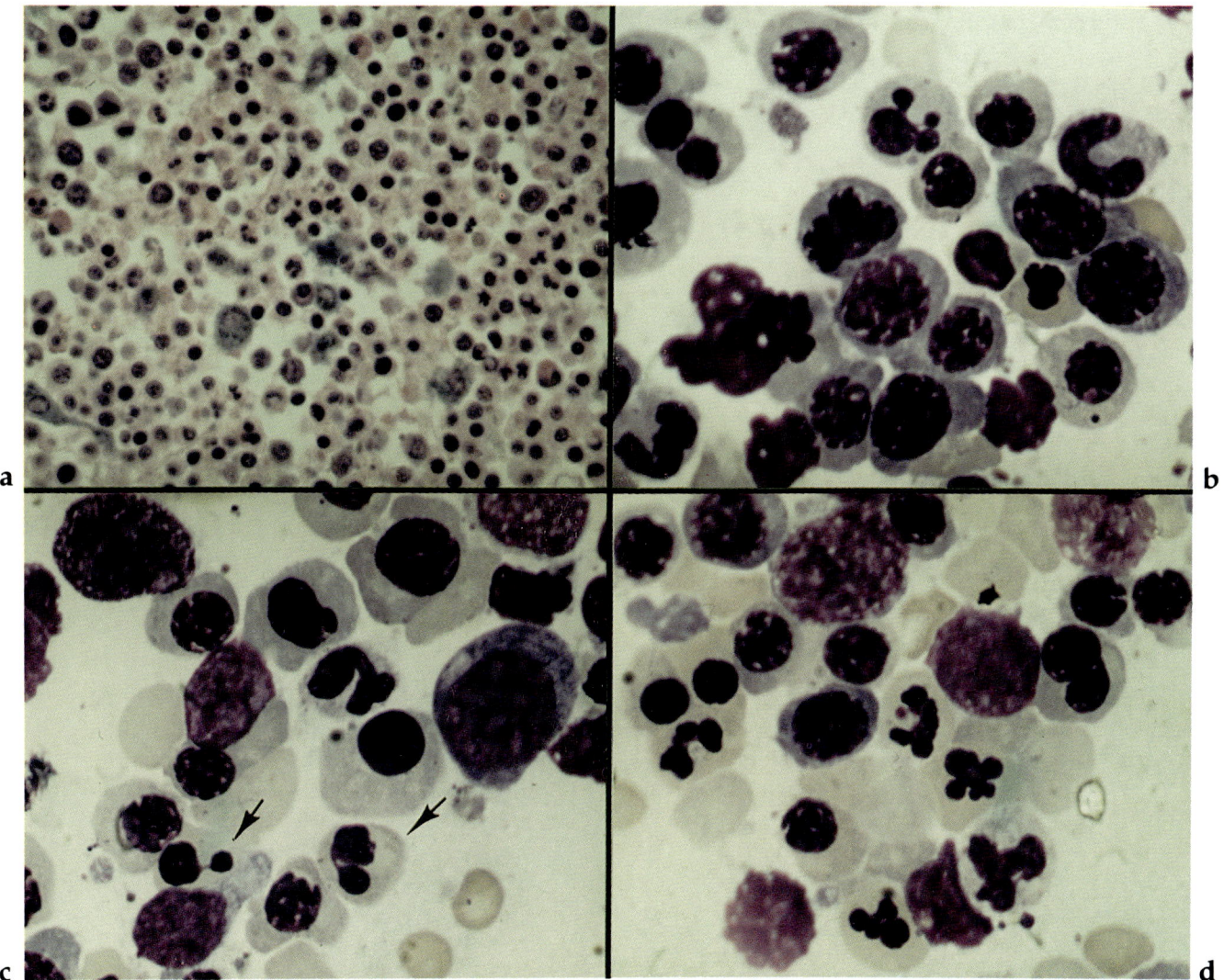

Figure 9-2. Bone marrow from a patient with congenital dyserythropoietic anemia type II demonstrating erythroid hyperplasia and dysplasia: (a) biopsy section; (b–d) marrow smears. Erythroid progenitor cells, particularly orthochromatic nucleated red cells, show bi- and multilobular nuclei. Cells with bilobed nuclei show unequal lobes (arrows).

tient's own serum. This feature is in contrast to PNH, in which red cells are lysed by the patient's own acidified serum.[32] Also, the sucrose hemolysis test, which is positive in PNH, is negative in HEMPAS.[32] HEMPAS cells are agglutinated and lysed by cold-reacting and anti-i and anti-I antibodies (Table 9-4).

Congenital Dyserythropoietic Anemia Type III

CDA type III is an autosomal dominant defect characterized by a mild to moderate macrocytic anemia associated with bone marrow erythroid hyperplasia and the presence of dysplastic, very large, multinucleated erythroid precursor cells (gigantoblasts).[33,34] The erythrocytes may react with anti-i and/or anti-I sera, but the acid serum test is negative (Table 9-4).

DISTURBANCE OF DNA SYNTHESIS (MEGALOBLASTIC ANEMIAS)

Megaloblastic anemias are a group of anemias characterized by megaloblastic erythropoiesis and RBC macrocytosis.

Etiology and Pathogenesis

The underlying defect in megaloblastic anemias is a decline in the rate of DNA synthesis in all the proliferating cells and, consequently, a delay in cell division. Megaloblastic anemia is due either to abnormal purine or pyrimidine metabolism or to inhibition of DNA polymerization.[35,36] The major etiologic factors in megaloblastic anemia include: (1) dietary insufficiency and acquired or congenital disorders, which lead to folic acid or vitamin B_{12} deficiency, and (2) congenital or acquired defects of purine or pyrimidine metabolism.

Folic Acid Deficiency

Folic acid (folate) is absorbed primarily within the upper third of the small intestine and is transported to the cells mainly as 5-methyl tetrahydrofolate (5-methyl THF). Methyl THF is required in the methylation of deoxyuridine monophosphate (dUMP) to deoxythymidine monophosphate (dTMP) in the presence of thymidylate synthetase. Folate deficiency leads to decreased synthesis of dTMP and increased levels of dUMP. The imbalance between thymidine and uridine residues apparently leads to a severe derangement of DNA synthesis and a delay in cell proliferation.[35,37-39] The end result of this slowed DNA synthesis is inappropriate enlargement of the cells (megaloblasts), which contain more than the normal amount of DNA but not enough for cell division.[35]

Folate deficiency is caused by decreased intake, malabsorption, excess losses, increased requirements, drugs and metabolic defects (Table 9-5). The principal cause of folate deficiency anemia is dietary, which is frequently observed in low-income, elderly people and in alcoholics.[40] Folate deficiency is also common in pregnancy and lactation.[41-43] However, pregnancy-associated anemias are usually compound and are caused by several deficiencies, including

Table 9-5 Major Causes of Folate Deficiency

1. Decreased intake
    Malnutrition (poverty, old age, alcoholism)
    Hyperalimentation
    Special diets, goat's milk
2. Malabsorption
    Gluten-induced enteropathy
    Tropical sprue
    Other diseases of the small intestine
3. Excess loss
    Dialysis
    Congestive heart failure
4. Increased requirements
    Pregnancy
    Premature infants
    Excess marrow turnover (e.g., hemolytic anemia)
    Malignancies (e.g., myeloma, carcinoma)
    Inflammatory diseases (e.g., rheumatoid arthritis, exfoliative dermatitis)
5. Drugs
    Antifolate drugs (e.g., methotrexate)
    Anticonvulsants
    Barbiturates
6. Congenital defects
    Congenital folate malabsorption
    Dihydrofolate reductase deficiency
    Homocysteine methyltransferase deficiency

Disorders of Red Blood Cells: Anemias

those of folate, vitamin B_{12} and iron. Folate is heat labile and is present in a variety of green vegetables, yeast, mushrooms, kidney and liver.

Vitamin B_{12} Deficiency

Vitamin B_{12} (cobalamin) derivatives act as coenzymes in a number of biochemical pathways[44,45] Vitamin B_{12} is involved in the conversion of 5-methyl THF to THF, which is required for the methylation of dUMP to dTMP. Vitamin B_{12} deficiency, similar to folate deficiency, leads to disturbance of DNA synthesis and, consequently, megaloblastic anemia.[35] Vitamin B_{12} is heat resistant and is abundant in animal proteins. The most common cause of vitamin B_{12} deficiency is impaired intestinal absorption. Other less frequent causes include inadequate intake and metabolic defects (Table 9-6).

In the gastrointestinal tract, vitamin B_{12} attaches to salivary and gastric vitamin B_{12} binders (*R binders*). When the R–B_{12} complexes are exposed to the pancreatic enzymes, the R binders are digested and the released vitamin B_{12} binds to the intrinsic factor (IF), a glycoprotein secreted by the gastric parietal cells.[46] The IF–B_{12} complex is then carried to the ileum, where it binds to the specific receptors. The IF is then dissociated from vitamin B_{12}, and the free vitamin B_{12} is absorbed. The absorbed vitamin B_{12} enters the portal circulation and binds to transcobalamins, mainly transcobalamin II. Decreased production of IF (e.g., in pernicious anemia or gastrectomy) or decreased absorption of vitamin B_{12} in the ileum (e.g., in ileal resection, Crohn's disease, blind-loop syndrome) leads to vitamin B_{12} deficiency and megaloblastic anemia.

IF deficiency (*pernicious anemia*) is either congenital or acquired. The congenital form is uncommon and appears to be the result of a defective gene involved in IF secretion. Symptomatic patients are presumably homozygous and usually demonstrate megaloblastic anemia during the first 2 years of life.[47,48]

Acquired pernicious anemia, in most cases, is an autoimmune disorder characterized by chronic atrophic gastritis and deficiency of IF production. The autoimmune etiology is based of the presence of autoantibodies against gastric antigens in patients with pernicious anemia and coexistance of pernicious anemia with other autoimmune disorders. Autoantibodies against gastric parietal cells (both surface and cytoplasmic), IF, and IF-B_{12} complexes have been detected in patients with acquired pernicious anemia[49,50]

Disturbance in Purine and Pyrimidine Metabolism

The defects of purine and pyrimidine metabolism are either congenital or acquired (Table 9-7). Hereditary orotic aciduria and Lesch-Nyhan syndrome represent the congenital deficiencies, and antimetabolite drugs (purine and pyrimidine analogs) are the major causes of acquired defects in purine and pyrimidine metabolism.

Hereditary orotic aciduria is an autosomal recessive disorder of pyrimidine metabolism characterized by an orotidylic decarboxylase deficiency, often associated with a pyrophosphorylase deficiency.[51,52]

Lesch-Nyhan syndrome is an X-linked disorder caused by a deficiency of hypoxanthine-guanine phosphoribosyltransferase.[53]

Pathology

The impaired DNA synthesis in megaloblastic anemia slows nuclear replication and cell division and leads

Table 9-6 Major Causes of Vitamin B_{12} Deficiency

1. Impaired absorption
   A. Gastric causes
      (1) Pernicious anemia
          Acquired (autoimmune)
          Congenital
      (2) Partial or total gastrectomy
      (3) Zollinger-Ellison syndrome
   B. Intestinal causes
      (1) Ileal resection or disease
      (2) Blind loop syndrome
      (3) Chronic tropical sprue
      (4) Fish tapeworm
      (5) Drugs (e.g., metformin)
   C. Pancreatic insufficiency
2. Inadequate diet (veganism)
3. Metabolic defects
   A. Congenital
      (1) Transcobalamin II deficiency
      (2) Homocystinuria with methylmalonic aciduria
   B. Acquired
      (1) Nitrous oxide
      (2) Anesthesia
4. Others
   A. Congenital transcobalamin II deficiency
   B. Congenital R-binder deficiency

Table 9-7 Causes of Megaloblastic Anemia Due to Disturbance of Purine and Pyrimidine Metabolism

1. Congenital
   A. Hereditary orotic aciduria
   B. Lesch-Nyhan syndrome
2. Drug-induced
   A. Purine analogs
      6-Mercaptopurine
      6-Thioguanine
      Azathioprine
      Acyclovir
   B. Pyrimidine analogs
      5-Fluorouracil
      5-Fluorodeoxyuridine
      6-Azauridine
      Azidothymidine (AZT)
   C. Inhibitors of ribonucleotide reduction
      Cytosine arabinoside
      Hydroxyurea

to an ineffective erythropoiesis and early destruction of the RBCs (hemolysis). Megaloblastic erythroid precursors are larger than their normal counterparts and have more cytoplasm relative to the size of the nucleus. These megaloblastic features are most striking in the intermediate and late stages of erythroid maturation and are demonstrated as unevenly speckled nuclear chromatin and abundant hemoglobin-filled cytoplasm[54] (Figures 9-3 and 9-4). Final condensa-

Figure 9-3. Bone marrow in megaloblastic anemias. A biopsy section (a) showing hypercellularity, erythroid hyperplasia and an increased number of large, early erythroid progenitor cells (arrow). Bone marrow smears (b–d) demonstrating early and late megaloblasts. The late megaloblasts show abundant well-hemoglobinized cytoplasm and speckled nuclear chromatin. Nuclear fragments are noted in several cells (arrows). ↓

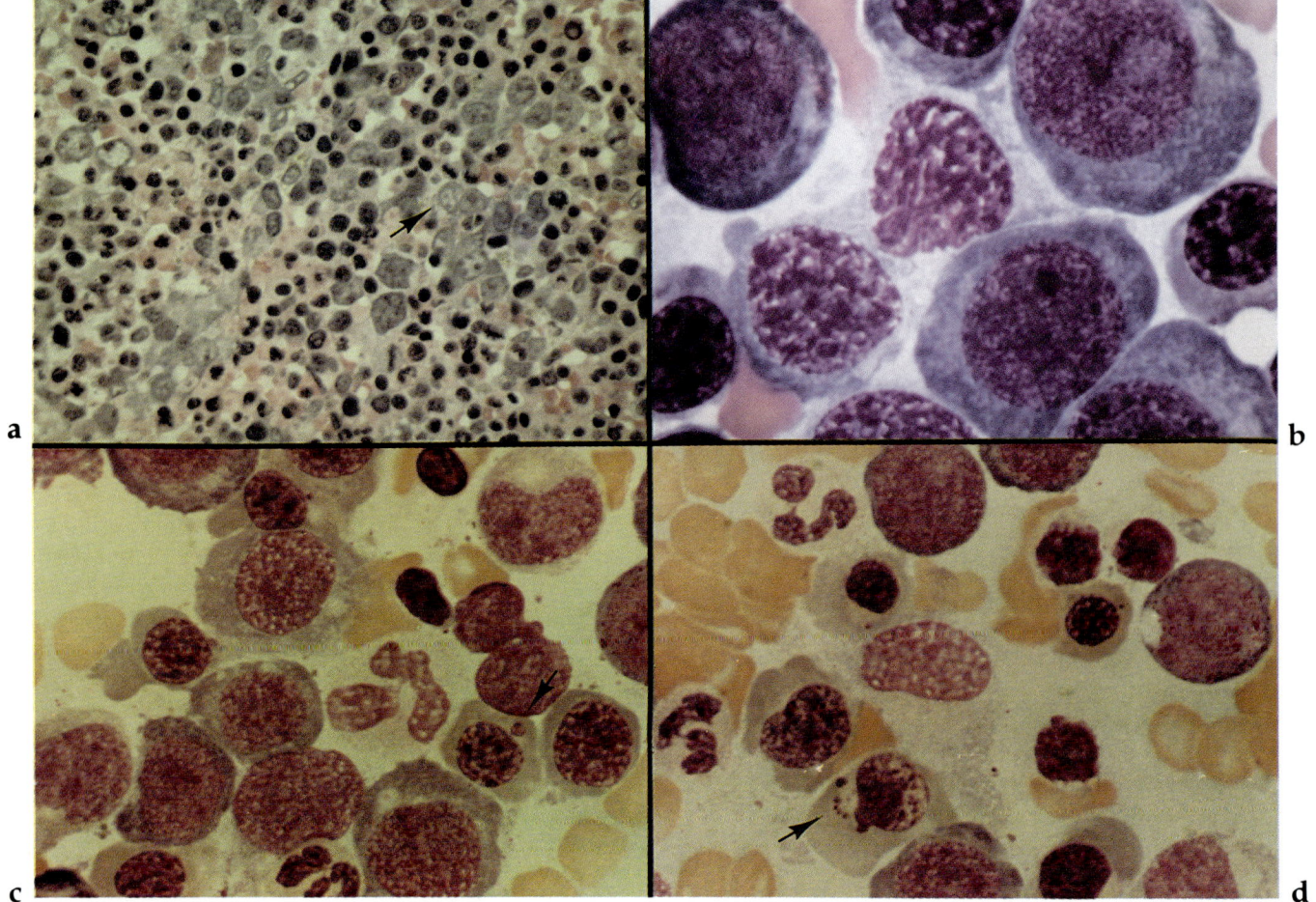

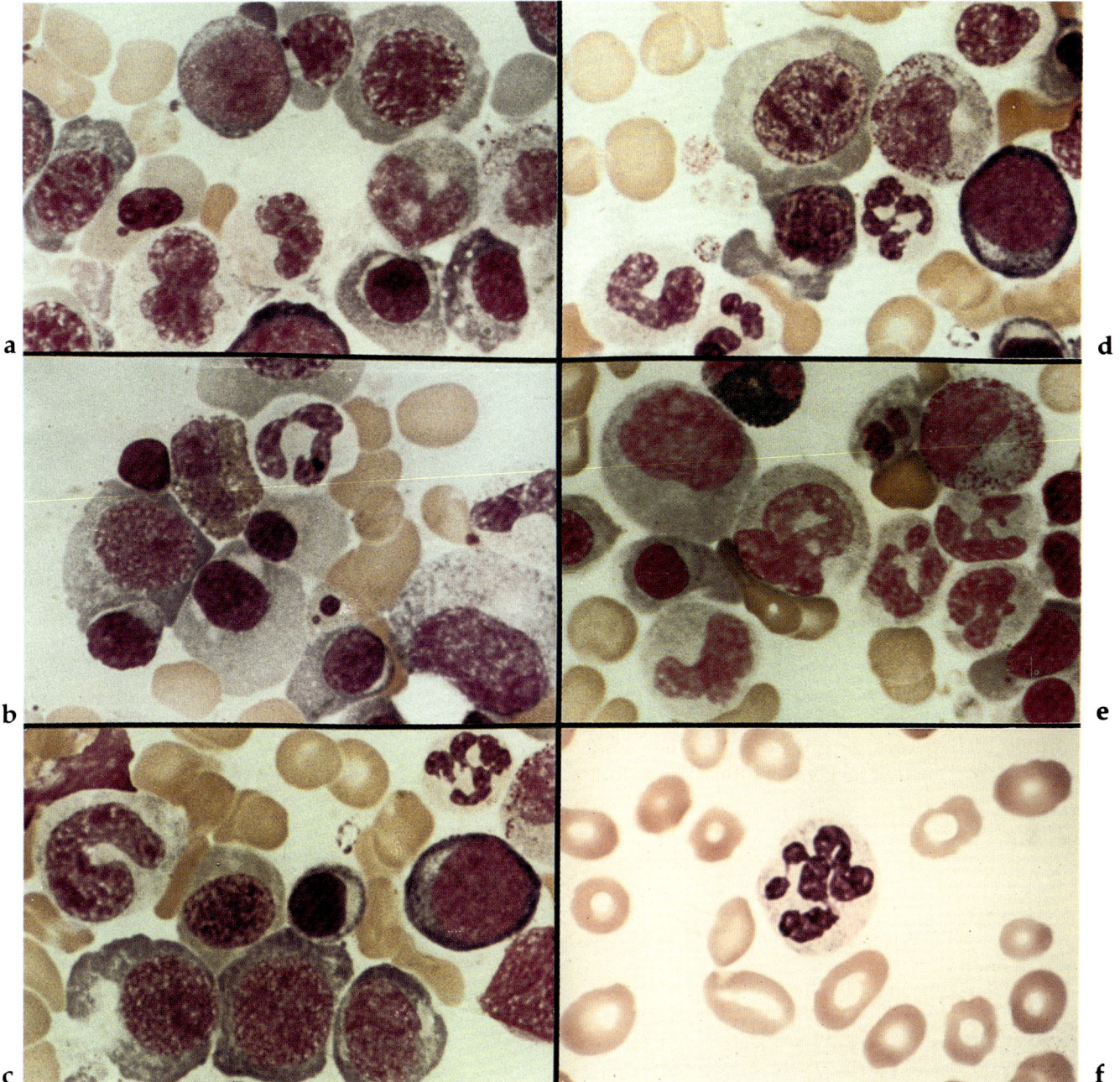

Figure 9-4. Bone marrow smears (a–e) from a patient with megaloblastic anemia demonstrating megaloblastic changes in both erythroid and granulocytic series. There are giant myelocytes, metamyelocytes, bands and segmented cells with nuclear hypersegmentation. (f) A peripheral blood smear with a large, hypersegmented neutrophil and several macroovalocytes.

tion of chromatin (pyknosis), which is seen in late orthochromatic normoblasts, is either delayed or fails to occur. Dysplastic changes such as nuclear irregularity or lobulation and nuclear fragmentation are common. The granulocytic series are also affected and show nuclear-cytoplasmic asynchrony, with the presence of giant metamyelocytes, giant bands and hypersegmented neutrophils (Figure 9-3 and 9-4).

Mild to moderate myeloid left shift is a common feature. Changes in the megakaryocytic lineage include nuclear hypersegmentation, megakaryocytic fragments and giant platelets. The megaloblastic maturation returns to normoblastic after 2–3 days of therapy, but neutrophilic hypersegmentation may persist for 10–14 days.

Bone marrow sections and smears are hypercellular and reveal erythroid predominance with an M:E ratio of usually <1. There is often a shift to the left, with numerous megaloblasts and frequent mitotic figures, particularly in severe cases. The megaloblastic changes and the erythroid left shift may simulate a leukemic process, especially in H&E sections, where clusters immature cells with open nuclear chromatin and prominent nucleoli are found.

Peripheral blood examination reveals pancytopenia with increased MCV of usually >115 fl and a reduced reticulocyte count. Smears show anisopoikilocytosis, macro-ovalocytes and hypersegmented (six or more nuclear segments) neutrophils. Other features include basophilic stippling, Howell-Jolly bodies and occasionally Cabot's rings. In severe cases, numerous nucleated RBCs are present. Serum levels of vitamin B_{12} or folate or both are low.

Megaloblastic changes are frequently present in myelodysplastic syndromes and erythroleukemia. However, unlike megaloblastic anemias, these conditions often display cytogenetic abnormalities and show normal or elevated levels of serum vitamin B_{12} a folate.

Clinical Aspects

Folic acid and vitamin B_{12} deficiencies are the second and third most frequent causes of nutritional anemia in the world (iron deficiency is the first).[35] The major clinical differences between folate and vitamin B_{12} deficiency are the neurologic symptoms associated with vitamin B_{12} deficiency. These symptoms result from degenerative changes of the dorsal and lateral columns of the spinal cord (subacute combined system disease) and have been attributed to the impairment of myelin synthesis due to the accumulation of methylmalonyl CoA,[55] or the impairment of methyl group metabolism.[56]

Folate deficiency is characterized by absence of neurologic symptoms and a full clinical response to physiologic doses of folic acid.

DISTURBANCE OF HEMOGLOBIN SYNTHESIS (HYPOCHROMIC ANEMIA)

Iron Deficiency Anemia

Iron deficiency is the most common cause of anemia in the world.[57,58] Infants, particularly premature ones, women of reproductive age and pregnant women are the groups with the highest frequency of iron deficiency.

Etiology and Pathogenesis

The common causes of iron deficiency anemia are inadequate dietary iron intake, blood loss, intravascular hemolysis with hemoglobinuria, iron malabsorption, dialysis treatment of renal failure, or a combination of two or more of these causes.

Inadequate dietary intake is the major cause of iron deficiency anemia in infants fed unsupplemented milk diets. Milk and milk products are low in iron, and prolonged breast- or bottle feeding (for more than 6 months) without iron supplementation often leads to iron deficiency anemia. Premature infants may become iron deficient as early as 10–12 weeks after birth if their diet is not supplemented with iron.

Iron dietary requirements increase during pregnancy and lactation. During pregnancy and delivery, approximately 300 mg iron is utilized by the fetus, 30–170 mg is drained into the placenta and 100–250 mg is lost during delivery. Approximately 1 mg/day iron is lost during lactation.

Blood loss, particularly in the form of chronic bleeding, is one of the major causes of iron deficiency in adults. Chronic gastrointestinal bleeding due to peptic ulcer, gastritis, ulcerative colitis, amebiasis, hiatal hernia, hemorrhoids, esophageal and gastric varices, and neoplasms are the most frequent causes of iron depletion in men and postmenstrual women. Intestinal parasites, such as hookworm, may also cause gastrointestinal blood loss. Genitourinary tract bleeds such as hematuria (kidney stone, cancer, Goodpasture syndrome), menstruation and menorrhage, and loss of iron in the urine in the form of hemoglobin, hemosiderin and ferritin (paroxysmal nocturnal hemoglobinuria and other hemolytic disorders), often lead to iron deficiency anemia. Similarly, respiratory tract blood loss secondary to infections, epistaxis, idiopathic pulmonary hemosiderosis and Goodpasture syndrome may cause iron deficiency anemia.

Other causes of blood loss include self-inflicted bleeding (factitious anemia), iatrogenic phlebotomy (nosocomial anemia) and blood donation. Iron deficiency associated with dialysis therapy of chronic renal disease is primarily caused by entrapment and loss of RBCs in the dialyzing equipment.

Iron malabsorption is relatively uncommon and may occur in association with malabsorption syndromes or in patients who undergo subtotal gastrectomy. Iron absorption is retarded by phosphate and phytates from cereals and is enhanced by vitamin C.[54]

Iron deficiency is associated with the depletion and disappearance of hemosiderin and ferritin from bone marrow and other storage sites, and with decreased concentration and/or reduced activity of several iron-containing proteins such as hemoglobin, myoglobin, cytochrome c, cytochrome oxidase, and xanthine oxidase. Approximately 10% of the total dietary iron (1–2 mg/day) is absorbed through the digestive system. Meat, eggs and liver are rich in iron. Individuals living predominantly on a vegetarian diet may develop iron deficiency anemia. All vegetables except legumes and all fruits are either poor in iron or contain unabsorbable iron chelates.

Pathology

Bone marrow examination often reveals an erythroid preponderance and a mild to moderate hypercellularity. But these findings are not consistent and do not correlate with the severity of anemia. Erythroid precursors, particularly intermediate and late normoblasts, are small and show scanty, ragged rims of poorly hemoglobinized cytoplasm (Figure 9-5). Bone marrow hemosiderin (demonstrated with Prussian blue stain) is decreased or absent. However,

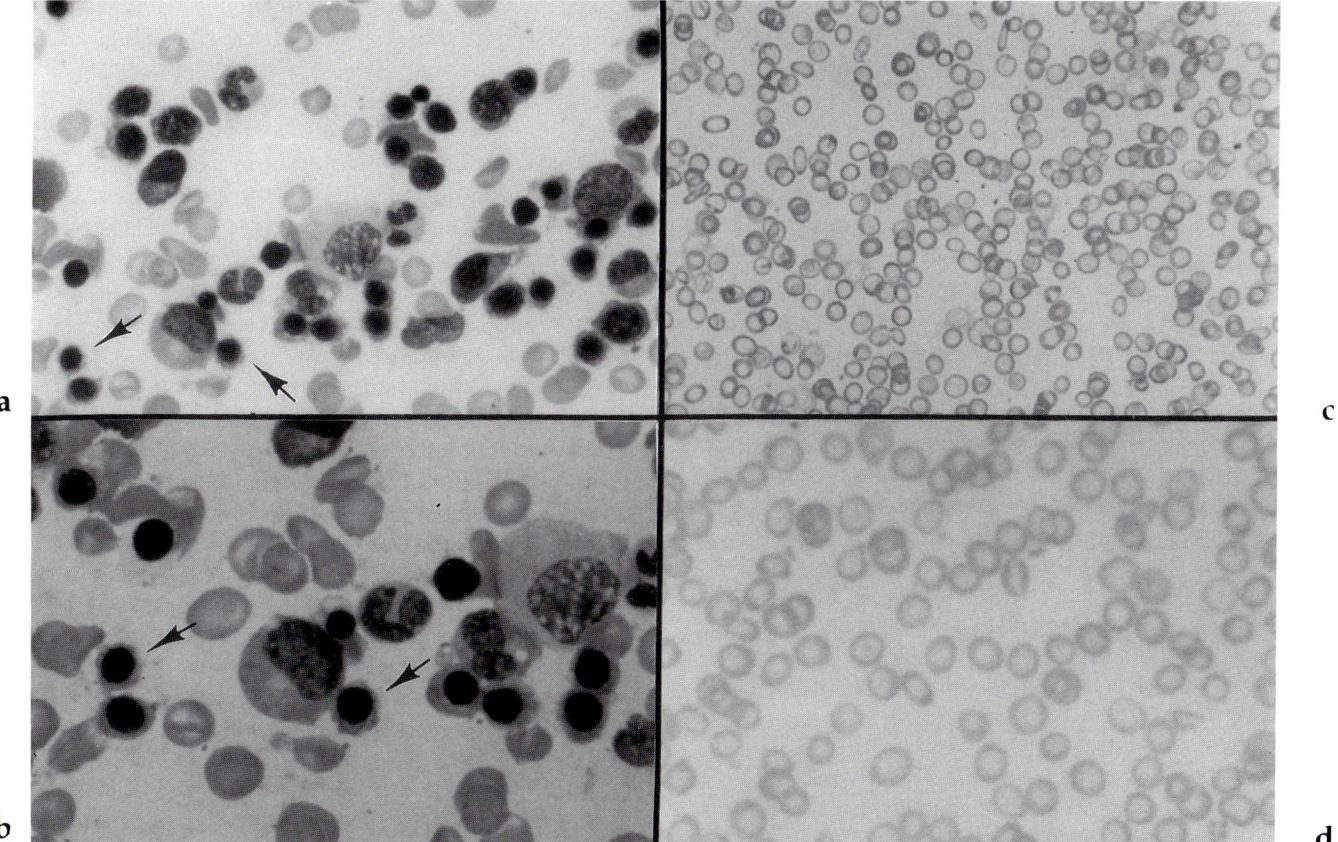

Figure 9-5. Severe iron deficiency anemia. Bone marrow smears showing small normoblasts with scanty, ragged rims of poorly hemoglobinized cytoplasm (a, b, arrows) and peripheral blood smears demonstrating hypochromasia (c, d).

lack of stainable iron has been noted in some patients with chronic myelogenous leukemia and myelofibrosis, probably due to the inability of bone marrow to store iron. These patients usually lack other evidences of iron deficiency and do not respond to iron therapy.

Peripheral blood examination in the early stages of iron deficiency anemia reveals a mild anisocytosis with a slightly elevated RDW, mild ovalocytosis, and decreased MCV (<80 fl). In the more severe forms, RBCs are clearly hypochromic and microcytic, and show pronounced anisocytosis with the presence of target cells. The RDW is markedly elevated, and the MCV, MCH and Hb levels are much lower than normal (Figure 9-5). Serum iron and ferritin levels are low and total iron binding capacity (TIBC) is elevated, as is the concentration of erythrocyte protoporphyrin (Table 9-8).

Serum ferritin measurements provide valuable information regarding the diagnosis and clinical assessment of iron-deficient patients. In all forms of anemia except iron deficiency, a decline in serum hemoglobin is accompanied by an increase in the serum ferritin level.[59] Serum ferritin is invariably low in a pure iron deficiency anemia. It is elevated in chronic inflammation, liver disease and malignancy.[60]

Clinical Aspects

Symptoms of anemia such as fatigue, headache, paresthesia and a burning sensation of the oropharyngeal mucosa are often preceded by the depletion of iron stores. There is a poor correlation between the severity of the symptoms and the blood Hb level, suggesting that some of the symptoms are caused by a deficiency of iron-containing enzymes or proteins rather than by a low concentration of hemoglobin. Impaired learning ability and growth in children, defects in cell-mediated immunity and the bactericidal function of leukocytes, increased frequency of premature contractions during pregnancy, and possibly an increased rate of premature births have been reported in association with iron deficiency.[61-65] A few days after initiation of iron therapy, most of the symptoms abate. The reticulocyte count reaches its peak at about 1–2 weeks and then gradually levels off. The Hb level begins to improve after 2 weeks and usually comes back to a normal level after 2 months of adequate therapy.

Thalassemias

Thalassemia syndromes are a group of disorders caused by inherited defects in the synthesis of one or more of the globin chains and are characterized by a microcytic anemia. These disorders are associated with a change in the proportion of Hb A ($\alpha 2\ \beta 2$), Hb A2 ($\alpha 2\ \delta 2$) and Hb F ($\alpha 2 \gamma 2$), which constitute >95%, >3% and <2% of the hemoglobin in normal persons, respectively. The reduction in the synthesis of certain globin chain(s) is also associated with a relative excess of the nonaffected globin chain(s) which leads to instability of Hb and RBC lysis. Depending on the affected globin chains, these disorders are divided into β-, δ-, βδ-, and α-thalassemias. δ-Thalassemia has no clinical significance.

The main β- and α-globin gene clusters are located on chromosomes 11 and 16, respectively[66,67a,67b] (Figure 9-6). The β-globin gene cluster encodes globin subunits specific for the embryonic, fetal, and adult developmental stages. This cluster includes ε, γ (Gγ and Aγ), δ and β genes.[68] The α-globin gene cluster encodes for two globin proteins: ζ for the embryonic period and α (α1 and α2) for the fetal-adult period. In normal conditions a balance is maintained between α-cluster and β-cluster gene expression so that functional Hb tetramers are assembled. In thalassemias this balance is lost.[67]

β-Thalassemias

ETIOLOGY AND PATHOGENESIS: β-Thalassemias are caused by a decrease or absence in production of the β-chain of Hb A.[69] The abnormal β-globin gene ex-

Table 9-8 Laboratory Findings in Iron Deficiency Anemia

Test	Diagnostic range
Hb	<13 g/dl in men
	<12 g/dl in women
MCV	<80 fl
Erythrocyte protoporphyrin	> 7μg/dl RBC
Serum iron	<75 μg/dl in men
	<65 μg/dl in women
TIBC	>450 μg/dl
Serum ferritin	<10 μg/l
Transferrin saturation	<16%
Serum transferrin receptor	>9 mg/dl
Bone marrow iron stain	Negative

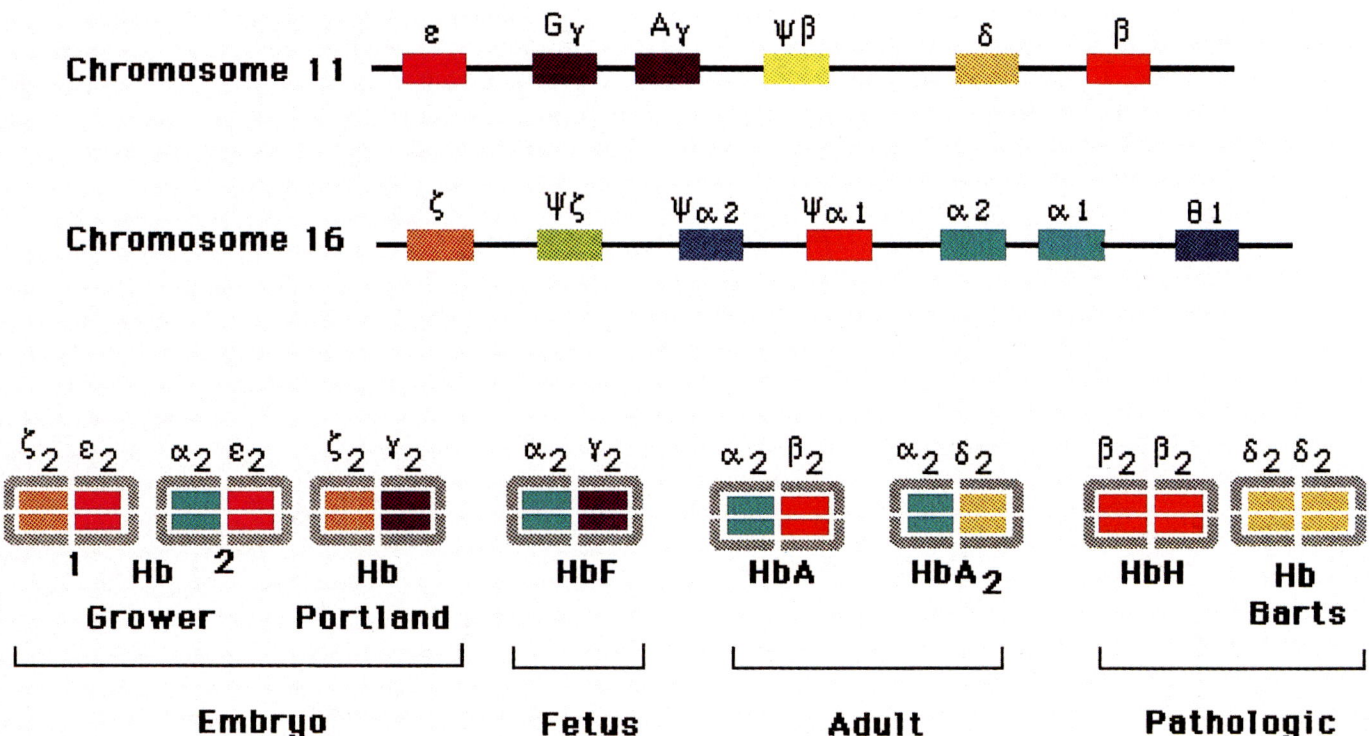

Figure 9-6. Schematic demonstration of globin genes on chromosomes 11 and 16.

pression is primarily the result of point mutations, but it may also be due to deletion of long stretches of nucleotides, or to substitution of a small number of nucleotides within or close to the β-globin gene.[66] So far, over 50 different mutations have been found in β-thalassemia, including gene deletions, transcriptional mutations, RNA-processing mutations, mutations to termination codons and frame-shift mutations,[70-81] (Figure 9-7). The decreased production of β-globin chains results in the accumulation of unpaired α-globin chains which form insoluble aggregates. These aggregates disrupt erythrocyte membranes and may have a direct toxic effect on normoblasts.[82,83] β-thalassemia has been divided into two major states: homozygous (β0) and heterozygous (β+), though it has considerable phenotypic variation, depending on the nature of the mutations.

CLINICAL AND PATHOLOGIC FEATURES: β-thalassemias are widespread in the Mediterranean basin, the Middle East and Southeast Asia. The clinicopathologic features of β-thalassemia vary from a severe, transfusion-dependent anemia to a very mild, asymptomatic anemia. β-Thalassemias with severe anemia are in general the result of either a homozygous state or of a compound heterozygous for two different thalassemia mutations. The most severe transfusion-dependent form is called β-*thalassemia major*. β-*thalassemia minor* is a term used to describe the asymptomatic heterozygous state, and β-*thalassemia intermediate* refers to a clinical condition that is less severe than thalassemia major and more severe than thalassemia minor.

β-*Thalassemia major* (β0-thalassemia) is usually demonstrated within the first year of life and is characterized by a severe anemia (Hb 2.5–6 g/dl), progressive hepatosplenomegaly, mild jaundice and recurrent attacks of fever. Affected children who are not maintained on an adequate blood transfusion program will subsequently show retarded growth and skeletal deformities due to the massive expansion of the erythropoietic tissue.

The bone marrow is hypercellular, with marked erythroid hyperplasia and increased stainable iron. Iron-laden macrophages are abundant, and scattered macrophages may contain phagocytosed normoblasts. The polychromatophilic normoblasts are poorly hemoglobinized, show ragged cytoplasm and contain precipitated α-chains.

The overall RBC life span is shortened. There is a marked microcytic and hypochromic anemia, with low MCV and MCH and elevated RDW and

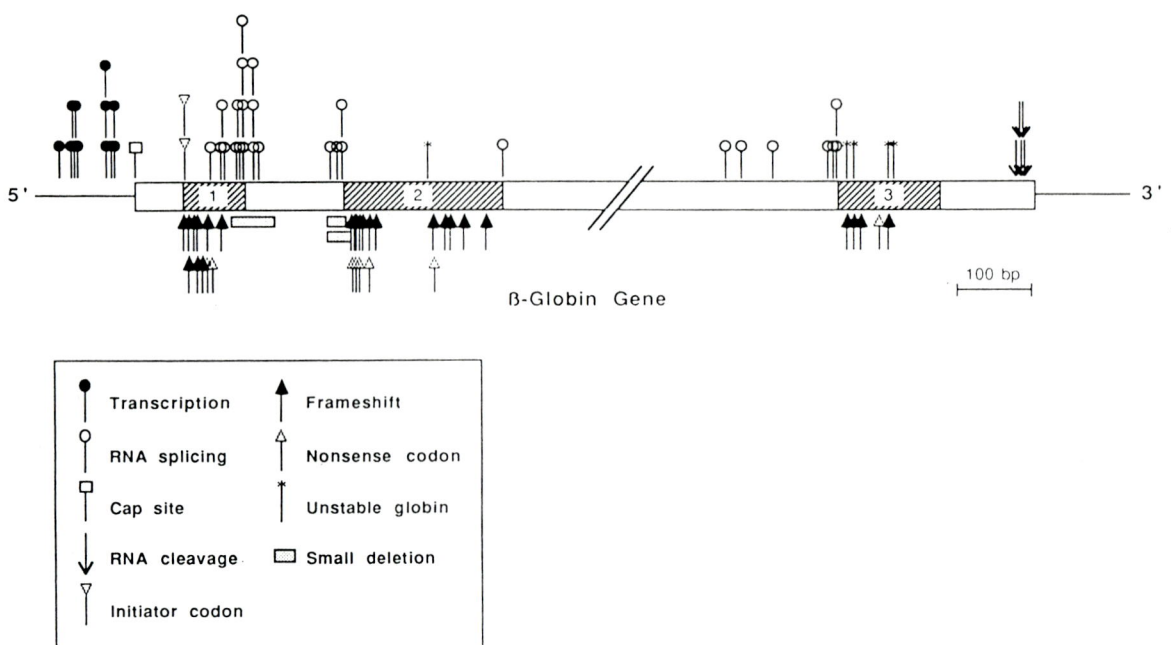

Figure 9-7. Point mutations in β-thalassemia. From Kazazian HH Jr: The thalassemia syndromes: Molecular basis and prenatal diagnosis in 1990. *Semin Hematol* 27:209, 1990, with permission.

reticulocyte count. Anisocytosis is prominent and there is a variable degree of poikilocytosis, target cell formation and basophilic stippling (Figure 9-8). One of the characteristic features of thalassemia major (β0-thalassemia) is an elevated level of fetal Hb (ranging from >10% to >90%). The acid elution test shows a heterogenous distribution of Hb F among the red cells. The proportion of Hb A2 to Hb A is elevated, though the overall Hb A2 level may be low, normal or high.

Thalassemia minor is usually associated with a very mild anemia which may worsen during stressful conditions, such as severe infection or pregnancy. The Hb level is about 9–11 g/dl, but the MCV and MCH values are markedly low. The bone marrow shows slight erythroid hyperplasia. The Hb A2 level is increased (3.5–7%).

Thalassemia intermediate refers to a wide range of clinical conditions that are between thalessemia minor and major.

δβ-Thalassemias

δβ-Thalassemias are the result of deletions of the δ- and β-globin genes or crossover between part of the δ locus on one chromosome and part of the β locus on the complementary chromosome. Deletions may extend into or beyond the Aγ gene on the 5′ side, leading to (AγδΒ)0 thalassemia, or may be limited to the δ- and β-genes, resulting in (δβ)0 thalassemia. The δβ-gene crossovers are apparently caused by misalignment of chromosome pairing during meiosis, resulting in a δβ fusion gene. The gene product is an abnormal Hb called *hemoglobin Lepore (Hb Lepore)*.[84,85] In a condition called *hereditary persistence of fetal hemoglobin (HPFH)*, the decreased production of Hb A and Hb A2 due to δβ-thalassemia is almost completely compensated for by increased produciton of Hb F. HPFH consists of a heterogeneous group of inherited conditions which are divided into deletion and nondeletion forms based on their genetic defects, and into pancellular and heterocellular types based on the intracellular distribution of Hb F. Clinical manifestations of these thalassemias are usually similar to thalassemia minor or intermediate.

α-Thalassemias

ETIOLOGY AND PATHOGENESIS: α-thalassemia results from deletion of one or more α-globin genes.[86] The single α-globin gene deletion is probably the most common mutation worldwide and can occur

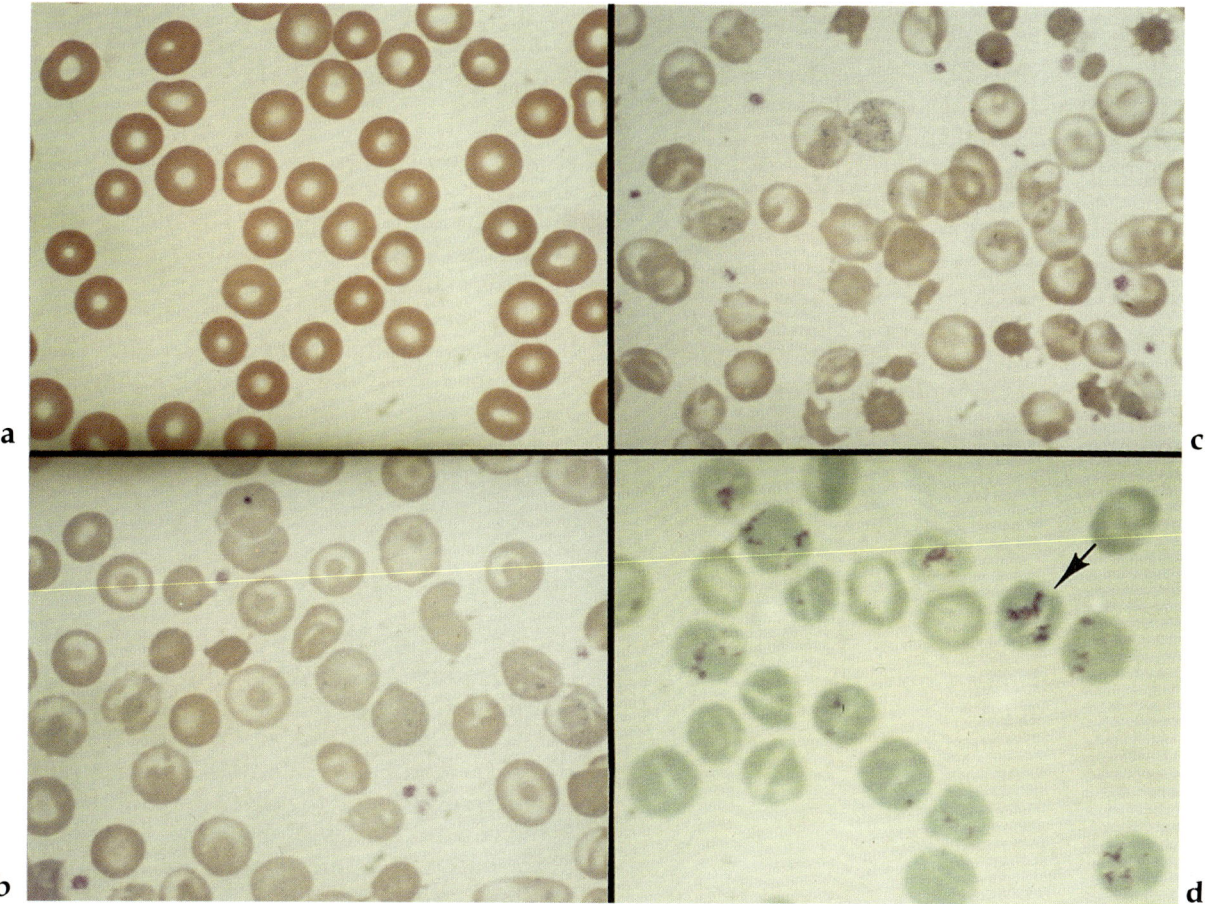

Figure 9-8. β-Thalassemia. Peripheral blood smears demonstrating normochromic, normocytic RBCs (a), target cells and basophilic stippling (b and c), and numerous reticulocytes (d, arrow).

with a greater than 80% frequency in some populations.[87,88] So far, the size and position of at least 14 deletions have been defined.[67] The nondeletion mutations may fall into three major categories: RNA processing defect, RNA translation defect and post-translational instability.[67,80,81]

The deficiency in α-chain production results in the accumulation of excessive γ- and/or β-globin in α-thalassemias. Excess β- and γ-chains may assemble into homotetramers β4 (Hb H) and γ4 (Hb Bart's). Precipitation of the Hb Bart's and Hb H in the red cells causes red cell damage and premature clearance by the mononuclear phagocytic system.[89,90] The severity of α-thalassemia is related to the number of genes affected, the extent of functional loss resulting from specific mutations and the affected gene (α1 or α2). The α2-globin is expressed at 2.6-fold higher levels than the α1-globin gene and thus plays a more significant clinical role.[67] There are four α-thalassemia phenotypes: (1) a silent carrier with three functional α-genes, (2) α-thalassemia trait with two functional genes, (3) Hb H disease with one functional α-gene and (4) Bart's hydrops or α0 thalassemia with no functional α-gene.[80]

CLINICAL AND PATHOLOGIC FEATURES: The silent carrier form of α-thalassemia (three functional α-genes) is prevalent in the Mediterranean basin, the Middle East, India, Southeast Asia and Indonesia, and affects approximately 30% of black Americans.[91] The affected persons display unremarkable hematologic parameters except for a borderline low MCV and MCH.

Patients with α-thalassemia trait usually have no clinical symptoms but have a low MCV (70–75 fl) with a normal Hb A2 concentration. α-Thalassemia trait affects approximately 3% of black Americans.[91]

In Hb H disease, formation and precipitation of the homotetramers lead to red cell membrane damage and hemolysis, which is often associated with bone marrow erythroid hyperplasia and hepatosplenomegaly. The anemia is moderate to severe, with Hb levels ranging from 3 to 11 g/dl. The anemia is microcytic and hypochromic, with very low MCV and MCH levels. Anisocytosis, poikilocytosis and target cells are present, and there is a mild to moderate reticulocytosis. Diagnosis is made by the demonstration of Hb Bart's (15–30%) in the cord blood at birth or by detection of Hb H (Heinz bodies). The Hb H-containing red cells, stained with brilliant crystal blue, have a "golf ball" appearance.

Bart's hydrops fetalis, or α0-thalassemia, is a disorder with no functional α-gene and the formation of γ4 homotetramers accounting for about 80–90% of the hemoglobin. Small amounts of embryonic Hb Portland (ζ2 γ2) (about 10%) and traces of Hb H are also present. This condition is incompatible with extrauterine life. The result is either a stillbirth or death shortly after birth. Hb Bart's and Hb H move faster than Hb A on electrophoresis at alkaline pH, Hb H running slightly faster than Hb Bart's.

Other Variants

In addition to the classical α- and β-thalassemia syndromes, there are a variety of phenotypes which are mostly similar to thalassemia intermediate or thalassemia minor in their clinical presentation. β-thalassemia associated with β structural Hb variants such as sickle cell, Hb C and Hb E thalassemias are examples.

ANEMIAS CAUSED BY RBC INTRINSIC ABNORMALITIES

The intrinsic RBC abnormalities are divided into three major groups: abnormal globin synthesis, membrane defects and enzyme deficiencies. These abnormalities lead to an early destruction of red cells and are often associated with a compensatory bone marrow erythroid hyperplasia and peripheral blood reticulocytosis.

Sickle Cell Diseases and Related Disorders (Abnormal Globin Synthesis, Hemoglobinopathies)

Sickle cell disease refers to a family of hemoglobinopathies with inheritance of the sickle β-globin gene (Hb S) from at least one parent. The most severe form of the disease is sickle cell anemia, which results from the inheritance of Hb S from both parents (homozygous state). Hb SC disease and sickle cell β-thalassemia are milder disorders, and Hb SD disease is the mildest in the group. Hb C and E diseases, similar to Hb S disease, are the result of β-chain gene mutations. Hb D disease is the result of either β- or α-chain gene mutation.

Etiology and Pathogenesis

The Hb S mutation is a single base change in the DNA codon (GAG to GTG) which results in the substitution of the amino acid valine for glutamic acid at the sixth amino acid position in the β-globin chain. Deoxygenated Hb S molecules align in liquid crystals (tactoids) and distort the RBCs into rigid sickle shapes. Reoxygenation disassembles the tactoids, and the RBCs become discoid and flexible again. Repeated sickling and unsickling causes RBC membrane changes and inability of cells to unsickle on reoxygenation (irreversible sickling). Membrane alterations in sickled RBCs include changes in membrane phospholipid composition and dynamics, perturbation of the interaction between membrane phospholipids and skeletal proteins, and perturbation of the translocase protein.[92-94] The irreversible sickle cells have a high Hb concentration, a high calcium and potassium content and a low ATP level.[92] These cells have a short intravascular life span and, because of their rigid shape, may cause small vessel blockage, leading to ischemia and endothelial cell damage.[95]

In *hemoglobin C* glutamic acid in the sixth position of the β-chain is replaced by lysine.[96] Hb C-containing RBCs are more rigid than normal RBCs and may show rod-like crystals in hypoxic conditions. RBC damage and fragmentation may result in the formation of microspherocytes. Formation of crystals is inhibited by the presence of Hb F.[97]

Hemoglobin D involves either the β- or the α-chain. In the β-chain variant, glutamate is substituted for

Disorders of Red Blood Cells: Anemias

lysine at the 121th, and in the α-chain variant, also known as $Hb\ G_{philadelphia}$, asparagine is replaced by lysine at the 68th position.[98]

Hemoglobin E is the result of a β-chain mutation in which glutamine is substituted for by lysine at the 26th position.[99]

Clinical and Pathologic Features

The prevalance of Hb S is greatest in Africa, with a heterozygote frequency of about 20%. In American blacks, sickle cell trait occurs in approximately 8% of the population.

The clinical symptoms of sickle cell disease are usually manifested in the affected infants 8–10 weeks after birth. Prior to this period, the newborn is protected by the high concentration of Hb F in the red cells. Patients have a steady-state course, which is periodically interrupted by a sudden onset of a severe clinical course (crisis). The most common cause of sickle cell crisis is ischemia and subsequent infarction of the ischemic tissues (frequently bone and spleen). This type of crisis is often associated with severe pain in the bones, chest and abdomen. Other crisis-associated clinical problems include the development of aplastic and megaloblastic anemias, acute hemolytic anemia, and massive pooling of the red cells in the spleen (sequestration crisis).

Affected children have growth retardation and skeletal abnormalities. Retinal damage, cerebrovascular accidents, leg ulcers, papillary necrosis of the kidney and recurrent infections are common complications.

Other forms of sickle cell disease and related disorders such as sickle cell trait, Hb SC, Hb C, Hb D, Hb E, Hb S–β-thalassemia and Hb C–β-thalassemia cause either no clinical symptoms or mild anemia.

Bone marrow changes usually correlate with the severity of the anemia; the more severe the anemia, the more extensive the bone marrow response and the erythroid hyperplasia (Figure 9-9). Bone marrow smears display marked erythroid hyperplasia and may show sickled RBCs. The erythroid hyperplasia and bone marrow hypercellularity may cause skeletal deformities. For example, bone marrow hyperplasia in the vertebrae and consequent reduction in the bone mass may cause partial vertebral collapse. Marrow spaces such as the femoral shaft, which in normal conditions are not actively involved in hematopoiesis, may become the site of active hematopoiesis. In addition, extramedullary hematopoiesis may occur.

Peripheral blood examination in a steady-state homozygous sickle cell anemia patient reveals a normochromic, normocytic anemia with an Hb level ranging from 5 to 11 g/dl and an elevated reticulocyte count (10–20%). There is anisopoikilocytosis with the presence of sickle cells, target cells and nucleated RBCs (Figure 9-9). A slight increase in WBCs and a left shift is common. There is an elevated indirect bilirubin level and an increased immunoglobulin level. Target cells are more prominent in Hb C disease and sickle cell β-thalassemia. Rod-like crystals may occasionally be present in the RBCs of patients with Hb C disease.

Diagnosis of sickle cell disease is based on the demonstration of Hb S by the sickle cell test and on hemoglobin electrophoresis. The principle of the sickle cell test is that the reducing agents, such as sodium metabisulfite, are able to induce precipitation of Hb S and sickle cell formation (Figure 9-9). In alkaline Hb electrophoresis, Hb S moves more slowly than Hb A and occupies a position between HbA and Hb A2; Hb C moves more slowly than Hb S; Hb D has a mobility similar to that of Hb S; and Hb E and Hb O occupy the same position as Hb C. These variants are distinguished further by an agar gel electrophoresis at an acid pH[100,101] (Figure 9-10).

Molecular biology techniques such as Southern blot analysis and PCR have been used for the diagnosis of sickle cell anemia and related disorders (see Chapter 2)

Unstable Hbs

Unstable Hbs are autosomal dominant disorders associated with a variety of amino acid substitutions or deletions in the tetrameric Hb molecule. These alterations weaken the stability of the Hb structure and result in the precipitation of Hb within the RBC[102-104] (Figure 9-11). The precipitated Hb structures, called *Heinz bodies*, are bound to the RBC membrane and are pitted from red cells by splenic macrophages. The removal of Heinz bodies in the spleen leads to membrane damage and shortening of the RBC life span. The pitting process also results in the reduction of MCH and MCHC. In addition, presence of the

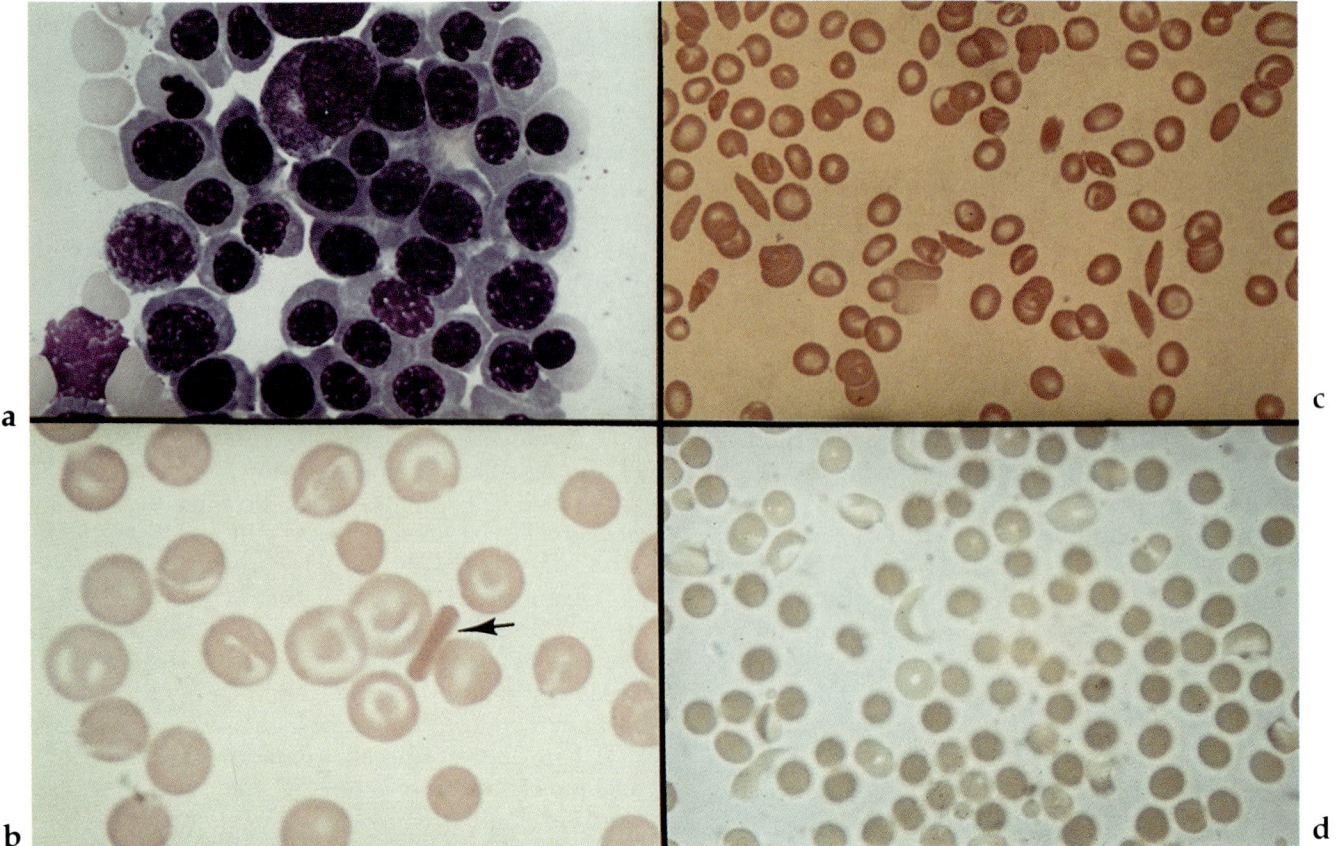

Figure 9-9. Hemoglobinopathies. Bone marrow smear demonstrating erythroid hyperplasia (a) and peripheral blood smears demonstrating target cells and a hemoglobin C crystal (b, arrow), numerous sickle cells (c), and a positive sickle cell test (d).

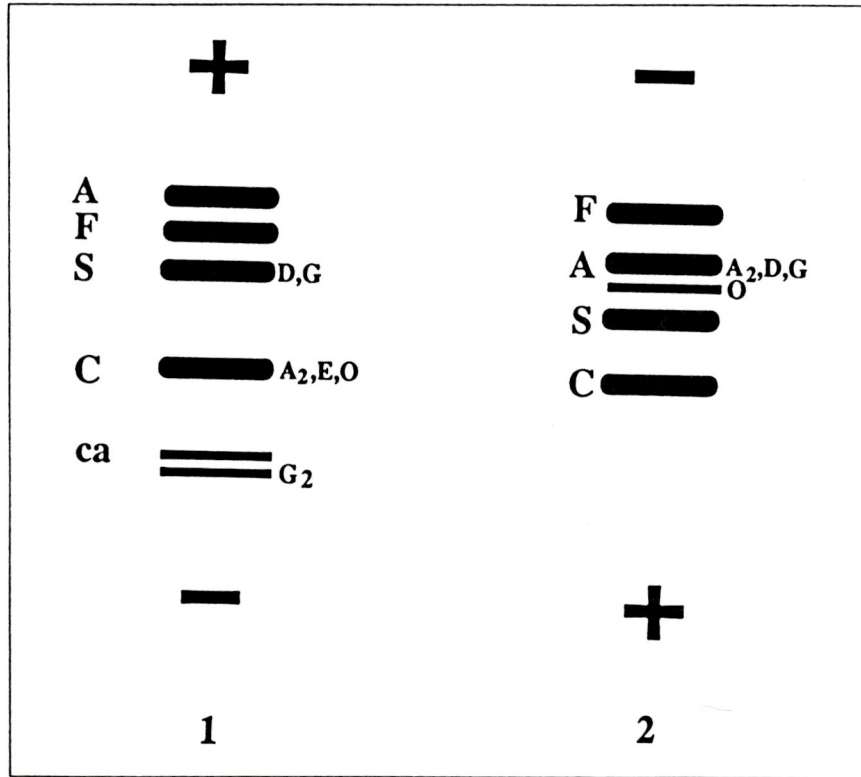

Figure 9-10. Diagrams of the electrophoretic patterns obtained on cellulose acetate at pH 8.6 (1) and in agar at pH 6.0 (2). From Hoffman GC: The sickling disorders. *Lab Med* 21:797, 1990, with permission.

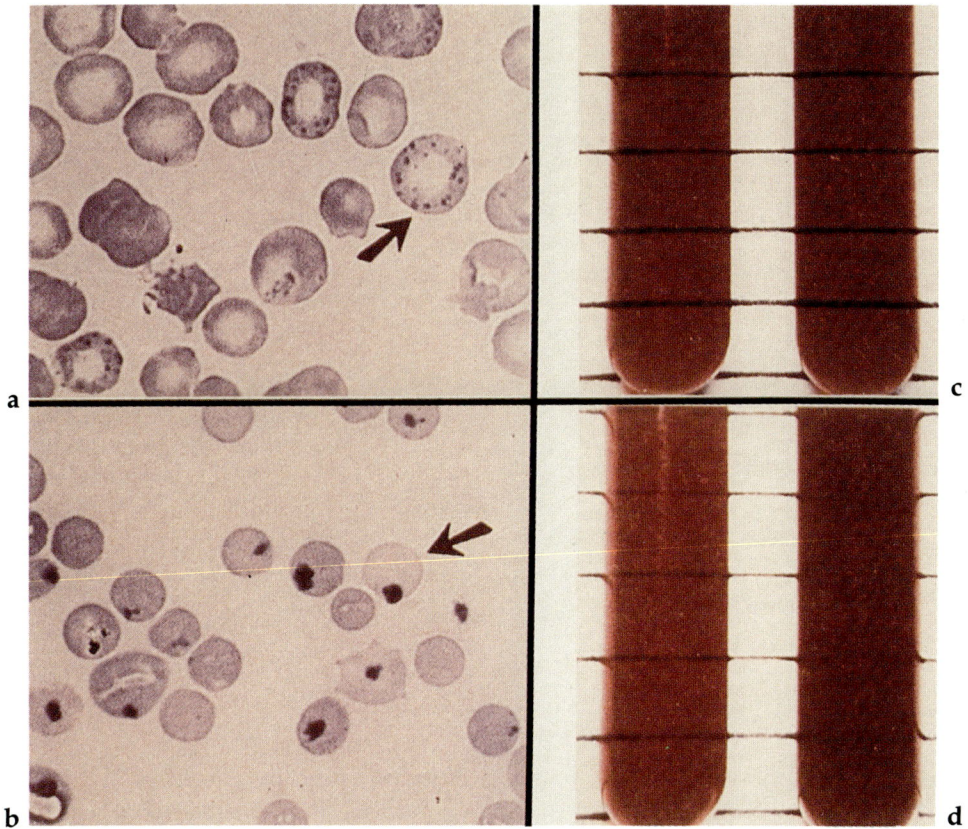

Figure 9-11. Unstable hemoglobins. Peripheral blood smears demonstrating basophilic stippling (a) and Heinz bodies (b). Isopropranol stability test at the beginning (c) and after 15 minutes of incubation (d); after incubation, the black lines in the background have been obliterated by the formation of the precipitate in the sample containing unstable hemoglobin (right tube). From Zinkham WH, Winslow RM: Unstable hemoglobins: Influence of environment on phenotypic expression of a genetic disorder. *Medicine (Baltimore)* 68:309, 1989, with permission.

Heinz bodies decreases RBC deformability and impedes RBC passage through the narrow splenic sinusoids.[105,106]

Heinz body formation appears to be an oxidative process.[103] Three consequences of Heinz body formation have been proposed: an increased propensity for the unstable Hb to oxidize, decreased globin heme affinity, and finally, conversion of the unstable methemoglobin into a hemichrome.[103] The presumed common sequence of events leading to the formation of Heinz bodies is presented in Figure 9-12.[103,107] Heinz bodies are detected by staining blood smears with supravital stains such as methyl violet or brilliant cresyl blue or by performing heat or isopropranol stability testing.[108]

Over 100 unstable Hbs have been identified; some with increased and others with decreased oxygen affinity.[109] Hb H (homotetramer of normal β-chains) and Hb Barts (homotetramer of normal γ-chains), which are subtypes of thalassemias, are also unstable.

Patients with unstable Hb demonstrate a broad spectrum of clinical manifestations ranging from normal Hb levels to severe anemia. Jaundice and splenomegaly may be present. In some cases, high oxygen affinity may cause polycythemia. Peripheral blood smears show aniso- and poikilocytosis, reticulocytosis, and often microcytosis and hypochromia. Bone marrow is usually hypercellular and shows erythroid hyperplasia. In severe cases, Heinz bodies may also be detected in the normoblasts. Clinical manifestations may be aggravated by infections or by administration of certain drugs such as sulfonamides, nitrofurans, aminoquinolines and analgesics.

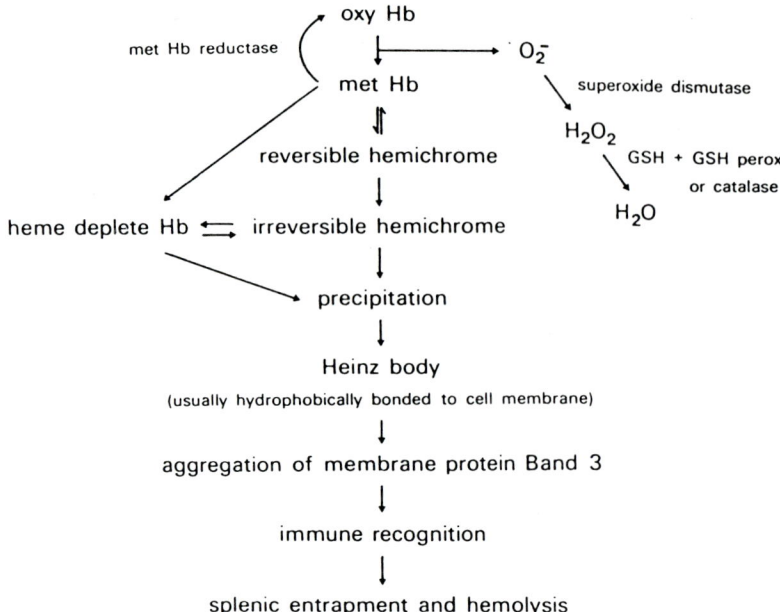

Figure 9-12. Proposed sequence of events in the oxidation and precipitation of unstable hemoglobins as Heinz bodies. From Winterbourne CC: Oxidative denaturation in congenital hemolytic anemias. The unstable hemoglobins. *Semin Hematol* 27:41, 1990, with permission.

Other Hemoglobinopathies

Approximately 250 Hb variants with abnormal α-, β- or γ-chains are known.[109] These variants are rare and generally do not present significant clinical symptoms or abnormal bone marrow morphology.

Erythrocyte Membrane Skeleton Defects

A group of hereditary hemolytic anemias are caused by defects of the red cell membrane skeleton. These anemias are relatively common (affecting approximately 1 in 5000 in Western populations) and are characterized by abnormal shape and decreased deformability of the erythrocytes.[110,111a,111b]

Etiology and Pathogenesis

The principal skeletal structure beneath the lipid bilayer of the erythrocyte membrane is spectrin (Figure 9-13). Spectrin consists of α and β subunits which are bound together as heterodimers arranged in a head-to-head configuration to produce tetramers and higher oligomers.[110] Spectrin is a highly flexible structure, and to a large extent is responsible for the deformability of the red cell membrane. The spectrin subunits bind to oligomers of actin, and this binding is facilitated by protein 4.1. There are a number of proteins, such as tropomyosin, protein 4.9, ankyrin and calmodulin, which bind to the spectrin-actin-protein 4.1 complex. This protein meshwork is responsible for the bioconcave shape of the normal erythrocytes. The erythrocyte membrane contains two major cytoskeleton-associated glycoproteins: protein 3 and glycophorin (Figure 9-13). Defects in spectrin and other membrane-associated skeletal proteins are associated with membrane lipid loss and surface area deficiency, alteration in cation content and permeability, and decreased deformability of the erythrocytes. The affected red cells are not able to pass through the Billroth cords to the splenic sinuses, and stagnate in an environment which has a lower pH and a decreased level of glucose. The erythrocytes lose more surface area and are eventually hemolyzed or removed by the splenic macrophages. The skeletal defects and their associated clinical disorders are summarized in Table 9-9.

Clinical and Pathologic Features

Hereditary disorders of the erythrocyte membrane skeleton include clinicopathologic entities such as spherocytosis, elliptocytosis, acanthocytosis and stomatocytosis.

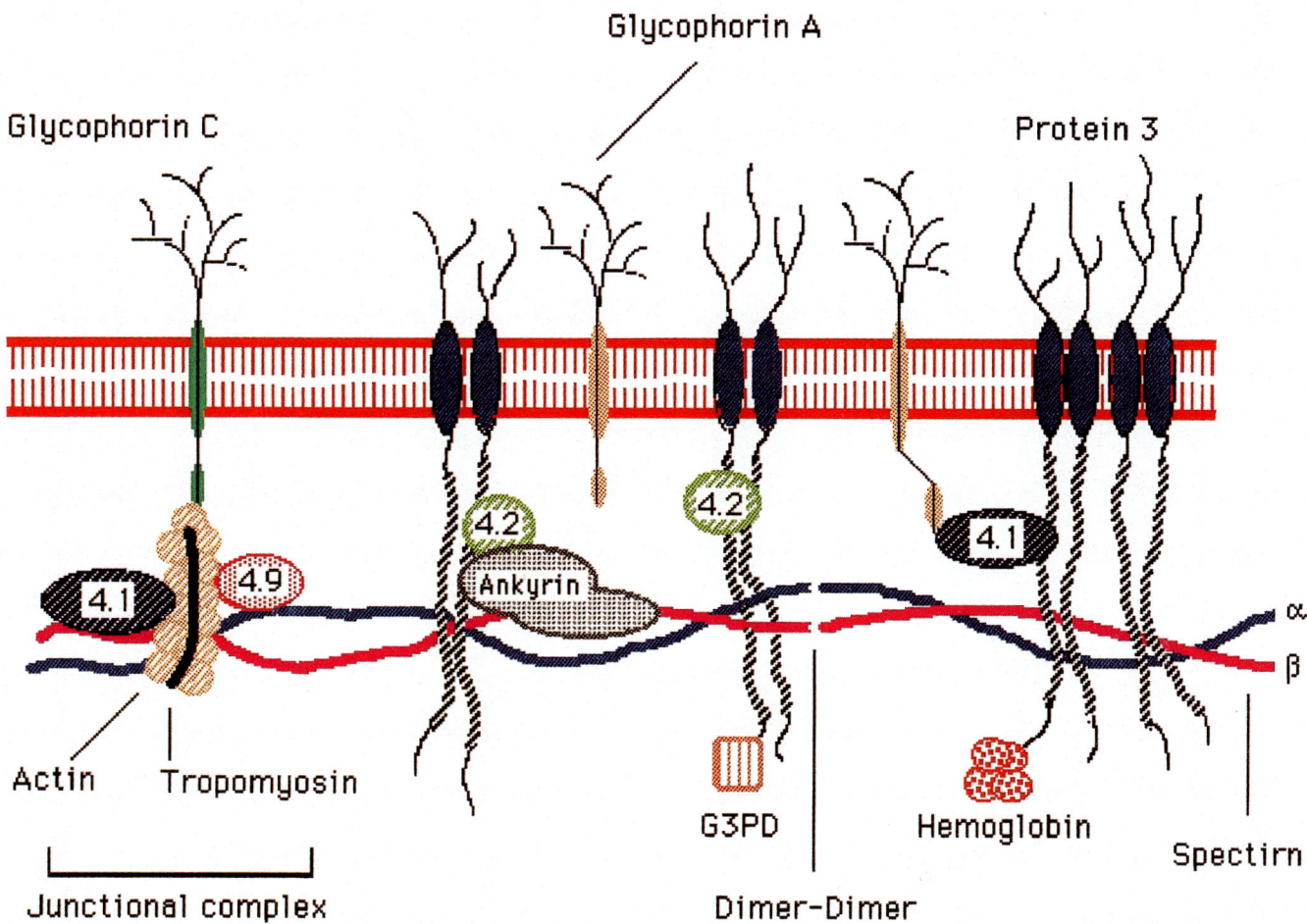

Figure 9-13. Schematic demonstration of the erythrocyte membrane and associated cytoskeleton. Adapted from Davies KA, Lux SE: Hereditary disorders of the red cell membrane skeleton. *Trends Genet* 5:222, 1989.

HEREDITARY SPHEROCYTOSIS: Hereditary spherocytosis (HS) is the most common hereditary hemolytic anemia. The autosomal dominant form is the most frequent one and accounts for approximately 75% of the HS cases. In this form, β-spectrin synthesis is defective.[112] Homozygous recessive HS is caused by deficiency in α-spectrin synthesis and has a more severe clinical course.[112]

Most patients with HS show mild to moderate, well-tolerated anemia, mild jaundice, and a palpable spleen with a family history of anemia involving one or more siblings or parents. However, the clinical manifestation of HS may range from no symptoms to a severe anemia. Peripheral blood examination reveals spherocytosis (Figure 9-14) and increased osmotic fragility of the RBCs. In severe cases, there is an increased reticulocyte count. HS is occasionally complicated by a bone marrow hypoplasia called *aplastic crisis*. The cause of aplastic crisis appears to be human parvovirus B19.[113,114]

HEREDITARY ELLIPTOCYTOSIS: Hereditary elliptocytosis (HE) constitutes a diverse group of hemolytic anemias characterized by the presence of numerous oval, elliptical or elongated erythrocytes (Figure 9-14). HE occurs throughout the world, with a prevalence of about 1 in 2000.[111] A variant known as *stomatocytic elliptocytosis* has been reported in up to 30% of the population of Malayan aborigines in Southeast Asia.[115] The most prominent molecular abnormalities are related to the structure of the spectrin, characterized by either a partial deficiency of spectrin or a mutation in the spectrin gene which results in a defective dimer-dimer association.[116,117] Protein 4.1 and glycophorin C deficiencies are other molecular abnormalities (Table 9-9).

Table 9-9 Disorders of Red Cell Membrane Skeletal Proteins*

Locus	Chromosomal Localization	Clinical Disorder	Protein Abnormality
α-Spectrin	1q22–q25	HS (recessive)	Quantitative spectrin deficiency (30–75% normal); αII domain proteolytic defect
		HE$_c$/HPP	Defective α-subunit self-association; abnormal proteolytic domains, e.g., αI/78, αI/74, αI/65, αI/50a, αI/50b, αI/46, αI/43; partial spectrin deficiency (predominantly blacks)
β-Spectrin	14q23–24.2	HS (dominant)	Quantitative spectrin deficiency (60–85% normal)
			Oxidative changes, impaired binding to 4.1
		HE$_c$	Diminished spectrin tetramer self-association (European)
			Impaired binding to ankyrin, impaired spectrin self-association
Ankyrin	8p11–21.1	HS	Quantitative deficiency (50% normal)
			Unstable ankyrin (and reduced spectrin)
			Reduced spectrin only
Protein 3	17q21–17qter	Acanthocytosis	High molecular weight variant; reduced ankyrin binding (50% normal)
Protein 4.1	1p32–1pter	HE$_c$	Partially or fully deficient (French/North African)
			High/low molecular weight variants (caucasians)
Protein 4.2	?	HE$_s$	Complete deficiency, or small amount of high molecular weight species: decreased ankyrin stability (Japanese)
Protein 4.9	?	Spheroacanthocytosis, neurodegenerative disease	Abnormal phosphorylation
Protein 7	?	Stomatocytosis	Quantitative deficiency; elevated membrane ion permeability; reduced osmotic resistance
Glycophorin C	2q14–2q21	HE$_c$	Weakened 4.1 association with membrane

* Adapted from Davies KA, Lux SE, Hereditary disorders for the red cell membrane skeleton. *Hematol Pathol* 2:1, 1988.
HS: hereditary spherocytosis; HE$_c$: hereditary elliptocytosis, common type.
HPP: hereditary pyropoikilocytosis; HE$_s$: hereditary elliptocytosis, stomatocytic type.

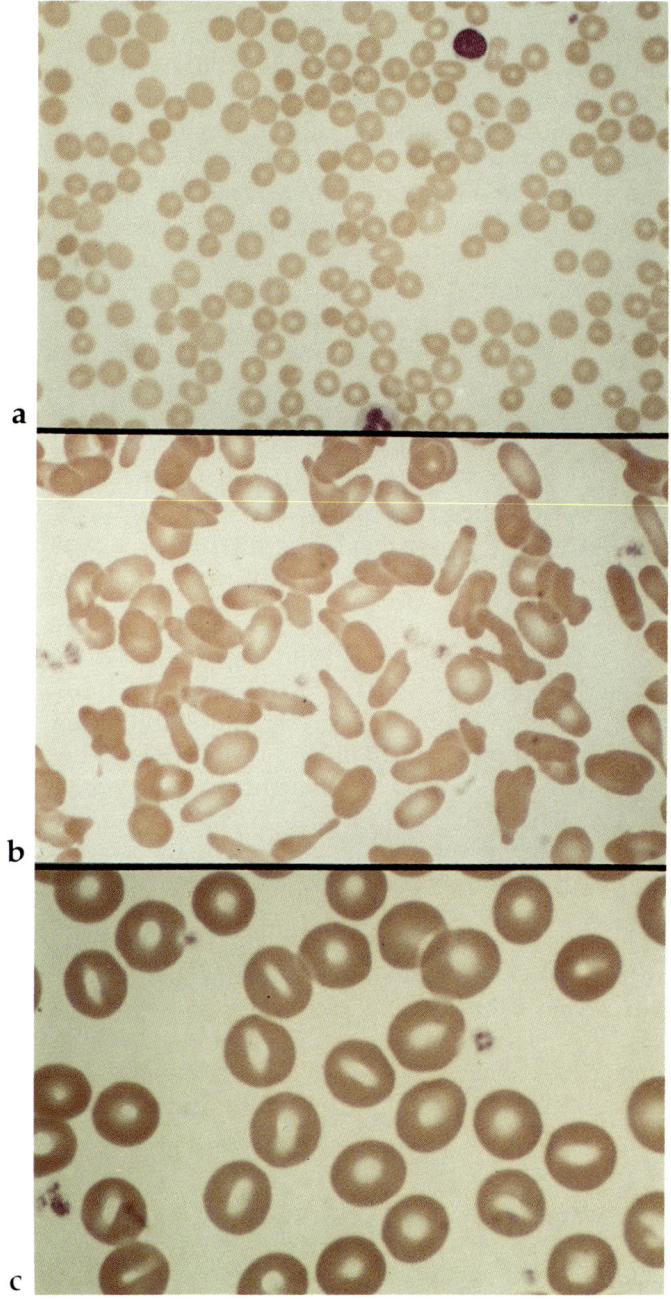

Figure 9-14. Peripheral blood smears demonstrating spherocytosis (a), elliptocytosis (b), and stomatocytosis (c).

HE has been divided into three groups: common HE, spherocytic HE (hereditary ovalocytosis) and stomatocytic HE.

Common HE in most instances is an autosomal dominant disorder, often with mild or no clinical manifestations. However, some cases may demonstrate reticulocytosis, jaundice and splenomegaly. A variant of common HE, hereditary pyropoikilocytosis (HPP), is an autosomal recessive disorder characterized by a severe hemolytic anemia and a marked poikilocytosis and spherocytosis. The affected RBCs are microcytic and show thermal instability.[118] HPP is found predominantly in the black population.[119]

Spherocytic HE is a variant in which the affected erythrocytes are rounder than the typical elliptocytes and show increased osmotic fragility. Occasional spherocytes are also present. The heterozygous HE is associated with a mild clinical course, and the homozygous form demonstrates severe hemolytic anemia.

Stomatocytic HE, or Melanesian ovalocytosis, is characterized by spoon-shaped erythrocytes and is found in up to 30% of certain aboriginal populations of Malaysia and Melanesia.[115] Clinical manifestations are mild or absent.

Other Membrane-Associated Erythrocyte Abnormalities

ACANTHOCYTOSIS: Acanthocytes, or spur cells, are erythrocytes with multiple irregularly shaped and randomly distributed cytoplasmic projections. These abnormal RBCs are seen in severe liver disease, abetalipoproteinemia, amyotrophic chorea, Kell antigen defects (McLeod phenotype), anorexia nervosa, cystic fibrosis and hypothyroidism.[120] A suggested molecular mechanism for acanthocytosis in severe liver disease is cholesterol accumulation in the outer layer of the membrane, causing overexpansion of the surface area of the outer half relative to the inner half of the erythrocyte membrane bilayer.[121-123] In abetalipoproteinemia, there is an increase in the proportion of sphingomyelin in the outer half of the membrane bilayer, leading to expansion of the outer surface and, persumably, to irregular projections.[120,124]

Acanthocytosis should be differentiated from echinocytosis (burr cells). Echinocytes are RBCs with short, blunt, evenly distributed projections. Several conditions are associated with echinocytosis such as uremia, hypomagnesemia and hypophosphatemia. Echnincytosis has also been noted in athletes after heavy physical exercise.[120] Echinocytosis is a common laboratory artifact caused by blood storage, contact with glass or elevated pH.[120,125]

STOMATOCYTOSIS: Stomatocytes are cup- or bowl-shaped erythrocytes which appear in blood smears as cells with a wide transverse slit or stoma (an artifact due to folding of the RBCs in the blood-smearing process)(Figure 9-14). Stomatocytosis may be hereditary or acquired.

In hereditary stomatocytosis (hereditary hydrocytosis) the primary lesion appears to be deficiency of Protein 7 (Table 9-9). This disorder is associated with an increase in erythrocyte membrane permeability to sodium, leading to increased intracellular sodium and water contents and red cell swelling.[126] In this condition, osmotic fragility is increased and cellular deformability is decreased. Hereditary stomatocytosis in most instances is an autosomal dominant disorder.

Acquired stomatocytosis has been described in alcoholism, malignancies, hepatobiliary diseases and cardiovascular disorders. The mechanism of the formation of stomatocytes in the acquired form is not known, but it has been shown that expansion of the inner half of the erythrocyte membrane bilayer may change the normal red cells to stomatocytes in vitro.[127]

Hemolytic Anemias Secondary to Erythrocyte Enzyme Abnormalities

Numerous enzymes are involved in erythrocyte metabolic activities including the Embden-Meyerhof glycolytic pathway, the Rapoport-Luebering shunt, the pentose phosphate pathway, and glutathione synthesis and metabolism. These metabolic activities maintain the functional and structural integrity of the RBCs, such as control of the ATPase-dependent cation pump, membrane flexibility and the erythrocyte shape. Abnormal levels of red cell enzymes may lead to a hemolytic anemia (Table 9-10). These hemolytic anemias are characteristically associated with an unremarkable red cell morphology and therefore are known as *hereditary nonspherocytic hemolytic anemias*.[128-130] The two most prominent red cell enzyme deficiencies, glucose-6-phosphatase dehydrogenase deficiency and pyruvate kinase deficiency, are briefly discussed below.

Glucose-6-Phosphatase Dehydrogenase Deficiency

Glucose-6-phosphatase dehydrogenase (G-6-PD) deficiency results from a variety of mutations in the G-6-PD gene located on the X chromosome. Over 350 variants of this enzyme deficiency have been described.[130-134] The A-type G-6-PD is the most common abnormal variant among black populations of all countries, and the G-6-PD Mediterranean is the most frequent abnormal type among white populations of all countries.[132] The G-6-PD deficiency affects about 10% of American blacks and West Africans, 15–45% of Kurds and 3–35% of Sardinians.[133,134] The G-6-PD deficiency is more severe in the Mediterranean type than

Table 9-10 Enzyme Abnormalities that may lead to Hematologic Disorders

Enzyme	Additional Clinical Features	Inheritance	Chromosome
Hexokinase	—	AR	10q22
Glucose phosphate isomerase	—	AR	19q13.1
Phosphofructokinase	Muscle glycogen storage disease	AR	Muscle: 1q Liver: 21q22.3 Platelet: 10p
Aldolase	Liver glycogen storage disease	AR	16q22-q24
Triosephosphate isomerase	Neuromascular disease	AR	12p13
Phosphoglycerate kinase	Myoglobinuria, behavioral Disturbances	SL	Xp13
Pyruvate kinase	—	AR	1q21
Glucose-6-phosphate dehydrogenase	Drug- and infection-induced hemolysis, favism	SL	Xq25
Diphosphoglycerate	Polycythemia	AR	?
Glutathione reductase	Drug- and infection-induced hemolysis, favism		8p21.1
γ-glutamylcysteine synthetase	Drug- and infection-induced hemolysis, spinocerebellar lesions	AR	?
Glutathione synthetase	Drug- and infection-induced hemolysis, neurologic lesions	AR	?
Adenylate kinase	—	AR	9p
5'-nucleotidase	? Mental retardation	AR	6q14-q21
Adenosine diaminase	—	AD	20q13

AR: Autosomal recessive; AD: Autosomal dominant; SL: Sex-linked

in the G-6-PD A-type. The mechanism of hemolysis in this condition is not well understood; however, the generation of hydrogen peroxide may play a role in the hemolytic process.[135] G-6-PD deficiency is associated with a failure to generate NADPH and low levels of reduced glutathione, and consequently with increased vulnerability of the Hb to oxygen and certain oxidant drugs, leading to the formation of denatured Hb (Heinz bodies).[136,137]

The vast majority of G-6-PD–deficient patients do not demonstrate hematologic abnormalities if they are not suffering from viral or bacterial infections or are not receiving medication.[138-140] Certain drugs (Table 9-11), fava beans (particularly in patients with the Mediterranean type) and infections may cause moderate to severe hemolysis. Reticulocytes and younger RBCs have relatively higher enzyme activity than older erythrocytes and therefore are more resistant to hemolysis. The hemolytic episode stimulates erythropoiesis and leads to bone marrow erythroid hyperplasia and peripheral blood reticulocytosis.

Pyruvate Kinase Deficiency

Pyruvate kinase (PK) deficiency is an autosomal recessive disorder with clinical manifestations of hemolytic anemia in homozygotes or double heterozygotes.[129,130] PK is involved in the conversion of phosphoenolpyruvate to pyruvate and the generation of ATP in the Embden-Meyerhof pathway.

Table 9-11 Drugs and Chemicals Reported to Cause Hemolysis in G-6-PD–deficient Patients*

Acetanilid	Pamaquine
Acetylphenylhydrazine	Pentaquine
Aspirin, high dose	Phenacetin
Aminosalicylates†	Phenasopyridine
Chloroqine†	Primaquine
Chloramphenicol†	Probenecid
Dimercaprol	Sulfacetamide
Doxorubicin	Sulfafurazole
Furanzolidone	Sulfamethazole
Methylene blue	Sulfanilamide
Nalidixic acid	Sulfapyridine
Naphthalene	Tuloidine blue
Neoarsphenamine	Trinitrotoluene
Nitrofurantoin	Vitamine K (water-soluble
Nitrofurazone	analogs)

* Refs. 138–140.
† Do not cause hemolysis in blacks.

Clinical manifestations of PK deficiency are the result of chronic hemolysis, which varies considerably from case to case. The red cell morphology is usually unremarkable, and there is some degree of reticulocytosis. In a group of PK-deficient patients studied by Hirono and associates,[141] the mean Hb concentration was 8.7 g/dl, the mean reticulocyte count was 9.4% and over 80% of the patients had hepatosplenomegaly.

IMMUNE RELATED HEMOLYTIC ANEMIAS

Autoimmune Hemolytic Anemia

Autoimmune hemolytic anemia (AIHA) is the result of RBC destruction due to autoantibody production. AIHA is characterized by (1) evidence of autoimmunity against erythrocytes (2) shortened in vivo red cell survival and (3) evidence of bone marrow erythroid hyperplasia.[142]

Etiology and Pathogenesis

The reasons for autoimmune disorders are not completely understood. Several etiologic factors have been proposed, such as altered self-antigen, abnormalities in antigen presentation, B-cell hyperactivity and aberrations in suppressor T-cell number and function.[142-146] One or a combination of these immunologic changes in association with genetic and environmental factors (drugs, infections, malignancies) lead to an autoimmune disorder (Table 9-12).

In AIHA, red cell destruction is either extravascular or intravascular. In extravascular hemolysis the antibody-coated red cells are damaged or removed by the mononuclear phagocytic system (macrophages). Intravascular hemolysis is a complement-induced hemolysis within the vascular space, without involvement of the macrophages.

EXTRAVASCULAR HEMOLYSIS: In extravascular hemolysis, the IgG-coated red cells adhere to the Fc receptors of macrophages and are damaged either by erythrophagocytosis or by lysosomal enzymes released during antibody-dependent cellular cytotoxicity (ADDC). Erythrophagocytosis is either complete or incomplete. Incomplete erythrophagocytosis leads to the formation of spherocytes. The efficacy of red cell-macrophage interaction depends on a number of factors such as the Ig class and subclass, the antibody concentration bound to RBCs, the thermal range of the antibody and the concentration of the Fc receptors on the macrophages.[142] Infection, probably due to the action of γ-interferon, activates macrophages and leads to increased affinity of Fc receptors.[147] IgG1 and IgG3 (warm-reactive antibodies) are the most predominant Ig subtypes involved in macrophage-induced autoimmune hemolysis. Approximately 2–3% of patients with severe autoimmune hemolysis have erythrocytes predominantly coated with IgA.[146,148,149] The erythrocyte-bound IgA may also induce macrophage activation and erythrophagocytosis. The C3b-coated erythrocytes can also bind to macrophages and undergo complete phagocytosis. Splenic macrophages are the most efficient effector cells and play a major role in extravascular RBC destruction in autoimmune conditions. Hepatic macrophages are relatively poor mediators of extravascular hemolysis.[146]

INTRAVASCULAR HEMOLYSIS: In the majority of patients with intravascular hemolysis, the autoantibody is of the IgM class (cold-reactive antibodies). The IgM autoantibodies at low temperature activate the complement cascade and lead to the binding of C8 and C9 to the erythrocyte membrane, causing small holes in the RBC membrane and consequently hemolysis.

Table 9-12 Distribution of Autoimmune Hemolysis (AIH) Based on Disease Association

Type	Approximate Incidence of AIH (%)			
	Warm	Cold	Mixed	Total
Idiopathic	24	15	4	43
Secondary to other diseases				
Lymphoid malignancies	9	4	2	15
Other malignancies	4	2	1	7
Infections	1	7	<1	8
Connective tissue disorders	2	1	2	5
Others	4	2	1	7
Drug-related	15	0	<1	15

* Adapted from Sokol RJ, Hewitt S, Stamps BK: Autoimmune hemolysis: A critical review. CRC Crit Rev Oncol Hematol 4: 125, 1985.

Clinical and Pathologic Features

AIHA WITH WARM-REACTING ANTIBODIES: This type of AIHA anemia occurs at any age, but the majority of patients are over age 40 and the peak incidence of the disease occurs at around age 70. A considerable proportion of the cases are idiopathic; others are associated with a wide variety of disorders such as connective tissue diseases, lymphoproliferative disorders and other malignancies. Most drug-related immune hemolytic anemias are also caused by warm-reacting antibodies (Table 9-12).

Clinical features are highly variable, ranging from a very mild chronic anemia with no clinical symptoms to a severe acute form with jaundice, splenomegaly and hepatomegaly. Most cases have a mild clinical course.

Peripheral blood examination shows various degrees of anisopoikilocytosis with reticulocytosis (sometimes over 30%), spherocytosis and the presence of nucleated red cells (Figure 9-15). In severe cases, peripheral blood monocytes may occasionally show erythrophagocytosis. Neutrophil granulocytosis and thrombocytosis may occur, and some severe cases may show a leukoerythroblastic blood picture. Serum bilirubin is elevated. The bone marrow shows erythroid hyperplasia.

Demonstration of IgG and/or complement bound to the patient's erythrocytes is the diagnostic test for AIHA. The use of a polyclonal antiglobulin (Coombs') reagent, which contains antibodies against IgG and complement components, is a routine screening procedure. In the direct antiglobulin test (DAGT), or direct Coombs' test, the patient's RBCs are examined for the presence of bound Ig and/or complement. In the indirect antiglobulin test, the patient's serum is screened for the presence of autoantibodies. Monospecific antisera are used for further characterization of the autoantibody and the nature of the hemolytic process. The combined IgG and complement (C3) is the most frequent red cell binding pattern in warm-reacting AIHA and accounts for about 50% of the cases. In over 70% of the cases, the autoantibodies are against the Rh complex.[148,150]

AIHA WITH COLD-REACTING ANTIBODIES (CRYOPATHIC HEMOLYTIC SYNDROMES): Cryopathic hemolytic syndromes are caused by autoantibodies which have enhanced activity below 37°C and usually below 20°C. These syndromes account for about 30% of AIHA and in 50% of the cases are idiopathic (Table 9-12). Two major syndromes are recognized in this group: cold hemagglutinin disease and paroxysmal cold hemoglobinuria.

Cold hemagglutinin disease (CHAD) is characterized by a positive DAGT due to the presence of complement (C3d and C4d) and high-titer anti-RBC antibodies with maximum erythrocyte agglutination at 0–5°C. In cold weather, the cold-reacting antibodies bind to the erythrocytes and mediate complement fixation with cooler peripheral circulation, leading to hemolysis. Hemolysis is mainly intravascular, resulting a mild to moderate anemia with hemoglobinuria and hemosiderinuria. Acrocyanosis and splenomeg-

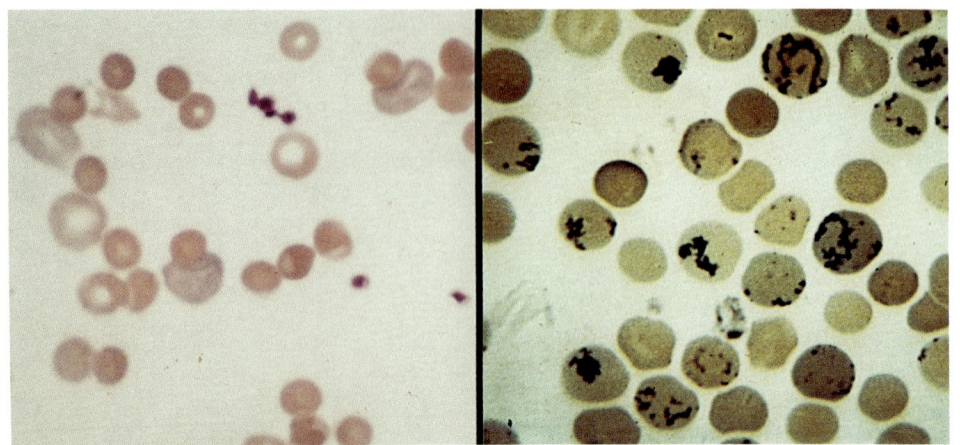

Figure 9-15. Peripheral blood smears from a patient with autoimmune hemolytic anemia demonstrating (a) spherocytes and polychromatophilic red cells (Wright stain) and (b) reticulocytosis (reticulin stain).

aly may be present. CHAD occasionally develops as a self-limiting complication of infections with *Mycoplasma pneumoniae* and Epstein-Barr virus, lasting for 1 to 3 weeks.[148] In such cases, the cold agglutinins are polyclonal IgM antibodies, often with anti-I or anti-i reactivity. A chronic form of CHAD is associated with lymphoproliferative disorders and is characterized by a monoclonal IgMk with anti-I specificity. This form may show bone marrow lymphoplasmacytosis or lymphoma.

Cold agglutinins are able to agglutinate saline-suspended RBCs at low temperature, particularly at 0–5° C. The agglutination is a reversible process and disappears by warming. In CHAD the serum titers are commonly 1/10,000 or higher (normal, 1/32 or less).

Paroxysmal cold hemoglobinuria (PCH) is a rare form of AIHA which was originally characterized by episodes of massive intravascular hemolysis and hemoglobinuria initiated by exposure to cold. However, PCH in recent years has been less severe, and many affected children show only one self-limited hemolytic attack with a favorable prognosis. PCH may be secondary to a number of viral infections (such as measles, chickenpox, mumps and influenza) or congenital and tertiary syphilis.[151-153] However, hemolysis associated with nonsyphlitic forms is often transient and unrelated to cold exposure.[154] Clinical features include muscle pains, headache, vomiting, diarrhea, fever, urticaria and acrocyanosis. The antibody responsible for the hemolysis is of the IgG class (usually with anti-P specificity) and is able to bind complement components at low temperature.

Other Immune Related Hemolytic Anemias

Hemolytic Transfusion Reactions

Hemolytic transfusion reactions occur when the recipient's plasma contains antibody against the transfused RBCs. In rare instances, it also occurs when plasma with a high titer of antibody is transfused to a patient whose erythrocytes bear the relevant antigen.

Transfusion reactions may occur during or immediately after transfusion. These reactions are typically due to ABO incompatibility and to anti-A or anti-B reactivity with RBCs bearing A or B antigens, respectively. Rapid intravascular hemolysis leads to hemoglobinemia, hemoglobinuria and jaundice, and may be complicated by disseminated intravascular coagulopathy (DIC) and renal failure. Chest pain, dyspnea, hypotension, rigors, fever, vomiting and diarrhea are among the initial clinical features.

Transfusion reactions may occur in a previously immunized patient 6–8 days after transfusion (delayed reactions). Rh incompatibility is a classical example of delayed transfusion reactions. In these reactions RBC destruction is predominantly extravascular, with a positive DAGT, causing anemia, fever, jaundice and often spherocytosis.

Hemolytic Disease of the Newborn

Hemolytic disease of the newborn is the result of interaction of maternal IgG (crossed placenta) and incompatible fetal erythrocytes in the fetal circulation. ABO and Rh incompatibilities are the first and second most common causes, respectively. The ABO type is less severe and occurs predominantly in group A or B infants and group O mothers. Rh-related hemolysis is more severe and may lead to intrauterine death or a hydropic fetus.

Drug-Induced Immune Hemolytic Anemia

Certain drugs may initiate an immunologically mediated erythrocyte destruction. Three possible mechanisms have been suggested for drug-induced immune hemolysis[142,155] (Figure 9-16).

1. The drug (or one of its metabolites) binds to the red cell membrane (carrier) and acts as a hapten to generate antibodies. The antibody-coated red cells are then subject to extravascular clearance by the mononuclear phagocytic system. Penicillin and other cephalosporins are examples.

2. A drug-antibody complex formed in plasma leads to complement activation at the erythrocyte surface and, consequently, RBC destruction. Examples are quinine, phenacetin, para-aminosalicylic acid and some sulfonamides. This mechanism has been challenged by recent studies demonstrating that, for example, in quinine-induced antibody production, the antibody recognizes the drug only in combination with a particular cell membrane structure.[156,157]

3. Certain drugs, such as α-methyldopa, initiate the formation of autoantibodies against RBCs. Approximately 10–35% of patients on long-term α-methyldopa therapy develop IgG anti-red cell autoantibodies, though less than 1% develop overt hemolytic anemia.[155,158] These antibodies are considered true autoantibodies, and their presence is not dependent on the presence of the drug. A mechanism suggested by Kirtland and associates is that production of anti-erythrocyte autoantibodies is due to the reduced suppression of autoreactive lymphocytes.[159] These investigators demonstrated that methyldopa inhibits activation and/or maturation of the suppressor T lymphocytes. Another mechanism, suggested by Owens et al., is based on the interaction of drug metabolites with RBC peptides and, thus, with the formation of new autoantigens.[160] The DAGT and the indirect antiglobulin test are usually positive in this condition.

NONIMMUNE ACQUIRED HEMOLYTIC ANEMIAS

Hemolysis may occur in a variety of nonimmune acquired conditions, such as damage to the RBCs by mechanical trauma and heat, drugs and other chemicals, infection and hypersplenism, and acquired dyserythropoiesis.

Hemolysis Induced by Mechanical Trauma and Heat

Traumatic injury to the erythrocytes may cause RBC fragmentation and hemolysis. RBC fragmentation has been observed in patients with cardiac valve prostheses (particularly aortic valves) and aortic valve disease, DIC, thrombotic thrombocytopenic purpura, malignant hypertension, generalized vasculitis and carcinomatosis. Traumatic rupture of the RBC and hemoglobinuria have been reported soon after walking or running long distances, bongo-drumming or karate exercises. Thermal damage is often associated with spherocytosis and generation of microvesicles.

Hemolysis Caused by Drugs and other Chemicals

As discussed earlier, certain oxidant drugs may cause hemolysis in G-6-PD-deficient patients (see Table 9–11). The same drugs may also cause oxidative hemolysis in patients with renal failure or in normal persons if given in very high doses. Drug-induced hemolysis unrelated to enzyme deficiencies is noted in various conditions such as exposure to arsenic hydride or nitrobenzene derivatives, copper, certain nitrites (used as recreational drugs by homosexuals), water-soluble vitamin K analogues and naphthalene.

Acute alcoholism may be associated with stomatocytosis and a transient hemolytic episode.[161] Patients with alcohol-induced fatty liver may develop a syndrome (Zieve's syndrome) characterized by episodes of hypercholesterolemia and hypertriglyceridemia with hemolysis, upper abdominal pain and fever.[162] Alcoholic cirrhosis is sometimes associated with acanthocytic hemolytic anemia.[163] Bone marrow may show erythroid hyperplasia with vacuolated normoblasts (Figure 9-17).

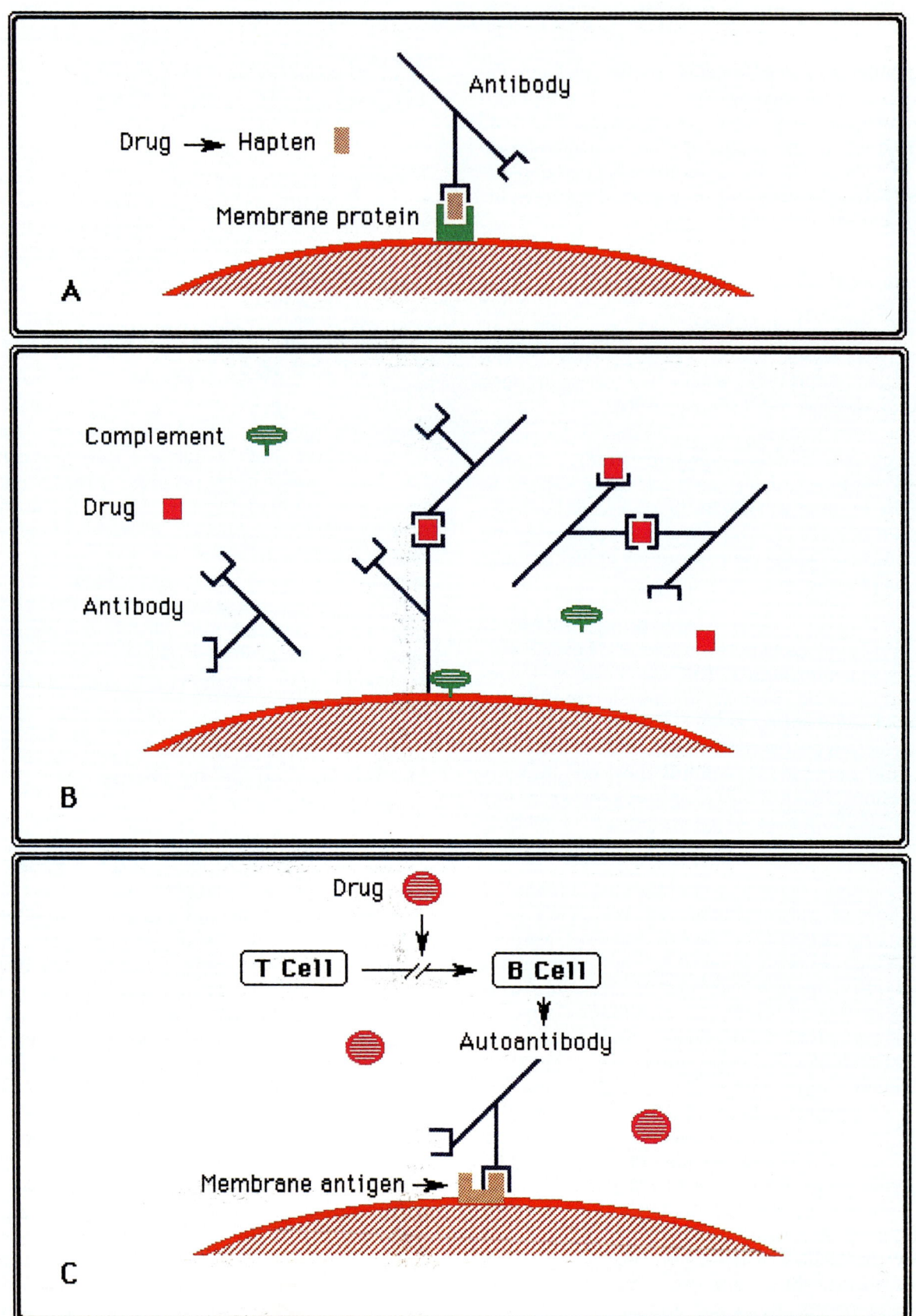

Figure 9-16. Possible mechanisms of drug-induced immune hemolytic anemia. (A) Drug as hapten; (B) drug–antibody complex formation; (C) inhibition of suppressor T cells leading to production of autoantibodies.

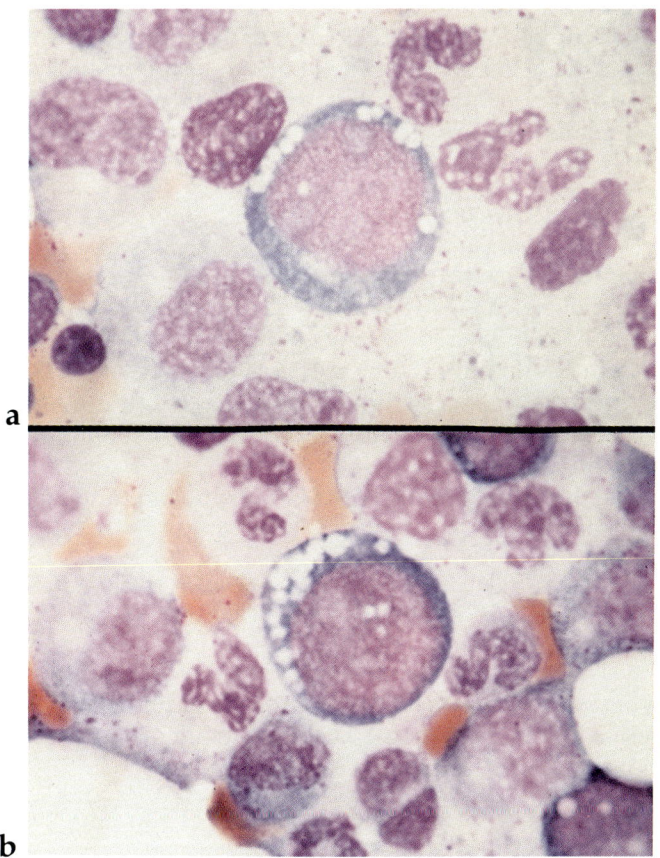

Figure 9-17. Bone marrow smears demonstrating vacuolated normoblasts in alcoholic liver disease (a) and copper deficiency (b).

Venoms of certain species of snakes, bees, spiders and wasps may cause hemolysis, probably due to the direct lytic effects of their enzymes.[164]

Hemolysis Caused by Infections

In general, infections to some extent may cause depression of erythropoiesis. They may also initiate or provoke hemolytic episodes in patients suffering from red cell enzyme deficiencies or hemoglobinopathies, presumably due to the generation of oxidant substances. Certain microorganisms may damage erythrocyte membrane and cause hemolysis by the release of substances such as phospholipases (*Clostridium perfringens*) and hemolysins (*Streptococcus pyogenes*). Activation of macrophages in some viral infections is associated with extensive erythrophagocytosis and anemia. Acute malaria, particularly due to *Plasmodium falciparum*, may cause hemolysis.

Hypersplenism

One of the main functional roles of the spleen is to serve as a filter by removing foreign materials, cell debris and defective blood cells.[165] This is accomplished by a slow, continuous flow of about 5–10% of the splenic blood supply through the nonendothelialized, macrophage-containing spaces present in the red pulp, functioning as a filter bed.[166] The bulk of the blood supply travels rapidly through the regular endothelialized vessels without filtration. The slow passage of the blood through the nonendothelial spaces of the red pulp puts the blood content in close contact with the macrophages and facilitates the removal of defective cells, antibody- and/or complement-coated cells and foreign materials by the macrophages. In splenomegaly, the proportion of the blood channeled through the red pulp and the filter bed increases, causing an inappropriate sequestration of both normal and abnormal blood cells, particularly RBCs, because of their limited, self-sufficient metabolic resources.[167,168] The increase in splenic sequestration is more pronounced when the splenomegaly is caused by congestion than by an infiltrative process (e.g., leukemia, myeloid metaplasia, amyloidosis).

Acquired Dyserythropoiesis

In many acquired dyserythropoietic anemias such as deficiency anemias, anemia of chronic diseases, sideroblastic anemias, and anemias associated with myeloproliferative disorders and leukemias, there is a mild to moderate reduction in the erythrocyte life span. However, in these conditions the primary cause of anemia is impaired bone marrow function and not hemolysis. These conditions are discussed elsewhere in this chapter and in Chapters 5 and 6.

Anemia Caused by Acute Blood Loss

The clinical manifestations of hemorrhage depend on the volume and speed of blood loss. A rapid, massive hemorrhage $\geq 40\%$ of the total blood volume causes cardiovascular collapse and shock, which may lead to death. When the blood loss is gradual, sufficient restoration of plasma volume can occur to prevent the cardiovascular collapse, even in extensive hemorrhages. It takes 20 to 60 hours to restore a sudden loss of 20% of the total blood volume. The restoration of plasma is primarily from the extravascular resources.[169] The bone marrow response to blood loss is a gradual process. The proliferating erythroid precursor cells take 2 to 5 days for complete maturation and delivery to the circulation. The bone marrow response is evidenced by erythroid hyperplasia and a drop in the M:E ratio, and by an increase in the peripheral blood reticulocyte count. The marrow response reaches its full extent after 8 to 10 days.

OTHER TYPES OF ANEMIA

Deficiency Anemias Other Than Vitamin B_{12} and Folate Deficiencies

Copper Deficiency

This has been described in malnourished children and in patients receiving parenteral alimentation. Excessive and chronic administration of zinc may also cause copper deficiency.[170] Copper deficiency is associated with microcytic anemia and neutropenia. The erythroid precursors in the bone marrow are often vacuolated (Figure 9-17).

Vitamin Deficiencies

Vitamin deficiencies such as vitamin A and vitamin B6 deficiencies may lead to a microcytic hypochromic anemia. Riboflavin deficiency may cause pure red cell aplasia.[171] Vitamin C deficiency is usually normocytic and normochromic, and is associated with a moderate reticulocytosis. Vitamin E deficiency, a common deficiency in patients with cystic fibrosis, is usually associated with abnormal RBC morphology and hemolysis.[172]

Anemia of Protein Deficiency (Kwashiorkor)

This anemia is usually normochromic and normocytic, with some anisopoikilocytosis and reticulocytopenia. The bone marrow is normocellular or slightly hypocellular, with an elevated M:E ratio.

Anemia of Chronic Disorders

Anemia of chronic disorders is characterized by a modest shortening of the erythrocyte life span, a low serum iron and iron-binding capacity, an increased bone marrow iron store and relatively ineffective erythropoiesis. The mechanism(s) of anemia in chronic disorders is not well understood, but it has been suggested that the excessive macrophage sequestration of iron and iron-binding protein, increased red cell destruction in the spleen and decreased erythropoietin production are the major contributing pathophysiologic factors.[173,174]

Bone marrow examination reveals a normo- to moderately hypocellular marrow with an M:E ratio of 3–4:1 and no evidence of erythroid hyperplasia. Stainable iron is present in the machrophages and in a high proportion of the nucleated red cells (sideroblasts).

Anemia of Endocrine Disorders

The endocrine glands, such as the pituitary, the thyroid and adrenal glands, and the gonads, may influence the production of erythropoietin, may directly stimulate erythroid progenitor cells, or may play a role in the synthesis of Hb and other red cell biochemical components. In most endocrine disorders, anemia is normocytic and normochromic. However, in hypothyroidism, anemia is often microcytic and sometimes macrocytic due to the associated iron deficiency or vitamin B_{12}/folate deficiencies, respectively.

Anemia of Chronic Renal Failure

Anemia in chronic renal failure is caused by a complex multifactorial process. Decreased erythropoietin production, the suppressive effects of uremia and other uremic toxins on erythropoiesis, plasma inhibitors of heme synthesis and erythroid progenitor cell proliferation, and erythropoietic unresponsiveness are among the possible mechanisms of anemia in patients with chronic renal failure.[175-178] The anemia is normocytic and normochromic, with a normal or decreased number of reticulocytes. Echinocytes or burr cells may be present. The bone marrow is normo- to hypocellular and may show severe erythroid hypoplasia.[179]

Anemia Associated with Marrow Infiltration (Myelophthisic Anemia)

The most common cause of marrow infiltration is a metastatic neoplasm, and the most frequent sources of marrow metastases are carcinomas of the lung, breast and prostate. Other causes of marrow infiltration are hematopoietic malignancies, marrow fibrosis, lipid storage diseases and inflammatory responses such as granulomas. The infiltrative process disrupts the bone marrow's microenvironment and reduces hematopoietic activities by replacement of the hematopoietic cells and/or release of inhibitory mediators. Myelophthisic anemia is often associated with anisocytosis and poikilocytosis, presence of the teardrop RBCs and a leukoerythroblastic peripheral blood picture. Bone marrow sections are the most reliable source for the definitive diagnosis of marrow infiltration.

References

1. Wickramasinghe SN: *Blood and Bone Marrow*. London, Churchill Livingstone, 1986, p 5.
2. Erslev AJ: Erythrocyte disorders: Classification and manifestations, in Williams WJ, Beutler E, Erslev AJ, et al (eds), *Hematology*, ed 4. New York, McGraw-Hill, 1990, p 423.
3. Tsukada T, Koike T, Koike R, et al: Epidemic of aplastic crisis in patients with hereditary spherocytosis in Japan. *Lancet* 1:1401, 1985.
4. Takahishi M, Koike T, Moryama Y, et al: Inhibition of erythropoiesis by human parvovirus-containing serum from a patient with hereditary spherocytosis in aplastic crisis. *Scand J Haematol* 37:118, 1986.
5. Pattison JR, Jones SE, Hadgson J, et al: Parvovirus infections and hypoplastic crisis in sickle cell anemia. *Lancet* 1:664, 1981.
6. Rao KRP, Patel AR, Anderson MJ, et al: Infection with parvovirus-like virus and aplastic crisis in chronic hemolytic anemia. *Ann Intern Med* 98:930, 1983.
7. Van Horn DK, Mortimer PP, Young N, et al: Human parvovirus associated red cell aplasia in the absence of underlying hemolytic anemia. *Am J Pediatr Hematol Oncol* 8:235, 1986.
8. Duncan JR, Cappellini MD, Anderson MJ, et al: Aplastic crisis due to parvovirus infection in pyruvate kinase deficiency. *Lancet* 2:14, 1983.
9. Young N: Hematologic and hematopoietic consequences of B19 parvovirus infection. *Semin Hematol* 25:159, 1988.
10. Dessypris EN, Krantz SB, Roloff JS, et al: Mode of action of Ig inhibitor of erythropoiesis in transient erythroblastopenia of childhood. *Blood* 59:114, 1982.
11. MacCulloch D, Jackson JM, Venerys J: Drug induced red cell aplasia. *Br Med J* 4:163, 1974.
12. Itoh K, Wong P, Asai T, et al: Pure red cell aplasia induced by alpha-methyldopa. *Am J Med* 84:1088, 1988.
13. Nathan DG, Clarke BJ, Hillman DG, et al: Erythroid precursors in congenital hypoplastic (Diamond-Blackfan) anemia. *J Clin Invest* 61:489, 1978.
14. Lipton JM, Kudisch M, Gross R, et al: Defective erythroid progenitor differentiation system in congenital hypoplastic (Diamond-Blackfan) anemia. *Blood* 67:962, 1986.
15. Tiber C, Casimir M, Nogeir B, et al: Thymoma with pure red cell aplasia and hemolytic anemia. *South Med J* 74:1164, 1981.
16. Clark DA, Dessypris EN, Lrantz SB: Studies on red cell aplasia. XI. Results of immunosuppressive treatment of 37 patients. *Blood* 63:277, 1984.
17. Cassileth PA, Myers AR: Erythroid aplasia in systemic lupus erythematosus. *Am J Med* 55:706, 1973.
18. Dessypris EN, Baer MR, Sergent GS, et al: Rheumatoid arthritis and pure red cell aplasia. *Ann Intern Med* 44:590, 1984.
19. Yoo D, Pierce LE, Lessin L: Acquired pure red cell

aplasia associated with chronic lymphocytic leukemia. *Cancer* 51:844, 1983.
20. Akard LP, Brandt J, Lu L, et al: Chronic T cell lymphoproliferative disorders and pure red cell aplasia. *Am J Med* 83:1069, 1987.
21. Krantz SB, Moore WH, Zaentz SD: Studies on red cell aplasia. V. Presence of erythroblast cytotoxicity in γG globin fraction of plasma. *J Clin Invest* 52:324, 1973.
22. Krantz SB, Dessypris EN: Pure red cell aplasia, in Golde DW, Takaku F (eds), *Hematopoietic Stem Cells*. New York, Marcel Dekker, 1985, p 229.
23. Ammus SS, Yunis AA: Acquired pure red cell aplasia. *Am J Hematol* 24:311, 1987.
24. Alter BP: The bone marrow failure syndrome, in Nathan D, Oski FA (eds), *Hematology of Infancy and Childhood*, ed 3. Philadelphia, WB Saunders, 1987, p 159.
25. Heimpel H, Wandt F: Congenital dyserythropoietic anemia with karyorrhexis and multinuclearity of erythroblasts. *Helv Med Acta* 34:103, 1968.
26. Heimpel H: Congenital dyserythropoietic anemia type 1, in Lewis SM, Verwilghen RL (eds), *Dyserythropoiesis*. London, Academic Press, 1976, p 135.
27. Vainchenker W, Guichard J, Bouguet J, et al: Congenital dyserythropoietic anaemia type 1: Absence of clonal expression in the nuclear abnormalities of cultured erythroblasts. *Br J Haematol* 46:33, 1980.
28. Heimpel H, Forteza-Vila J, Dueisser W: Electron and light microscopic study of the erythroblasts of patients with congenital dyserythropoietic anemia. *Blood* 37:299, 1971.
29. Verwilghen RL: Congenital dyserythropoietic anemia type II (HEMPAS), in *Congenital Disorders of Erythropoiesis*. CIBA Foundation Symposium 37. Amsterdam, Elsevier, 1976, p 151.
30. Fukuda MN, Dell A, Scartezzini P: Primary defect of congenital dyserythropoietic anemia type II: Failure in glycosylation of erythrocyte lactosaminoglycan proteins caused by lowered N-acetylglucosaminyltransferase II. *J Biol Chem* 262:7195, 1987.
31. Lewis SM, Frisch B: Congenital dyserythropoietic anemias: Electron microscopy, in *Congenital Disorders of Erythropoiesis*. CIBA Foundation Symposium 37. Amsterdam, Elsevier, 1976, p 171.
32. Crookston MC: HEMPAS: Congenital dyserythropoietic anemia (type II). *Q J Med* 66:257, 1973.
33. Goudsmith R: Congenital dyserythropoietic anemia, type III, in Lewis SM, Verwilghen RL (eds), *Dyserythropoiesis*. London, Academic Press, 1977, p 83.
34. Vainchenker W, Breton-Gorius J, Guichard J, et al: Congenital dyserythropoietic anemia type III. Studies on erythroid differentiation of blood erythroid progenitor cells (BFU-E) in vitro. *Exp Hematol* 8:1057, 1980.
35. Herbert V: Megaloblastic anemia. *Lab Invest* 52:3, 1985.
36. Chanarin I: Megaloblastic anemia, cobalamin and folate. *J Clin Pathol* 40:978, 1987.
37. Wickramasinghe RG, Hoffbrand AV: Conversion of partially single-stranded DNA to double-stranded DNA is delayed in megaloblastic anemia. *Biochem Biophys Acta* 607:411, 1980.
38. Lindahl T: New class of enzymes acting on damaged DNA. *Nature* 259:64, 1976.
39. Killman SA: Effects of deoxyuridine on incorporation of tritiated thymidine: Difference between normoblasts and megaloblasts. *Acta Med Scand* 175:483, 1964.
40. Gough KR, Read AE, McCarthy CF, et al: Megaloblastic anemia due to nutritional deficiency of folic acid. *Q J Med* 32:243, 1963.
41. Gross S, Kamen B, Fanaroff A: Folate compartments during gestational maturation. *J Pediatr* 96:842, 1980.
42. Landon MJ, Eyre DH, Hytten FE: Transfer of folate to the fetus. *Br J Obstet Gynecol* 82:12, 1975.
43. Shapiro J, Alperts HW, Welch P, et al: Folate and vitamin B_{12} deficiency associated with lactation. *Br J Haematol* 11:498, 1965.
44. Hogenkamp HPC: Enzymatic reactions involving corrinoids. *Ann Rev Biochem* 37:225, 1968.
45. Babior BM: *Cobalamin: Biochemistry and Pathophysiology*. New York, Wiley, 1975.
46. Herzlich B, Herbert V: The role of pancreas in cobalamin (vitamin B_{12}) absorption. *Am J Gastroenterol* 79:489, 1984.
47. Waters AH, Murphy MEB: Familial juvenile pernicious anemia. *Br J Haematol* 9:1, 1963.
48. Callender ST, Denborough MA: A familial study of pernicious anemia. *Br J Haematol* 3:88, 1957.
49. De Aizpurua HJ, Cosgrove LH, Toh BH: Autoantibodies cytotoxic to gastric parietal cells in serum of patients with pernicious anemia. *N Engl J Med* 309:625, 1983.
50. Schade SG, Abels J, Schining RF: Studies on antibody to intrinsic factor. *J Clin Invest* 46:615, 1967.
51. Fox RM, O'Sullivan WJ, Firkin BG: Orotic aciduria: Differing enzyme patterns. *Am J Med* 47:332, 1969.
52. Fox RM, Wood MH, Royse-Smith D, et al: Hereditary orotic aciduria: Types I and II. *Am J Med* 55:791, 1973.
53. Van der Zee SPM: Megaloblastic anemia in Lesch-Nyhan syndrome. *Lancet* 1:1427, 1968.
54. Krouse JR: The bone marrow in nutritional deficiencies. *Hematol Oncol Clin North Am* 2:557, 1988.
55. Cardinale GJ, Carty TJ, Abeles RH: Effect of methylmalonyl coenzyme A, a metabolite which accumulates in vitamin B_{12} deficiency, on fatty acid synthesis. *J Biol Chem* 247:4270, 1972.
56. Beck WS: Cobalamin and the nervous system. *N Engl J Med* 318:1752, 1988.

57. DeMaeyer E, Adiels-Tegman M: The prevalence of anemia in the world. *World Health Stat Q* 38:302, 1985.
58. Woods S, de Marco T, Friedland M: Iron metabolism. *Am J Gastroenterol* 85:1, 1990.
59. Cook JD, Skikne BS: Iron deficiency: Definition and diagnosis. *J Intern Med* 226:349, 1989.
60. Lipschitz DA, Cook JD, Finch CA: A clinical evaluation of serum ferritin as an index of iron stores. *N Engl J Med* 290:1213, 1974.
61. Soemantri AG, Pollitt E, Kim I: Iron deficiency anemia and educational achievement. *Am J Clin Nutr* 42:1221, 1985.
62. Chwang LC, Soemantri AG, Pollitt E: Iron supplementation and physical growth of rural Indonesian children. *Am J Clin Nutr* 47:496, 1988.
63. Dallman PR: Iron deficiency and the immune response. *Am J Clin Nutr* 46:329, 1987.
64. Goepel E, Ulmer RD, Neth RD: Premature labor contractions and value of serum ferritin during pregnancy. *Gynecol Obstet Invest* 26:265, 1988.
65. Lieberman E, Ryan KJ, Monson RR, et al: Association of maternal hematocrit with premature labor. *Am J Obstet Gynecol* 159:107, 1988.
66. Schwartz E, Cohen A, Surrey S: Overview of the β-thalassemias: Genetic and clinical aspects. *Hemoglobin* 12:551, 1988.
67. Leibhaber SA: α Thalassemia. *Hemoglobin* 13:685, 1989.
68. Jones RW, Old JM, Trent RJ, et al: Major rearrangement in the human β-globin gene cluster. *Nature* 291:39, 1981.
69. Stamatoyannopoulos G, Nienhuis AW, Leder P, et al: *The Molecular Basis of Blood Diseases*. Philadelphia, WB Saunders, 1987.
70. Weatherall DJ: The thalassemias, in Williams WJ, Beutler E, Erslev AJ, et al (eds), *Hematology*, ed 4. New York, McGraw-Hill, 1990, p 510.
71. Spritz RA, Orkin SH: Duplication followed by deletion accounts for the structure of an Indian deletion β-thalassemia gene. *Nucleic Acid Res* 10:8025, 1982.
72. Gilman JG: The 12.6 kilobase DNA deletion in Dutch β-thalassemia. *Br J Haematol* 67:369, 1987.
73. Orkin SH, Sexton JP, Cheng TC, et al: TATA box transcription mutation in β-thalassemia. *Nucleic Acid Res* 11:4727, 1983.
74. Antonarakis SE, Orkin SH, Cheng TC, et al: β-Thalassemia in American blacks: Novel mutations in the TATA box and IVS-2 acceptor splice site. *Proc Natl Acad Sci USA* 81:1154, 1984.
75. Wong C, Dowling CE, Saiki RK, et al: Characterization of β-Thalassemia mutations using direct genomic sequencing of amplified single copy DNA. *Nature* 330:384, 1987.
76. Treisman R, Orkin SH, Maniatis T: Specific transcription and RNA splicing defects in five cloned β-thalassemia genes. *Nature* 302:591, 1983.
77. Atweh GF, Anagnou NP, Shearin J, et al: β-Thalassemia resulting from a single nucleotide substitution in a receptor splice site. *Nucleic Acid Res* 13:777, 1985.
78. Nagel RL, Ranney HM: Genetic epidemiology of structural mutations of the β-globin gene. *Semin Hematol* 27:342, 1990.
79. Orkin SH, Cheng TC, Antonarakis SE, et al: Thalassemia due to a mutation in the cleavage-polyadenylation signal of the human β-globin gene. *EMBO J* 4:453, 1985.
80. Kazazian HH Jr: The thalassemia syndromes: Molecular basis and prenatal diagnosis in 1990. *Semin Hematol* 27:209, 1990.
81. Adams JG, Coleman MB: Structural hemoglobin variants that produce the phenotype of thalassemia. *Semin Hematol* 27:229, 1990.
82. Wickramasinghe SN, Letsky E, Moffat B: Effect of α-chain precipitates on bone marrow function in homozygous β-thalassemia. *Br J Haematol* 25:123, 1973.
83. Rachmilewitz EA, Lubin BH, Shohet SB: Lipid membrane peroxidation in β-thalassemia major. *Blood* 47:495, 1976.
84. Bunn HF, Forget BG: *Hemoglobin: Molecular, Genetic and Clinical Aspects*. Philadelphia, WB Saunders, 1986.
85. Gianni AM, Bregni M, Cappellini MD, et al: A gene controlling fetal hemoglobin expression in adults is not linked to the non-α globin cluster. *EMBO J* 2:291, 1983.
86. Higgs DR, Weatherall DJ: Alpha-thalassemia. *Curr Top Hematol* 4:37, 1983.
87. Yenchitsomanus PT, Summers KM, Bhatia KK, et al: Extremely high frequencies of α-globin gene deletion in Madang and on Kar Island, Papua, New Guinea. *Am J Hum Genet* 37:778, 1985.
88. Hill AVS, Flint J, Weatherall DJ, et al: Alpha-thalassemia and the malaria hypothesis. *Acta Haematol* 78:173, 1987.
89. Nathan DG, Stossel TB, Gunn RB, et al: Influence of hemoglobin precipitation on erythrocyte metabolism in alpha and beta thalassemia. *J Clin Invest* 48:33, 1969.
90. Schory M, Ramot B: Globin chain synthesis in the marrow and reticulocytes of beta thalassemia, hemoglobin H disease, and beta delta thalassemia. *Blood* 40:105, 1972.
91. Dozy AM, Kan YW, Embury SH, et al: α-Globin gene organization in blacks precludes the severe form of α-thalassemia. *Nature* 280:605, 1979.
92. Eaton JW, Jacob HS, White JM: Membrane abnor-

malities of irreversibly sickle cells. *Semin Hematol* 16:52, 1979.
93. Lubin B, Kuypers F, Chiu D: Lipid alteration and cellular properties of sickle red cells. *Ann NY Acad Sci* 565:86, 1989.
94. McGuire M, Agre P: Clinical disorders of the erythrocyte membrane skeleton. *Hematol Pathol* 2:1, 1988.
95. Brozovic DM: The presentation, management and prophylaxis of sickle cell disease. *Blood Rev* 3:29, 1989.
96. Hunt JA, Ingram VM: Allelomorphism and chemical differences of the human hemoglobins A, S, and C. *Nature* 181:1062, 1958.
97. Hirsch RE, Lin MJ, Nagel RL: The inhibition of hemoglobin C crystallization by hemoglobin F. *J Biol Chem* 263:5936, 1988.
98. Beutler E; The sickle cell diseases and related disorders, in Williams WJ, Beutler E, Erslev AJ, et al (eds), *Hematology*, ed 4. New York, McGraw-Hill, 1990, p 613.
99. Hunt JA, Ingram VM: Abnormal human haemoglobins. VI. The chemical difference between hemoglobins A and E. *Biochem Biophys Acta* 49:520, 1961.
100. Schmidt RM, Borsious EF: *Basic Laboratory Methods of Hemoglobinopathy Detection*, ed 6. HEW Pub. No. (CDC) 77-8266. Atlanta, U.S. Department of Health, Education and Welfare, Center for Disease Control, 1976.
101. Schneider RG: Methods for detection of hemoglobin variants and hemoglobinopathies in the routine clinical laboratory. *CRC Crit Rev Clin Lab Sci* 9:243, 1978.
102. Carrell RW, Lehmann H: The unstable haemoglobin hemolytic anemias. *Semin Hematol* 6:116, 1969.
103. Winterbourn CC: Oxidative denaturation in congenital hemolytic anemias: The unstable hemoglobins. *Semin Hematol* 27:41, 1990.
104. Zinkham WH, Winslow RM: Unstable hemoglobins: Influence of environment on phenotypic expression of a genetic disorder. *Medicine (Baltimore)* 68:309, 1989.
105. Reinhart WH, Sung LA, Chein S: Quantitative relationship between Heinz body formation and red blood cell deformability. *Blood* 68:1376, 1986.
106. Weiss L: A scanning electron microscopic study of the spleen. *Blood* 43:665, 1974.
107. Winterbourn CC, Carrell RW: Studies of hemoglobin denaturation and Heinz body formation in the unstable hemoglobins. *J Clin Invest* 54:678, 1974.
108. Kim IIC, Schwartz E: Unstable hemoglobin, in Williams WJ, Beutler E, Erslev AJ, et al (eds), *Hematology*, ed 4. New York, McGraw-Hill, 1990, p 1707.
109. Beutler E: Hemoglobinopathies associated with unstable hemoglobin, in Williams WJ, Beutler E, Erslev AJ, et al (eds), *Hematology*, ed 4. New York, McGraw-Hill, 1990, p 644.
110. Davies KA, Lux SE: Hereditary disorders of the red cell membrane skeleton. *Trends Genet* 5:222, 1989.
111a. McGuire M, Agre P: Clinical disorders of the erythrocyte membrane skeleton. *Hematol Pathol* 2:1, 1988.
111b. Palek J, Lambert S: Genetics of the red cell membrane skeleton. *Semin Hematol* 27:290, 1990.
112. Agre P, Asimos A, Casella JF, et al: Inheritance pattern and clinical response to splenectomy as a reflection of erythrocyte spectrin deficiency in hereditary spherocytosis. *N Engl J Med* 315:1579, 1986.
113. Rappaport ES, Quick G, Ranson D, et al: Aplastic crisis in occult hereditary spherocytosis caused by human parvovirus (HPV B19). *South Med J* 82:247, 1989.
114. Green DH, Bellingham AJ, Anderson MJ: Parvovirus infection in a family associated with aplastic crisis in an affected sibling pair with hereditary spherocytosis. *J Clin Pathol* 37:1144, 1984.
115. Lie-Injo LE: Hereditary ovalocytosis and haemoglobin E—ovalocytosis in Malayan aborigines. *Nature* 208:1329, 1965.
116. Liu SC, Palek J, Prchal JT: Defective spectrin dimer-dimer association in hereditary elliptocytosis. *Proc Natl Acad Sci USA* 79:2072, 1982.
117. Marchesi SL, Letsinger JT, Speicher DW, et al: Mutant forms of spectrin α-subunits in hereditary elliptocytosis. *J Clin Invest* 80:191, 1987.
118. Palek J: Hereditary elliptocytosis, spherocytosis and related disorders: Consequence of a deficiency or a mutation of membrane skeletal proteins. *Blood Rev* 1:147, 1987.
119. Palek J: Hereditary elliptocytosis and related disorders, in Williams WJ, Beutler E, Erslev AJ, (eds), *Blood*, ed 4. New York, McGraw-Hill, 1990, p 569.
120. Palek J: Acanthocytosis, stomatocytosis, and related disorders, in Williams WJ, Beutler E, Erslev AJ, et al (eds), *Hematology*, ed 4. New York, McGraw-Hill, 1990, p 582.
121. Cooper RA: Hemolytic syndromes and red cell membrane abnormalities in liver disease. *Semin Hematol* 17:103, 1980.
122. Flamm M, Schachter D: Acanthocytosis and cholesterol enrichment decrease lipid fluidity of only the human erythrocyte membrane leaflet. *Nature* 298:290, 1982.
123. Lange Y, Culter HB, Steck TL: The effect of cholesterol and other interrelated amphipaths on the contour and stability of the isolated red cell membranes. *J Biol Chem* 255:9331, 1980.
124. Cooper RA, Durocher JR, Leslie M: Decreased fluidity

of red cell membrane lipids in abetalipoproteinemia. *J Clin Invest* 60:115, 1977.
125. Bessis M: *Living Blood Cells and Their Ultrastructure.* New York, Springer Verlag, 1973, p 146.
126. Oski FA, Naiman JL, Blum SF, et al: Congenital hemolytic anemia with high-sodium, low potassium red cells: Study of three generations of a family with a new variant. *N Engl J Med* 280:909, 1969.
127. Sheetz MP, Singer SJ: Biological membranes as bilayer couples: A molecular mechanism of drug–erythrocyte interactions. *Proc Natl Acad Sci USA* 71:4457, 1974.
128. Beutler E: Hereditary nonspherocytic hemolytic anemia: Pyruvate kinase deficiency and other abnormalities, in Williams WJ, Beutler E, Erslev AJ, et al (eds), *Hematology*, ed 4. New York, McGraw-Hill, 1990, p 606.
129. Miwa S: Molecular basis of red cell enzymopathies associated with hereditary nonspherocytic hemolytic anemia. *Haematologica* 22:215, 1989.
130. Beutler E: Red cell enzyme defects. *Hematol Pathol* 4:103, 1990.
131. Beutler E, Yoshida A: The current status of genetic variations of glucose-6-phosphate dehydrogenase. *Medicine* 67:311, 1988.
132. Kirkman HN, Schettini F, Pickard BM: Mediterranean variant of glucose-6-phosphate dehydrogenase. *J Lab Clin Med* 63:726, 1964.
133. Beutler E: The genetics of glucose-6-phosphatase dehydrogenase deficiency. *Semin Hematol* 27:137, 1990.
134. Wickramasinghe SN: Disorders of erythron, in Wickramasinghe SN (ed), *Blood and Bone Marrow*. London, Churchill Livingstone, 1986, p 108.
135. Mager J, Glaser G, Razin A, et al: Metabolic effects of pyrimidines derived from fava bean glycosides on human erythrocytes deficient in glucose-6-phosphate dehydrogenase. *Biochem Biophys Res Commun* 20:235, 1965.
136. Cohen G, Hochstein P: Generation of hydrogen peroxide in erythrocytes by hemolytic agents. *Biochemistry* 3:895, 1964.
137. Itano HA, Hosokawa K, Hirato A: Induction of hemolytic anemia by substituted phenylhydrazines. *Br J Haematol* 32:99, 1976.
138. De Gruchy GC: *Drug-Induced Blood Disorders*. Oxford, Blackwell Scientific, 1975.
139. Doll DC: Oxidative haemolysis after administration of doxorubicin. *Br Med J* 287:180, 1983.
140. Tishler M: Phenazopyridine-induced hemolytic anemia in a patient with G-6-PD deficiency. *Acta Haematol* 70:208, 1983.
141. Hirono A, Forman L, Beutler E: Enzymatic diagnosis in non-spherocytic hemolytic anemia. *Medicine* 67:110, 1988.
142. Gibson J: Autoimmune hemolytic anemia: Current concepts. *Aust NZ J Med* 18:625, 1988.
143. Smith HR, Steinberg AD: Autoimmunity—a perspective. *Annu Rev Immunol* 1:175, 1983.
144. Gibson J, Basten A, Walker KZ, et al: A role for suppressor T cells in induction of self tolerance. *Proc Natl Acad Sci USA* 82:5150, 1985.
145. Dorf ME, Benaceraff B: Suppressor cells and immunoregulation. *Ann Rev Immunol* 2:127, 1984.
146. Sokol RJ, Hewitt S: Autoimmune hemolysis: A critical review. *CRC Crit Rev Oncol Hematol* 4:125, 1985.
147. Unanue ER: Antigen presenting function of the macrophage. *Annu Rev Immunol* 2:395, 1984.
148. Petz LD, Garratty G: *Acquired Immune Hemolytic Anemia*. New York, Churchill Livingstone, 1980.
149. Clark DA, Dessypris EN, Jenkins DE, et al: Acquired immune hemolytic anemia associated with IgA erythrocyte coating: Investigation of hemolytic mechanisms. *Blood* 64:1000, 1984.
150. Vos GH, Petz LD, Fundenberg HH: Specificity and immunoglobulin characteristics of autoantibodies in acquired hemolytic anemia. *J Immunol* 106:1172, 1971.
151. Nordhagen R, Stensvold K, Winsnes A, et al: Paroxysmal cold hemoglobinuria. The most frequent autoimmune hemolytic anemia in children? *Acta Paediatr Scand* 73:258, 1984.
152. Wolach B, Heddle N, Barr RD, et al: Transient Donath-Landsteiner hemolytic anemia. *Br J Haematol* 48:425, 1981.
153. Sokol RJ, Hewitt S, Stamps BK: Autoimmune hemolysis associated with Donath-Landsteiner antibodies. *Acta Haematol* 68:268, 1982.
154. Petz DL: Drug-induced immune haemolytic anaemia. *Clin Haematol* 9:455, 1980.
155. Worlledge SM: Immune drug-induced hemolytic anemia. *Semin Hematol* 10:327, 1973.
156. Berndt MC, Chong BH, Bull HA, et al: Molecular characterization of quinine/quinidine drug dependent antibody platelet interaction using monoclonal antisera. *Blood* 66:1292, 1985.
157. Salama A, Mueller-Eckhardt C: On the mechanisms of sensitization and attachment of antibodies to RBC in drug-induced immune hemolytic anemia. *Blood* 69:1006, 1987.
158. Carstairs KC, Worlledge SM, Dollery CT, et al: Methyldopa and haemolytic anaemia. *Lancet* 1:201, 1986.
159. Kirtland HH, Mohler DN, Horowitz DA: Methyldopa inhibition of suppressor-lymphocyte function. A proposed cause of autoimmune hemolytic anemia. *N Engl J Med* 313:469, 1980.
160. Owens NA, Hui HL, Green FA: Induction of direct Coombs' positivity with a methyldopa in chimpanzees. *J Med* 13:473, 1982.

161. Douglass CC, Twomey JJ: Transient stomatocytosis with hemolysis: A previously unrecognized complication of alcoholism. *Ann Intern Med* 72:159, 1970.
162. Zieve L: Jaundice, hyperlipemia and hemolytic anemia: An unrecognized syndrome associated with alcoholic fatty liver and cirrhosis. *Ann Intern Med* 48:471, 1958.
163. Fossaluzza V, Rossi P: Flunarizine treatment for spur cell anemia. *Br J Haematol* 55:715, 1983.
164. Schulte K-L, Kochen MM: Hemolytic anemia in an adult after a wasp sting. *Lancet* 2:478, 1981.
165. Rosse WF: The spleen as a filter (editorial). *N Engl J Med* 317:704, 1987.
166. Weiss L: The reticuloendothelial basis of the clearance of blood by the spleen, in Pochedly C, Sills R, Schwartz A (eds), *Disorders of the Spleen: Pathophysiology and Management*. New York, Marcel Dekker, 1989, p 431.
167. Bowdler AJ: Splenomegaly and hypersplenism. *Clin Haematol* 12:467, 1983.
168. Christensen BE: Quantitative determination of splenic red blood cell destruction in patients with splenomegaly. *Blood* 47:629, 1976.
169. Adamson J, Hillman RS: Blood volume and plasma protein replacement following acute blood loss in normal man. *JAMA* 205:609, 1968.
170. Hoffman HN, Phyliky RL, Fleming CR: Zinc-induced copper deficiency. *Gastroenterology* 94:508, 1988.
171. Lane M, Alfrey CP: The anemia of human riboflavin deficiency. *Blood* 22:811, 1963.
172. Oski FA, Barness LA: Hemolytic anemia in vitamin E deficiency. *Am J Clin Nutr* 21:45, 1968.
173. Reizenstein P: The hematological stress syndrome. *Br J Haematol* 43:329, 1979.
174. Cavill I, Bantley DP: Erythropoiesis in the anemia of rheumatoid arthritis. *Br J Haematol* 50:583, 1982.
175. Radtke HW, Claussner A, Erbes PM, et al: Serum erythropoietin concentration in chronic renal failure: Relationship to degree of anemia and excretory function. *Blood* 54:877, 1979.
176. Fisher JW: Mechanism of the anemia of chronic renal failure. *Nephron* 25:106, 1980.
177. Ohno Y, Rege AB, Fisher JW, et al: Inhibitors of erythroid colony forming cells (CFU-E and BFU-E) in sera of azotemic patients with anemia of renal disease. *J Lab Clin Med* 92:916, 1978.
178. Caro J, Erslev AJ: Uremic inhibitors of erythropoiesis. *Semin Nephrol* 5:128, 1985.

10 DISORDERS OF MEGAKARYOCYTES AND PLATELETS

Megakaryocytopoiesis is a complex process which includes proliferation of committed CFU-Meg cells, size growth and nuclear polyploidization during terminal differentiation, and finally, production of platelets. This proliferation and differentiation process is regulated by a number of cytokines, such as IL-3, GM-CSF, erythropoietin and thrombopoietin, and is characterized by generation of several differentiation-associated antigens[1-4] (Figure 10-1).

Megakaryocytes are located predominantly in parasinusoidal regions and are rare in paratrabecular areas of the bone marrow. In addition to platelet production, megakaryocytes are involved in facilitating cellular exchange between bone marrow and blood (see Chapter 2).

Quantitative and qualitative megakaryocytic abnormalities are prominent features of pluripotent stem cell defects such as aplastic anemia, myelodysplastic syndromes, myeloproliferative disorders and leukemias. These conditions are discussed in Chapters 4, 5 and 6. In this chapter, megakaryocytic and platelet disorders which are not caused by pluripotent stem cell defects are discussed.

AMEGAKARYOCYTOSIS

Amegakaryocytosis is one of the features of congenital or acquired aplastic anemias. Marked decrease in or lack of production of megakaryocytes without marrow aplasia is rare, and has been attributed to chronic alcoholism and prolonged administration of prednisone, estrogens, interferon and chlorothiazide.[5,6] Virus-induced amegakaryocytosis has been reported in measles, varicella, infectious mononucleosis, dengue, cytomegaly and viral hepatitis.[5-7]

CONGENITAL MEGAKARYOCYTIC HYPOPLASIA

Congenital megakaryocytic hypoplasia (thrombocytopenia with absent radii, TAR syndrome) is characterized by thrombocytopenic purpura, bilateral aplasia of the radii and cardiac and/or renal malformations.[8] An intrauterine disturbance (? rubella) during the 6–8 weeks of gestation may play a role in the etiology of this disorder.[9] Thrombocytopenia is usually severe and is sometimes associated with a transient granulocytic leukemoid reaction. Platelets may demonstrate abnormal function.[10] Bone marrow examination reveals a marked decrease in the number of megakaryocytes.

MEGAKARYOCYTOSIS

Bone marrow metastasis is one of the most frequent nonhematologic causes of reactive megakaryocytosis.[11] Increased bone marrow megakaryocytes in malignancy may be related to the release of a thrombopoietin-like substance by tumor cells.[12] Other conditions associated with megakaryocytosis and thrombocytosis are acute infections, iron deficiency and postsplenectomy status. Platelet destruction or consumption may also induce a compensatory megakaryocytosis. The major causes of thrombocytopenia with subsequent bone marrow megakaryocytosis are antibodies or immune complexes. The most prominent example is autoimmune thrombocytopenic purpura, in which platelet destruction is due to the effect of an antiplatelet autoantibody[5,13] (see below).

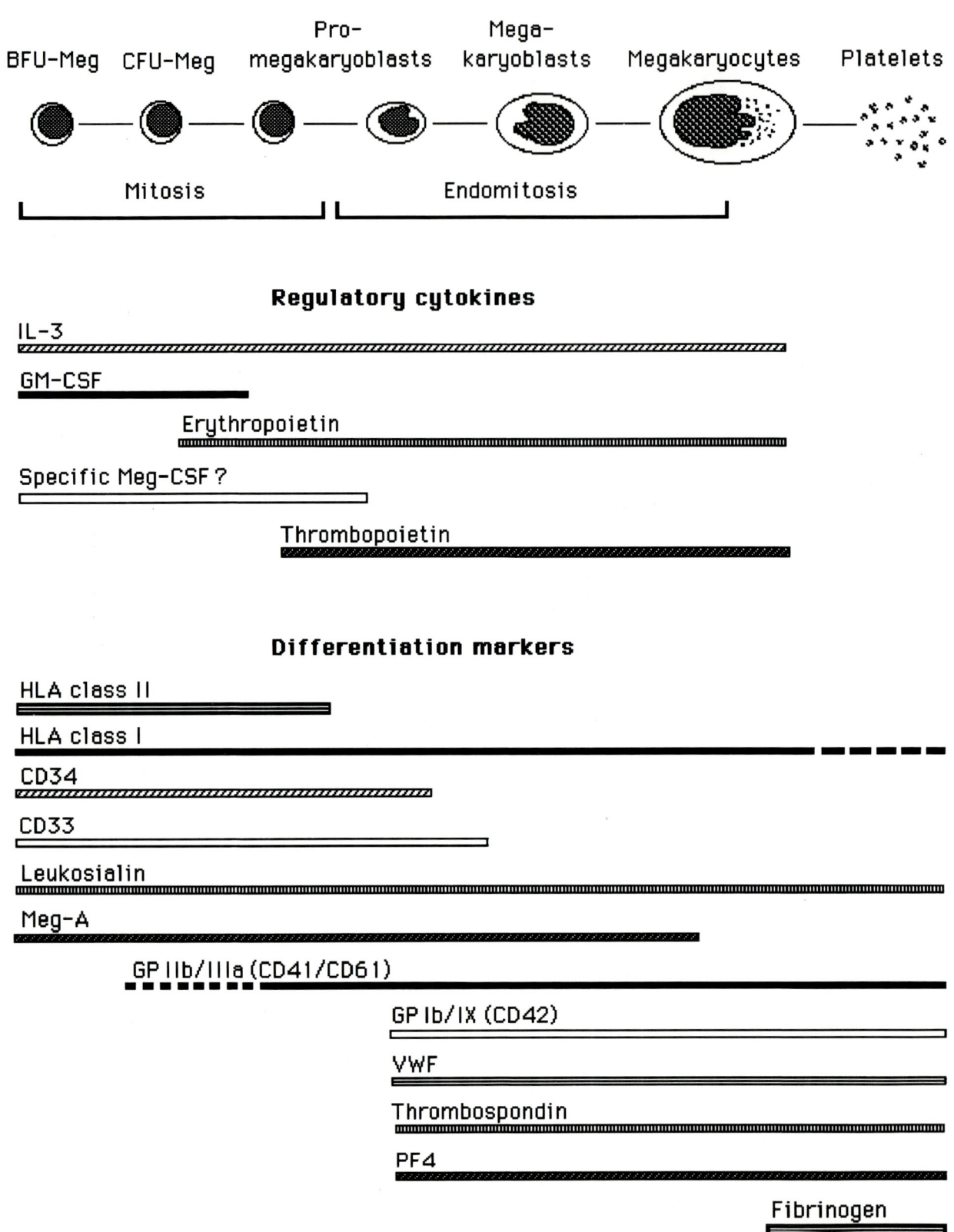

Figure 10-1. Schematic demonstration of regulation in megakaryocytopoiesis and expression of the differentiation markers in megakaryocytes and platelets. Adapted from Vainchenker W, Kieffer N: Human megakaryocytopoiesis: In vitro regulation and characterization of megakaryocytic precursor cells by differentiation markers. *Blood Rev* 2:102, 1988.

Disorders of Megakaryocytes and Platelets

Megakaryocytosis associated with myeloproliferative disorders, myelodysplastic syndromes and AML-M7, unlike reactive megakaryocytosis, is often characterized by marked dysplastic changes and the arrangement of megakaryocytes in clusters or sheets (Figures 10-2, 10-3) (see Chapters 5 and 6).

THROMBOCYTOPENIA

Thrombocytopenia is due either to impaired platelet production or to increased platelet destruction. Impaired platelet production is caused by congenital and acquired aplastic anemias, paroxysmal nocturnal hemoglobinuria, congenital deficiency of megakaryocytes, infiltration of bone marrow by neoplastic cells, myelofibrosis, drugs, radiation, certain infections and malnutrition. Increased platelet destruction may occur by either immunologic or nonimmunologic mechanisms.

AUTOIMMUNE THROMBOCYTOPENIC PURPURA (ATP)

Etiology and Pathogenesis

ATP, or idiopathic thrombocytopenic purpura (ITP), is an antibody-mediated thrombocytopenia[14,15] The vast majority of patients appear to have an antiplatelet antibody that binds to platelet membrane

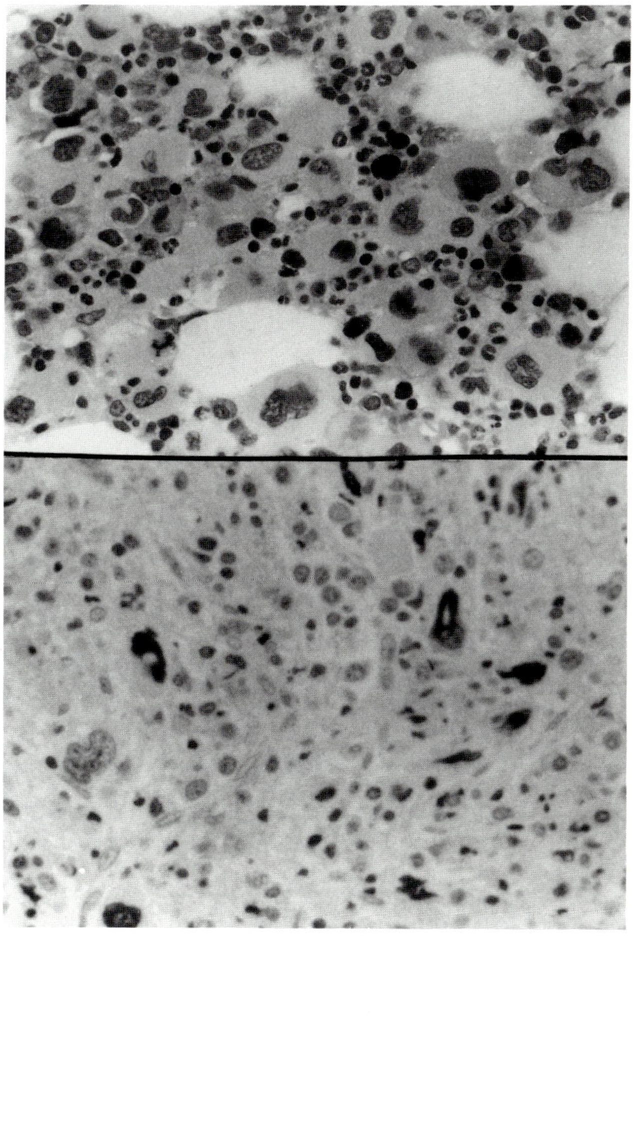

Figure 10-2. Megakaryocytosis in myeloproliferative disorders. (a) Bone marrow biopsy section from a patient with essential thrombocythemia. (b) Bone marrow biopsy section from a patient with myelofibrosis.

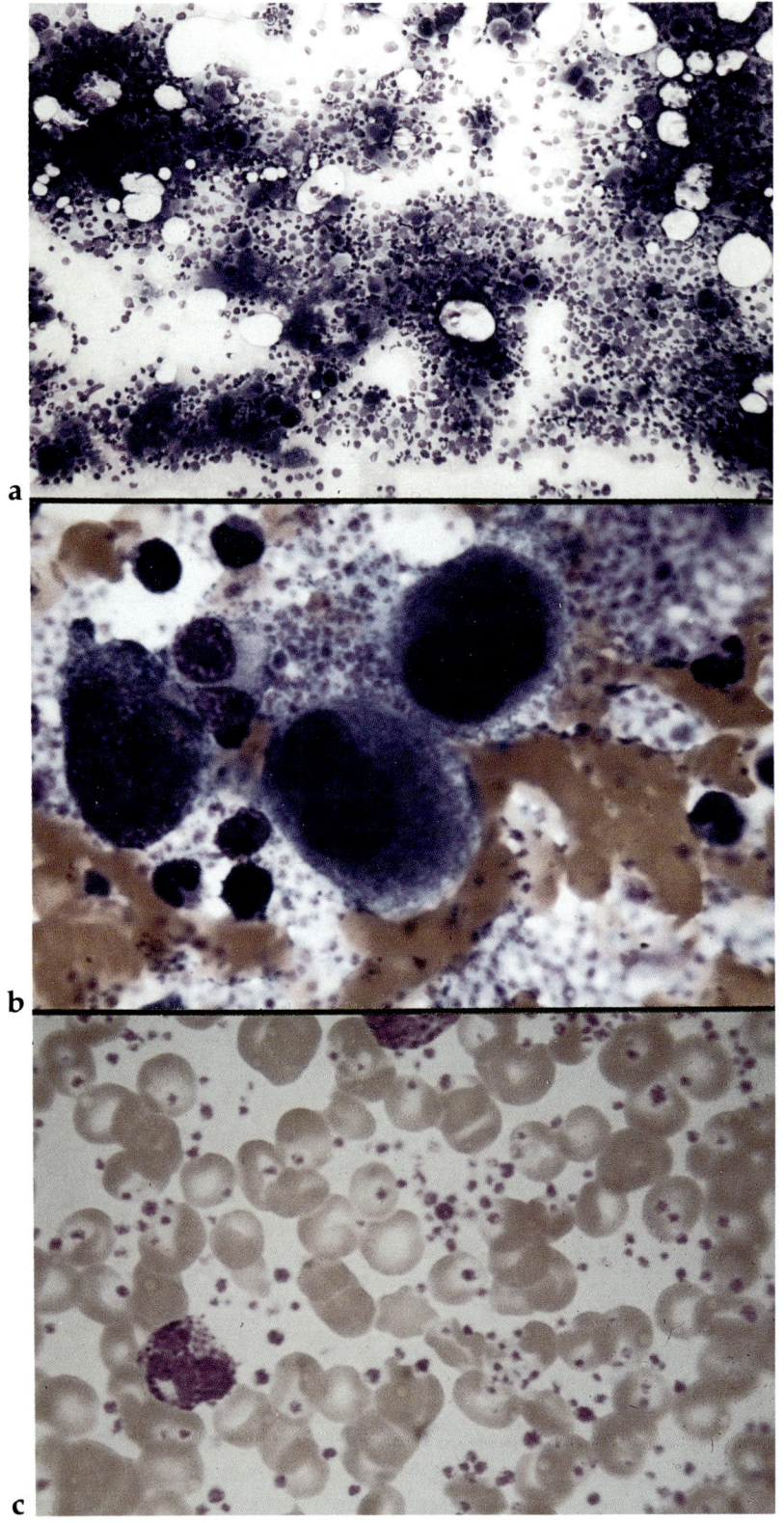

Figure 10-3. Bone marrow megakaryocytosis (a, b) and peripheral blood thrombocytosis (c) in a patient with essential thrombocythemia.

glycoproteins.[16-19] Glycoprotein (GP) IIb/IIIa and GP1b/IX are the two major target antigens in approximately two-thirds of ATP patients.[17,18,20] The antiplatelet antibody is usually of the IgG class, is stable at 56°C and is transferred across the placenta.[21]

ATP may be associated with other diseases (secondary ATP) such as systemic lupus erythematosus, rheumatoid arthritis, systemic sclerosis, Hashimoto's thyroiditis, ulcerative colitis, Crohn's disease, biliary cirrhosis, myasthenia gravis, pernicious anemia, sarcoidosis, Gaucher's disease, CLL, other lymphoproliferative disorders and AIDS.[22-32] Panhypogammaglobulinemia and IgA deficiency are strongly associated with ATP.[15]

Clinical and Pathologic Features

Clinical manifestations of ATP are acute or chronic. Acute ATP is observed predominantly in children between 2 and 9 years old, and is characterized by the onset of severe thrombocytopenia and spontaneous remission within 6–12 months of onset in at least 80% of the affected children. Symptoms include petechiae, purpura, and frequently, gastrointestinal and/or urinary tract bleeds. Intracranial hemorrhage occurs in 0.5–1.0% of the affected children.[33] Acute ATP is often preceded by a history of infection, usually of viral origin, such as chickenpox, rubeola and rubella, or sometimes following immunization with live vaccine for measles, smallpox, chickenpox and mumps.[34-37] Splenomegaly is rare.

Chronic ATP occurs primarily in adults, usually between 20 and 50 years of age; the female:male ratio is about 3, and there is less of a tendency toward spontaneous recovery. Clinical manifestations vary from scattered petechiae to purpuric and ecchymotic lesions, epistaxis, and even intracranial hemorrhage. Splenomegaly is usually not present. In HIV-infected patients, the incidence of immune-mediated thrombocytopenia ranges from 5% to 12% in ARC patients and reaches as high as 30% in patients with AIDS.[38-40]

Peripheral blood examination reveals thrombocytopenia, with marked variation in the shape and size of the platelets. The platelet count may reach <30,000 µl, with prolongation of the bleeding time. Chronic bleeding may lead to an iron deficiency anemia. Rare patients with ATP may also demonstrate an autoimmune hemolytic anemia (Evans syndrome).[41]

Serum and platelet-bound IgG antibodies are of two major types: (1) α-granule IgG, which comprises well over 95% of the total platelet-bound IgG and does not seem to function as an antiplatelet antibody, and (2) platelet surface IgG, which accounts for the remaining platelet-bound IgG and, in the majority of ATP patients, reacts with platelet membrane GP IIb/IIIa and GP Ib/IX complexes.[42] Thus, the measurement of platelet surface IgG, and not the total platelet-bound IgG, is important in establishing the diagnosis of ATP.

Bone marrow examination usually reveals an increased number of megakaryocytes, which are diffusely distributed in the bone marrow. Giant megakaryocytes, as well as micromegakaryocytes with bi- or trilobed nuclei, are present. Megakaryocytes with more basophilic and less granular cytoplasm and little or no platelet budding have been described[5,13] (Figure 10-4). Cross-reactivity of antiplatelet antibodies with megakaryocytes has been demonstrated, which may explain the decreased level of platelet production in some patients with chronic ATP.[43,44]

DRUG-INDUCED IMMUNE THROMBOCYTOPENIA

A wide variety of drugs have been implicated as the cause of immune-mediated thrombocytopenia. The major immunologic mechanisms proposed for drug-induced thrombocytopenia are as follows: (1) The drug binds to one or several components of the platelet membrane and induces a structural change. This drug-platelet structural modification acts as a new antigen and provokes antibody formation in certain individuals. (2) The drug or its metabolites bind to a plasma protein, and antibodies are generated against the drug-protein complexes. Platelet membrane glycoproteins such as GPIb/IX and GPIIb/IIIa appear to be the prime targets. Antibody-binding sites are Fab regions.[45,46]

Quinine, quinidine, sulfonamides, organic arsenicals, sulfisoxazole, para-aminosalicylate, alphamethyldopa, rifampicin, oxprenolol and gold salts are among the drugs that have caused immune thrombocytopenia in certain patients.[45-50]

Heparin-induced thrombocytopenia is one of the most important drug-induced thrombocytopenias

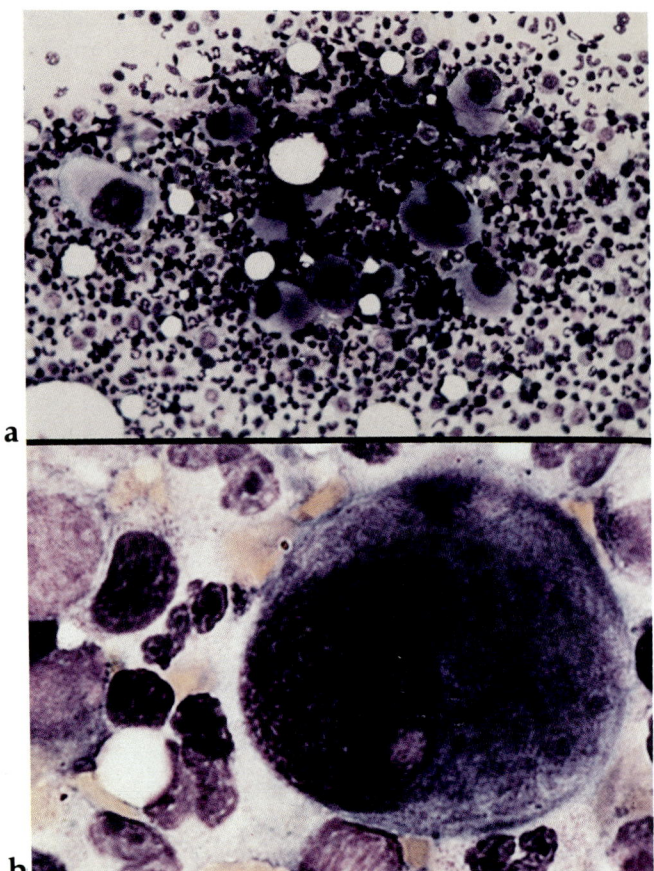

Figure 10-4. A bone marrow smear from a patient with ATP demonstrating increased numbers of megakaryocytes (a). A megakaryocyte with a basophilic cytoplasm and no platelet budding is shown (b).

because of its frequent association with thromboembolism. The majority of cases of heparin-induced thrombocytopenia are caused by immunologic mechanisms.[51-54]

Drug-induced immune thrombocytopenia typically has an acute onset, with a markedly low platelet count (usually <10,000/µl), manifestations of petechiae, purpura, and sometimes gastrointestinal and urinary tract hemorrhages. The bleeding episodes usually appear within 6–12 hours after medication is taken. Other associated symptoms are fever, joint pain and urticaria. Symptoms usually disappear 3–4 days after discontinuation of the medication.

Bone marrow examination reveals a normocellular marrow with a normal or increased number of megakaryocytes.

NEONATAL IMMUNE THROMBOCYTOPENIA

Neonatal immune thrombocytopenia develops when maternal antiplatelet antibodies cross the placenta and bind to fetal platelets. Antiplatelet antibody production in the mother is due either to feto-maternal incompatibility in platelet antigens (alloimmune thrombocytopenia) or to maternal ATP.

Alloimmune Thrombocytopenia

Alloimmune thrombocytopenia occurs when maternal IgG alloantibodies are formed against fetal platelets. In addition to class 1 HLA and ABO antigens, platelets express specific alloantigens (P1^A) which show biallelic autosomal inheritance.[55-59] The most common cause of neonatal alloimmune thrombocytopenia is feto-maternal P1^{A1} incompatibility between P1^{A1}-positive babies and P1^{A1}-negative mothers. This incompatibility accounts for 50-90% of the proven cases of neonatal alloimmune thrombocytopenia.[60,61] The risk of maternal sensitization in feto-maternal P1^{A1} incompatibility strongly correlates with the maternal HLA type and is virtually confined to HLA-B8 and -DR3 mothers.[62] Platelets express class 1 HLA antigens, and there are reports of maternal sensitization and antibody production against fetal platelet HLA antigens due to feto-maternal HLA incompatibility.[63,64] However, whether HLA incompatibility can cause alloimmune thrombocytopenia is controversial. The consensus is that anti-HLA antibodies are absorbed into the placental tissue and do not reach the fetal circulation.[64] ABO incompatibility does not seem to result in thrombocytopenia.

Affected children usually demonstrate scattered, generalized petechial and purpuric hemorrhages at birth or soon after delivery. Intracranial hemorrhage is the most serious complication, occurring in up to 25% of the affected infants.[58,61,62] Thrombocytopenia usually persists for 2–3 weeks, with a platelet count of around 30,000/μl or even lower. Bone marrow examination usually demonstrates a normal or elevated number of megakaryocytes, though amegakaryocytosis secondary to antimegakaryocytic effects of alloantibodies has also been reported.[59]

Thrombocytopenia Associated with Maternal ATP

This disorder is observed in approximately 50% of neonates born to mothers with ATP. The maternal IgG autoantibody crosses the placenta and binds to fetal platelets.[63,64] Thrombocytopenia may last for 1 to 6 months. The incidence of spontaneous abortion is increased in mothers with ATP.[65]

POSTTRANSFUSION PURPURA

Posttransfusion purpura is the result of platelet alloantigen incompatibilities between the recipient and the donor, and is observed approximately 7–10 days after blood or platelet transfusion. The alloantibodies are raised against one of the platelet-specific alloantigens, particularly P1^{A1}(ZWa).[66] This alloimmunization, similar to neonatal alloimmune thrombocytopenia, is associated with certain recipients' class II HAL antigens such as HLA-DR3, -DR3/DRw52 and -DR6/DRw52.[67]

THROMBOCYTOPENIA IN ALLERGIC AND ANAPHYLACTIC REACTIONS

Allergic and anaphylactic reactions are frequently associated with thrombocytopenia. Thrombocytopenia in these conditions may be related to binding of IgE to the platelet membrane.[68,69] In anaphylactic shock, the development of disseminated intravascular coagulation (DIC) intensifies the severity of thrombocytopenia.

THROMBOTIC THROMBOCYTOPENIC PURPURA (TTP)

TTP is characterized by thrombocytopenia, microangiopathic hemolytic anemia, fever, neurologic symptoms and renal involvement.[70] The peak incidence is in the third decade, and the female:male ratio is about 3:2.[71,72]

Etiology and Pathogenesis

The etiology and pathogenesis of TTP are not well understood. Several etiologic factors have been proposed which are related primarily to endothelial cell damage. TTP has been associated with collagen vascular disorders such as systemic lupus erythematosus, rheumatoid arthritis, Sjögren's syndrome and polyarteritis nodosa[71,73-75]; abnormalities of endothelial cell function such as production of large plasma vWF molecules,[76] defects in prostacyclin metabolism,[77,78] deficiency of plasminogen activator[79,80] and production of a platelet-aggregating protein[81] have been demonstrated in some cases. Pregnancy may trigger the onset of TTP.[82,83] Reports of the hereditary forms of TTP suggest a genetic predisposition in the pathogenesis of this disorder in some patients.[83,84]

Certain viruses and bacteria such as HIV, coxsackie A and B, *Mycoplasma pneumoniae*, and *Legionella pneumophila* have been associated with TTP and have been suggested as predisposing factors.

Clinicopathologic Features

Thrombocytopenia is often manifested as purpura, but epistaxis, hemoptysis, hematuria, menorrhagia and gastrointestinal bleeding may also be present. Approximately 40% of the patients may display a prodromal phase resembling a virus-like disease.[71] Fever is a common finding, and neurologic symptoms are present in up to 90% of the patients. The clinical course may be acute or chronic.[70] The acute form is a fulminant disorder with a grave outcome, usually ending in death if treatment is not effective. The chronic form is less common than the acute form, symptoms develop gradually and patients survive for many years.

Peripheral blood examination demonstrates a moderate to severe anemia with marked red blood cell fragmentation, reticulocytosis and often the presence of nucleated RBCs. Thrombocytopenia is marked and in some patients is <20,000/μl.

The most prominent pathologic feature of TTP is disseminated hyaline thrombi in the capillaries and arterioles of various tissues. These microthrombi apparently represent a form of DIC and are commonly observed in the brain, kidney, pancreas, adrenal glands and heart.[71,85] Microthrombi are rarely detected in bone marrow biopsy specimens. Bone marrow examination reveals normocellular marrow with adequate or increased numbers of megakaryocytes.

HEMOLYTIC UREMIC SYNDROME (HUS)

HUS is a TTP-related disorder which is observed primarily in infancy and early childhood and is characterized by thrombocytopenia, acute renal failure and microangiopathic hemolytic anemia, often preceded by a febrile diarrhea or a respiratory disorder. The clinical symptoms, similar to those of TTP, are the result of the formation of microthrombi in the capillaries and arterioles.[86] Bacterial and viral cytotoxins appear to play an important role in the pathogenesis of this process. Evidence of verocytotoxin-producing *Escherichia coli* has been demonstrated in up to 75% of children with HUS.[87,88] Other microorganisms reported in association with HUS are *Pneumococcus pneumoniae*, *Yersinia pseudotuberculosis*, *Campylobacter jejuni*, *Salmonella typhi*, varicella, coxsackie enteroviruses and ECHO virus.[89-95] Cytotoxins released by microorganisms appear to damage the vascular endothelium and initiate intravascular coagulation in the capillaries and arterioles, particularly in the kidney. The presence of familial forms suggests a genetic predisposition in the pathogenesis of the disease in certain patients.[96,97]

Adult HUS is clinically similar to TTP, except for its more prominent renal involvement and less frequent neurologic symptoms. It is found more frequently in women, especially in association with eclampsia, the use of oral contraceptives or the postpartum period. Chemotherapy, particularly with mitomycin C, may induce HUS in cancer patients.[98-100]

OTHER CONDITIONS ASSOCIATED WITH THROMBOCYTOPENIA

Numerous pathologic conditions are associated with thrombocytopenia, such as a wide variety of infections, glomerulonephritis, renal transplant rejection, renal vein thrombosis, DIC, giant cavernous hemangioma, burns, snake bites, aortic valvular disease, primary pulmonary hypertension,[101] and Wiscott-Aldrich syndrome. Certain drugs induce thrombocytopenia by their direct action on circulating platelets such as hematin, protamine sulfate and bleomycin.[102-105] Administration of antithymocyte globulin may cause thrombocytopenia, probably due to the formation of immune complexes and their effects on the platelet surface.[106] Thrombocytopenia observed in hypersplenism and in prolonged occlusion of the venous return in an extremity is due to platelet sequestration.

QUALITATIVE PLATELET DISORDERS

Platelets are involved in complex interrelated interactions with vessel walls and with coagulation factors.

Adhesion of the platelets with the subendothelial matrix of the injured blood vessels leads to activation of platelets and subsequently to platelet aggregation and secretion of the contents of platelet granules. In the initial process of adhesion, a family of platelet membrane glycoproteins (GPs), which are known as *adhesion receptors* or integrins, adhere to various components of the subendothelial matrix. For example, the GP 1b/IX complex adheres to vWF, GP 1a/IIa is a receptor for collagen and the GP 1c/IIa complex adheres to fibronectin and laminin.[107] Following initial platelet adhesion and activation, the GP IIb/IIIa complex becomes the major component of the adhesion process, and by binding to vWF and fibronectin, it helps the spreading of platelets on the subendothelial matrix.[107] A number of soluble agonists such as adenosine diphosphate (ADP), vasopressin, epinephrine, serotonin and thrombin can also activate platelets.[107] Activated platelets attach to each other (aggregation) by converting GP IIb/IIIa into a receptor for fibrinogen and other adhesive proteins such as vitronectin and vWF.[108] The dimeric fibrinogen molecule, by binding to the GP IIb/IIIa complex on the adjacent platelets, causes platelet aggregation.[107,109] Another major role of platelets in hemostasis is their interaction with coagulation factors and activation of the coagulation cascade. Several enzymatic coagulation reactions occur on the membrane of activated platelets.

Qualitative platelet defects affect hemostasis by altering platelet interactions with blood vessels and/or coagulation factors. These defects are either congenital or acquired.

CONGENITAL QUALITATIVE PLATELET DISORDERS

Disorders of Platelet Adhesion (Bernard-Soulier Syndrome)

This syndrome is characterized by deficiency of platelets GP 1b, GP IX and GP V.[110-112] The affected platelets are not able to bind vWF and the subendothelium.[113-115] In the majority of the cases, inheritance appears to be autosomal recessive. Common clinical manifestations are purpura, epistaxis, gingival bleeding and menorrhagia. Hematuria and gastrointestinal bleeding may occur, but bleeding into muscles and joints is uncommon.

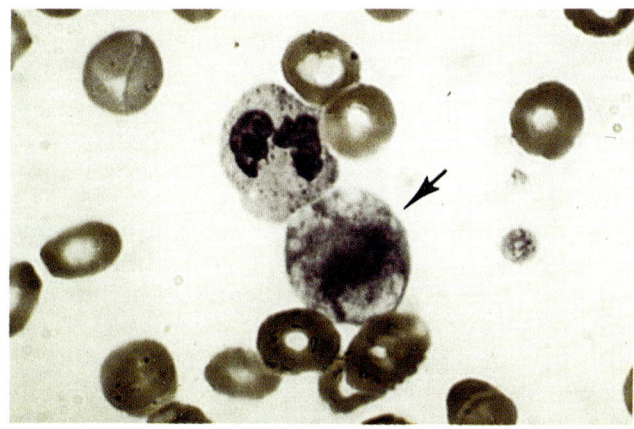

Figure 10-5. Peripheral blood smear demonstrating a giant platelet (arrow).

Peripheral blood examination reveals a normal to moderately reduced platelet count. Platelets are large, averaging two to five times their normal size (Figure 10-5). Abnormal ultrastructural defects have not been observed in transmission electron microscopy, but freeze-fracture studies have demonstrated an abnormal distribution of intramembranous particles.[116,117] It has been demonstrated that GP 1b-IX complexes are attached to the platelet membrane-associated cytoskeleton through an actin-binding protein.[118] One speculation is that interruption of GP-cytoskeleton binding is a factor in altered platelet morphology in Bernard-Soulier syndrome.[110,119] Platelet aggregation studies demonstrate normal aggregation with ADP, collagen and epinephrine and lack of aggregation in the presence of ristocetin.[120-122]

Bone marrow examination is unremarkable. Megakaryocytes are adequate in number and display a normal morphology by light microscopic examination. However, at the ultrastructural level, megakaryocytes may show numerous membrane complexes, an irregular appearance of the demarcation membrane system and many vacuoles.[110] Absence of the expression of GP 1b and reduced expression of GP IX have been demonstrated in the megakaryocytes of patients with Bernard-Soulier syndrome.[123]

Disorders of Platelet Aggregation: Glanzmann Thrombasthenia

Glanzmann thrombasthenia is a rare autosomal recessive disease caused by a deficiency or abnormality of the GP IIb/IIIa complex and is characterized by a normal platelet count and morphology, prolonged bleeding time and defective platelet aggregation.[122,124-127] The GP IIb/IIIa complex is necessary for the binding of platelets to fibrinogen and for platelet aggregation. The GP IIa/IIIb complex also binds to vWF, fibronectin and vitronectin.[128-130] The thrombasthenic platelets fail to aggregate in response to ADP, thrombin, collagen and epinephrine but aggregate in the presence of ristocetin. The most frequent clinical symptoms are menorrhagia, easy bruising, purpura, epistaxis and gingival bleeding.[101] Gastrointestinal bleeding and hematuria are less frequent. Bone marrow examination is unremarkable.

Other Platelet Receptor Defects

Selective impairments of platelet responsiveness to certain proteins (defects in platelet–agonist interaction) such as epinephrine, collagen and thromboxane A_2 may be due to a defect in the structure or expression of a specific platelet receptor. The outcome is often an abnormality in the aggregation-secretion responses.

Defect in Response to Epinephrine

Epinephrine, through platelet α_2-adrenergic receptors, induces platelet aggregation and secretion, and inhibits adenylate cyclase activity in platelets.[109,131,132]

Defect in Response to Collagen

Collagen promotes platelet spreading and adhesion to the subendothelial matrix. Studies related to the specific platelet receptors for collagen are still inconclusive, though there are reports suggesting GP 1a.[133,134]

Defect in Response to Thromboxane A2

Platelet abnormal function in some patients is due to a defect in the thromboxane A_2 receptor or to impairment of the platelet response to thromboxane A_2.[135,136] However, the response to thromboxane A_2 appears to be ADP dependent, and a defect in platelet ADP secretion can cause impairment of the platelet response to thromboxane A_2.[137]

Deficiency of Secretory Granules and Disorders of Platelet Secretion

In these congenital disorders, either platelet granules or their contents are reduced or there is a defect in the ability of the platelets to release their contents. Dense granules contain serotonin, pyrophosphate, calcium, ADP and ATP. Approximately 65% of the platelet adenine nucleotides are stored in dense granules, with an ATP:ADP ratio of 2:3. The dense granule pool is metabolically inactive. The α-granules contain numerous proteins including fibrinogen, platelet factor 4, platelet-derived growth factor, β-thromboglobulin, factor V, vWF, high molecular weight kininogen, ATP and ADP (the ATP:ADP ratio is 8–10:1). The α-granule contents are metabolically active. In addition to dense and α-granules, platelets contain vesicles with acid hydrolases. These vesicles are involved in the arachidonic acid pathways and in thromboxane A_2 production.

Dense Granule Deficiency (δ-Storage Pool Disease)

This syndrome is characterized by a marked decrease in or absence of dense granules in the affected platelets. The total platelet and dense granule contents of ADP and ATP are reduced.[138,139] Similarly, there is evidence of a decline in other dense granule contents such as calcium, serotonin and pyrophosphate.[140,141] Platelets are normal in size and number and demonstrate unremarkable ultrastructural features, except for a marked deficiency or absense of dense granules.[142,143]

Patients with dense granule deficiency demonstrate a mild to moderate bleeding diathesis such as easy bruising, epistaxis, gingival bleeding and menorrhagia. The bleeding time is usually prolonged, and platelet aggregation studies reveal absence of the second wave of aggregation with ADP and epinephrine and an impaired aggregation response to collagen.[109] Dense granule deficiency has been associated with a number of other congenital abnormalities such as the Hermansky-Pudlak syndrome (oculocutaneous albinism and increased ceroid in the mononuclear phagocytic system), CHS, the Wiscott-Aldich syndrome and the thrombocytopenia–absent-radii syndrome.[144,149]

α-Granule Deficiency (Gray Platelet Syndrome, α-Storage Pool Disease)

This syndrome is due to reduction or absence of platelet α-granules.[150-152] Affected patients have a history of bleeding diathesis and show a mild thrombocytopenia. Platelets appear gray in peripheral blood smears stained with Wright's stain. Ultrastructural studies of the affected platelets reveal absent or markedly decreased α-granules, presence of numerous vacuoles, normal numbers of dense granules and mitochondria and a prominent open canalicular system.[143,153] Affected megakaryocytes also show absence or decreased numbers of α-granules and presence of small granules which are assumed to be the precursors of α-granules.[154] The basic abnormality in gray platelet syndrome appears to be a megakaryocytic defect in transferring endogenously synthesized proteins into α-granule precursors.[155] The bone marrow fibrosis observed in this condition may be the direct result of the release of the platelet-derived growth factor into the bone marrow stroma due to the inability of the affected megakaryocytes to store this growth factor in α-granules.[155]

Patients show a prolonged bleeding time and variable responses in platelet aggregation studies. The platelet response to collagen is decreased or absent in some patients and normal in others.[150-152,156] The most consistent finding in this disorder is impairment of thrombin-induced aggregation and secretion.[109] The aggregation pattern of gray platelets following stimulation with ADP, epinephrine and arachidonic acid varies from normal to abnormal.[151,155]

Abnormalities in Platelet Arachidonic Acid Pathways

Liberation of arachidonic acid and formation of thromboxane A_2 is one of the major responses of platelets during activation. Thromboxane A_2 is necessary for platelet secretion during stimulation of platelets with ADP, epinephrine, and low concentrations of collagen and thrombin.[109]

Abnormalities in arachidonic acid pathways are extremely rare and include (1) a defect in the liberation of arachidonic acid from phospholipids and (2) deficiencies of cyclooxygenase and thromboxane synthetase.[109,157-159] Most of the reported patients with these defects have been adults with a mild to moderate bleeding diathesis.[109]

Platelet Secretion Defects with Normal Granule Stores and Normal Thromboxane Synthesis

Several patients have been reported with mild to moderate bleeding manifestations and abnormal platelet secretion without evidence of a defect in arachidonic acid pathways or abnormal granule stores. The mechanism of the impaired secretion is not well understood, though the possibility of a defect in calcium mobilization has been entertained.[160]

ACQUIRED QUALITATIVE PLATELET DISORDERS

Acquired platelet dysfunctions are very common and are observed in association with a large number of drugs, a variety of foods, and many pathologic conditions such as cardiopulmonary bypass, chronic renal disease and hematologic disorders.[107]

Drug- and Food-Induced Platelet Dysfunction

Aspirin

Aspirin irreversibly inactivates cylcooxygenase, inhibits the production of thromboxane A_2 from arachidonic acid and impairs platelet secretion. The end result is abnormal platelet aggregation and a prolonged bleeding time. In approximately 50% of normal subjects, after administration of 650 mg aspirin the bleeding time increases beyond the normal range which may last for 4 days.[161,162] Ethanol ingestion may enhance prolongation of the bleeding time in individuals who take aspirin.[163]

β-Lactam Antibiotics

Abnormal platelet aggregation and prolongation of the bleeding time have been demonstrated in association with the use of many β-lactam–containing antibiotics such as penicillin and cephalosporin derivatives.[107,164-166] These antibiotics appear to interfere with the function of a variety of platelet membrane integrins. The effect is dose and duration dependent.

Other Drugs and Foods

Many drugs and foods may induce abnormal platelet aggregation, often without prolongation of the bleeding time or significant bleeding. For example, dextran can increase the bleeding time in normal persons but does not increase operative or postoperative bleeding, and therefore has been used in the prevention of postsurgical thromboembolic complications.[167] Excessive garlic ingestion may induce platelet dysfunction.[168] Diets rich in marine oils reduce the platelet content of arachidonic acid, and may cause abnormal platelet aggregation and slight prolongation of the bleeding time.[107,169]

Platelet Dysfunction Associated with Pathologic Conditions

Cardiopulmonary Bypass

Prolonged bleeding time, abnormal platelet aggregation and thrombocytopenia are some of the common features of cardiopulmonary bypass.[170] During bypass surgery, platelets adhere to fibrinogen absorbed by the bypass circuit. Bypass procedures also enhance thrombin and ADP generation and complement activation.[107] In uncomplicated bypass surgery, abnormal platelet function usually returns to normal within 1 hour after the operation.

Chronic Renal Failure

The primary hemostatic defect in chronic renal failure and uremia appears to be platelet dysfunction, evi-

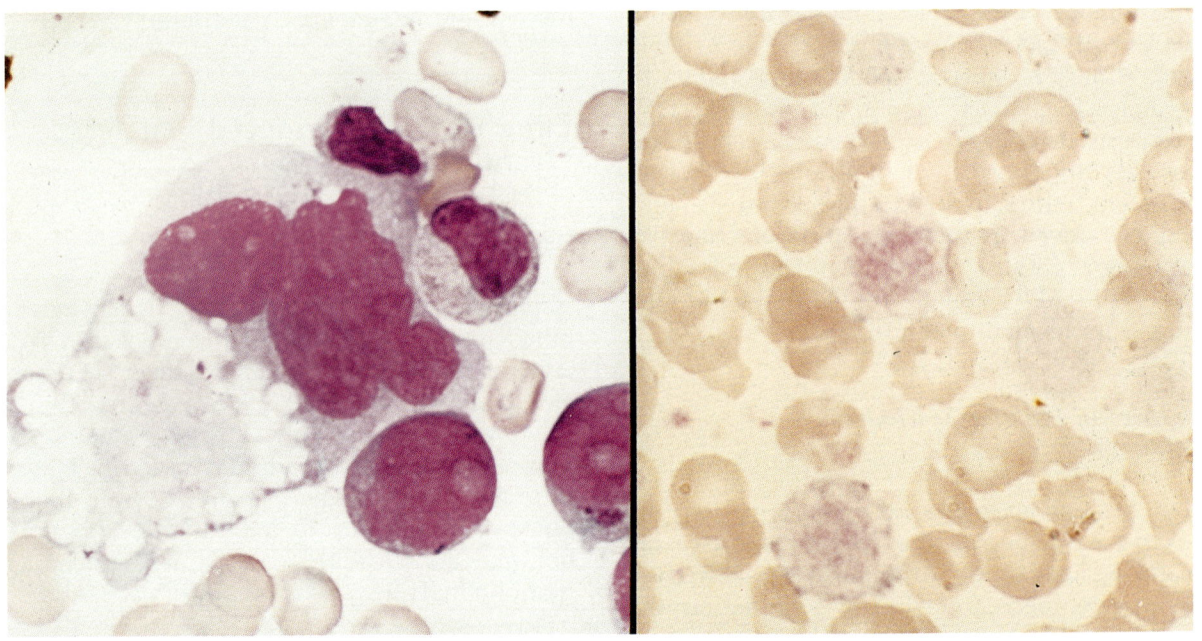

Figure 10-6. Megakaryocyte and platelet abnormalities in a patient with myelodysplastic syndrome (refractory anemia with excess blasts). A bone marrow smear (a) demonstrates a vacuolated megakaryocyte, and a peripheral blood smear (b) shows micro- and giant platelets. Several hypogranular platelets are present.

denced by abnormal secretion and aggregation.[171,172] The bleeding time is frequently prolonged, and there may be bleeding manifestations such as purpura, epistaxis, menorrhagia, gastrointestinal hemorrhage and hematuria. Abnormal platelet function may improve after the uremia is corrected.

Hematologic Disorders

Abnormal platelet function and morphology may occur in myelodysplastic syndrome, myeloproliferative disorders, acute myelogenous leukemia and hairy cell leukemia.[173-176] Morphologic changes in platelets include abnormal shapes, marked variation in size with giant forms, and hypogranularity (Figure 10-6). Abnormal functions include a decline in platelet procoagulant activities and decreased aggregation and secretion in response to ADP, epinephrine and collagen. Abnormal platelet function also occurs in a significant proportion of patients with IgA or IgG myeloma and in patients with Waldenstrom's macrogammaglobulinemia.[177]

References

1. Vainchenker W, Kieffer N: Human megakaryocytopoiesis: In vitro regulation and characterization of megakaryocytic precursor cells by differentiation markers. *Blood Rev* 2:102, 1988.
2. Hegyi E, Navarro S, Debili N, et al: Regulation of human megakaryocytopoiesis: Analysis of proliferation, ploidy and maturation in liquid cultures. *Int J Cell Cloning* 8:236, 1990.
3. Gewirtz AM: Human megakaryocytopoiesis. *Semin Hematol* 23:27, 1986.
4. Long MW: Regulation of human megakaryocytopoiesis. *Ann NY Acad Sci* 554:192, 1989.
5. Burkhardt R: Bone marrow in megakaryocytic disorders. *Hematol Oncol Clin North Am* 2:695, 1988.
6. Jandl JH: Disorders of platelets, in Jandl JH (ed), *Textbook of Hematology*, Boston, Little, Brown, 1987, p 1041.
7. Slater LM, Katz J, Walter B, et al: Aplastic anemia occurring as a megakaryocytic thrombocytopenia with and without an inhibitor of granulocytopoiesis. *Am J Hematol* 18:25, 1985.
8. Hall JG: Thrombocytopenia and absent radius (TAR) syndrome. *J Med Genet* 24:79, 1987.
9. Berge T, Brunnhage F, Nisson LR: Congenital thrombocytopenia in rubella embryopathy. *Acta Pediatr Scand* 52:349, 1963.
10. Day HJ, Holmsen H: Platelet adenine nucleotide storage pool deficiency in thrombocytopenic absent radii syndrome. *JAMA* 221:1053, 1972.
11. Levin J, Conley CL: Thrombocytosis associated with malignant disease. *Arch Intern Med* 114:497, 1964.
12. Liebelt RA, Gehring G, Delmonte L, et al: Paraneoplastic syndrome in experimental animal systems. *Ann NY Acad Sci* 230:547, 1974.
13. McMillan R: Chronic idiopathic thrombocytopenic purpura. *N Engl Med* 304:1135, 1983.
14. Mueller-Eckhardt C, Kayser W, Mersch-Baumert K, et al: The clinical significance of PAIgG. A study of 298 patients with various disorders. *Br J Haematol* 46:123. 1980.
15. Bussel JB: Autoimmune thrombocytopenic purpura. *Hematol Oncol Clin North Am* 4:179, 1990.
16. Van Leeuwen EF, van der Van JTH, Engelfriet CP, et al: Specificity of autoantibodies in autoimmune thrombocytopenia. *Blood* 59:23, 1982.
17. Beardsley DS, Spiegel JE, Jacobs MM, et al: Platelet membrane glycoprotein IIIa contains target antigens that bind anti-platelet antibodies in immune thrombocytopenias. *J Clin Invest* 74:1701, 1984.
18. Nugent D, Kunicki TJ, Furihata K, et al: Human monoclonal antibodies to platelet glycoprotein Ib (GPIb). *Blood* 70:356a, 1986.
19. Woods VL Jr, Kurata Y, Montgomery RR, et al: Autoantibodies against platelet glycoprotein Ib in patients with chronic immune thrombocytopenic purpura. *Blood* 64:156, 1984.
20. McMillan R, Tani P, Millard F, et al: Platelet-associated and plasma antiglycoprotein autoantibodies in chronic ITP. *Blood* 70:1040, 1987.
21. Karpatkin M, Siskind GW, Karpatkin S: The platelet factor 3 immunoinjury technique reevaluated. Development of a rapid test for anti-platelet antibody. Detection in various clinical disorders, including immunologic drug-induced and neonatal thrombocytopenias. *J Lab Clin Med* 89:400, 1977.
22. Field SK, Poon M-C: Sarcoidosis presenting as chronic thrombocytopenia. *West J Med* 146:481, 1987.
23. Waddell CC, Cimo PL: Idiopathic thrombocytopenic purpura occurring in Hodgkin's disease after splenectomy: Report of two cases and review of the literature. *Am J Hematol* 7:381, 1979.
24. Merl SA, Theodorakis ME, Goldberg J, et al: Splenectomy for thrombocytopenia in chronic lymphocytic leukemia. *Am J Hematol* 15:253, 1983.
25. Agai E, Quitt M, Lurie M, et al: Primary hepatic lym-

phoma presenting as symptomatic immune thrombocytopenic purpura. *Cancer* 60:2308, 1987.
26. Budman DR, Steinberg AD: Hematologic aspects of systemic lupus erythematosus: Current concepts. *Ann Intern Med* 86:220, 1977.
27. Harris EN, Asherson RA, Gharavi AE, et al: Thrombocytopenia in SLE and related autoimmune disorders: Association with anticardiolipin antibody. *Br J Haematol* 59:227, 1985.
28. Kurata Y, Nishioed Y, Tsubakio T, et al: Thrombocytopenia in Graves' disease: Effect of T3 on platelet immunoglobulin G in Graves' disease and Hashimoto's thyroiditis. *Ann Intern Med* 94:27, 1981.
29. Gupta S, Saverymuttu SH, Marsh JCW, et al: Immune thrombocytopenic purpura, neutropenia and sclerosing angiitis associated with ulcerative colitis in an adult. *Clin Lab Haematol* 8:67, 1986.
30. Lester TJ, Grabowski GA, Goldblatt J, et al: Immune thrombocytopenia and Gaucher's disease. *Am J Med* 77:569, 1984.
31. Kosmo MA, Bordin G, Tani P, et al: Immune thrombocytopenia and Crohn's disease (letter). *Ann Intern Med* 104:136, 1986.
32. Selinger S, Tsai J, Pulini M, et al: Autoimmune thrombocytopenia and primary biliary cirrhosis with hypoglycemia and insulin receptor autoantibodies. A case report. *Ann Intern Med* 107:686, 1987.
33. Woerner SJ, Abildgaard CF, et al: Intracranial hemorrhage in children with idiopathic thrombocytopenic purpura. *Pediatrics* 67:453, 1981.
34. Lusher JM, Lyer R: Idiopathic thrombocytopenic purpura in children. *Semin Thromb Hemost* 3:175, 1977.
35. McClure PD: Idiopathic thrombocytopenic purpura in children: Diagnosis and management. *Pediatrics* 55:68, 1975.
36. Yeager AM, Zinkham WH: Varicella-associated thrombocytopenia: Clues to the etiology of childhood idiopathic thrombocytopenic purpura. *Johns Hopkins Med J* 146:270, 1980.
37. Carpentieri U, Haggard ME: Thrombocytopenia and viral diseases. *Tex Med* 71:81, 1975.
38. Aboulafia DM, Mitsuyasu RT: Hematologic abnormalities in AIDS. *Hematol Oncol Clin North Am* 5:195, 1991.
39. Murphy MF, Metcalf P, Walters AH, et al: Incidence and mechanism of neutropenia and thrombocytopenia in patients with human immunodeficiency virus infection. *Br J Haematol* 66:337, 1987.
40. Karpatkin S: HIV-1-related thrombocytopenia. *Hematol Oncol Clin North Am* 4:193, 1990.
41. Ciaffoni S, Ferro I, Potenza R, et al: Evans syndrome: A case of autoimmune thrombocytopenia and autoimmune hemolytic anemia caused by anti-JK. *Haematologica* 72:245, 1987.
42. George JN: Platelet IgG: Measurement, interpretation, and clinical significance. *Prog Hemost Thromb* 10:97, 1991.
43. McKenna JL, Pisciotta AV: Fluorescence of megakaryocytes in ITP stained with fluorescent antiglobulin serum. *Blood* 19:664, 1962.
44. McMillan R, Luiken GA, et al: Antibody against megakaryocytes in ITP. *JAMA* 239:2460, 1978.
45. Christie DJ, Mullen PC, Aster RH: Fab-mediated binding of drug-dependent antibodies to platelets in quinidine- and quinine-induced thrombocytopenia. *J Clin Invest* 75:310, 1985.
46. Smith ME, Reid DM, Jones CE, et al: Binding of quinine- and quinidine-dependent drug antibodies to platelets is mediated by the Fab domain of the immunoglobulin G and is not Fc dependent. *J Clin Invest* 79:912, 1987.
47. Lerner W, Caruso R, Faig D, et al: Drug-dependent and non-drug-dependent antiplatelet antibody in drug-induced immunologic thrombocytopenia. *Blood* 66:306, 1985.
48. Van dem Borne AEG Jr, Pegels JG, van der Stadt RJ, et al: Thrombocytopenia associated with gold therapy: A drug-induced autoimmune disease? *Br J Haematol* 63:509, 1986.
49. Marcus GJ, Stevenson M, Brown T: Alpha-methyldopa–induced immune thrombocytopenia. Report of a case. *Am J Clin Pathol* 64:113, 1975.
50. Murphy MF, Riordan T, Minchinton RM, et al: Demonstration of an immune-mediated mechanism of penicillin-induced neutropenia and thrombocytopenia. *Br J Haematol* 55:155, 1983.
51. Warkentin TE, Kelton JG: Heparin and platelets. *Hematol Oncol North Am* 4:243, 1990.
52. Lynch DM, Howe SE: Heparin-associated thrombocytopenia: Antibody binding specificity to platelet antigens. *Blood* 66:1176, 1985.
53. Sheridan D, Carter C, Kelton JA: A diagnostic test for heparin-induced thrombocytopenia. *Blood* 67:27, 1986.
54. Warkentin TE, Kelton JG: Heparin-induced thrombocytopenia. *Prog Hemost Thromb* 10:1, 1991.
55. Skacel PO, Conteras M: Neonatal alloimmune thrombocytopenia. *Blood Rev* 3:174, 1989.
56. Van dem Borne AEC Jr, van Leeuwen E, von Riesz LE, et al: Neonatal alloimmune thrombocytopenia: Detection and characterization of the responsible antibodies by platelet immunofluorescence test. *Blood* 57:649, 1981.
57. Muller-Eckhardt C, Kiefel V, Grubert A, et al: 348 cases of suspected neonatal alloimmune thrombocytopenia. *Lancet* 1:363, 1989.
58. Reznikoff-Etievant MF, Muller JY, Julien F, et al: An immune response gene linked to HLA in man. *Tissue Antigens* 22:312, 1983.

59. Evans DIK: Immune amegakaryocytic thrombocytopenia of the newborn: Association with anti-HLA-A2. *J Clin Pathol* 40:258, 1987.
60. Sternbach MS, Malette M, Nadon F, et al: Severe alloimmune neonatal thrombocytopenia due to specific HLA antibodies. *Cur Stud Hematol Blood Trans* 52:97, 1986.
61. Naidu S: Central nervous system lesions in neonatal isoimmune thrombocytopenia. *Arch Neurol* 40:552, 1983.
62. Morales JW, Stroup M: Intracranial haemorrhage in utero due to isoimmune neonatal thrombocytopenia. *J Paediatr* 97:695, 1985.
63. Territo M, Finkelstein J, Oh H, et al: Management of autoimmune thrombocytopenia in pregnancy and in the neonate. *Obstet Gynecol* 41:579, 1973.
64. Hedge UM: Immune thrombocytopenia in pregnancy and the newborn (letter). *Br J Obstet Gynecol* 92:657, 1985.
65. Kelton JG, Inwood MJ, Barr RM, et al: The prenatal prediction of thrombocytopenia in infants of mothers with clinically diagnosed immune thrombocytopenia. *Am J Obstet Gynecol* 144:449, 1982.
66. Muller-Eckhardt C: Post-transfusion purpura. *Br J Haematol* 64:419, 1986.
67. De Waal LP, van Dalen CM, Engelfriet CP, et al: Alloimmunization against the platelet-specific ZWa antigen resulting in neonatal alloimmune thrombocytopenic purpura or post-transfusion purpura is associated with the supertypic DRw52 antigen including DR3 and DRw6. *Hum Immunol* 17:45, 1986.
68. Capron A, Joseph M, Ameisen JC, et al: Platelets as effectors in immune and hypersensitivity reactions. *Int Arch Allergy Appl Immunol* 82:307, 1987.
69. Cines DB, van der Keyl H, Levinson AI: In vitro binding of an IgE protein to human platelets. *J Immunol* 136:3433, 1986.
70. Ruggenenti P, Giuseppe R: Thrombotic thrombocytopenic purpura and related disorders. *Hematol Oncol North Am* 4:219, 1990.
71. Amorosi EL, Ultmann JE: Thrombotic thrombocytopenic purpura: Report of 16 cases and review of the literature. *Medicine* 45:139, 1966.
72. Kennedy SS, Zachrski LR, Beck JR: Thrombotic thrombocytopenic purpura: Analysis of 48 unselected cases. *Semin Thromb Haemost* 6:341, 1980.
73. Dekker A, O'Brien ME, Cammarata RJ: The association of thrombotic thrombocytopenic purpura with systemic lupus erythematosus. *Am J Med Sci* 267:243, 1974.
74. Steinberg AD, Green WT, Talal N: Thrombotic thrombocytopenic purpura complicating Sjögren's syndrome. *JAMA* 215:757, 1971.
75. Benitez L, Mathews M, Mallory GK: Platelet thrombosis with polyarteritis nodosa: Report of a case. *Arch Pathol* 77:116, 1964.
76. Moake JL, Rudy CK, Troll JH, et al: Unusually large plasma factor VIII: Von Willebrand factor multimers in chronic relapsing thrombotic thrombocytopenic purpura. *N Engl J Med* 307:1432, 1982.
77. Chen Y-C, Hall ER, McLeod B, et al: Accelerated prostacyclin degradation in thrombotic thrombocytopenic purpura. *Lancet* 2:267, 1981.
78. Wu KK, Hall ER, Rossi EC, et al: Serum prostacyclin binding defects in thrombotic thrombocytopenic purpura. *J Clin Invest* 75:168, 1985.
79. Glas-Greenwalt P, Hall JM, Panke TW, et al: Fibrinolysis in health and disease: Abnormal levels of plasminogen activator, plasminogen activator inhibitor, and protein C in thrombotic thrombocytopenic purpura. *J Lab Clin Med* 108:415, 1986.
80. Kwaan HC: Role of fibrinolysis in thrombotic thrombocytopenic purpura. *Semin Hematol* 24:101, 1987.
81. Siddiqui FA, Lian EC-Y: Novel platelet agglutinating protein P37 from a thrombotic thrombocytopenic purpura plasma. *J Clin Invest* 76:1330, 1985.
82. Holdrinet RSG, de Pauw BE, Hannen C: Hormonal dependent thrombotic thrombocytopenic purpura. *Scand J Haematol* 30:250, 1983.
83. Bukowski RM: Thrombotic thrombocytopenic purpura: A review, in Spaet TH (ed), *Progress in Hemostasis and Thrombosis*. New York, Grune and Stratton, 1982, p 287.
84. Fuchs WE, George JN, Dotin LN, et al: Thrombotic thrombocytopenic purpura. Occurrence two years apart during late pregnancy in two sisters. *JAMA* 235:2126, 1976.
85. Berkowitz LR, Dalldorf FG, Blatt PM: Thrombotic thrombocytopenic purpura: A pathologic review. *JAMA* 241:1709, 1979.
86. Moake JL: Recent observations on the pathophysiology of thrombotic thrombocytopenic purpura and the hemolytic-uremic syndrome. *Hematol Pathol* 4:197, 1990.
87. Karmali MA, Steele BT, Petrie M, et al: Sporadic cases of haemolytic uremic syndrome associated with faecal cytotoxin and cytotoxin producing *Escherichia coli* in stools. *Lancet* 1:619, 1983.
88. Karmali MA, Petrie M, Lim C, et al: The association between idiopathic hemolytic-uremic syndrome and infection by verotoxin-producing *Escherichia* coli. *J Infect Dis* 151:775, 1985.
89. Moorthy B, Makker SP: Hemolytic-uremic syndrome associated with pneumococcal sepsis. *J Pediatr* 95:558, 1979.
90. Prober CG, Tune B, Hoder L: *Yersinia pseudotuberculosis* septicemia. *Am J Dis Child* 133:623, 1979.
91. Delans RD, Biuso JD, Saba SR: Hemolytic-uremic

syndrome after *Campylobacter*-induced diarrhea in an adult. *Arch Intern Med* 144:1074, 1984.
92. Baker NM, Mills AG, Rachman I: Haemolytic-uremic syndrome in typhoid fever. *Br Med J* 2:84, 1974.
93. Sharman VL, Goodwin FJ: Hemolytic-uremic syndrome following chicken pox. *Clin Nephrol* 14:49, 1980.
94. Austin TW, Ray CG; Coxsackie virus group B infections and hemolytic-uremic syndrome. *J Infect Dis* 127:698, 1973.
95. O'Regan S, Robitaille P, Mongeau J-G, et al: The hemolytic-uremic syndrome associated with ECHO 22 infection. *Clin Pediatr* 19:125, 1980.
96. Kaplan BS, Chesney RW, Drummond KN: Hemolytic-uremic syndrome in families. *N Engl J Med* 292:1090, 1975.
97. Pirson Y, Lefebvre C, Arnout C, et al: Hemolytic-uremic syndrome in 3 adult siblings: A familial study and evolution. *Clin Nephrol* 28:250, 1987.
98. Cantrell JE Jr, Phillips TM, Schein PS: Carcinoma-associated hemolytic-uremic syndrome: A complication of mitomycin C chemotherapy. *J Clin Oncol* 3:723, 1895.
99. Sheldon R, Slaughter D: A syndrome of microangiopathic hemolytic anemia, renal impairment, and pulmonary edema in chemotherapy-related patients with adenocarcinoma. *Cancer* 58:1428, 1986.
100. Jackson AM, Rose BD, Graff LG, et al: Thrombotic microangiopathy and renal failure associated with antineoplastic chemotherapy. *Ann Intern Med* 101:41, 1984.
101. George JN, Aster RH: Thrombocytopenia due to enhanced platelet destruction by nonimmunologic mechanisms, in Williams WJ, Beutler E, Erslev AJ, et al (eds), *Hematology*, ed 4. New York, McGraw-Hill, 1990, p 1351.
102. Glueck R, Green D, Cohen I, et al: Hematin: Unique effects on hemostasis. *Blood* 61:243, 1983.
103. Wakefield TW, Bouffard JA, Spauding SA, et al: Sequestration of platelets in the pulmonary circulation as a consequence of protamine reversal of the anticoagulant effects of heparin. *J Vasc Surg* 5:187, 1987.
104. Hilgard H, Hossfeld DK: Transient bleomycin-induced thrombocytopenia: A clinical study. *Eur J Cancer* 14:1261, 1978.
105. Verwey J, Breed WPM, Hillen HFP: Bleomycin-induced early-onset transient decrease in platelet counts. *Neth J Med* 27:202, 1984.
106. Spiegel JE, Levey AS: Life-threatening thrombocytopenia complicating antithymocyte globulin therapy for acute kidney transplant rejection. Evidence for in situ immune complex formation on the platelet surface. *Transplantation* 45:647, 1988.
107. George JN, Shattil SJ: The clinical importance of acquired abnormalities of platelet function. *N Engl J Med* 324:27, 1991.
108. Ginsberg MH, Loftus J, Plow EF: Platelets and the adhesion receptor superfamily, in Jamieson GA (ed), *Platelet Membrane Receptors: Molecular Biology, Immunology, Biochemistry, and Pathology: Proceedings of the 19th Annual Scientific Symposium of the American Red Cross. Progress in Clinical and Biological Research*, Vol 238, New York, Alan R Liss, 1988, p 171.
109. Rao KA: Congenital disorders of platelet function. *Hematol Oncol North Am* 4:65, 1990.
110. Nurden AT, Pico M, Heilmann E, et al: Inherited disorders of platelets and megakaryocytes. *Prog Clin Biol Res* 356:333, 1990.
111. Berndt MC, Gregory C, Chong BH, et al: Additional glycoprotein defects in Bernard-Soulier's syndrome: Confirmation of genetic basis by parenteral analysis. *Blood* 62:800, 1983.
112. Clemetson KL, McGregor JL, James E, et al: Characterization of the platelet membrane glycoprotein abnormalities in Bernard-Soulier syndrome and comparison with the normal by surface-labeling techniques and high resolution two dimensional gel electrophoresis. *J Clin Invest* 70:304, 1982.
113. Caen JP, Nurden AT, Jeannaeu C, et al: Bernard-Soulier syndrome: A new platelet glycoprotein abnormality. Its relationship with platelet adhesion to subendothelium and with the factor VIII von Willebrand protein. *J Lab Med* 87:586, 1976.
114. Weiss HJ, Tschopp TB, Baumgartner HR: Decreased adhesion of giant (Bernard-Soulier) platelets to subendothelium. Further implications on the role of the von Willebrand factor in hemostasis. *Am J Med* 57:920, 1974.
115. Weiss HJ, Turitto VT, Baumgartner HR, et al: Platelet adhesion and thrombus formation on subendothelium in platelets deficient in glycoproteins IIb–IIIa, Ib and storage granules. *Blood* 67:322, 1986.
116. White JG: Structural defects in inherited and giant platelet disorders. *Adv Hum Genet* 19:133, 1990.
117. Chevalier J, Nurden AT, Thiere JM, et al: Freeze-fracture studies on the plasma membranes of normal human, thrombasthenic and Bernard-Soulier platelets. *J Lab Clin Med* 94:232, 1979.
118. Fox JEB, Boyles JK, Steffen PK, et al: Identification of a membrane skeleton in platelets. *J Cell Biol* 106:1525, 1988.
119. White JG, Burris SM, Hasegawa D, et al: Micropipette aspiration of human blood platelets: A defect in Bernard-Soulier syndrome. *Blood* 63:1249, 1984.
120. Evensen SA, Solum NO, Grottum KA, et al: Familial bleeding disorder with a moderate thrombocytopenia and giant blood platelets. *Scand J Haematol* 13:203, 1974.
121. Howard MA, Hutton RA, Hardisty RM: Hereditary giant platelet syndrome: A disorder of a new aspect of platelet function. *Br Med J* 4:586, 1973.

122. McEver RP: The clinical significance of platelet membrane glycoproteins. *Hematol Oncol North Am* 4:87, 1990.
123. Nurden AT, Jallu V, Hourdille P: GP Ib and Bernard-Soulier platelets. *Blood* 73:2225, 1989.
124. Weiss HJ, Kochwa S: Studies on platelet function and proteins in three patients with Glanzmann's thrombasthenia. *J Lab Clin Med* 71:153, 1968.
125. Nurden AT, Caen JP: An abnormal platelet glycoprotein pattern in three cases of Glanzmann's thrombasthenia. *Br J Haematol* 28:233, 1974.
126. Phillips DR, Agin PP: Platelet membrane defects in Glanzmann's thrombasthenia. *J Clin Invest* 60:535, 1977.
127. George JN, Caen JP, Nurden AT: Glanzmann's thrombasthenia: The spectrum of clinical disease. *N Engl J Med* 75:1383, 1990.
128. Ginsberg MH, Forsyth J, Lightsey A, et al: Reduced surface expression and binding of fibronectin by thrombin-stimulated thrombasthenic platelets. *J Clin Invest* 71:619, 1983.
129. Ruggeri ZM, Bader R, Demarco L: Glanzmann thrombasthenia: Deficient binding of von Willebrand factor. *J Clin Invest* 72:1, 1983.
130. Pytela R, Pierschbacher MD, Ginsberg MH, et al: Platelet membrane glycoprotein IIb/IIIa: Member of a family of Arg-Gly-Asp–specific adhesion receptors. *Science* 231:1559, 1986.
131. Rao AK, Willis J, Kowalska MA, et al: Differential requirements for platelet aggregation and inhibition of adenylate cyclase by epinephrine. Studies of a familial alpha-2-adrenergic receptor defect. *Blood* 71:494, 1988.
132. Tamponi G, Pannocchia A, Arduino C, et al: Congenital deficiency of alpha-2-adrenoreceptors on human platelets: Description of two cases. *Thromb Haemost* 58:1012, 1987.
133. Nieuwenhuis HK, Akkerman JW, Houdijk WPM, et al: Human platelets showing no response to collagen fail to express surface glycoprotein Ia. *Nature* 318:470, 1985.
134. Nieuwenhuis HK, Sakariassen KS, Houdijk WPM, et al: Deficiency of platelet membrane glycoprotein Ia is associated with a decreased platelet adhesion to subendothelium: A defect in platelet spreading. *Blood* 68:692, 1986.
135. Wu KK, LeBreton GC, Thai HH, et al: Abnormal platelet response to thromboxane A_2. *J Clin Invest* 67:1801, 1981.
136. Samama M, Lecrubier C, Conrad J, et al: Constitutional thrombocytopathy with subnormal response to thromboxane A_2. *Br J Haematol* 48:293, 1981.
137. Rao AK, Willis J, Holmsen H: A major role of ADP in thromboxane transfer experiments: Studies in patients with platelet secretion defects. *J Lab Clin Med* 104:116, 1984.
138. Holmsen H, Weiss HJ: Hereditary defect in the release reaction caused by a deficiency in the storage pool of platelet adenine nucleotides. *Br J Haematol* 19:643, 1970.
139. Holmsen H, Weiss HJ: Further evidence for a deficient storage pool of adenine nucleotides in platelets from some patients with thrombocythopathia—"storage pool disease." *Blood* 39:197, 1972.
140. Lages B, Scrutton M, Holmsen H, et al: Metal ion content of gel-filtered platelets from storage pool disease. *Blood* 46:119, 1975.
141. Weiss HJ, Witte LD, Kaplan KL, et al: Heterogeneity in the storage pool deficiency: Studies of granule-bound substances in 18 patients including variants deficient in α-granules, platelet factor-4, β-thromboglobulin and platelet-derived growth factor. *Blood* 54:1296, 1979.
142. White JG: Platelet granule disorders. *Crit Rev Oncol Hematol* 4:337, 1986.
143. White JG: Structural defects in inherited and giant platelet disorders. *Adv Hum Genet* 19:133, 1990.
144. Hardisty RM: Mills DCB, Ketsa-Ard K: The platelet defect associated with albinism. *Br J Haematol* 23:672, 1972.
145. Logan LJ, Rapaport SI, Mather I: Albinism and abnormal platelet function. *N Engl J Med* 284:1340, 1971.
146. Buchanan GR, Handin RI: Platelet function in the Chediak-Higashi syndrome. *Blood* 47:941, 1976.
147. Boxer GJ, Holmsen H, Robkin L, et al: Abnormal platelet function in Chediak-Higashi syndrome. *Br J Haematol* 35:251, 1977.
148. Grottum KA, Hovig T, Holmsen H, et al: Wiscott-Aldrich syndrome: Quantitative platelet defects and short platelet survival. *Br J Haematol* 17:373, 1969.
149. Day HJ, Holmsen H: Platelet adenine nucleotide "storage pool deficiency" in thrombocytopenia absent radii syndrome. *JAMA* 221:1053, 1972.
150. Raccuglia G: Gray platelet syndrome: A variety of qualitative platelet disorder. *Am J Med* 51:818, 1971.
151. Gerrard JM, Phillips DR, Rao GHR, et al: Biochemical studies of two patients with gray platelet syndrome: Selective deficiency of platelet alpha granules. *J Clin Invest* 66:102, 1980.
152. Levy-Toledano S, Caen JP, Breton-Gorius J, et al: Gray platelet syndrome: α-Granule deficiency: Its influence on platelet function. *J Lab Clin Med* 98:831, 1981.
153. White JG: Ultrastructural studies of gray platelet syndrome. *Am J Pathol* 95:445, 1979.
154. Breton-Gorius J, Vainchenker W, Vinci G, et al: Defective α-granule production in megakaryocytes from gray platelet syndrome: Ultrastructural studies of bone marrow cells and megakaryocytes growing in culture from blood precursors. *Am J Pathol* 102:10, 1981.
155. Bennet JS, Shattil SJ: Congenital qualitative platelet disorders, in Williams WJ, Beutler E, Erslev AJ, et al,

(eds), *Hematology*, ed 4. New York, McGraw-Hill, 1990, p 1401.
156. Brendt MC, Castaldi PA, Gordon S, et al: Morphological and biochemical confirmation of gray platelet syndrome in two siblings. *Aust NZ J Med* 13:387, 1983.
157. Rao AK, Koke K, Willis J, et al: Platelet secretion defect associated with impaired liberation of arachidonic acid and normal myosin light chain phosphorylation. *Blood* 64:914, 1984.
158. Ehara H, Yoshimoto T, Yamamoto S, et al: Enzymological and immunological studies on a clinical case of platelet cyclooxygenase abnormality. *Biochem Biophys Acta* 960:35, 1988.
159. Mestel F, Oatlike O, Beck E, et al: Severe bleeding associated with defective thromboxane synthetase. *Lancet* 1:157, 1980.
160. Hardisty RM, Machin SJ, Nokes TJC, et al: A new congenital defect of platelet secretion: Impaired responsiveness of the platelets to cytoplasmic calcium. *Br J Haematol* 53:543, 1983.
161. Mielke CH Jr, Kaneshiro MM, Maher IA, et al: The standardized normal ivy bleeding time and its prolongation by aspirin. *Blood* 34:204, 1969.
162. Mielke CH Jr: Aspirin prolongation of the template bleeding time: Influence of venostasis and direction of incision. *Blood* 60:1139, 1982.
163. Deykin D, Janson P, McMahon L: Ethanol potentiation of aspirin-induced prolongation of the bleeding time. *N Engl J Med* 306:852, 1982.
164. Fass RJ, Copelan EA, Brandt ML, et al: Platelet-mediated bleeding caused by broad-spectrum penicillins. *J Infect Dis* 155:1242, 1987.
165. Natelson EA, Brown CH III, Bradshaw MW, et al: Influence of cephalosporin antibiotics on blood coagulation and platelet function. *Antimicrob Agents Chemother* 9:91, 1976.
166. Brown RB, Klar J, Lemeshow S, et al: Enhanced bleeding with coeoxitin or moxolactam: Statistical analysis within a defined population. *Arch Intern Med* 146:2159, 1986.
167. Gruber UF, Hughes LE, Campbell H, et al: Prevention of postoperative thromboembolism by Dextran 40, low dose heparin, or xantinol nicotinate. *Lancet* 1:207, 1977.
168. Rose KD, Croissant PD, Parliment CF, et al: Spontaneous spinal epidural hematoma with associated platelet dysfunction from excessive garlic ingestion: A case report. *Neurosurgery* 26:880, 1990.
169. Von Schacky C, Weber PC: Metabolism and effects on platelet function of the purified eicosapentaenoic and docosahexaenoic acids in humans. *J Clin Invest* 75:2446, 1985.
170. Holloway DS, Summaria L, Sandesara J, et al: Decreased platelet number and function and increased fibrinolysis contribute to postoperative bleeding in cardiopulmonary bypass patients. *Thromb Haemost* 59:62, 1988.
171. Di Minno G, Cerbone A, Usberti M, et al: Platelet dysfunction in uremia. II. Correction by arachidonic acid of the impaired exposure of fibrinogen receptors by adenosine diphosphate or collagen. *J Lab Clin Med* 108:246, 1986.
172. Escolar G, Cases A, Bastida E, et al: Uremic platelets have functional defect affecting the interaction of von Willebrand factor with glycoprotein IIb/IIIa. *Blood* 76:1336, 1990.
173. Meschengieser S, Blanco A, Maugeri N, et al: Platelet function and interplatelet von Willebrand factor antigen and fibrinogen in myelodysplastic syndromes. *Thromb Res* 46:601, 1987.
174. Schafer AI: Bleeding and thrombosis in the myeloproliferative disorders. *Blood* 64:1, 1984.
175. Cowan DH, Graham RR Jr, Baunach D: The platelet defect in leukemia: Platelet ultrastructure, adenine nucleotide metabolism, and the release reaction. *J Clin Invest* 56:188, 1975.
176. Rosove MH, Naeim F, Harwig S, et al: Severe platelet dysfunction in hairy cell leukemia with improvement after splenectomy. *Blood* 55:903, 1980.
177. Lackner H: Hemostatic abnormalities associated with dysproteinemias. *Semin Hematol* 10:125, 1973.

11 BONE MARROW TRANSPLANTATION

Faramarz Naeim, Robert Peter Gale

During the last decade, there has been considerable progress in using bone marrow transplants to treat neoplastic and nonneoplastic diseases such as aplastic anemia, severe combined immunodeficiency, leukemias, and solid tumors (Table 11-1). This chapter discusses recent advances in bone marrow transplantation in hematologic disorders.

PRINCIPLES OF BONE MARROW TRANSPLANTATION

Bone marrow transplantation is based on the principle of restoring hematopoiesis in patients who receive high-dose chemotherapy and/or radiation therapy or who have defective hematopoiesis.[1-4]

Three sources of bone marrow cells are used: syngeneic (identical twin) transplants, allogeneic transplants, and autologous transplants using the recipient's own bone marrow.

Syngeneic transplants cannot be rejected or cause graft-versus-host disease (GVHD). However, most persons do not have twin donors. Allogeneic grafts, usually from an HLA-identical donor, are the most common transplants.[5-9] Their applicability is limited to about 30–40% of patients with a suitable donor.[5] Selected patients have received transplants from HLA-partially matched, related donors.[10] Patients receiving transplants from a phenotypically identical parent or related donor mismatched for only HLA-A, -B or -D locus have results comparable to those receiving transplants from an HLA-identical sibling. Acceptable family member donors are found for about 10% of patients.[5] Results are less satisfactory in recipients of transplants mismatched for two or more HLA loci. A small number of patients receive transplants from unrelated, HLA-identical donors.[11] Preliminary results suggest a higher risk of GVHD and a lower survival rate.

Table 11-1 Applications of Bone Marrow Transplantation

Congenital disorders
   severe combined immunodeficiency
   Wiskott-Aldrich syndrome
   Fanconi anemia
   Ataxia telangiectasia
   Infantile agranulocytosis
   Chronic granulomatous disease
   Osteopetrosis
   CHS
   Congenital red cell aplasia
   Lysosomal storage diseases
   Cartilage-hair aplasia
   Thalassemia major
Aplastic anemia
Leukemias
   Acute lymphoblastic leukemia
   Acute myelogenous leukemia
   Chronic myelogenous leukemia
Other hematologic malignancies
   Lymphoma
   Multiple myeloma
   Hairy cell leukemia
   Malignant histiocytosis
Myelodysplastic syndromes
Solid tumors
   Breast carcinomas
   Neuroblastomas
   Others

Autologous bone marrow transplantation is sometimes used to treat patients who do not have an HLA-identical sibling. Bone marrow is collected and cryopreserved when the patient is in remission. The patient then receives high-dose chemotherapy and/or radiation therapy followed by reinfusion of the autologous bone marrow.[12-14] Graft rejection and GVHD do not occur with autotransplants, and the incidence of cytomegalovirus infection, usually associated with interstitial pneumonitis, is decreased. The major concern in autotransplants is contamination of the cryopreserved bone marrow with malignant cells. Several different methods are used to eliminate the residual malignant cells from the bone marrow, including density centrifugation, monoclonal antibodies and pharmacologic techniques.

APLASTIC ANEMIA

Bone marrow transplantation is the most effective treatment of aplastic anemia, with 5-year disease-free survival of >50%. Graft rejection is a relatively modest problem, occurring in about 10% of the patients at risk. Graft rejection seems to be related to blood transfusions received by the patient prior to transplantation and is decreased by adding radiation therapy to the conditioning regimen[15-18] (Table 11-2). Other factors contributing to graft rejection include a low dose of marrow cells and a positive relative response in mixed lymphocyte culture.[19,20] Incorporating these observations, modern conditioning regimens result in rejection rates as low as 10%.[21-24] However, radiation therapy results in increased toxicity, especially interstitial pneumonia.

Table 11-2 Results of Allogeneic Bone Marrow Transplantation for Severe Aplastic Anemia*

		Actuarial Survival (%)	
Center	Graft Rejection	CY	CY + TBI
HLA-identical			
Seattle†	10	82	
Seattle	11	73	
IBMTR	11	52–70	54
EBMTR	17	62	40
HLA-mismatched			
Seattle	43	32	50
EBMTR	33	15	30

* Adapted from Sullivan KM, Witherspoon RP, Storb R, et al: Long-term results of allogeneic bone marrow transplantation. *Transplantation Proc* 2: 2928, 1989.
† Untransfused patients only.
CY: Cyclophosphamide
TBI: Total body irradiation

GVHD is one of the major complications of allogeneic bone marrow transplantation. The five-year actuarial probability of survival for patients with moderate to severe acute GVHD is about 35% compared to about 80% for patients with no or only mild acute GVHD.[18]

Recent updated reports by two large transplant registries, IBMTR (International Bone Marrow Transplant Registry) and EBMTR (European Bone Marrow Transplant Registry), show an impressive improvement in the survival rate of HLA-identical transplants for severe aplastic anemia (about 60%) at 4 to 6 years.[18,25] The results of HLA-mismatched transplants are less encouraging: 25% for one HLA-antigen mismatched grafts and 11% for grafts mismatched at more than one HLA-locus.[26]

ACUTE LYMPHOBLASTIC LEUKEMIA (ALL)

Bone marrow transplantation in patients with advanced ALL results in 10–20% long-term survival. This outcome is clearly superior to that achieved with chemotherapy.[1,2,27] Even better results are reported in patients receiving transplants in the first or second remission (Table 11-3). There is considerable debate over whether high-risk subtypes of ALL [B- or T-cell ALL, age <1 or >20 years, WBC >50 × 10/liter, CNS involvement, t(9;22) or t(4;11) chromosome translocations] should receive an allogeneic transplant in the first remission. Preliminary data from the IBMTR on high-risk subtypes of ALL demonstrate an actuarial 60% survival for persons transplanted in the first remission compared with 25% for similar patients transplanted in the second remission.[28] Actuarial relapse rates are 20% and 60%, respectively. Transplant-related complications account for 25–35% of the failures.

The results of autotransplants in ALL are less impressive. Relapse rates for autotransplants in persons with advanced ALL range from 60% to 100%.[29] Various techniques have been used to eliminate residual ALL cells from the cryopreserved bone marrow sample; monoclonal antibodies are used most commonly.[30,31] The outcome is better for patients with favorable prognostic factors such as those relapsing after a long first remission. However, these patients are also expected to respond favorably to chemotherapy.

Table 11-3 Results of Chemotherapy and Allogeneic Bone Marrow Transplantation from HLA-identical Siblings for Acute Leukemia*

Disease Status	Survival (%)†	
	Bone Marrow Transplant	Chemotherapy
ALL		
Advanced	15 (10–20)	0
2nd remission	35 (25–45)	5 (0–10)
1st remission	50 (30–60)	30 (10–60)
AML		
Advanced	15 (10–30)	0
2nd remission or initial relapse	30 (15–50)	<5
1st remission		
<20 years	50 (40–70)	30 (20–60)
20–50 years	35 (30–47)	20 (10–45)

* Adapted from Champlin R, Gale RP: Bone marrow transplantation: Its biology and roles as treatment for acute and chronic leukemias *Ann NY Acad Sci* 511: 447, 1987.
† >3 year leukemia-free survival

ACUTE MYELOGENOUS LEUKEMIA (AML)

The results of bone marrow transplantation in AML have improved significantly (Table 11-3). The outcome depends primarily on the patient's age and the remission state. Results of transplants in AML in the first remission are comparable or possibly superior to those achieved with chemotherapy, especially in children.[32-35] Data from the IBMTR and several transplant centers indicate that 20–30% of patients with AML, transplanted in the second to fourth complete remission, have a >3 year leukemia-free survival[35]; this is clearly superior to the results achieved with chemotherapy.

There is controversy over whether patients with AML in the first remission should receive bone marrow transplants or whether transplantation should be delayed until the second relapse. Several prospective controlled trials compared the efficacy of chemotherapy in this setting.[36-38] These studies confirm a decreased risk of leukemia relapse following bone marrow transplantation. Survival is also often better in transplant recipients.

The available data indicate that for persons <20–30 years of age with an HLA-identical sibling donor, survival is likely to be equivalent or superior with a transplant than with postremission chemotherapy. However, bone marrow transplantation during remission, even if potentially useful, is limited by age and donor availability. The median age of patients with AML is approximately 55 years, and only 30–40% of these have an HLA-identical sibling donor.

Several factors contribute to the efficacy of bone marrow transplantation in hematologic malignancies. Although the eradication of tumor cells is largely related to high-dose chemotherapy and radiation therapy, there is considerable evidence of an immune-mediated graft-versus-leukemia effect. This antitumor effect is documented in animals and in persons with acute and chronic GVHD receiving transplants for leukemia[39-41] and by the fact that the incidence of leukemia relapse is significantly increased if GVHD is prevented by T-cell depletion of the graft.[42] In addition, persons with AML in the first remission transplanted from a genetically identical twin, have a threefold higher relapse rate than those transplanted from an HLA-identical sibling.[43]

Autotransplants in patients with advanced AML are associated with relapse rates exceeding 90%.[29] These relapses may occur from residual leukemia in the patient, occult leukemia cells in the cryopreserved bone marrow, or both. The actuarial relapse rate for syngeneic (identical twin) bone marrow transplants in the first remission is approximately 60% for AML. Immune-mediated antileukemia effects (graft-versus-leukemia) observed in allogeneic bone marrow transplants do not seem to operate in autotransplants or syngeneic transplants.

Various approaches are used to eliminate residual leukemia cells in bone marrow to be used for autotransplants, such as treatment with 4-hydroperoxycyclophosphamide or with monoclonal antibodies to leukemia cells, or maintaining bone marrow cells in long-term cultures under conditions unfavorable for the growth of leukemia cells.[44,45] These approaches have not been investigated in controlled trials, and it is not possible to comment on their efficacy.

CHRONIC MYELOGENOUS LEUKEMIA (CML)

Bone marrow transplantation is the only effective approach currently available for CML.[46-48] Results depend primarily on age and the disease state. The best results are obtained in younger patients transplanted in the chronic phase, 55–70% of whom achieve 3- to 5-year leukemia-free survival (Table 11-4). There is a high risk of recurrent leukemia if the transplant is delayed until the accelerated or acute phase; actuarial leukemia-free survival rates are about 25% and 10%, respectively. In contrast, the risk of leukemia recurrence is only about 10% in transplants in the chronic phase. Transplants can also reverse the myelofibrosis that accompanies CML.

Another transplant prognostic factor for allogeneic bone marrow transplantation in CML is age. The best results are reported in children and young adults; most centers do not consider persons older than 45–50 years. Approximately 30% of the recipients die of transplantation-related complications.

Autologous transplants are also used to treat CML. Stem cells are collected from the blood or bone marrow during the chronic phase of the disease and cryopreserved. When CML progresses to the acute phase, these persons receive intensive chemotherapy, with or without total body radiation, followed by reinfusion of the cryopreserved autologous cells. The object of this approach is to restore the chronic phase. Surprisingly, some persons have transiently recovered hematopoiesis with Ph^1 chromosome-negative cells. However, Ph^1 chromosome-positive leukemia cells recover rapidly.[49-51] The major limitation of this approach is resistance of cells in the blast crisis to high-dose chemotherapy. Most patients achieve a brief second chronic phase, but fewer than 30% survive for 1 year.

OTHER HEMATOPOIETIC MALIGNANCIES

Patients with hematologic malignancies, such as lymphoma, multiple myeloma, hairy cell leukemia and CLL, have been treated with allogeneic, syngeneic or autologous bone marrow transplantation.[5,7,13,14] The benefit of transplantation compared to the risks of transplantation-related complications and the frequency of posttransplant relapses in these disorders is still uncertain; further studies are required.

COMPLICATIONS OF BONE MARROW TRANSPLANTATION

Allogeneic bone marrow transplantation is associated with serious complications, summarized in Table 11-5.[52,53] One of the major complications is GVHD. This is mediated by T lymphocytes present in the donor bone marrow that react against host tissue. Morbidity and mortality from GVHD are major problems, particularly in older persons. Several studies have evaluated T-cell depletion from the donor marrow ex vivo before transplantation to prevent GVHD. This approach decreases GVHD but is associated with increased graft failure and recurrent leukemia; survival is not improved[41] (Table 11-6).

Interstitial pneumonitis occurs in 20–40% of allogeneic bone marrow recipients.[54] It is related to drug and radiation toxicity, as well as to opportunistic infections in the setting of posttransplant immunodeficiency. Cytomegalovirus (CMV) is the most

Table 11-4 Actuarial Rates of Relapse and Survival at 4 or More Years of Bone Marrow Transplantation in CML*

Disease Status	Relapse (%)	Survival (%)
Chronic	7–12	55–70
Accelerated	40	15–35
Acute	40–60	10
Second chronic†	40–60	20–50

* Adapted from Champlin R, Gale RP, Bone marrow transplantation: Its biology and roles as treatment for acute and chronic leukemias. *Ann NY Acad Sci* 511: 447, 1987.
† Patients who had developed blast crisis but responded to chemotherapy and entered a second chronic phase.

Table 11-5 Complications of Bone Marrow Transplantation

Toxicity of the pretransplant conditioning
Graft rejection or failure
GVHD
Posttransplant immunodeficiency
Opportunistic infections
Interstitial pneumonia
Recurrent malignancy
Immunosuppression-related lymphoproliferative disorder

Table 11-6 Incidence of GVHD Among Recipients of Allogeneic Non-T-cell–depleted and T-cell–depleted Bone Marrow Transplants for Early Leukemia*

GVHD	Non-T-cell Depleted (%)	T-cell Depleted (%)
Acute GVHD		
None	31	57
Mild	26	22
Moderate	22	13
Moderately severe	10	4
Severe	11	4
Chronic GVHD		
None	60	72
Mild	20	17
Moderate	14	8
Severe	6	9

*Adapted from Horowitz MM, Gale RP, Sondel PM, et al: Graft-versus-leukemia reaction after bone marrow transplantation, *Blood* 75:555, 1990.

frequent pathogen. There is no effective treatment for CMV interstitial pneumonia. CMV infection is often acquired via blood product transfusion. The risk of interstitial pneumonitis can be reduced in previously uninfected persons by using blood products from CMV-seronegative donors or by treatment with intravenous immunoglobulin with high antibody levels against CMV.[54,55] Other opportunistic infections such as *Pneumocystis carinii* and fungi also complicate the outcome of bone marrow transplants.

MORPHOLOGIC EVALUATION OF BONE MARROW BEFORE AND AFTER TRANSPLANTATIONS

Pretransplant Considerations

Bone marrow donors for allogeneic and syngeneic transplants are normal persons without evidence of infection or malignancy. Donor bone marrow samples should be normocellular, with all the hematopoietic elements present and without significant dysplasia or evidence of primary or metastatic malignancies or infections (e.g., granulomas). The recipient's bone marrow should be carefully examined prior to transplantation to confirm the clinical diagnosis and to evaluate the bone marrow structure. Assessment of lymphoplasmacytic aggregates and mast cells in the bone marrow of recipients prior to transplantation may be of value. There is some evidence that persons with aplastic anemia who have intensely lymphoplasmacytic bone marrow infiltrates may respond to immunosuppressive therapy with anti-thymocyte globulin (ATG).[56] This may suggest an alternative approach in persons lacking an HLA-matched sibling donor. It has also been suggested that increased mast cells in pretransplanted bone marrows are associated with an increased risk of graft rejection or failure, though this is controversial.[57,58] The assessment of pretransplant bone marrow fibrosis is important. Bone marrow fibrosis is present in acute and chronic myelofibrosis, and may be associated with myelodysplastic syndromes, CML, acute leukemias, and bone marrow hypoplasia secondary to radiation therapy and/or chemotherapy. Mild to moderate bone marrow fibrosis is not significantly associated with decreased engraftment, and in malignancies it correlates with tumor levels and usually disappears following remission.[59,60]

Bone marrow samples from patients with severe pancytopenia and a diagnosis of aplastic anemia should be carefully examined for conditions such as hairy cell leukemia, hypocellular acute leukemia and myelodysplastic syndrome, which occasionally may display hypoplastic marrow simulating aplastic anemia. The bone marrow transplantation approach in these conditions is different from that of aplastic anemia and is similar to bone marrow transplantation in leukemias.

Bone marrow evaluation prior to transplantation is also important in patients with hematopoietic malignancies or solid tumors. In patients with a diagnosis of leukemia, the stage of relapse or remission must be confirmed and characterized by immunophenotypic and cytochemical studies prior to bone marrow transplantation. In patients with lymphoma or solid tumors, it is extremely important to assess for the presence or absence of bone marrow tumor involvement by careful examination of the pretransplant recipient marrow. In these conditions, bilateral bone marrow biopsy and aspiration are recommended, and all marrow sections, smears and touch preparations should be screened carefully.

In autologous transplantation, bone marrow specimens for cryopreservation should be free of tumor cells.

Posttransplant Evaluation of the Bone Marrow

Examination of the bone marrow after transplantation at selected intervals is common. These evaluations provide information regarding engraftment, rejection and disease recurrence.

Recovery

During the first week after transplantation the bone marrow is markedly hypocellular. There may be extensive marrow damage, evidenced by fat necrosis, edema and an increased number of foamy macrophages (lipophages). Occasional hematopoietic precursors and scattered lymphocytes and plasma cells are seen. Samples obtained 1 to 3 weeks after transplantation reveal regenerating hematopoietic cells (Figure 11-1). The engrafted bone marrow contains small clusters of erythroid and granulocytic cells. Erythroid cells usually appear in small, solid aggregates with a minimum of intercellular space, often in the middle of fatty bone marrow space (Figures 11-2, 11-3 and 11-4). In contrast, granulocytic foci tend to spread around fatty tissue and are often concentrated in paratrabecular areas. Foci of mixed hematopoietic cells such as granulocytic and erythroid precursors and megakaryocytes are rare before 2–3 weeks. During this period, erythroid precursors are usually more predominant than granulocytic ones. Dysplastic changes, such as nuclear irregularity and fragmentation, as well as megaloblastic changes, are

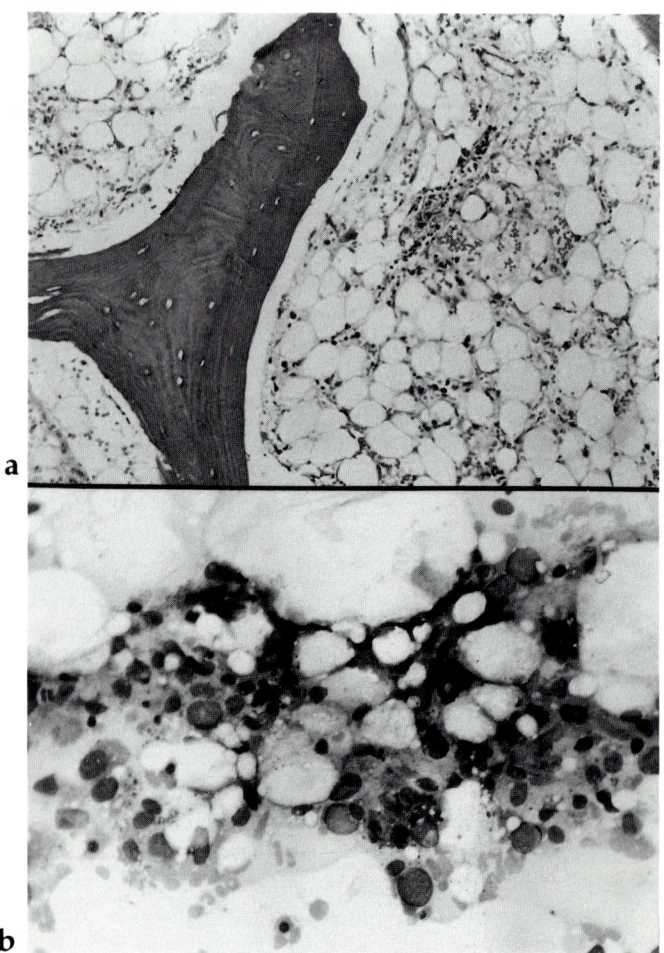

Figure 11-1. Bone marrow 1 week following transplantation. (a) A biopsy section demonstrating marked hypocellularity with small clusters of hematopoietic cells. (b) A bone marrow smear shows scattered early myeloid precursors. From Naeim F, Smith G and Gale RP, Morphologic aspects of bone marrow transplantation in patients with aplastic anemia. *Hum Pathol* 9:295, 1978, with permission.

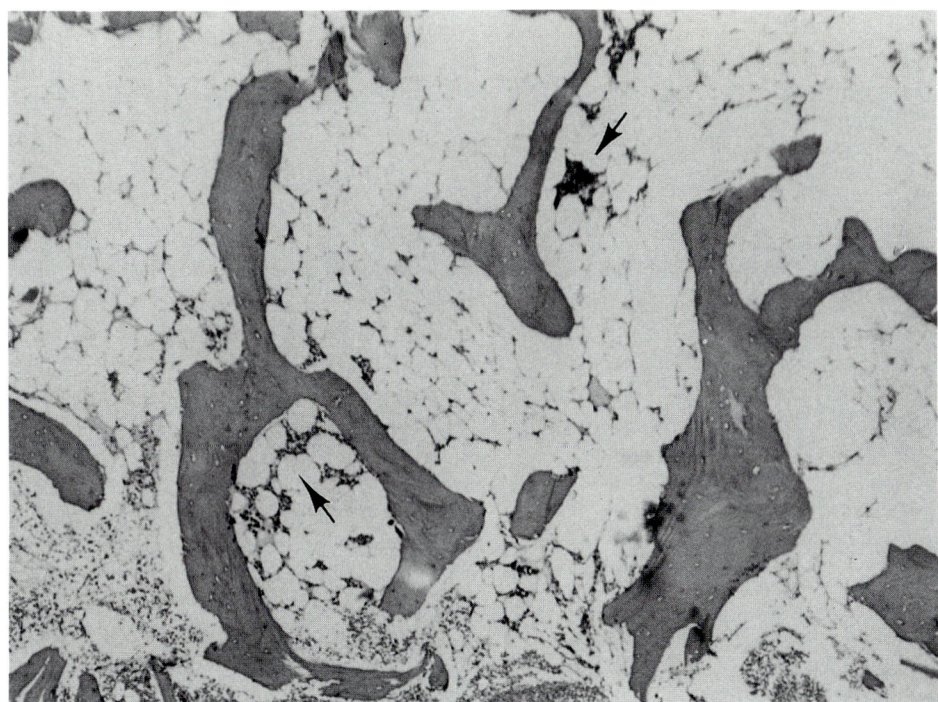

Figure 11-2. Bone marrow biopsy section obtained 2 weeks following marrow transplantation. Small foci of erythroid cells (upper right arrow) and myeloid cells (lower left arrow) are present in a markedly hypocellular marrow. From Naeim F, Smith G and Gale RP, Morphologic aspects of bone marrow transplantation in patients with aplastic anemia. *Hum Pathol* 9:295, 1978, with permission.

frequently seen. Both erythroid and granulocytic lines may show a moderate to marked left shift. The left shift in the granulocytic lineage may be associated with a marked increase in the number of myeloblasts and promyelocytes, which may resemble acute leukemia in some instances. This makes the diagnosis of residual AML in early posttransplant marrow samples very difficult. Transplant patients with bone marrow morphology suggestive of leukemia in the early posttransplant period should be followed carefully, with repeated bone marrow examinations before a definitive diagnosis of residual leukemia is made. In leukemias associated with chromosomal aberration, cytogenetic and/or DNA hybridization techniques may help to establish residual leukemia (see Chapter 2).

Bone marrow samples obtained 4 to 8 weeks after transplantation show increasing cellularity, with large clusters of hematopoietic cells composed of mixed-lineage cellular elements (Figure 11-5). Dysplastic changes are minimal. No significant left shift is present. Along with the improvement in bone marrow cellularity, peripheral blood displays a progressive increase in hemoglobin concentration and in white cell and platelet counts. Platelets are the last peripheral blood cellular elements to increase. Normocellularity is usually achieved 8 to 12 weeks following transplantation.

A transient appearance of "small blastoid cells" was recently reported in some bone marrow transplant patients.[61a] The peak percentage of these immature cells ranged from 4% to 21% and occurred between days 55 and 365 after transplant. These cells were of a precursor B-cell phenotype and expressed TdT, HLA-DR, CD10, CD19 and cytoplastic μ heavy chain.

Although morphologic evaluation of the posttransplant marrow and the presence of hematopoietic precursors are consistent with engraftment in most cases, rare transplant recipients show recovery of autologous hematopoiesis. The most common way to determine the genetic origin of cells after transplantation is to search for Barr bodies or perform cytogenetic analysis. Recent advances in molecular biology techniques and the development of DNA "fingerprinting" make it possible to distinguish do-

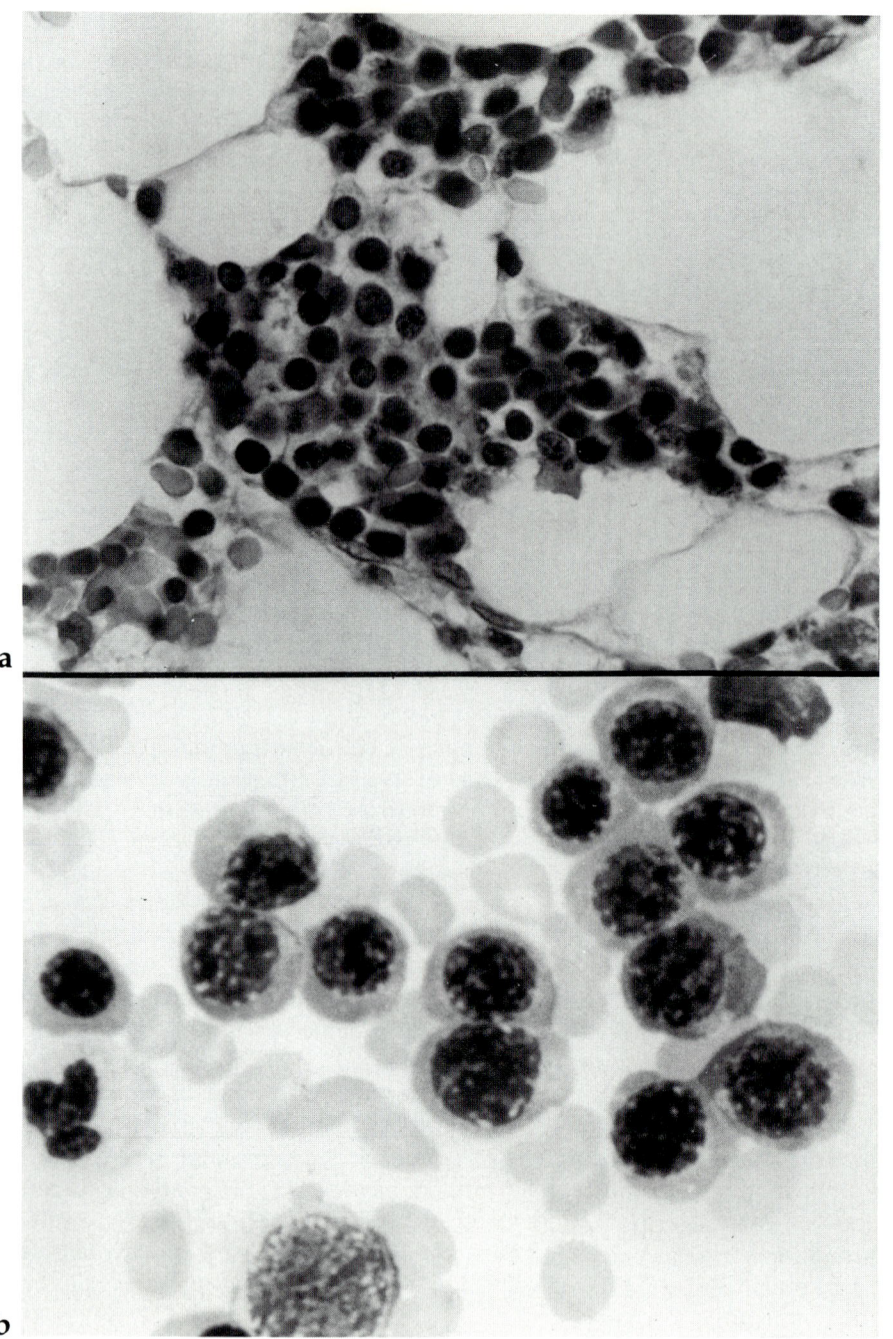

Figure 11-3. Clusters of erythroid precursors in bone marrow 2 weeks following transplantation; biopsy (a) and smear (b). From Naeim F, Smith G and Gale RP, Morphologic aspects of bone marrow transplantation in patients with aplastic anemia. *Hum Pathol* 9:295, 1978, with permission.

nor from recipient cells, except when the donor and recipient are identical twins. This technique can detect early bone marrow engraftment even before morphologic evidence of engraftment is noted. It also provides information regarding the proportion of donor and recipient cells in the bone marrow sample.

The principle of DNA fingerprinting, or restriction-fragment length polymorphism (RFLP), is based on comparing the DNA polymorphisms of the donor and the recipient. Certain areas of the human genome vary so greatly between people that they have been designated *hypervariable regions*. DNA probes derived from these regions reveal many variations in restriction fragment sizes on Southern blot analysis.

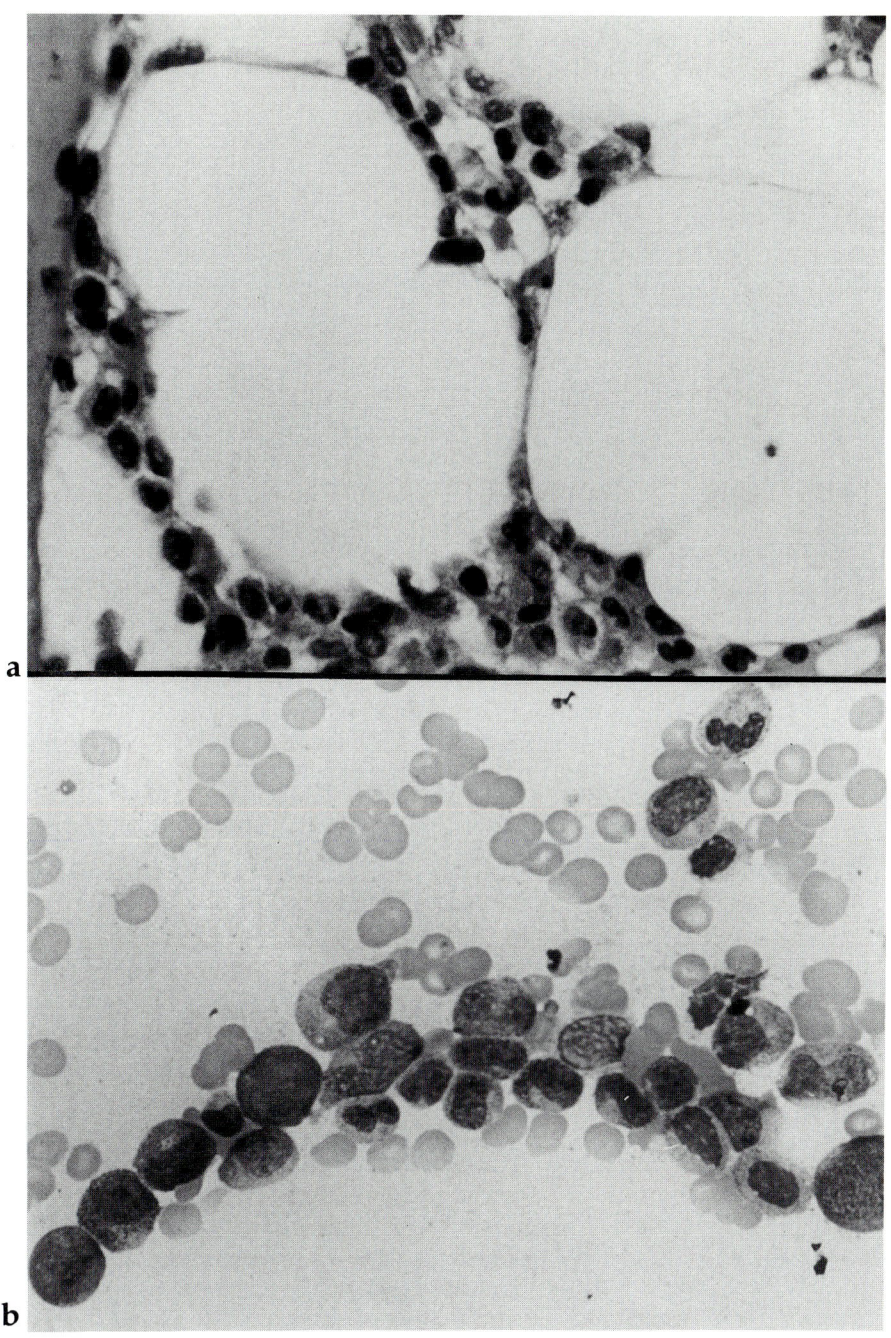

Figure 11-4. Clusters of myeloid precursors in bone marrow 2 weeks following transplantation; biopsy (a) and smear (b). From Naeim F, Smith G and Gale RP, Morphologic aspects of bone marrow transplantation in patients with aplastic anemia. *Hum Pathol* 9:295, 1978, with permission.

These hypervariable regions consist of long stretches of oligonucleotide sequences repeated in tandem. This results in high-frequency gain or loss of variable numbers of the unit repeat elements between individuals. The resulting patterns are so complex that essentially no two persons, except for identical twins, will demonstrate the same pattern (Figure 11-6).

Rejection

Approximately 10–20% of persons transplanted for aplastic anemia have graft failure. This is also a problem after T-cell-depleted transplants for leukemia. There are no specific morphologic criteria for bone marrow rejection. However, bone marrow cellularity

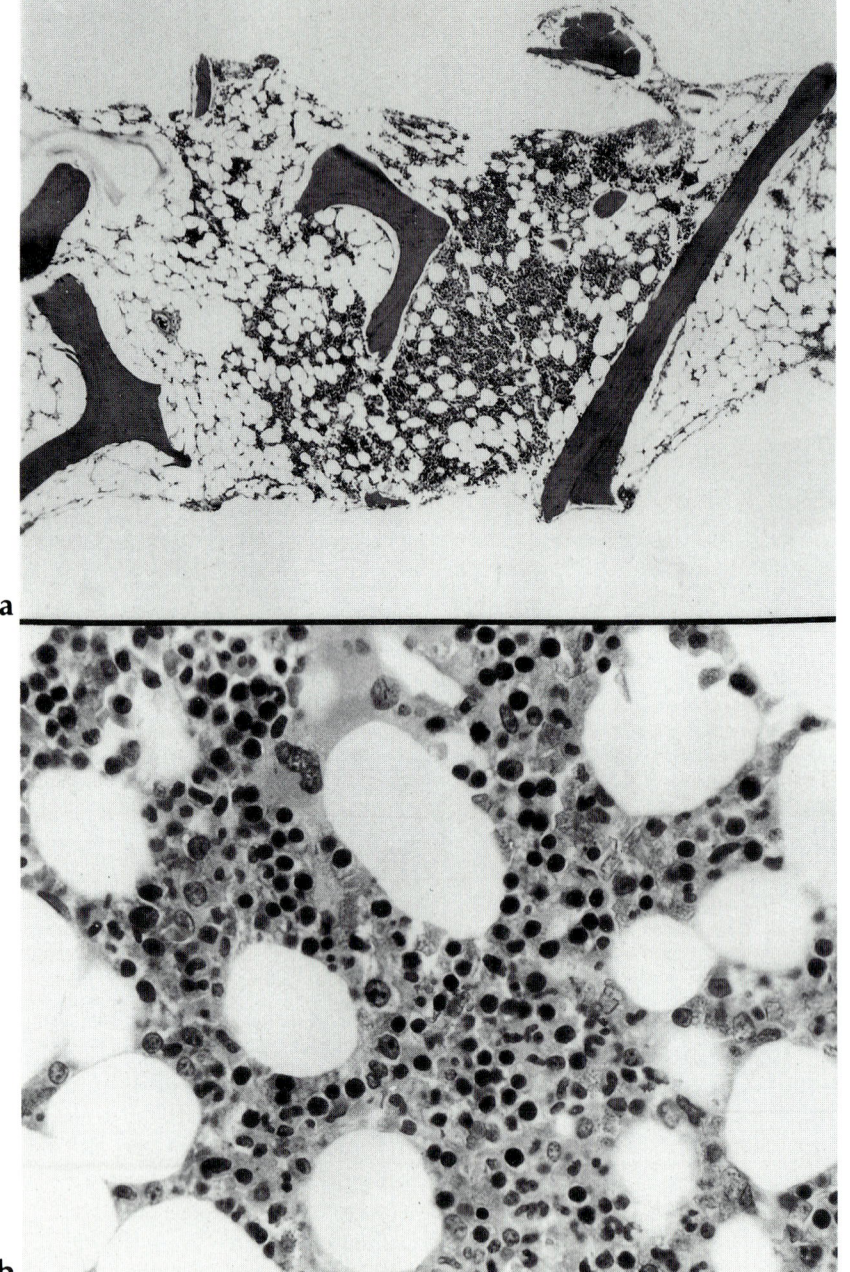

Figure 11-5. Bone marrow biopsy section 6 weeks following transplantation reveals a patchy cellularity with a large cellular area composed of a mixture of hematopoietic cells. (a) Low-power view and (b) high-power view. From Naeim F, Smith G and Gale RP, Morphologic aspects of bone marrow transplantation in patients with aplastic anemia. *Hum Pathol* 9:295, 1978, with permission.

decreases, and some nonspecific changes, such as a relative increase in the number of plasma cells, lymphocytes and macrophages with evidence of fat necrosis, may be observed. Graft failure is distinguished from no graft acceptance by evidence of marrow engraftment (by morphologic examination or other methods such as molecular biology) prior to graft failure.

Relapse

Detection of leukemia relapse in the bone marrow in early posttransplant bone marrow samples is difficult. According to Harrison et al.[61b] persistence of blasts in bone marrow on days 7–14 after transplantation is correlated with relapse. However, detection of relapse or residual acute leukemia in transplant recip-

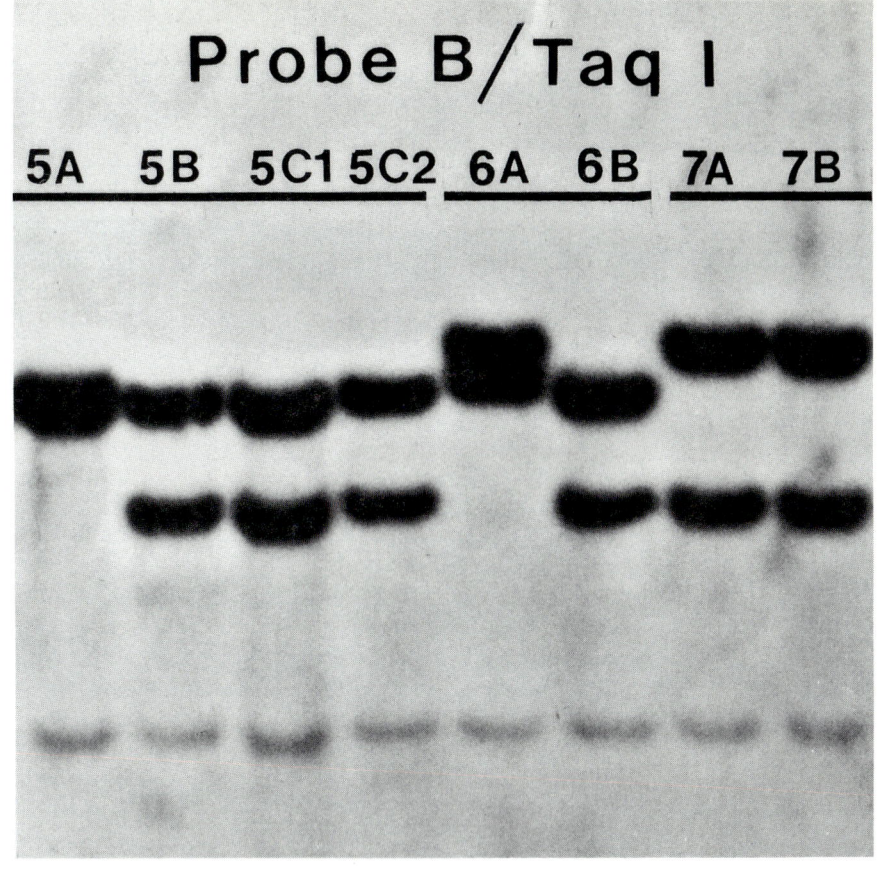

Figure 11-6. Identification of donor from recipient hematopoietic cells in bone marrow transplantation by RFLP analysis. For each numbered family: A, transplant recipient's DNA, B, donor's DNA, and C, DNA isolated from the recipient's marrow cells at 30 and 60 days after transplantation. The donor pattern is present in both posttransplant specimens of families 5 and 6, indicating successful engraftment. The donor and recipient in family 7 are identical twins and therefore give no informative polymorphism. From Grody WW, Gatti, RA, Naeim F: Diagnostic molecular pathology. *Modern Pathol* 2:553, 1988, with permission.

ients is difficult because of the high percentage of lymphoid cells in the bone marrow of children and the presence of a myeloid left shift in adults in the early posttransplant period. As suggested, in this period it is best to follow these cases with serial bone marrow sampling before reaching a conclusion.

Immunosuppression-Mediated Lymphoproliferative Disorders

Bone marrow transplant recipients who receive immunosuppressive therapy are at risk for the development of EBV-associated lymphoproliferative disorders.[62,63] These cases are often associated with GVHD. The problem is greatest in those receiving T-cell-depleted transplants, cyclosporine and/or anti-T-cell antibodies.[62-64] The lymphoid lesions in such cases resemble either immunoblastic or Burkitt's lymphoma and may display a monoclonal or polyclonal lymphoproliferative process. Withdrawal of immune suppression or initiation of antiviral therapy may initiate tumor regression in some cases. Other cases may respond to acyclovir.

References

1. Champlin RE, Gale RP: Bone marrow transplantation for acute leukemia: Recent advances and comparison with alternative therapies. *Semin Hematol* 24:55, 1987.
2. Gale RP, Champlin RE: *Recent Progress in Bone Marrow Transplantation.* New York, Alan R Liss, 1987.
3. Thomas ED, Storb R, Clift RA, et al: Bone marrow transplantation. *N Engl J Med* 292:832, 1973.
4. O'Reilly RJ: Allogeneic bone marrow transplantation: Current status and future directions. *Blood* 62:941, 1983.
5. Storb R, Buckner CD: Human bone marrow transplantation. *Eur J Clin Invest* 20:119, 1990.
6. Sullivan KM, Witherspoon RP, Storb R, et al: Long-term results of allogeneic bone marrow transplantation. *Transplant Proc* 21:2928, 1989.
7. Santos GW: Bone marrow transplantation in hematologic malignancies. Current status. *Cancer* 65:786, 1990.
8. Champlin R, Gale RP: Bone marrow transplantation: Its biology and roles as treatment for acute and chronic leukemias. *Ann NY Acad Sci* 511:447, 1987.

9. Champlin RE: Bone marrow transplantation for aplastic anemia: Recent advances and comparisons with alternative therapies. *Cancer Treat Res* 50:185, 1990.
10. Ash RC, Horowitz MM, Gale RP, et al: Bone marrow transplantation from related donors other than HLA-identical siblings: Effect of T-cell depletion. *Bone Marrow Transplant* 7:443, 1991.
11. Gingrich R, Howe C, Goekin N, et al: Successful bone marrow transplantation with partially matched unrelated donors. *Transplant Proc* 17:450, 1985.
12. Chao NJ, Blume KG: Bone marrow transplantation. Part II—autologous. *West J Med* 152:46, 1990.
13. Phillips GL: Autologous bone marrow transplantation for hematologic cancer. *Prog Clin Biol Res* 354B:171, 1990.
14. Armitage JO: Bone marrow transplantation in the treatment of patients with lymphoma. *Blood* 73:1749, 1989.
15. Storb R, Epstein RB, Rudolph RH, et al: The effect of prior transfusions on marrow grafts between histocompatible canine siblings. *J Immunol* 105:627, 1970.
16. Storb R, Floersheim GL, Weiden PL, et al: Effects of prior blood transfusion on marrow grafts: Abrogation of sensitization by procarbazine and antithymocyte serum. *J Immunol* 112:1508, 1974.
17. Storb R, Thomas ED, Buckner CD, et al: Marrow transplantation for aplastic anemia. *Semin Hematol* 21:27, 1984.
18. Gluckman E: Current status of bone marrow transplantation for severe aplastic anemia: A preliminary report from the International Bone Marrow Transplant Registry. *Transplant Proc* 19:2597, 1987.
19. Deeg HJ, Self S, Storb R, et al: Decreased incidence of marrow graft rejection in patients with severe aplastic anemia: Changing impact of risk factors. *Blood* 68:1363, 1986.
20. Niederwieser D, Pepe M, Storb R, et al: Improvement in rejection, engraftment rate and survival without increase in graft-versus-host disease by high marrow cell dose in patients transplanted for aplastic anemia. *Br J Haematol* 69:23, 1988.
21. Storb R, Thomas ED, Appelbaum FR, et al: Marrow transplantation for severe aplastic anemia: The Seattle experience, in Young N, Humphreys K, Levine A (eds), *Aplastic Anemia: Stem Cell Biology and Advances in Treatment*. New York, Alan R Liss, 1984, p 297.
22. Storb R, Witherspoon RP: Bone marrow transplantation: What determines success or failure of hematologic reconstitution? *Onkologie* 10:166, 1987.
23. Storb R, Witherspoon RP, Sullivan KM, et al: Allogeneic marrow transplants for treatment of severe aplastic anemia, in Gale RP (ed), *Recent Advances in Bone Marrow Transplantation*. New York, Alen R Liss, 1983, p 3.
24. Champlin RE, Horowitz MM, van Bekkum DW, et al: Graft failure following bone marrow transplantation for severe aplastic anemia: Risk factors and treatment results. *Blood* 73:606, 1989.
25. Bacigalupo A, Van Lint MT, Congiu M, et al: Bone marrow transplantation (BMT) for severe aplastic anemia (SAA) in Europe: A report of the EBMT-SAA Working Party. *Bone Marrow Transplant* 3:44, 1988.
26. Gordon-Smith EC, Hows J, Bacigalupo A, et al: Bone marrow transplantation for severe aplastic anemia (SAA) from donors other than HLA-identical siblings: A report of the EBMT Working Party. *Bone Marrow Transplant* 2:100, 1987.
27. Gale RP, Kersey JH, Bortin MM, et al: Bone marrow transplantation for acute lymphoblastic leukemia. *Lancet* 2:663, 1983.
28. Barret AJ, Kendra JR, Lucas CF, et al: Bone marrow transplantation for acute lymphoblastic leukemia. *Br J Haematol* 52:181, 1983.
29. Dicke KA, Spitzer G: Evaluation of the use of high dose cytoreduction with autologous marrow rescue in various malignancies. *Transplantation* 41:4, 1986.
30. Ritz J, Sallan SE, Base RC, et al: Autologous bone marrow transplantation in CALLA positive acute lymphoblastic leukemia after in vitro treatment with J5 monoclonal antibody and complement. *Lancet* 2:60, 1982.
31. Ramsay N, LeBien T, Nesbit M, et al: Autologous bone marrow transplantation for patients with lymphoblastic leukemia in second or subsequent remission: Results of bone marrow treated with BA-1, BA-2, and BA-3 with complement. *Blood* 66:508, 1985.
32. Champlin RE, Gale RP: Treatment of acute myelogenous leukemia: Recent advances. *Blood* in press.
33. Witherspoon RP, Schubach W, Neiman P, et al: Donor cell leukemia developing six years after marrow grafting for acute leukemia. *Blood* 65:1172, 1985.
34. Thomas ED, Buckner CD, Clift RA, et al: Marrow transplantation for acute nonlymphoblastic leukemia in first remission. *N Engl J Med* 301:597, 1979.
35. Gale RP, Kay EMH, Rimm AA, et al: Bone marrow transplantation for acute leukemia in first remission: Report of the International Bone Marrow Transplant Registry. *Lancet* 2:1006, 1982.
36. Powels RL, Clink HM, Bandini G, et al: The place of bone marrow transplantation in acute myelogenous leukemia. *Lancet* 1:1047, 1980.
37. Appelbaum FR, Dahlberg S, Thomas ED, et al: Bone marrow transplantation or chemotherapy after remission induction for adults with acute non-lymphoblastic leukemia. A prospective study. *Ann Intern Med* 101:581, 1984.
38. Champlin RE, Ho WG, Gale RP, et al: Treatment of acute myelogenous leukemia: A prospective controlled

trial of bone marrow transplantation versus consolidation chemotherapy. *Ann Intern Med* 102:285, 1985.
39. Champlin RE, Gale RP: The role of bone marrow transplantation in the treatment of hematologic malignancies and solid tumors: A critical review of syngeneic, autologous and allogeneic transplants. *Cancer Treat Rep* 68:145, 1984.
40. Weiden PL, Sulivan KM, Flournoy N, et al: Anti-leukemic effect of chronic graft-versus-host disease: Contribution to improved survival after allogeneic marrow transplantation. *N Engl J Med* 304:1529, 1981.
41. Horowitz MM, Gale RP, Sondel PM, et al: Graft-versus-leukemia reaction after bone marrow transplantation. *Blood* 75:555, 1990.
42. Marmont AM, Horowitz MM, Gale RP, et al: T-cell depletion of HLA-identical transplants in leukemia. *Blood* 78:2120, 1991.
43. Gale RP, Champlin RE: How does bone marrow transplantation cure leukemia? *Lancet* 2:28, 1984.
44. Yeager AM, Kaiser H, Santos GW, et al: Autologous bone marrow transplantation in patients with acute nonlymphocytic leukemia using ex vivo marrow treatment with 4-hydroperoxycyclophosphamide. *N Engl J Med* 315:141, 1986.
45. Ball ED, Bernier BM, Cornwell GC, et al: Monoclonal antibodies to myeloid differentiation antigens: In vivo studies of three patients with acute myelogenous leukemia. *Blood* 62:1203, 1983.
46. Chang J, Coutinho L, Morgenstern G: Reconstitution of hemopoietic system with autologous marrow taken during relapse of acute myeloblastic leukemia and grown in long term culture. *Lancet* 1:294, 1986.
47. Champlin RE, Golde DW: Chronic myelogenous leukemia: Recent advances. *Blood* 65:1039, 1985.
48. Sokal JE, Cox BE, Baccarani M, et al: Prognostic discrimination in "good-risk" chronic granulocytic leukemia. *Blood* 63:789, 1984.
49. Champlin RE, Gale RP, Foon KAA, et al: Chronic leukemias: Oncogenes, chromosomes and advances in therapy. *Ann Intern Med* 104:671, 1986.
50. Thomas ED, Clift RA, Fefer A, et al: Marrow transplantation for the treatment of chronic myelogenous leukemia. *Ann Intern Med* 104:155, 1986.
51. Goldman JM, Apperly JS, Jones L, et al: Bone marrow transplantation for patients with chronic myelogenous leukemia. *N Engl J Med* 314:202, 1986.
52. Champlin RE, Gale RP: The early complications of bone marrow transplantation. *Semin Hematol* 21:101, 1984.
53. Sullivan KM, Deeg HJ, Sanders JE, et al: Late complications of bone marrow transplantation. *Semin Hematol* 21:53, 1984.
54. Meyers JD, Flournoy N, Thomas ED: Non-bacterial pneumonia after allogeneic marrow transplantation: A review of ten years' experience. *Rev Infect Dis* 4:1119, 1982.
55. Bowden RA, Sayers M, Flournoy N, et al: Cytomegalovirus immune globulin and seronegative blood products to prevent primary cytomegalovirous infection after bone marrow transplantation. *N Engl J Med* 314:1006, 1986.
56. Te Velde J, Haak HL: Histological investigation of methacrylate embedded bone marrow biopsy specimens; correlation with survival after conventional treatment in 15 adult patients. *Br J Haematol* 35:61, 1977.
57. Naeim F, Smith G, Gale RP: Morphologic aspects of bone marrow transplantation in patients with aplastic anemia. *Hum Pathol* 9:295, 1978.
58. Sale GE, Marmont P: Mast cell counts do not predict marrow graft rejection. *Hum Pathol* 12:605, 1981.
59. Rajantie J, Sale GE, Deeg HJ, et al: Adverse effect of severe marrow fibrosis on hematologic recovery after chemoradiotherapy and allogeneic bone marrow transplantation. *Blood* 67:1693, 1986.
60. Rajantie J, Sale GE: Course of marrow fibrosis and chronic myelogenous leukemia after marrow transplantation. *Lancet* 1:318, 1986.
61a. Kobayashi SD, Seki K, Suwa N, et al: The transient appearance of small blastoid cells in the marrow after bone marrow transplantation. *Am J Clin Pathol* 96:191, 1991.
61b. Harrison DT, Flournoy N, Ramberg R, et al: Relapse following marrow transplantation for acute leukemia. *Am J Hematol* 5:191, 1978.
62. Martin PJ, Shulman HM, Shubach WH, et al: Fatal Epstein-Barr-virus-associated proliferation of donor B-cells after treatment of acute graft-versus-host disease with a murine anti T-cell antibody. *Ann Intern Med* 101:310, 1984.
63. Gratama JW, Zutter MM, Minarovits J, Oosterveer MA, et al: Expression of Epstein-Barr virus-encoded growth-transformation-associated proteins in lymphoproliferations of bone-marrow transplant recipients. *Int J Cancer* 47:188, 1991.
64. Sale GE, Buckner DC: Pathology of bone marrow in transplant recipients. *Hematol Oncol Clin North Am* 2:735, 1988.

INDEX*

*Italic numbers are for primary entries.

A

Abl-bcr, 57, 62, 142, 147, 156, 187
ABO blood group, 314
Acid hydrolase, 11
Acid phosphatase, 12, 13, 15
Acute infectious lymphocytosis, 278
Acanthocytosis, 310
Acid phosphatase, 40
Acquired dyserythropoiesis, 318
Acquired immunodeficiency syndrome, (AIDS), 83, 90, 245, 255, *274–275*, 329
   bone marrow changes in, 88–89
Acquired qualitative platelet disorders, 335–337
Acute basophilic leukemia, 163
Acute leukemias, *143–168*
   hand-mirror cell type, 164
   hypocellular, 163
   mixed, 164–168
   transformation of chronic leukemias into, 164
Acute lymphoblastic leukemia (ALL), 37, 40, 57, 58, 61, *143–148*, 258
   ALL-L1, 143
   ALL-L2, 143
   ALL-L3, 143
   ALL, granular, 163
   ALL, common, 145, 147
   bone marrow transplantation as treatment for, 344–345
   clinical aspects, 147–148
   cytogenetics, 146–147
   immunologic classification, 143–146
   morphologic classification, 143
   See also Acute lymphoid leukemia of NK phenotype; Non-T-ALL; T-ALL
Acute lymphoid leukemia of NK phenotype, 161–163
Acute mixed leukemia, 164–168
   biclonal, 164
   bilineal, 164
   biphenotypic, 164
   hybrid, 164
Acute monocytic leukemia (M5), 151–152
Acute myelofibrosis, 155
Acute myelogenous leukemia (AML), 37, 57, 58, 75, 78, *148–160*, 258
   bone marrow transplantation as treatment for, 345
   classification, 148–157
   clinical aspects, 158–160
   cytogenetics, 156
Acute myelomonocytic leukemia (M4), 149–151, 245
Acute non-lymphoid leukemia (ANLL), 148–160
Acute promyelocytic leukemia (M3), 148–149

Adenosine, 333
Adenosine deaminase deficiency, 273
Adipocytes, 25–26
ADP, 334–336
Aggressive mastocytosis, 259
Adult T-cell leukemia/lymphoma, 181
Agammaglobulinemia
   common variable, 274
   X-linked, 274
Agnogenic myeloid metaplasia. *See* Myelofibrosis with extramedullary hematopoiesis
AIDS-related complex (ARC), 88
AIDS. *See* Acquired immunodeficiency syndrome
AIHA. *See* Autoimmune hemolytic anemias (AIHA)
AL, 241–242
Albinism, 250
Alcoholic cirrhosis, 315
Alcoholism, 73, 292
Alkaline phosphatase, 12, 15, *40*
Allergic reactions, thrombocytopenia associated with, 331
Allogeneic transplants, 343
Alloimmune thrombocytopenia, 330–331
ALL. *See* Acute lymphoblastic leukemia (ALL)
α-globin chain, 300
α granules, 19, 334, 335
α heavy chain disease, 241
α-methyldopa, 315
Alpha-naphthyl acetate esterease, 38–39
Alpha-naphthyl butyrate esterase, 38–39
Amegakaryocytosis, 325
AML. *See* Acute myelogenous leukemia (AML)
Amyloidosis, 95–96, 239
   light chain-associated, 241–242
Anaphylactic reactions, thrombocytopenia associated with, 331
Anemia
   characteristics and classification of, 287–288
   aplastic, 40, 73, 327
   congenital dyserythropoietic, 72
   hemolytic, 73
   iron deficiency, 73
   macrocytic, 287, 288
   megaloblastic, 76, 173
   microcytic, 287, 288
   normocytic, 287, 288
   refractory, 73
Angiocentric T-cell lymphoma, 207–210
Angiofollicular lymphadenopathy, 241
Angioimmunoblastic lymphadenopathy, 241
Angiotropic large cell lymphoma, 210

Anisocytosis, 74
Ankyrin, 306
ANLL. *See* Acute non-lymphoid leukemia (ANLL)
Anorexia nervosa, 89
Antiglobulin test, indirect, 313
Antiglobulin test, direct, 313
Aplasia. *See* Pure red cell aplasia
Aplastic anemia
   acquired, 102–107
      clinical aspects, 106–108
      etiology and pathogenesis, 103–104
      pathology, 104–106
   bone marrow transplantation as treatment for, 344
   constitutional, 102
Aplastic crisis, 289
Arachidonic acid pathways, abnormalities in, 335
ARC. *See* AIDS-related complex (ARC)
Aryl sulphatase, 12
Aspiration of bone marrow, 32
Aspirin, platelet disorders associated with, 35
Asymptomatic gammopathies, 234
ATLL, 181
ATP. *See* Autoimmune thrombocytopenic purpura (ATP)
Auer rods, 62, 75, 148, 149
Autoimmune disorders, neutropenia associated with, 254
Autoimmune hemolytic anemias (AIHA), 312–314
   with cold-reacting antibodies, 313–314
   with warm-reacting antibodies, 313
Autoimmune thrombocytopenic purpura (ATP), 327–329
   neonatal immune thrombocytopenia associated with, 331
Autologous transplants, 343, 345
Azidothymidine (AZT), 88, 275

B

B-ALL, 146–147
B-lymphocytes (B cells), 21
B-PLL, 173
Basopenia, 255
Basophilia, 259
Basophilic leukemia, 191
Basophilic stippling, 73
Basophils, 13–15
Bcl-1, *53*, 56, 239
Bcl-2, 56
B-CLL, 169–171
Bernard-Soulier syndrome, 333
Bence Jones protein, 234, 238, 240, 241
Benign gammopathy, 234
β-globin gene, 298, 299, 301

Index

β-thromboglobulin, 19
BFU-E, 128, 132, 143
Biclonal gammopathies, 245
Biclonal leukemia, 164
Biliary cirrhosis, 245, 329
Bilineal leukemia, 164
Biphenotypic leukemia, 164
Birbeck bodies (granules), 63, 214, 263, 267
Biopsy of bone marrow, 32
   sections, 34
   touch preparations, 34–35
Blood loss, anemia caused by, 296–297, 318
Bone disorders, bone marrow changes and, 96
Bone marrow, sample preparation, 32–35
Bone marrow cells
   abnormal, 80
   morphologic characteristics, 10–26
Bone marrow cellularity, 2
Bone marrow fibrosis, 81–83
Bone marrow infiltration, anemia associated with, 319
Bone marrow metastasis, 91–95
Bone marrow necrosis, 90–91
Bone marrow microenvironment, 4
Bone marrow stroma, 1
Bone marrow transplantation, 343–353
   autologous, 343, 345
   syngeneic, 343, 345
   allogeneic, 343, 345
Breast carcinoma, 93, 95
Burkitt's lymphoma, 88, *203*, 353
Burr Cells, 310, 319

C

C-abl, 56, 57
C-fos, 57
C-myb, 57
C-myc, 56, 57, 142, 147, 239
Cabot's ring, 73, 239
Calmodulin, 306
Castleman's disease, 241
Cardiopulmonary bypass, platelet disorders associated with, 336
Cathepsin, 11, 13
$CD11c^+$ CLL, 171
$CD4^+$ CLL, 172
$CD8^+$ CLL, 171
CDAs, 290–292
Cell cycle analysis, 48–49
Cell morphology, abnormal, 75–80
Ceroid lipofuscinosis, 78
CFU-Bas, 4
CFU-E, 4, 17, 132, 148
CFU-Eo, 4, 148, 257
CFU-G, 4
CFU-GM, 4, 148
CFU-M, 4
CFU-Meg, 4, 129, 148, 132
CFU-S, 148
CGD, 250–252
CHAD, 313–314

Chediak-Higashi syndrome, 74–75, *250*, 334
Chemicals
   hematopoietic malignancies and, 141–142
   hemolysis induced by, 315–316
Chickenpox, 259, 314, 329
Chloroma, 158
Chlorothiazide, 325
Chronic active hepatitis, 245
Chronic B-cell lymphocytosis, 278
Chronic disorders, anemia associated with, 318
Chronic granulomatous disease, 250–252
Chronic leukemias, 168–191
   blast transformation of, 164
Chronic lymphocytic leukemia (CLL), 40, *168–174*, 196, 241, 329
   B-CLL, 169–171
   $CD11c^+$ CLL, 171
   $CD4^+$ CLL, 172
   $CD8^+$ CLL, 171
   clinical aspects and prognostic factors, 173
   CLL/PL, 171
   cytogenetics, 172–173
   mixed CLL, 171
   transformation to aggressive lymphoid malignancy, 173–174
Chronic lymphoid leukemias, 168
Chronic monocytic leukemia (CMoL), 189
Chronic myelogenous leukemia (CML), 40, 53, 58, 61, 62, 78, 132, 138, *184–188*, 245, 258
   blast transformation, 187
   blast crisis, 187
   blast phase, 187
   bone marrow transplantation as treatment for, 345–346
   diagnosis using DNA hybridization techniques, 53
Chronic myelomonocytic leukemia, 119–120
Chronic neutrophilic leukemia, 189
Chronic renal disease, 89
CHS, 250
CLL. *See* Chronic lymphocytic leukemia (CLL)
CML. *See* Chronic myelogenous leukemia (CML)
CMML, 119–120
Cold hemagglutinen disease, 313–314
Cold reactive antibodies, 312
Collagen, 132, 269, 334
   defects in platelet response to, 334
Colony-forming unit (CFU), 4
Colony-stimulating factor (CSF), 4
Common ALL, 145, 147
Congenital dyserythropoietic anemias
   type I, 290
   type II, 290–292
   type III, 292

Congenital immunodeficiency syndromes, 272–274
Congenital megakaryocytic hypoplasia, 325
Congenital qualitative platelet disorders, 333–335
Congo red stain, 96
Coomb's test, 313
Copper defiency anemia, 318
Corticosteroids, 255, 257
Cryopathic hemolytic syndromes. *See* Autoimmune hemolytic anemias (AIHA), with cold-reacting antibodies
CSFs, 6–10
CTCL, 181–184
Culture procedures for bone marrow, 64–65
Cushing's syndrome, 255
Cutaneous T-cell lymphoma, 181–184
CVAG, 274
Cyclic neutropenia, 261
Cytochrome b, 250
Cytogenetic analysis, 58–63
Cytokines, hematopoietic effects, 9–10
Cytoplasmic granules, 74–75
   absence or reduction of, 75
Cytoplasmic inclusions, 74–75

D

Defensin, 11
Deficiency anemias, 292–293, 318–319
Dendritic histiocytes, malignant tumors of, 214
Dendritic reticulum cells, 17
Dengue fever, 255, 325
Dense granule deficiency, 334–335
Dialysis neutropenia, 255
Diet, iron deficiency anemia associated with, 296
Di George syndrome, 274
DiGuglielmo's syndrome. *See* Erythroleukemia (M6)
Diabetes mellitus, 259
Diamond-Blackfan anemia, 289
Diphteria, 90
Disseminated intravascular coagulopathy (DIC), 149, 314, 333
DNA
   aneuploidy, 48
   content assays, 48–49
   hybridization techniques, 49–56
   hyperdiploidy, 48
   hypodiploidy, 48
   index, 48
Dohle inclusion bodies, 74
Dot blot, for DNA hybridization, 50
Down's syndrome, 40, 153
   TMD in, 134–135
Drug-induced hemolytic anemia, 74, 315
Drugs
   hemolysis induced by, 315–316

immune thrombocytopenia induced by, 329–330
neutropenia induced by, 255
platelet disorders associated with, 335–336
Dutcher bodies, 21, 241
Dyserythropoiesis, 114
  acquired, 318
Dysgranulopoiesis, 114
Dysmyelopoietic syndromes. *See* Myelodysplastic syndromes

E
EBV, 277
Echinocytes, 319
Echinocytosis, 310
Elastase, 11
Electron microscopy, in diagnosis of hematologic disorders, 63
ELIZA, 275
Endocrine disorders, anemia associated with, 318–319
Endothelial cells, 27
Environmental inducing factors, for hematopoietic malignancies, 141–142
Eosinopenia, 255
Eosinophilia, 257–259
  associated with malignant tumors, 258
  conditions associated with, 258
Eosinophilic granulocytes, 12–13
Eosinophilic leukemia, 189
Eosinophilic leukocytosis. *See* Eosinophilia
Eosinophils, atypical, 75
Epinephrine, defects in platelet response to, 334
Epstein-Barr virus (EBV), 104, 142, 277, 314
Erythroblasts
  basophilic, 17
  orthochromic, 18
  polychromatophilic, 18
Erythrocyte abnormalities, membrane–associated, 310
Erythrocyte enzyme abnormalities, secondary hemolytic anemias, 310–312
Erythrocyte membrane skeleton defects
  clinical and pathologic features, 306–310
  etiology and pathogenesis, 306
Erythroid morphology, abnormal, 72–74
Erythroid precursors, 17–18
Erythroid progenitor cells, disturbancees in proliferation and differentiation, 289–292
Erythroleukemia (M6), 38, 72, *152–153*
Erythrophagocytosis, 76
Erythropoietin, 9
Essential thrombocythemia, 129–130
Esterase reactions, 38–40
Estrogen, 325
Evans syndrome, 329
Ewing's sarcoma, 94

Extramedullary hematopoiesis, 91
Extravascular hemolysis, 312

F
Familial hemophagocytic lymphohistiocytosis, 266–267
Fat cells. *See* Adipocytes
Felty syndrome, 254
Fetal hemoglobin, 300
Fibrinogen, 19
Fibroblast-like cells, 27
Fibronectin, 16, 19, 132
Fibrosis. *See* Bone marrow fibrosis
$5q^-$ syndrome, 125
Flow cytometry, 44–47
  in DNA analysis, 48–49
Flame cells, 72
Fluorescent microscopy, 47
Foamy histiocytes, 77
Folic acid deficiency, 292–293
Follicular, mixed, small cleaved and large cell lymphoma, 196–200
Follicular small cleaved lymphoma, 196–200
Foods, platelet disorders associated with, 335–336
French-American-British (FAB) Classification
  MDS, 114
  ALL, 143
  AML, 148

G
G-6-PD, 310–311
Gaucher cells, *77*, 269
Gaucher's disease, 77, 82, 239, 245, *269–272*
  type 1, 269
  type 2, 271–272
  type 3, 271–272
  acute neuropatic, 272
  chronic adult type, 271
  subacute neuropatic, 272
G-CSF, 7
Gelatinous transformation of bone marrow, 89–90
Gene rearrangements and translocations, diagnosis using DNA hybridization techniques, 52–53
Germ-cell tumors, 153
Giemsa stain, 34
Glanzmann thrombasthenia, 333–334
Globin synthesis, abnormal, 302–303
Glucose-6-phosphatase dehydrogenase deficiency, 310–311
Glycophorin c, 307
GM-CSF, *7*, 334
GP 1a, 333
GP 1a/IIa, 329
GP 1b/IX, 333
GP IIb/IIIa, 333
GP V, 333

Graft-versus-host disease (GVHD), 245, *343–345*, 353
Granular acute lymphoblastic leukemia, 163
α-Granula deficiency, 335
Granulocyte-CSF, 7
Granulocyte-macrophage-CSF, 7
Granulocytes
  disorders of, 250–261
  functional abnormalities, 250–253
Granulomas, 83–87
Gray platelet syndrome, 335
Growth factor, hematopoietic stem cells and, 4–10

H
H-ras, 239
Hairy cell leukemia (HCL), 175–181
  cytochemical and immunophenotypic features, 178–180
  cytogenetics, 180
  defective immune functions, 180–181
  T-cell, 179
  variant (HCL-V), 181
Hand-Schiller-Christian disease, 262
Hand-mirror cell leukemia, 164
Hashimoto's disease, 329
Hashimoto-Pritzker syndrome, 262
Hb. *See* Hemoglobin
Hb Bart's, 301
Hb Grower, 3
Hb H disease, 301, 302
Hb Portland, 3
Hb structure, unstable, 303–306
HCL. *See* Hairy cell leukemia (HCL)
HE, 307–310
Heat, hemolysis induced by, 315
Heavy chain disease, 242
Heinz bodies, 74, *302–306*, 311
Hematologic disorders
  DNA hybridization techniques in diagnosis of, 51–52
  molecular diagnosis of, 51
  monoclonal gammopathies associated with, 245
  platelet disorders associated with, 337
Hematopoiesis, regulatory mechanisms and, 3–10
Hematopoietic cells, 1–2
Hematopoietic growth factors, 6–10
Hematopoietic malignancies, 346
  etiology and pathogenesis, 141–142
Hematopoietic stem cells, growth factor and, 4–10
Hematoxylin and Eosin (H&E) stain, 34
Hemochromatosis, 36
Hemoglobin A, 298–300
Hemoglobin A2, 298–300
Hemoglobin C, 302
Hemoglobin D, 302–303
Hemoglobin E, 302–303
Hemoglobin F, 298
Hemoglobin G, 303

Index

Hemoglobin H, 301, 305
Hemoglobin Lepore, 300
Hemoglobin S, 302–303
Hemoglobin SC, 302–303
Hemoglobin, Bart's, 301
Hemoglobin, embryonic, 3
Hemoglobin, fetal, 290
Hemoglobinopathies, 74, 306
  sickle cell diseases, 302–303
Hemoglobin synthesis, disturbance of, 296–302
Hemolysis
  drug- and chemical-induced, 315–316
  heat-induced, 315
  infection-induced, 317
  trauma-induced, 315
Hemolytic anemias
  acantholytic, 315
  drug-induced, 74
  immune related, 312–315
  nonimmune acquired, 315–318
  secondary to erythrocyte enzyme abnormalities, 310–312
Hemolytic disease of the newborn, 314–315
Hemolytic transfusion reactions, 314–315
Hemolytic uremic syndrome, 332
Hemophagocytic lymphohistiocytosis, 266–267
Hemophagocytic macrophages, 76
Hemophagocytic syndromes, 266–268
  infection-associated, 268–269
Hemophilia A, diagnosis using DNA hybridization techniques, 52
Hemorrhage. See Blood loss
Hemosiderin, 17
HEMPAS, 290–292
Henoch-Schonlein purpura, 245
Heparin, 15
Hereditary elliptocytosis, 307–310
  stomatocytic, 307
  spherocytic, 309
Hereditary non-spherocytic hemolytic anemia, 310
Hereditary orotic aciduria, 293
Hereditary persistence of fetal hemoglobin (HPFH), 300
Hereditary pyropoikilocytosis (HPP), 309
Hermansky-Pudlak syndrome, 334
Histamine, 15
Hereditary spherocytosis, 307
Histiocytes. See Foamy histiocytes; Sea-blue histiocytes
Histiocytic disorders, 262–278
Histiocytic malignancies, 211–214, 269
  lymphomas, 211–212
Histiocytic medullary reticulosis. See Malignant histiocytosis
Histiocytosis, 262–272
  Class I. See Langerhans cell histiocytosis
  Class II. See Hemophagocytic syndromes
  Class III. See Histiocytic malignancies

Histiocytosis X, malignant, 214
Histoplasmosis, 90
HIV, 88, 104, *275*
HIV-I, 275
HIV-II, 275
Hodgkin's disease, 40, 83, 132, *192–195*
  lymphocyte depletion, 193
  lymphocyte predominant, 193
  mixed cellularity, 193
  nodular sclerosis, 193
Howell-Jolly bodies, 73, 296
HTLV-1, T-cell leukemia and. See Adult T-cell leukemia/lymphoma
HTLV-II, 179
Hybrid leukemia, 164
Hypercholesterolemia, 77, 315
Hypereosinophilic syndromes, 189, 257–258
Hyperparathyroidism, 82
Hypersplenism, 317–318
Hyperthyroidism, 255
Hypocellular acute leukemia. See Hypoplastic acute leukemia
Hypochromic anemia, 296–302
Hypoplastic acute leukemia, 163–164
Hypothyroidism, 73

I

Idiopathic gemmopathies, 234
Idiopathic hypereosinophilic syndromes. See Hypereosinophilic syndromes
Idiopathic myelofibrosis, 131–134
Idiopathic thrombocytopenic purpura (ITP). See Autoimmune thrombocytopenic purpura
IFN-α, 177
IGM monoclonal gammopathy, 240–241
IL-1, 9, 96
IL-2, 9
IL-3, 7–9
IL-4, 9–10
IL-5, 10
IL-6, 9
IL-7, 10
IM, 277–278
IMF, 131–134
Immune related hemolytic anemias, 312–315
Immune thrombocytopenia
  drug-induced, 329–330
  in newborns, 330–331
Immunoblastic lymphoma, *202*, 353
  with epithelioid cell component, 202
  clear cell, 202
  plasmacytoid, 202
  pleomorphic, 202
Immunodeficiency syndromes. See Congenital immunodeficiency syndromes
Immunoenzyme staining, 43
Immunofluorescent staining, 43–44
Immunogold technique, 47
Immunophenotyping, in MDS studies, 127

Immunosuppression-mediated lymphoproliferative disorders, 353
Infection-associated hemophagocytic syndrome, 268–269
Infections
  hemolysis induced by, 317
  neutropenia associated with, 255
Indolent mastocytosis, 259
Infectious mononucleosis (IM), 277–278
Influenza, 259, 314
Injury, hemolysis induced by, 315
In situ hybridization, for DNA, *50–51*, 58
Interdigitating cells, 17
Interferon, 16, 325
Inferferon-a, 177
Interleukin-1, 9
Interleukin-2, 9
Interleukin-3, 7–9
Interleukin-4, 9–10
Interleukin-5, 10
Interleukin-6, 9
Interleukin-7, 10
Intermediate lymphocytic lymphoma, 207
Internum in eosinophils, 13
Intrinsic factor, 293
Intravascular hemolysis, 312
Iron deficiency anemia, 73, 259, 296–298
  blood loss, 296
  inadequate dietary intake, 296
  iron malabsorption, 297
Iron stain. See Prussian blue reaction
ITP. See Autoimmune thrombocytopenic purpura

J

Juvenile chronic myelogenous leukemia (JCML), 188–189

K

Kaposi's sarcoma, 8
Kawasaki disease, 255
Ki-1$^+$ anaplastic large cell lymphoma, 207
Kwashiorkor, 318

L

β-Lactam antibiotics, platelet disorders associated with, 335–336
Lacunar cells, 193
Laminin, 132
Langerhans cell histiocytosis (LCH), 77, *262–266*
  clinical aspects, 264–266
  etiology and pathogenesis, 262
  pathology, 262–264
Langerhans cell sarcoma. See Malignant histiocytosis, Type X
Langerhans cells, 17, 63, *263*
Large cell lymphoma, 173
Large cell lymphoma, angiotropic, 210
Large granular lymphocytes (LGL), 21
Large granular lymphocytic leukemia, 171
Lazy-leukocyte syndrome, 255
LCH. See Langerhans cell histiocytosis (LCH)

Lead poisoning, 73
Legionnaires' disease, 83
Lennert's lymphomas, 200–201
Lepra bacilli, 84
Lesch-Nyhan syndrome, 293
Letterer-Siwe disease, 262
Leukemias
  bone marrow morphology in, 91
  granulocytic, 189–191
  main groups, 142
  true eosinophilic, 258
  See also Acute leukemia
Leukemic reticuloendotheliosis. See Hairy cell leukemia
Leukemoid reaction, 40, 257
Leukocyte adhesion deficiency, 253
Leukocyte morphology, abnormal, 74–80
Light chain-associated amyloidosis, 241–242
Lipocytes. See Adipocytes
Lipogranuloma, 84
Lithium salts, 257
Lutzner cell, 184
Lymphoblastic lymphomas, 202–203
Lymphoblasts, 21, 143
Lymphocytes, 21–24
  atypical, 78
  B cells, 21
  disorders of, 272–277
  large granular, 21
  NK cells, 21
  T cells, 21
Lymphocytopenia, 272
Lymphocytosis, 275–277
  chronic B-cell, 278
  idiopathic, 278
Lymphoid malignancies
  cytogenetic analysis of, 58–61
  diagnosis using DNA hybridization techniques, 52–53
Lymphomas
  angiocentric T-cell, 207
  angiotrophic, large cell, 210
  bone marrow morphology in, 91
  Burkitt's, 60–61, 88, 203
  follicular, 60, 196–200
  IgM gammopathies and, 241
  immunoblastic, 202, 253
  intermediate lymphocytic, 207
  Ki-1 positive, anaplastic large cell, 207
  large cell, 173
  large cell, diffuse, 200
  large cell, follicular, 200
  leukemic phases, 184
  mantle zone, 207
  mixed small and large cell, diffuse, 200
  mixed, small cleaved and large cell, follicular, 196
  monocytoid B-cell, 207
  small cleaved cell, follicular, 196
  small cleaved cell, diffuse, 200
  small lymphocytic, 196
  small noncleaved cell, 203

T cell, 60
T cell, with epithelioid cell component, 200
plasmacytoid, 196
See also Malignant lymphomas; Richter's syndrome; Splenic lymphoma
Lymphomatoid granulomatosis, 210
Lymphopenia. See Lymphocytopenia
Lysosomal storage diseases, 269
Lysozyme, 11

M
Macrocytosis, 73, 290–296
Macrophage-CSF, 7
Macrophages
  monocyte-macrophage lineage, 15–17
  phagocytosis of hematopoietic cells, 76
  See also Foamy histiocytes; Gaucher cells; Histiocytic disorders
Malignancies
  hematologic, main groups, 141
  See also Histiocytic malignancies; Lymphoid malignancies; Myeloid malignancies
Malignant eosinophilia, 189
Malignant histiocytosis, 212–214
Malignant lymphomas, 171–210. See also Lymphoma
  high-grade, 203–205
  intermediate-grade, 200–202
  low-grade, 196–200
Malignant myelofibrosis, 155
Malignant tumors, eosinophilia associated with, 258
Mantle zone lymphoma, 207
Marrow particle sections, 32–34
Mast cell growth factor, 9
Mast cell leukemia, 189–191
Mast cells, 13–15
Mastocytic eosinophilic fibrohistiocytic lesion, 259
Mastocytic leukemia, 250
Mastocytosis, 259–261
  aggressive, 259
  indolent, 259
Maximov's method, 34
May-Hegglin anomaly, 74
MCH, 298–299
MCV, 296–301
M-CSF, 7
MDS, 113–128
Measles, 255, 325, 329
Megakaryoblastic leukemia (M7), 153–155
Megakaryocytes,
  abnormal, 78, 114
  granular, 18–19
  group I, 18
  group II, 18
  group III, 18
Megakaryocytosis, 73, 76, 325–326
Megaloblastic anemias, 292–296
  clinical aspects, 296

etiology and pathogenesis, 292–293
pathology, 293–296
Megaloblastic changes, 72
Melanoma, 95
Metamyelocytes, 11
Metarubricyte, 18
Metastasis. See Bone marrow metastasis
Methyl green pyronine stain, 40
MGUS. See Monoclonal gammopathies, of undetermined significance
Microorganisms, detection by DNA hybridization techniques, 55–56
Mixed lineage leukemia, 164
Monoblasts, 15
Monoclonal antibodies, in bone marrow examination, 41–47
Monoclonal gammopathies
  association with hematologic and non-hematologic disorders, 245
  asymptomatic, 234
  benign, 234
  clinicopathologic features, 233–245
  etiology and pathogenesis, 232
  idiopathic, 234
  nonmyelomatous, 234
  of undetermined significance, 234
  See also IGM monoclonal gammopathy
Monocyte/macrophage-colony stimulating factor, 7
Monocyte-macrophage lineage, 15–17
Monocytes, 37, 38
Monocytic disorders, 261–262
Monocytoid B-cell lymphoma, 207
Monocytopenia, 261–262
Monocytosis, 261–262
Monosomy 7, 127
Monosomy 7q$^-$, 127
Mott cell, 21
MPO, 252–253
Mucopolysaccharoidosis, 74
Multiple myeloma (MM), 40, 78, 82, 234–240
  CD10$^+$ myeloma, 239
  cytogenetics and DNA alterations, 239
  pathology, 234–239
  prognostic factors, 239
Mumps, 329
Mycobacterium avium-intercellulare, 84
Mycoplasma pneumoniae, 314
Mycosis fungoides, 181
Myeloblastic leukemia with maturation (M2), 148
Myeloblastic leukemia without maturation (M1), 148
Myeloblasts, 10, 38
Myelocytes, 11
Myelodysplastic syndromes, 57, 72, 75, 82, 113–128
  clinical aspects and prognostic factors, 127–128
  cytogenetic studies, 121–127
  etiology and pathogenesis, 113
  pathology, 113–121

Index

primary, 113
therapy-related, 114
Myelofibrosis, 40, 78, 82, *131–134*, 327
Myelofibrosis with extramedullary hematopoiesis, 131–134
Myeloid malignancies, cytogenetic analysis of, 61–63
Myelokathexis, 255
Myelomonocytic leukemia with atypical eosinophilia, 151
Myeloperoxidase, 11
Myeloperoxidase deficiency, 252–253
Myelophthisic anemia, 319
Myeloproliferative disorders, 128–135

N
N-ras, 21
Naphthol AS-D acetate esterase, 39–40
Naphthol AS-D chloroacetate, 40
Natural killer (NK) cells, 21
Natural killer cell leukemia, 171
Necrosis. *See* Bone marrow necrosis
Neonatal immune thrombocytopenia, 330–331
Neuroblastoma, 91–93
Neutropenia, 253–255
  alloimmune (isoimmune neonatal), 254
  associated with infections, 255
  autoimmune, 254
  congenital, 253
  cyclic, 253–254
  drug-induced, 255
Neutrophilia, 255–257
Neutrophilic precursors of bone marrow cells, 10–12
  bands, 11–12
  segmented neutrophils, 11–12
Neutrophils, 11–12
  hypersegmentation of, 76
Newborns
  hemolytic disease of, 314–315
  neutropenia in, 234
  thrombocytopenia in, 330–331
NHL. *See* Non-Hodgkin's lymphoma
Niemann-Pick disease, 77, *272*
  group I, 272
  group II, 272
  infantile type, 272
  neuronopathic, 272
  visceral type, 272
Nitroblue tetrazolium test, 252
NK cells, 75, 254
Nodular sclerosing Hodgkin's disease,
  syncytial type, 193
  cellular phase, 193
Non-Hodgkin's lymphoma, 195–210
  classification, 196–205
  clinical aspects, 205–207
  leukemic phase, 184
Nonmyelomatous gammopathies, 234
Nonsecretory multiple myeloma (MM), 240
Non-T-ALL, 145–146

Northern blot technique, for DNA hybridization, 50
Null ALL, 145

O
Oil Red O stain, 40
Oncogenes, 56–58
Osmotic fragility, 309
Osteoblasts, 24–25
Osteoclasts, 24–25
Osteolysis. *See* Osteopenia
Osteopenia, associated conditions, 96–97
Osteopetrosis, 82, *97*
Osteoporosis. *See* Osteopenia
Osteosclerosis, associated conditions, 97
Osteosclerotic myeloma. *See* POEMS syndrome

P
p53 gene, 58
Paget's disease, 82
Para-aminosalicylic acid, 315
paraprotein, 234
Paroxysmal cold hemoglobniuria (PCH), 314
Paroxysmal nocturnal hemoglobinuria, 82, *108–109*, 327
Parvovirus B19, 104, 245, 293
PAS reaction, 36–38
PCR, for DNA hybridization, 50
Pegler-Huet anomaly, 75
Penicillin, 15
Periodic acid-Schiff (PAS) reaction, 36–38
Pernicious anemia, 245, 293
Peroxidase, 38
Phenacetin, 315
Philadelphia chromosome (Ph^1), 53, 147, 184
Phospholipase, 13
PK deficiency, 311–312
Plasma cell dyscrasia, *See also* Monoclonal gammopathies
Plasma cell leukemia, 240
Plasma cells, 21–24
  atypical, 78
  flame cells, 21
  Mott cells, 21
Platelet disorders, 332–337
  abnormal secretory granules, 334–335
  of adhesion, 333
  of aggregation, 333–334
  arachidonic acid pathway abnormalities, 335
  associated with pathologic conditions, 336–337
  receptor defects, 334
  secretion defects, 335
Platelet factor 4, 19
Platelet peroxidase (PPO), 38
Platelet-derived growth factor, 19, 83
Platelet precursors, 18–21
Platelets, *18–20*, 37–38, 75
  abnormal, 114

PLL, 174–175
PNH, 108–109
POEMS syndrome, 240
Poikilocytosis, 74
Polyarteritis nodosa, 331
Polycythemia rubra vera, 40, 78, 82, *128–129*
Polymerase chain reaction, for DNA hybridization, 50
Polymorphic reticulosis, 210
Posttransfusion purpura, 331
Pre-B ALL, 146–147
Pre-pre-B ALL, 145
Prednisone, 325
Pregnancy, 73, 255
Primary eosinophilia, 189
Primary megakaryocytosis, 78
Prolymphocytic leukemia, 174–175
Promegakaryoblast, 18
Promegakaryocyte, 18
Promyelocytes, 11, 21
Prorubricyte, 17
Prostatic carcinoma, 95
Protease, 15
Protein 4.1, 306–307
Protein 4.9, 306
Protein deficiency anemia, 318
Prussian blue reaction, 35–36
PRV, 128–129
Pseudo-Gaucher cells, 77, 291
Pseudo-Pelger-Huet, 114
Pure cutaneous histiocytosis, 262
Pure red cell aplasia, 245, *289–290*
Purine metabolism, disturbances in, 293
Pyrimidine metabolism, disturbances in, 293
Pyruvate kinase deficiency, 311–312

Q
Q fever, 83–84, 90
Qualitative platelet disorders, 332–333
Quinine, 315

R
RA, 117
Radiation, ionizing, hematopoietic malignancies and, 141
RAEB, 119
RAEB-T, 120–121
RARS, 117–119
RBC intrinsic abnormalities, anemias caused by, 302–312
Reed-Sternberg (RS) cells, 192
  L and H type, 193
  RS variants, 193
Refractory anemia (RA), 73, *117*
  with excess blasts, 119
  with excess blasts in transformation, 120–121
  with ringed sideroblasts, 117–119
Regulatory mechanisms, hematopoiesis and, 3–10
Rejection, after transplantation, 351–352

Relapse, after transplantation, 352–353
Renal failure, chronic
  anemia associated with, 319
  platelet disorders associated with, 336–337
Restriction fragment length polymorphism (RFLP), 55, 132
Reticulum cells. See Fibroblast-like cells
Reticulin fibers, 81, 132
Reticulin stain, 40, 81, 132
Reticulocytes, 18, 288, 300, 303, 307, 311, 313
Reticulum cells, 26
Retinoblastoma suppressor gene, 58
RFLP, 55, 350
Rh blood group, 315
Rhabdomyosarcoma, 91–93
Rheumatoid arthritis, 259, 329, 331
Ribonuclease, 13
Richter's syndrome, 173–174
Rieder cells, 169
Rider-Reilly anomaly, 74
Ringed sideroblast, 36, 73, 104
Romanovsky's method, 34
Rosai-Dorfman syndrome, 268–269
Rubella, 104, 329
Rubeola, 329
Rubricyte, 18
Russell bodies, 21

S
Sample preparation, 32–35
Schistocytes, 74
SCID, 273–274
Sea-blue histiocytes, 77–78
Secondary polycythemia, 129
Sections, bone marrow, 32–34
Self-healing reticulohistiocytosis, 262
Serotonin, 15, 333
Serum feritin, 298
Serum iron, 298
Severe combined immune deficiency (SCID), 273–274
Sezary-like cells, 184
Sezary syndrome, 181–184
Sickle cell disease, 51, 90, 302–303
  diagnosis using DNA hybridization techniques, 51–52
Sideroblast, 35
Sinus histiocytosis with massive lymphadenopathy, 268–269
Sjogrene's syndrome, 331
Smallpox, 259, 329
Small lymphocytic lymphoma, 196
Small noncleaved cell lymphomas, 203–205
Smears, bone marrow, 32
Smoking, 73, 262
Smoldering multiple myeloma, 240
Solitary plasmacytomas, 240
Southern blot technique, for DNA hybridization, 50
Spectrin, 306–307

Spielmeyer-Sjögren syndrome, 78
Spleen. See Hypersplenism
Splenic lymphoma, leukemic phase, 184
Staining
  in bone marrow examination, 35–41
  in MDS studies, 127
  See also Immunoenzyme staining; Immunofluorescent staining
Steel factor, 9
Stem cells. See Hematopoietic stem cells
Stomatocytic elliptocytosis, 307
Stomatocytosis, 310
Storage pool disease-α, 335
Storage pool disease-δ, 334–335
Sucrose hemolysis test, 292
Sudan black B, 38
Sulfonamides, 315
Suppressor genes ("anti-oncogenes"), 58
Syngeneic transplants, 343
Syphilis, 83, 314
Systemic lupus erythematosus, 329, 331
Systemic schlerosis, 329

T
T Cells. See T-lymphocytes
T-ALL, 145
T-cell lymphoma with epitheliod cell component, 200
T-cell growth factor, 2, 9
T-cell leukemia, HTLV associated, 181
T-cell lymphoma, angiocentric, 207
T-cell replacing factor (TRF), 10
T-CLL, 171–172
T-lymphocytes (T cells), 21
T-PLL, 175
Tangier disease, 77
Tartrate resistant acid phosphatase (TRAP), 40, 178
TGF-alpha, 96
Thalassemias, 298–302
  α-thalassemias, 300–302
  β-thalassemias, 298–300
    diagnosis using DNA hybridization techniques, 52
  $\delta\beta$-thalassemias, 300
Thrombin, 333
Thrombocytopenia, 327
  with absent radii (TAR syndrome), 325
  pathologic conditions associated with, 332
  See also Immune thrombocytopenia
Thrombopoietin, 325
Thrombospodin, 19
Thrombotic thrombocytopenic purpura, 90, 330–331
Thromboxane A2, defects in platelet response to, 334
TNF-α, 10
TNF-β, 10
Total iron binding capacity (TIBC), 298, 318
Touch preparations, 34–35
Toxic granulation, 74

Transcobalamin II, 16
Transferrin, 16
Transfusions,
  hemolytic transfusion reactions, 314–315
  posttransfusion purpura, 331
Transient myeloproliferative disorder in Down's syndrome, 134–135
Transplantation,
  complications of, 346–347
  detection of marrow origin by DNA, 53–55
  morphologic evaluation of bone marrow, 347–353
  posttransplant evaluation, 348–353
  pretransplant consideration, 347–348
  principles of, 343–344
Trichrome stain, 40, 81, 132
Triclonal gammopathies, 245
True eosinophilic leukemia, 258
Tryptophan-induced eosinophilia-myalgia syndrome, 258
TTP, 331–332
Tubercolosis, 89, 90, 259
Tumor necrosis factor-alpha, 10
Tumor necrosis factor-beta, 10
Typhoid fever, 83, 90

U
Ulcerative colitis, 89, 259
Unstable hemoglobins, 74

V
Varicella, 325
Vascular changes, in bone marrow, 96
Villous lymphocytes, 184
Viral hepatitis, 325
Viruses, hematopoietic malignancies and, 142
Vitamin B_{12} deficiency, 72, 293
Vitamin deficiency anemia, 293, 318
  vitamin B_6 deficiency, 318
  vitamin C deficiency, 318
  vitamin E deficiency, 318
  vitamin A deficiency, 318
Von Willebrand disease, diagnosis using DNA hybridization techniques, 52

W
Waldenstrom's macroglobulinemia, 82, 240–241
Warm-reactive antibodies, 312
Western blot, 275
Wiscott-Aldrich syndrome, 274, 334
Wolman's disease, 77
Wright's stain, 34

X
X-linked lymphoproliferative syndrome, 278

Z
Zieve's syndrome, 315